Pulmonary Fibrosis: Pathophysiology and Therapeutics

Pulmonary Fibrosis: Pathophysiology and Therapeutics

Edited by Kimberly Dawson

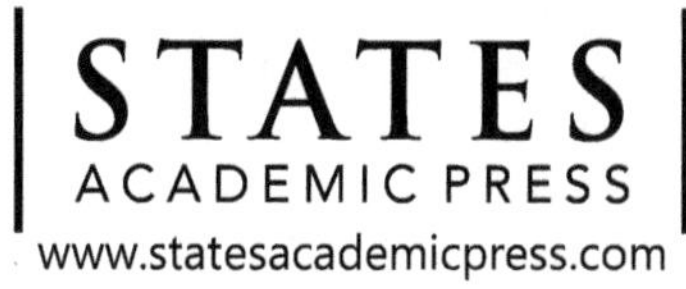

States Academic Press,
109 South 5th Street,
Brooklyn, NY 11249, USA

Visit us on the World Wide Web at:
www.statesacademicpress.com

ISBN: 978-1-63989-763-6

Cataloging-in-Publication Data

Pulmonary fibrosis : pathophysiology and therapeutics / edited by Kimberly Dawson.
p. cm.
Includes bibliographical references and index.
ISBN 978-1-63989-763-6
1. Pulmonary fibrosis. 2. Pulmonary fibrosis--Pathophysiology. 3. Pulmonary fibrosis--Treatment.
I. Dawson, Kimberly.

RC776.F5 P85 2023
616.24--dc23

Table of Contents

Preface

The main aim of this book is to educate learners and enhance their research focus by presenting diverse topics covering this vast field. This is an advanced book which compiles significant studies by distinguished experts in the area of analysis. This book addresses successive solutions to the challenges arising in the area of application, along with it; the book provides scope for future developments.

Fibrosis refers to an excessive deposition of extracellular matrix proteins and results in scarring and thickening of the affected tissue. It is, in essence, an exaggerated wound healing response that leads to organ malfunction. Fibrosis is commonly associated with high morbidity and mortality. Pulmonary fibrosis refers to a group of serious lung diseases that affect the respiratory system. It is caused by damage and scarring of the lung tissue. It cannot be cured, but its treatment involves management of symptoms through pulmonary rehabilitation and oxygen therapy. In some cases, lung transplantation can also help the patients. This book explores all the important aspects of pulmonary fibrosis. It presents researches and studies performed by experts across the globe on the pathophysiology and therapeutics for this medical condition. The extensive content of this book provides the readers with a thorough understanding of pulmonary fibrosis.

It was a great honour to edit this book, though there were challenges, as it involved a lot of communication and networking between me and the editorial team. However, the end result was this all-inclusive book covering diverse themes in the field.

Finally, it is important to acknowledge the efforts of the contributors for their excellent chapters, through which a wide variety of issues have been addressed. I would also like to thank my colleagues for their valuable feedback during the making of this book.

Editor

1

Mesoporous Polydopamine Loaded Pirfenidone Target to Fibroblast Activation Protein for Pulmonary Fibrosis Therapy

Qi Fang[1], Shaoyu Liu[1], Jiangyu Cui[2], Ruiyue Zhao[1], Qian Han[2], Peng Hou[1], Youcai Li[1], Jie Lv[1], Xiaoyao Zhang[1], Qun Luo[2] and Xinlu Wang[1]**

[1]Department of Nuclear Medicine, The First Affiliated Hospital of Guangzhou Medical University, Guangzhou, China, [2]State Key Laboratory of Respiratory Diseases, Guangzhou Institute of Respiratory Diseases, The First Affiliated Hospital of Guangzhou Medical University, Guangzhou, China

***Correspondence:**
Qun Luo
luoqunx@163.com
Xinlu Wang
71Lu@163.com

Recently, fibroblast activation protein (FAP), an overexpressed transmembrane protein of activated fibroblast in pulmonary fibrosis, has been considered as the new target for diagnosing and treating pulmonary fibrosis. In this work, mesoporous polydopamine (MPDA), which is facile prepared and easily modified, is developed as a carrier to load antifibrosis drug pirfenidone (PFD) and linking FAP inhibitor (FAPI) to realize lesion-targeted drug delivery for pulmonary fibrosis therapy. We have found that PFD@MPDA-FAPI is well biocompatible and with good properties of antifibrosis, when ICG labels MPDA-FAPI, the accumulation of the nanodrug at the fibrosis lung *in vivo* can be observed by NIR imaging, and the antifibrosis properties of PFD@MPDA-FAPI *in vivo* were also better than those of pure PFD and PFD@MPDA; therefore, the easily produced and biocompatible nanodrug PFD@MPDA-FAPI developed in this study is promising for further clinical translations in pulmonary fibrosis antifibrosis therapy.

Keywords: mesoporous polydopamine, fibroblast activation protein, fibroblast activation protein inhibitor, pulmonary fibrosis, antifibrosis therapy

1 INTRODUCTION

Pulmonary fibrosis is the terminal of many interstitial lung diseases (ILDs), it damages the normal lung structure, causes lung function decay, impairs the quality of life, and even leads to death by fibroblasts activated aberrantly and extracellular matrix (ECM) accumulated excessively (Rockey et al., 2015; Deng et al., 2020; Lai et al., 2021). Idiopathic pulmonary fibrosis (IPF) is a very common ILD, manifesting progressive pulmonary fibrosis with unclear etiology, the middle survival time of IPF is 2–5 years (Fernández Pérez et al., 2010; Ley et al., 2011; Nathan et al., 2011; Raghu et al., 2011). Nowadays, the critical treatment for IPF is antifibrosis therapy, for example, pirfenidone (PFD). PFD had finished the phase three trial, represented a good effect on patients with IPF, but often comes along with gastrointestinal (GI) adverse events (AE), which may be brought by the oral administration (King et al., 2014; Lancaster et al., 2017).

Activated fibroblast is a key cell in pulmonary fibrosis pathogenesis, and fibroblast activation protein (FAP), a 97 kDa type II transmembrane protein, with dipeptidyl peptidase activity as one kind of serine protease, only overexpressed on the membrane of aberrantly activated fibroblast, had been proved that could be found at the remolding area of IPF and cancer (Garin-Chesa et al., 1990; Acharya et al., 2006; Keane et al., 2013). So FAP has become the target of pulmonary fibrosis diagnosis and therapy, which

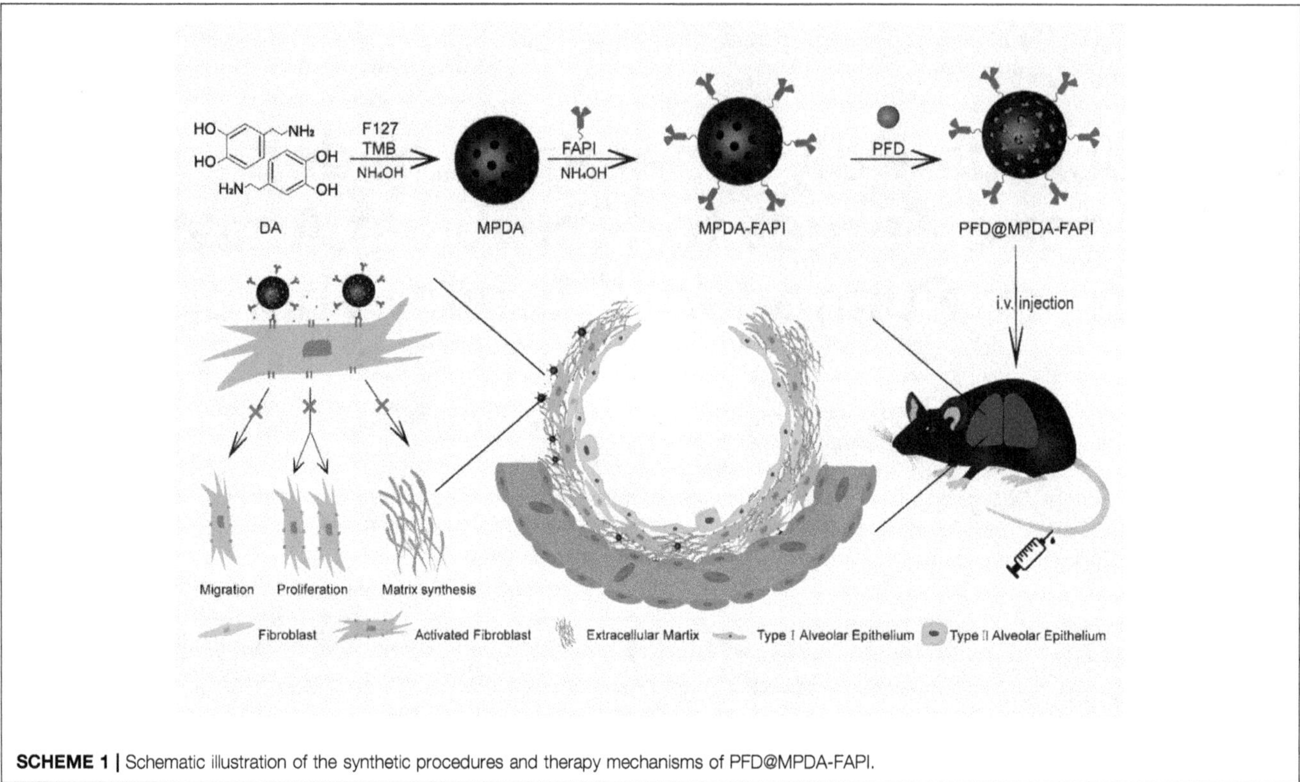

SCHEME 1 | Schematic illustration of the synthetic procedures and therapy mechanisms of PFD@MPDA-FAPI.

interests many researchers (Wenlong et al., 2015; Lin et al., 2019; Wu et al., 2020; Bergmann et al., 2021; Rohrich et al., 2022). It had been reported that FAP inhibitor (FAPI) labeled by radionuclide could reveal the FAP expression in patients with ILD, (Bergmann et al., 2021; Rohrich et al., 2022) positron emission tomography computed tomography (PET/CT) used FAPI as a tracer maybe is a promising imaging modality for ILDs to detect lesion earlier than CT, because CT only focuses on the change of structure, but FAPI PET/CT can observe the metabolism of the fibroblast before the change of anatomy. At the same time, Ma et al. have proved that bioluminescent probe target to FAP successfully indicated that the expression of FAP in the lung of the pulmonary fibrosis mice was increased (Lin et al., 2019). FAP is also has been proved that can play a role in antifibrosis therapy, Egger et al. (2017) reported that FAP inhibitor PT100 manifests antifibrosis properties in pulmonary fibrosis mice induced by bleomycin (BLM). Getting et al. found that FAP stimulates the activation of fibroblast (Wu et al., 2020). But in contrast, Kimura et al. found that the lack of FAP accelerates fibrosis. Meanwhile, Fan et al. (2016) found that FAP can accelerate the degradation and clearance of collagen. Therefore, the real role that FAP plays in fibrosis remains a mystery, but we may base the specific membrane protein to develop a class of target drug delivery nano.

There has been no nanodrug target to FAP for antifibrosis therapy before. Recently, nanodrugs that utilize nanoparticles as drug delivery carriers for targeting lesions, releasing drugs, improving pharmacokinetics, biocompatibility, and bioavailability interested people greatly (George et al., 2019; Altinoglu and Adali, 2020; Maghsoudi et al., 2020; Liu et al., 2021; Abd Al-Jabbar et al., 2022; Sultan et al., 2022). The mesoporous polydopamine (MPDA) is one of the most popular nanoparticles because of its intrinsic biocompatibility, facile preparation, and various easily modified surface groups (Seth et al., 2020; Lin et al., 2021; Zhu et al., 2021). Therefore, the nanodrug based on MPDA targets to FAP administrated by intravenous (IV) is one of the promising approaches for antifibrosis therapy without GI AE.

Here, we develop a nanodrug, PFD@MPDA-FAPI, based on MPDA, loading with PFD, and linking FAPI for antifibrosis therapy by FAP targeting drug delivery (**Scheme 1**), it is well biocompatibility and performs well at antifibrosis. MPDA was synthesized from dopamine hydrochloride with F127 and TMB as templates and then to remove template; NH_2-PEG_2-FAPI was conjugated to MPDA *via* condensation. PFD was loaded in the mesoporous on MPDA-FAPI. Compared to pure PFD and PFD@MPDA, PFD@MPDA-FAPI could target activated fibroblast *in vitro* and fibrosis lung *in vivo*, as well as improving the antifibrosis efficacy. This promising strategy demonstrates a new avenue for antifibrosis therapy.

2 EXPERIMENTAL SECTION

2.1 Materials

Dopamine hydrochloride (Aladdin, Shanghai, China) was used to synthesize MPDA; 1,3,5-trimethyl benzene (TMB) and F127 (Macklin, Shanghai, China) were used as the template. NH_2-PEG-FAPI (Tanzhenbio, Nanchang, China) was used for FAP targeting. Pirfenidone (Aladdin, Shanghai, China) is an antifibrosis drug. In immunohistochemical

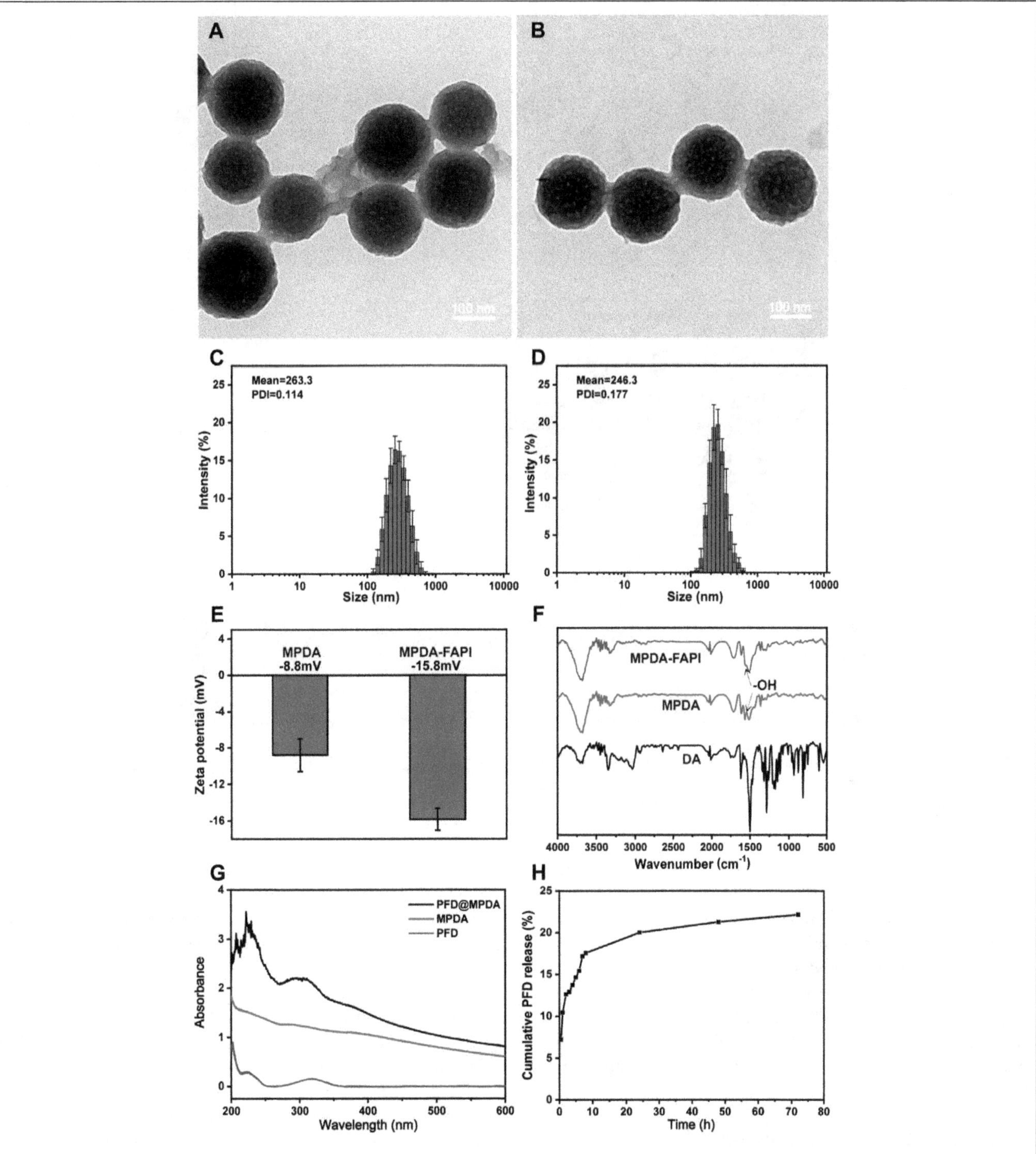

FIGURE 1 | TEM images of **(A)** MPDA and **(B)** MPDA-FAPI. Hydrodynamic diameters of **(C)** MPDA and **(D)** MPDA-FAPI. **(E)** Zeta potential of MPDA and MPDA-FAPI. **(F)** FTIR absorption spectrum of DA, MPDA, and MPDA-FAPI. **(G)** UV/Vis absorption spectrum of MPDA, PFD, and PFD@MPDA. **(H)** PFD released from PFD@MPDA at pH 7.4 for 72 h.

(IHC) staining, FN antibody (ab2413, Invitrogen) and FAP antibody (PA5-99458, Invitrogen) diluted 1:200, and α-SMA antibody (19245S, CST) diluted 1:800. For Western blot, FN antibody and FAP antibody diluted 1:1,000 was used. All other reagents were obtained from Aladdin.

2.2 Synthesis of MPDA and MPDA-FAPI

MPDA was synthesized by a facile approach. In short, 150 mg of dopamine hydrochloride was dissolved in 3 ml of deionized water, and 100 mg of F12 was dissolved in 3 ml of ethanol. The F127 solution was added to the dopamine solution, then

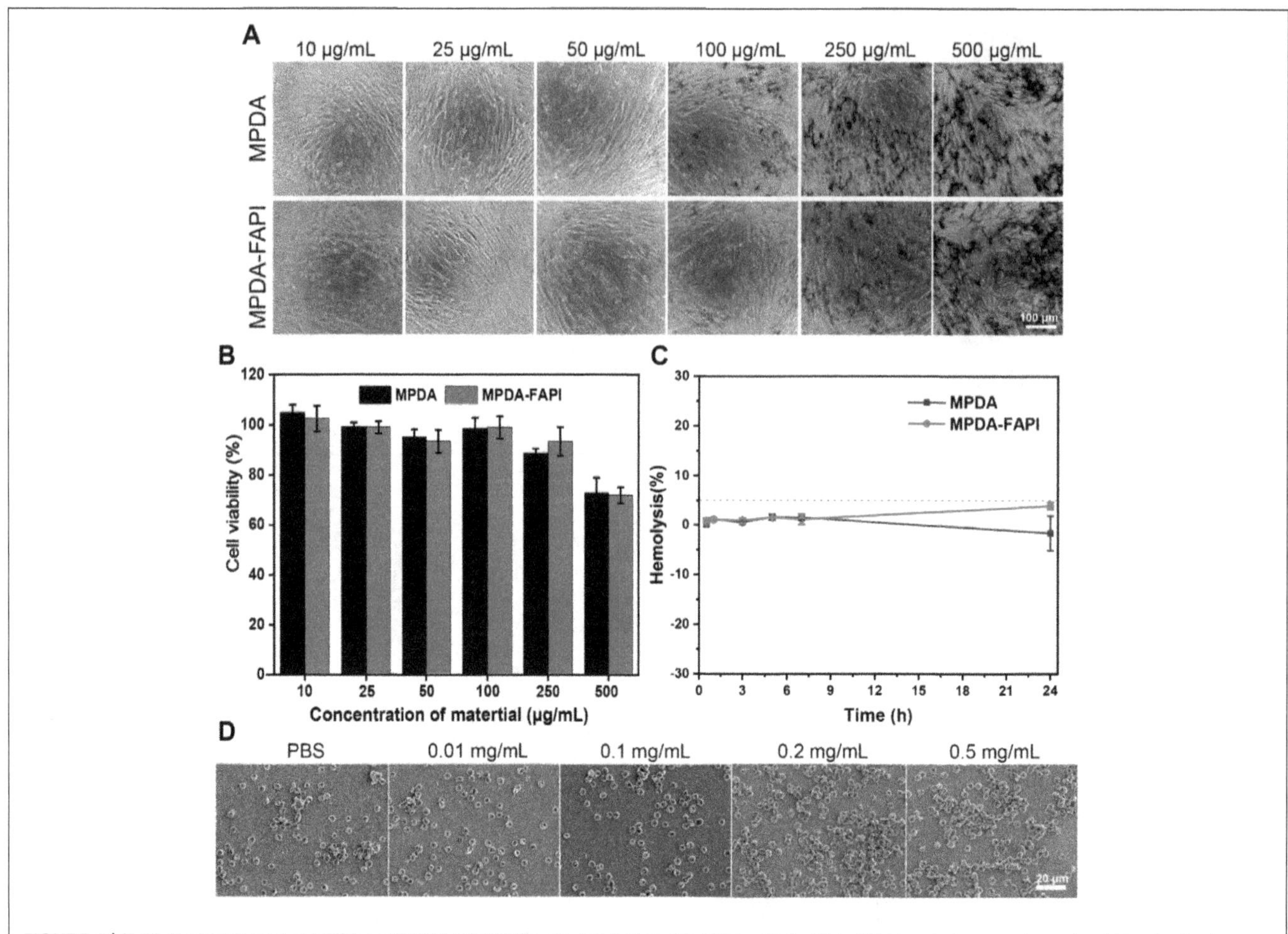

FIGURE 2 | (A,B) Cytotoxicity test of MPDA and MPDA-FAPI NPSs after incubation with HFL1 cells for 24 h. **(C)** Hemolysis percentage of red blood cells at 0.01 mg/ml of MPDA and MPDA-FAPI. **(D)** Morphology of red blood cell incubated with MPDA-FAPI.

added 160 μl of TMB, followed by 2 min of ultrasonic mixing, then 375 μl of 28% NH_4OH was added to the solution finally. After magnetic stirring for 2 h of the mixed solution, MPDA was obtained by centrifugal washing three times and resuspended in 1 ml deionized water. After drying, 1 ml MPDA solution weighs 1.5–2 mg. MPDA-FAPI was synthesized as follows. Then, 28% NH_4OH was used to adjust the pH of 3 ml MPDA solution to 9, then added 2 mg FAPI-NH_2-PEG, then the MPDA-FAPI was obtained by centrifugal washing after magnetic stirring at room temperature overnight.

2.3 Drug Loading and Release

First, 10 mg PFD was dissolved in 2 ml of methanol, then added PFD solution into 500 μl MPDA solution, magnetic stirring overnight and then centrifugally washing, finally resuspended the sediment in 1 ml deionized water to obtain MPDA@PFD. We tested the ultraviolet-visible (UV-Vis) absorbance of different concentrations of PFD to draw a standard curve of PFD, which is used for calculating the PFD concentration of nanodrug. The loading capacity is the weight ratio of PFD in MPDA@PFD. The 500 μl MPDA@PFD was sealed in a dialysis bag and put in a 15 ml tube with 2 ml PBS (pH 7.4) buffer solution, the mixture was shaken for 72 h a speed of 150 rpm. Periodically remove 0.5 ml of dialysate with a pipette gun and immediately add 0.5 ml of fresh PBS buffer to keep the constant total volume of the solution. After 72 h, the drug release was measured by the UV-Vis spectrophotometer.

2.4 Characterization

The morphology of MPDA and MPDA-FAPI were observed by using a transmission electron microscope (TEM). Firstly, prepared MPDA and MPDA-FAPI were dripped on the copper net, then dried and placed under the transmission electron microscope. The hydrodynamic diameter and the distribution of MPDA and MPDA-FAPI used dynamic light scattering (DLS) and zeta potential were measured by the laser nanometer particle size analyzer. The Fourier transform infrared (FTIR) spectrum and UV-vis spectrum of samples were obtained as follows. The proper amount of samples (DA, MPDA, and MPDA-FAPI) were grinded and pressed with KBr, respectively, then the prepared samples were detected by FTIR spectrometer, the scanning wavelength range was 500–4000 cm^{-1}. The appropriate number of samples (PFD, MPDA, and MPDA@ PFD) were uniformly dispersed in the deionized water, using

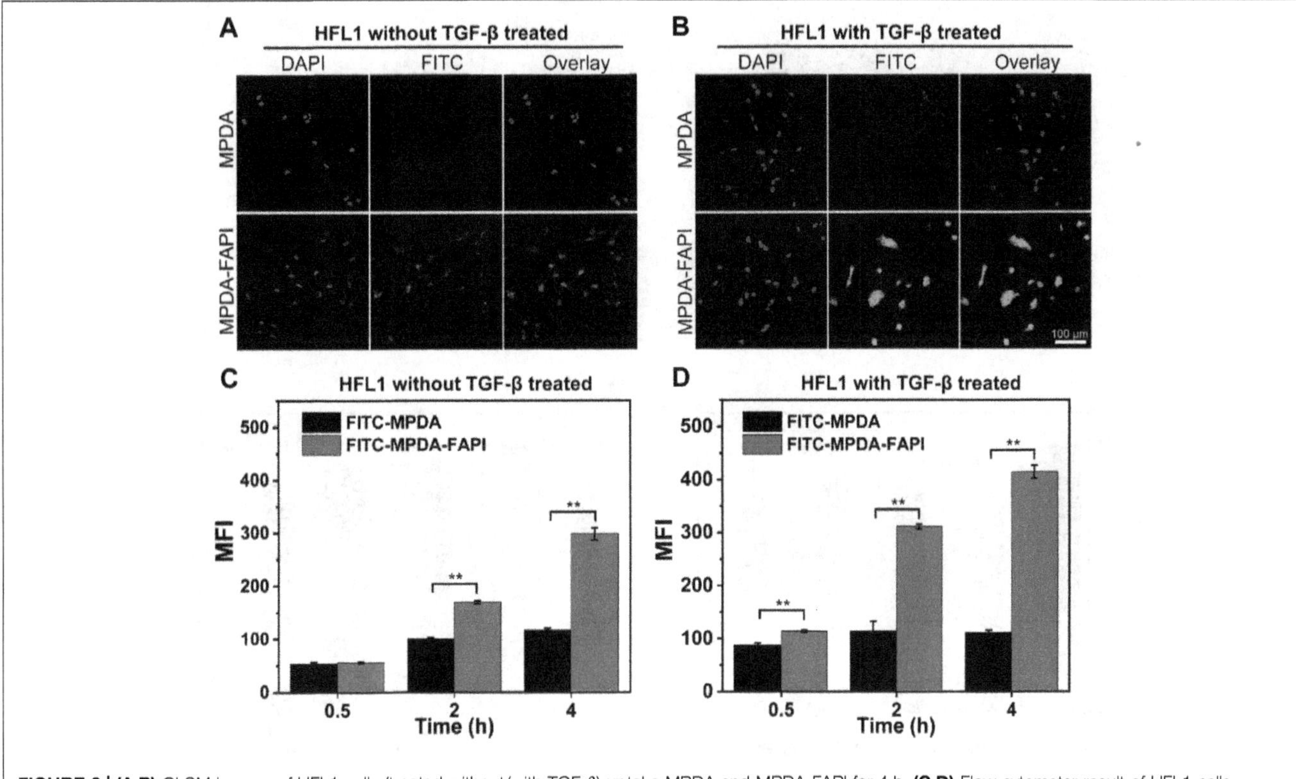

FIGURE 3 | (A,B) CLSM images of HFL1 cells (treated without/with TGF-β) uptake MPDA and MPDA-FAPI for 4 h. **(C,D)** Flow cytometer result of HFL1 cells (treated without/with TGF-β) uptake of MPDA and MPDA-FAPI (**$p < 0.01$).

the UV-Vis spectrophotometer to record the spectrum of samples within the range of 200–600 nm.

2.5 *In Vitro* Experience

2.5.1 Cell Culture

HFL1 (human fetal lung fibroblast, Procell CL-0106) was provided by Procell Life Science and Technology Co., cultured in Ham's F-12K with 10% fetal bovine serum (FBS) and 1% penicillin-streptomycin, cells were kept in a humidified atmosphere containing 5% CO_2 at 37°C.

2.5.2 Cytotoxicity and Blood Compatibility

For the cytotoxicity assay *in vitro*, HFL1 was first seeded into 96-well plates at a density of 5,000 cells per well overnight. Then, the original medium is then taken away and replaced with a fresh one containing various concentrations of nanoparticles and incubated for 24 h. The concentration of MPDA and MPDA-FAPI were 10–500 μg/ml. Finally, 100 μl, 0.1 μl/ml CCk8 solution was added to determine the relative cell viabilities among different concentration of nanoparticles treated groups as well as the untreated control.

Then, 200 μl 16% red blood cell suspension was incubated with MPDA and MPDA-FAPI (0.01 mg/ml), respectively, then centrifuged for 5 min, 1,000 × g at pre-set time points (1, 3, 6, 9, 18, and 24 h) to obtain supernatant. The Microplate Reader measured the absorbance of each supernatant at 540 nm to calculate the hemolysis rate. Whole blood was centrifuged with 1,000 × g for 5 min, then the lower red blood cells were collected, and incubated with MPDA-FAPI (0.01 mg/ml) for 15 min, then centrifuged to collect the red blood cell, then washed with PBS, and added 4% paraformaldehyde for 1 h. The fixed red blood cells were dehydrated with 70, 85, 95, and 100% ethanol, respectively, for 10 min. After the samples were dried, the samples were sprayed with gold, and the cell morphology was observed by scanning electron microscope (SEM).

2.5.3 Cellular Uptake Analyzed

FITC-MPDA and FITC MPDA-FAPI were prepared for cellular uptake experiment, obtained by stirring MPDA or MPDA-FAPI (1 ml) with FITC (300 μg) overnight, followed with centrifugally washed, and resuspended in 1 ml deionized water. Cellular uptake of FITC-MPDA and FITC-MPDA-FAPI were analyzed by endocytosis experiments. Specifically, HFL1 cells were seeded into a 24-well plate with a density of 5 × 10̂4 cells/holes, cultured overnight, and half of the holes were treated with 10 ng/ml TGF-β for 48 h. Then added to a complete medium containing 50 μg/ml FITC-MPDA or FITC-MPDA-FAPI. After incubating for 0.5, 2, and 4 h, the cells in each group were washed with PBS to remove the free material, digested with trypsin, and centrifuged to collect the cells. Finally, cells were resuspended by 200 μl PBS and detected by flow cytometry, the fluorescence intensity was measured by Flow JO 7.6.1 software.

The endocytosis of MPDA-FITC or MPDA-FAPI-FITC was also observed by confocal laser scanning. Specifically, HFL1 cells were first seeded in a cell culture dish with a density of 2 × 10̂5 cells per dish and then cultured overnight; then, two dishes of cells were treated with

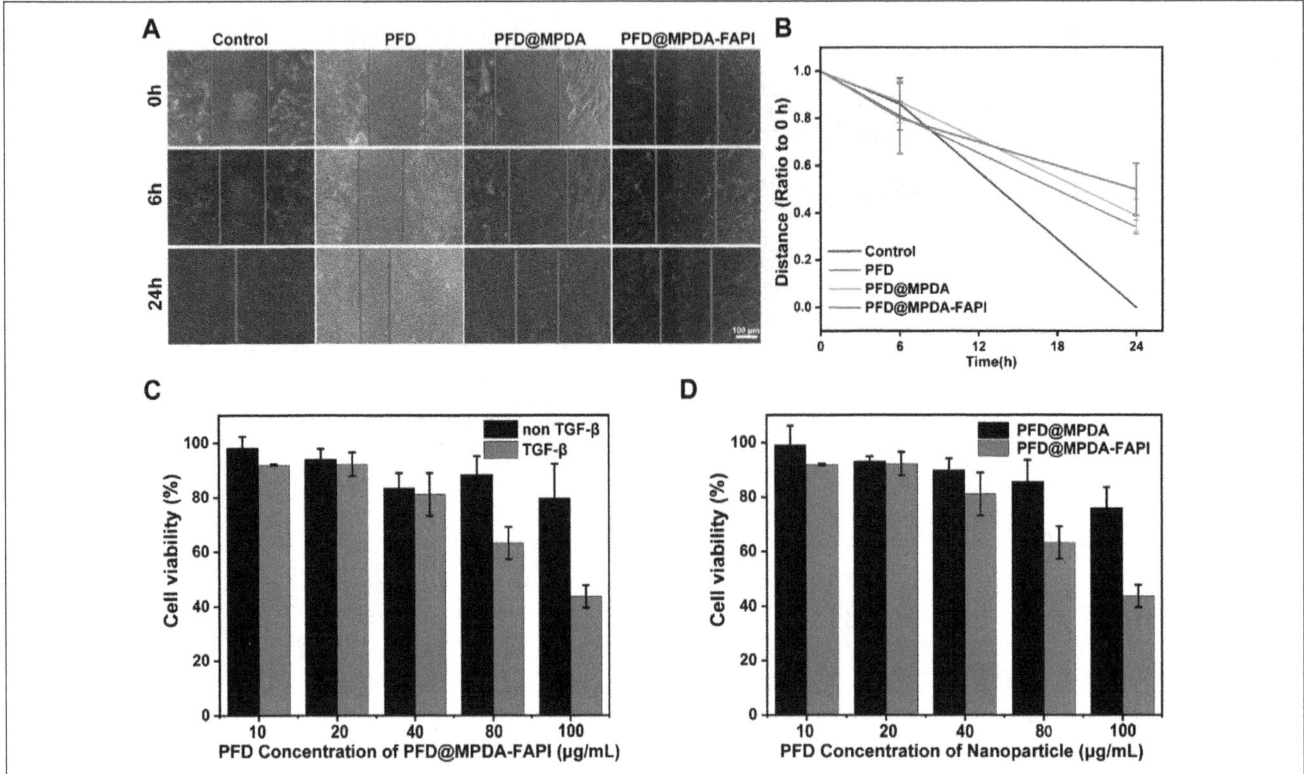

FIGURE 4 | (A,B) Scratch test results of HFL1-1 treated by TGF-β and incubated with PFD, PFD@MPDA, and PFD@MPDA-FAPI. **(C)** Proliferation test of PFD@MPDA-FAPI NPSs after incubation with HFL1 cells without/with TGF-β for 24 h. **(D)** Proliferation test of PFD@MPDA and PFD@MPDA-FAPI NPSs after incubation with HFL1-1 cells treated by TGF-β for 24 h (**$p < 0.01$).

TGF-β for 48 h and finally added to a complete medium containing 50 μg/ml FITC-MPDA or FITC-MPDA-FAPI. The cells were then washed with PBS after incubation for 4 h, then the cells were immobilized with 4% paraformaldehyde for 30 min and washed with PBS three times, the cell nucleus was stained with 1 ml DAPI in each dish for 15 min, and the cells were washed with PBS three times, and 2 ml PBS was added to each dish to keep the cell morphology, finally cells were observed and photographed with a laser confocal microscope.

2.5.5 Cell Proliferation Inhabitation

MTT assay was used to investigate the effects of MPDA@PFD and PFD@MPDA-FAPI on HFL1 with and without TGF-β treated. HFL1 cells were seeded into a 96-well plate at a density of 5,000 cells per hole and then cultured overnight. The original medium is then taken away and replaced with fresh complete media containing different concentrations of nanomaterials, the concentration of PFD in MPDA@PFD and MPDA-FAPII@PFD was in the range of 10–100 μg/ml, 50 μl, 1 mg/ml. MTT solution was then added to determine the relative cell viabilities among different concentration of nanoparticles treated groups as well as the untreated control.

2.5.6 Cell Scratches Experiment

HFL1 cells were seeded into a 24-well plate with a density of 5×10^4 cells per hole and cultured overnight, then treated with 10 ng/mg TGF-β for 48 h and scratched the bottom of the well to create artificial gaps in the cell. Then the cells were divided into three groups, incubated with 50 μg/ml MPDA@PFD, PFD@MPDA-FAPI, and PBS especially for 12 h, then washed with PBS, cultured in DMEM (serum-free), and photographed the gaps at the same position every different time (0, 6, and 24 h) by an inverted microscope, ImageJ software was used to measure and analyze the scratch area.

2.6 *In Vivo* Experience

2.6.1 Pulmonary Fibrosis Animal Model

C57BL/6 male mice (6–8 weeks, w ≈ 25 g) were used for the study. Animals were kept in a good environment. Drinking water and food were freely available. Mice were lightly anesthetized with 1.5% pentobarbital sodium, and BLM (2 mg/kg, YuanYe, Shanghai) was administered transtracheal *via* a laryngoscope (Yuyan, Shanghai). Micro CT (ALOKA LCT-200) was performed after 6 days to confirm the interstitial lung disease (**Supplementary Figure S5**).

2.6.2 *In Vivo* Imaging

MPDA and MPDA-FAPI are prepared for ICG/NIR imaging. The nanodrug labeled by ICG was obtained by stirring MPDA or MPDA-FAPI (1 ml) and 1 ml 1 mg/ml ICG overnight, followed by centrifugally washed and resuspended in 1 ml deionized water. ICG-MPDA and ICG-MPDA-FAPI were administrated *via* tail

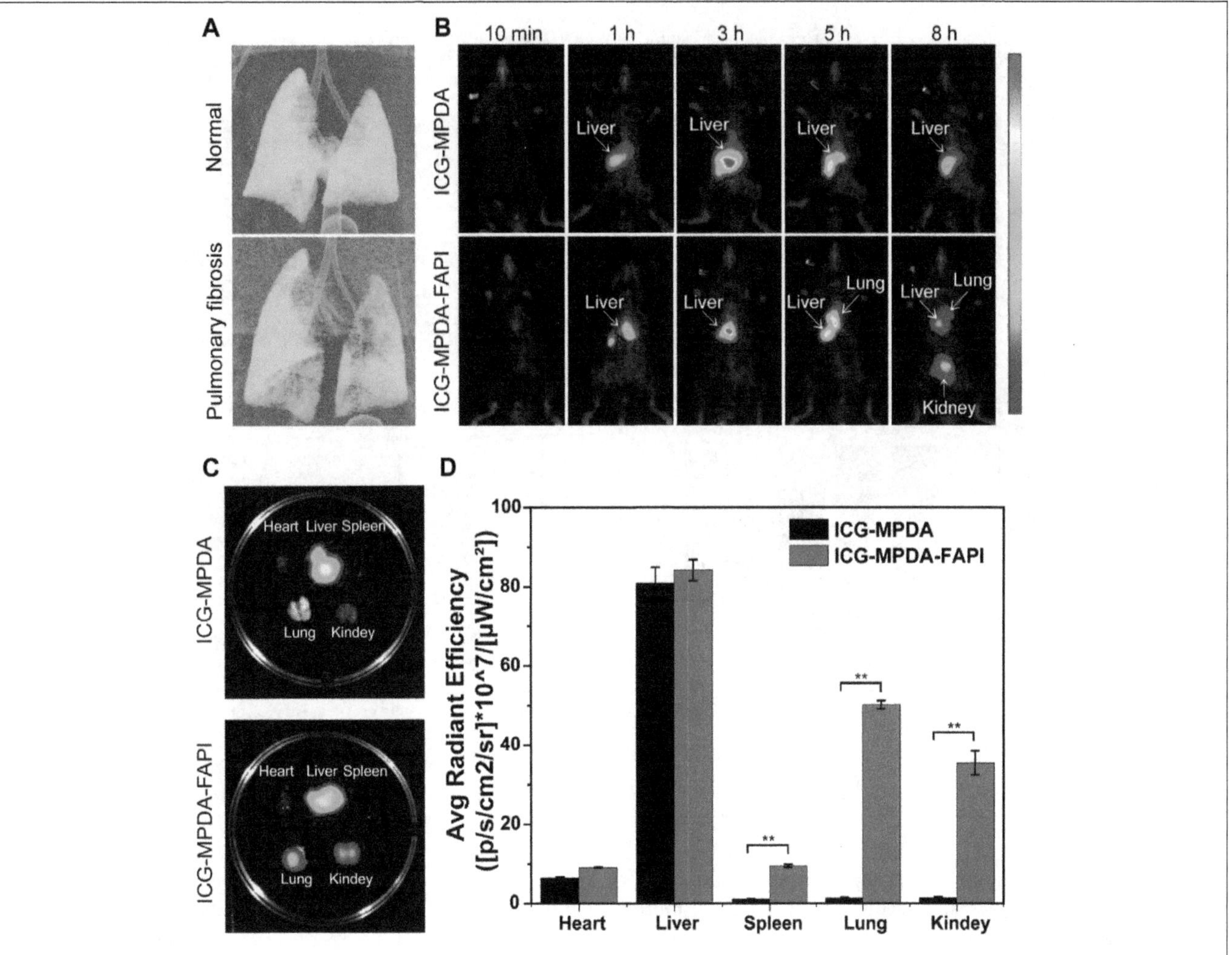

FIGURE 5 | (A) 3D CT of the normal lung and pulmonary fibrosis. **(B)** ICG-MPDA and ICG-MPDA-FAPI NIR fluorescence imaging *in vivo* of pulmonary fibrosis mice. **(C)** ICG-MPDA and ICG-MPDA-FAPI NIR fluorescence imaging of pulmonary fibrosis mice *in vitro*. **(D)** ICG-MPDA and ICG-MPDA-FAPI NIR fluorescence quantification of pulmonary fibrosis mice *in vitro*.

vein, and *in vivo* imaging was obtained after 10 min, 1, 3, 5, and 8 h administration of the pulmonary fibrosis mice. After 8 h imaging, the heart, liver, spleen, lungs, and kidneys were resected to quantify the radiant efficiency *in vitro*.

2.6.3 *In Vivo* Antifibrosis Therapy

Three healthy mice as the control group. Then, 15 pulmonary fibrosis mice were divided into five groups randomly, named NaCl, MPDA, PFD, PFD@MPDA, and PFD@MPDA-FAPI groups especially. Except for the control group, other groups of mice were pulmonary fibrosis, after 7 days induced by BLM, each group of mice was IV administrated with the corresponding drugs every 2 days regularly. In NaCl and MPDA groups, mice were IV injected with 120 μl NS and 120 μl MPDA solution, respectively. In the PFD, PFD@MPDA, and PFD@MPDA-FAPI groups, the dosage of PFD was 6 mg/kg. After three times of therapy, all the mice were sacrificed, right lungs were collected for WB analyses, and left lungs were collected for histological analyses.

2.6.4 Alveolitis and Fibrosis Grading

In histological analyses, HE staining and Masson staining were performed for grading alveolitis and fibrosis, the grading is according to the method of Szapiel et al. (1979). Alveolitis was evaluated with the HE stained sections and was graded using the criteria as follows: none (0), no alveolitis; mild (1+), thickening of the alveolar septum by a mononuclear cell infiltrate, with involvement limited to focal, pleural-based lesions occupying less than 20% of the lung and with good preservation of the alveolar architecture; moderate (2+), more widespread alveolitis involving 20–50% of the lung, although still predominantly pleural based; severe (3+), diffuse alveolitis involving more than 50% of the lung, with occasional consolidation of air spaces by the intra-alveolar mononuclear cells and some hemorrhagic areas within the interstitium and/or alveolus. The extent of fibrosis in these sections was graded using the following criteria: none (0), no evidence of fibrosis; mild (1+), focal regions of fibrosis involving less than 20% of the lung. Fibrosis involved

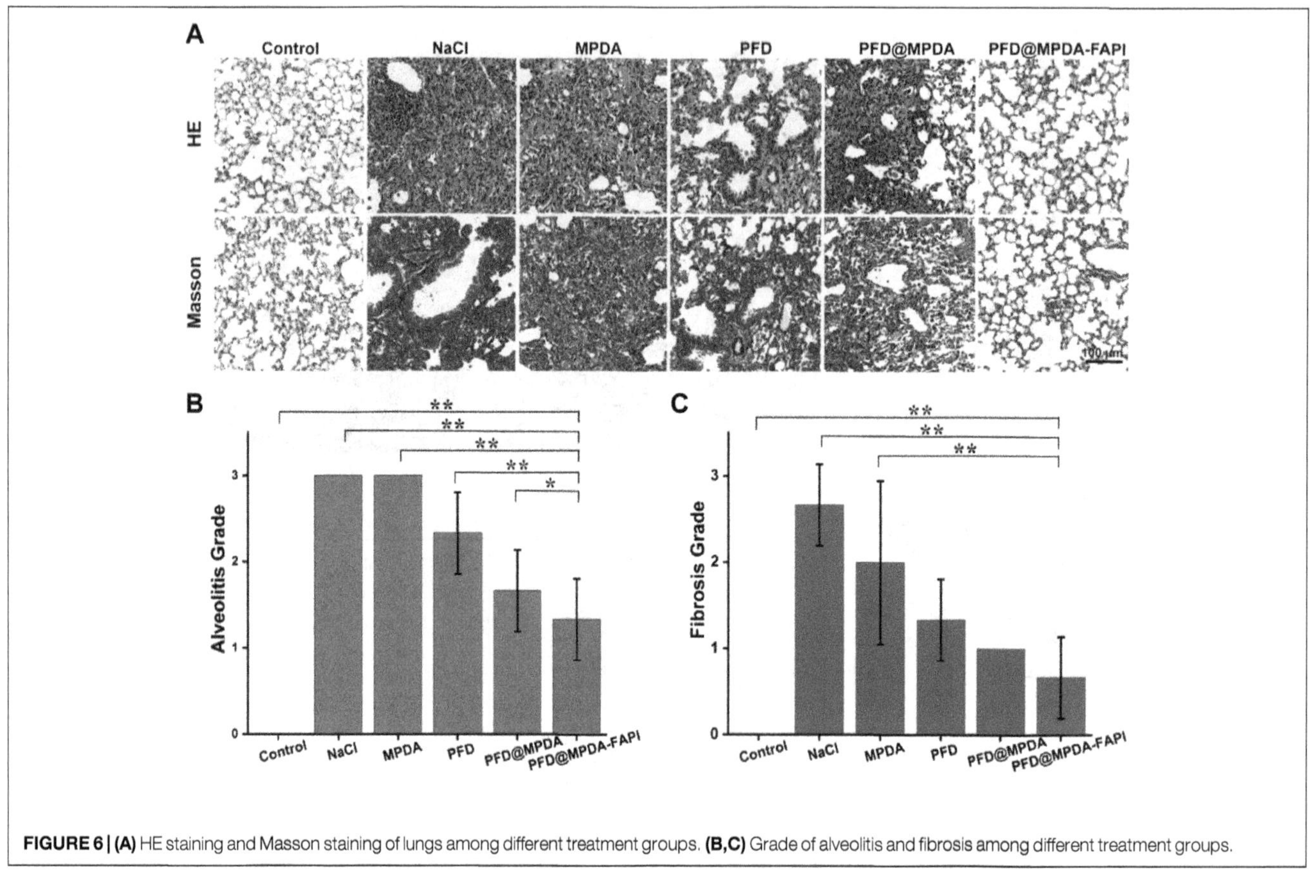

FIGURE 6 | (A) HE staining and Masson staining of lungs among different treatment groups. **(B,C)** Grade of alveolitis and fibrosis among different treatment groups.

the pleura and the interstitium of the subpleural parenchyma with some distortion of alveolar architecture; moderate (2+), more extensive fibrosis involving 20–50% of the lung and fibrotic regions mostly extending inward from the pleura and still focal; severe (3+), widespread fibrosis, involving more than 50% of the lung. Confluent lesions with extensive derangement of parenchymal architecture, including cystic air spaces lined by cuboidal epithelium.

2.6.5 IHC Staining

FN antibody and FAP antibody were diluted to 1:200, and α-SMA antibody was diluted to 1:800 for IHC staining. Image-Pro Plus was used to calculate the average optical density (AOD) of FN, FAP, and α-SMA among different groups.

2.6.6 Western Blot Analyses

The expression of FN and FAP in different groups was analyzed by WB. FN antibody and FAP antibody are diluted to 1: 1,000 for WB.

3 RESULT AND DISCUSSION

3.1 Synthesis and Characterization of MPDA, PFD@MPDA, and PFD@MPDA-FAPI

The synthetic procedures of MPDA, MPDA-FAPI, and PFD@ MPDA-FAPI nanoparticles are depicted in **Scheme 1**. First, the soft templating method was used to synthesize MPDA. All these nanoparticles were obtained in the aqueous solution. As for the production of MPDA, F127, and TBM were chosen as templates, ethanol, and ammonia solution were used for cosolvent and the catalyst in the polymerization of DA, then *via* the π–π stacking interactions, PDA was self-assembled on the templates, MPDA NPs were finally obtained by removing of templates (Wu et al., 2019; Lin et al., 2021). Second, NH_2-PEG_2-FAPI was conjugated to MPDA *via* condensation of the amine groups on NH_2-PEG_2-FAPI and the dihydroxy indole groups on MPDA to form MPDA-FAPI. Finally, PFD was loaded onto MPDA and MPDA-FAPI by magnetic stirring to form PFD@MPDA and PFD@MPDA-FAPI.

TEM observations confirmed that MPDA and MPDA-FAPI NPs manifest the well-defined spherical morphology and mesoporous structure, as well as uniform size distribution (**Figures 1A,B**), and the huge surface area created by mesoporous structure, is suitable for drug loading. The average diameters of MPDA and MPDA-FAPI NPs are all about 200 nm. DLS measurement also demonstrates that no aggregation occurs of these nanoparticles, the average hydrodynamic diameters of MPDA and MPDA-FAPI nanoparticles are ≈263 and 246 nm, respectively (**Figures 1C,D**). Compared to the diameter of the dried sample used in TEM measurement, the hydrodynamic diameter is larger. The tiny variety of the nanoparticles' diameter between TEM and DLS results may occur by swelling effect, which is

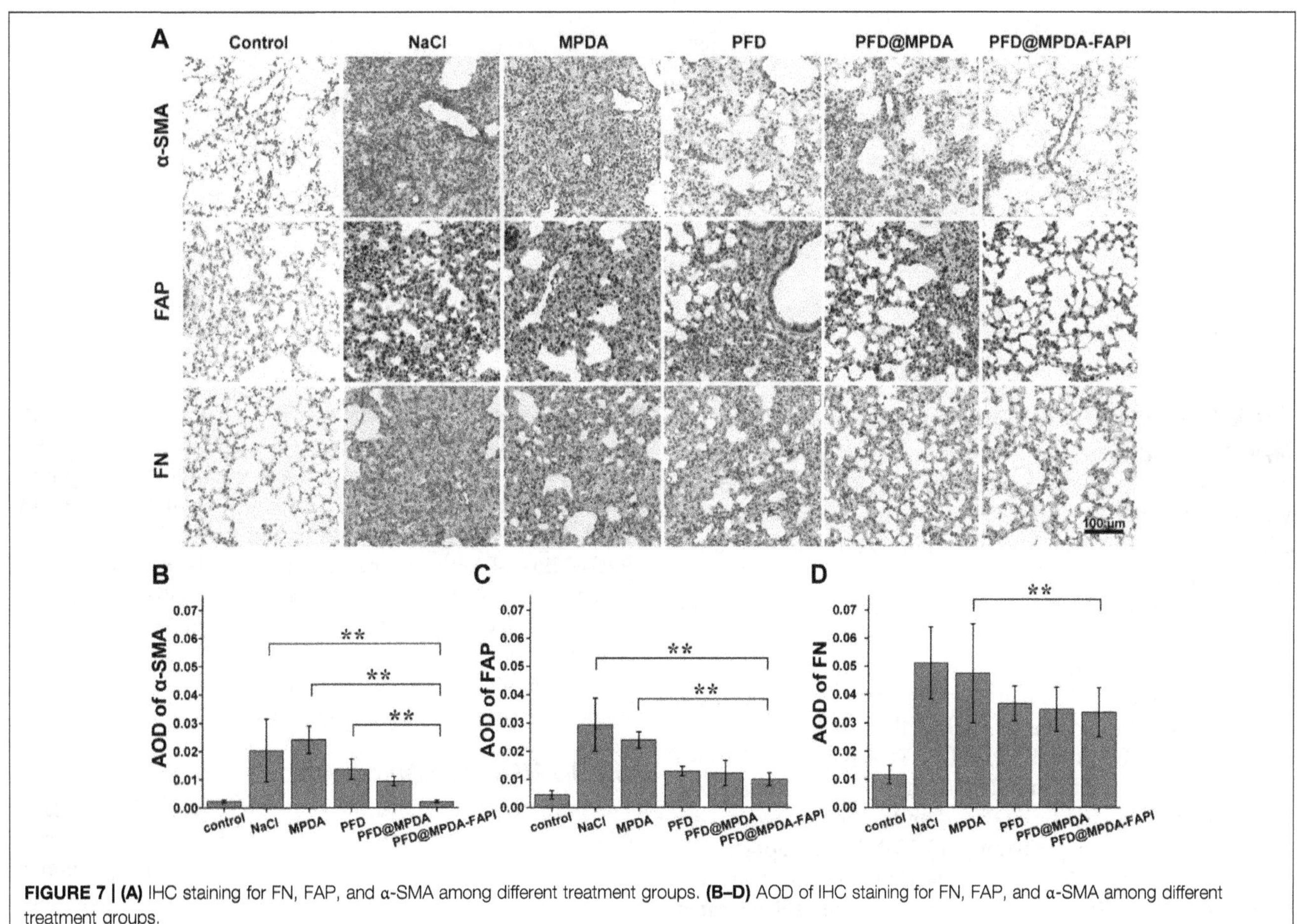

FIGURE 7 | (A) IHC staining for FN, FAP, and α-SMA among different treatment groups. **(B–D)** AOD of IHC staining for FN, FAP, and α-SMA among different treatment groups.

common in polymer material. The nanoscale diameter is safe for IV administration without pulmonary embolism risk. Meanwhile, the zeta potentials of MPDA and MPDA-FAPI nanoparticles are −8.8 and −15.8 mV, respectively (**Figure 1E**), the lower charge of MPDA-FAPI confirmed the conjugation of MPDA and the negatively charged NH_2-PEG_2-FAPI. FTNR spectrum can also prove the conjunction of MPDA and FAPI, the condensation of the amine groups on NH_2-PEG_2-FAPI with the hydroxy indole groups on MPDA, consuming the hydroxyl, because of hydroxyl on MPDA manifests a characteristic absorption band at 1,500 cm^{-1}, hence, the lower absorbance of MPDA-FAPI at 1,500 cm^{-1} proved the condensation of MPDA and NH_2-PEG_2-FAPI (**Figure 1F**).

3.2 Drug Loading and Release Properties

The UV-Vis absorption spectrum of PFD@MPDA clearly shows the characteristic absorption band of PFD at 319 nm (**Figure 1G**). Based on the standard curve of PFD (**Supplementary Figure S1**), the loading capacity (the weight ratio of PFD to MPDA) was calculated as 53% by measuring the PFD@MPDA absorbance at 319 nm. It is reported that the loading efficiency of MPDA is better than PDA without mesoporous (Chen et al., 2016; Peng et al., 2019), the satisfying loading efficiency of PFD@MPDA in our study may also be thanks to the large specific surface area brought by the mesoporous structure.

In vitro, the release of PFD from PFD@MPDA was investigated in PBS by a UV-Vis spectrophotometer. PFD released from PFD@MPDA was accumulated in a neutral solution (pH 7.4) mimicking *in vivo* environments. After 72 h, about 22% of PFD is released from PFD@MPDA at pH 7.4 (**Figure 1H**).

3.3 Cytotoxicity and Blood Compatibility

Biocompatibility is crucial for nanoparticles. Both MPDA and MPDA-FAPI nanoparticles of various concentrations (10–500 μg/ml) display negligible cytotoxicity after 24 h incubation with HFL1 cells. (**Figures 2A,B**), which proved that the nanoparticle does not harm normal HFL1 cells. After 72 h treated with MPDA and MPDA-FAPI (0.01 mg/ml), the hemolysis rate was less than 5% *in vitro* (**Figure 2C**). Also, the SEM result of RBC treated with MPDA-FAPI at various concentrations (10–500 μg/ml) shows normal morphology, consistent with the low hemolysis (**Figure 2D**). As expected, the biocompatibility of nanoparticle based on PDA is good because PDA is also the primary pigment of melanin, which naturally exist in the human body. Good biocompatibility allows nanoparticle utility in practice.

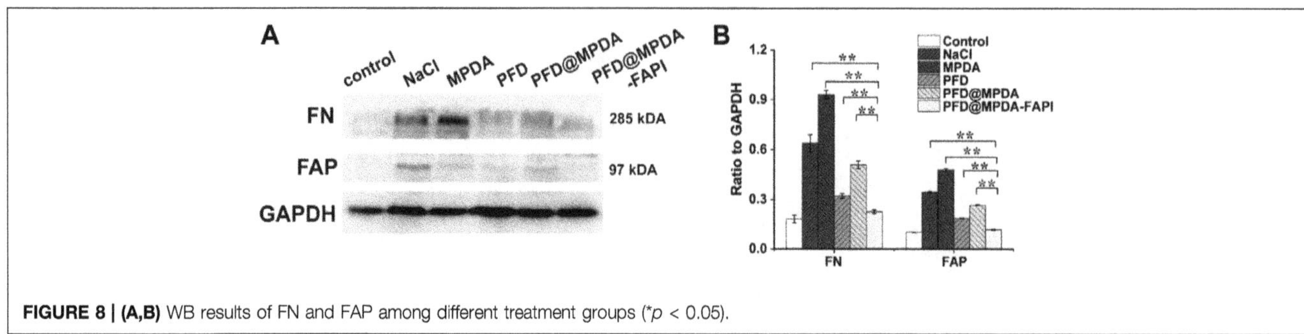

FIGURE 8 | (A,B) WB results of FN and FAP among different treatment groups (*$p < 0.05$).

3.4 Cellular Uptake and Localization of Nanoparticle

We observed the HFL1 treated without/with TGF-β uptake MPDA and MPDA-FAPI for 4 h by the confocal laser scanning microscope (CLSM), the highest cell uptake was observed for FITC-MPDA-FAPI in HFL1 with TGF-β treated (**Figures 3A,B**). The cellular uptake of MPDA and MPDA-FAPI for 0.5, 2, and 4 h were quantificationally investigated by a flow cytometer (**Figures 3C,D**). With the time changed, the uptake of nanodrug increased, and at each time point, the MFI of the FITC-MPDA-FAPI group is higher than FITC-MPDA no matter whether HFL1 was treated by TGF-β or not. We also found that the uptake of FITC-MPDA-FAPI is higher in HFL1 which is treated by TGF-β than the nontreated group, but the difference between FITC-MPDA uptake in HFL1 treated by TGF-β and nontreated groups was tiny (**Supplementary Figure S2**). As expected, the HFL1 treated with TGF-β and incubated with FITC-MPDA-FAPI for 4 h showed the highest MFI (414 ± 12), which is consistent with the CLSM result.

The higher uptake of MPDA-FAPI by HFL1 treated with TGF-β indicates that the MPDA-FAPI is successfully targeting the activated fibroblast and improving the uptake of nanodrug, which is beneficial for pulmonary fibrosis foci target drug delivery.

3.5 *In Vitro* Therapy of Nanoparticle

TGF-β is considered a key regulator in tissue fibrosis by promoting the overexpression of downstream fibrosis-related target genes. The HFL1 is activated *in vitro* and treated by TGF-β for 48 h, which can promote the proliferation and migration of HFL1, and also promote the expression of the biomarkers of fibrosis (such as FN and α-SMA). PFD can inhibit the activity of TGF-β and regulate the downstream signal of the TGF/Smad signal pathway, which has the properties of antifibrosis. Compared to pure PFD and PFD@ MPDA, PFD@MPDA-FAPI can promote the drug uptake of HFL1, which manifest the best antifibrosis properties.

The effects of NPS-loaded PFD on the proliferation of HFL1 were analyzed by MTT assay. The results showed that PFD@MPDA-FAPI could inhibit the proliferation of HFL1 treated by TGF-β, while HFL1 without TGF-β treatment had not been significantly inhibited (**Figure 4C**). In addition, PFD@MPDA-FAPI performs better than PFD@MPDA in inhibiting the proliferation of HFL1 treated with TGF-β (**Figure 4D**). According to the results of the MTT assay, the 100 μg/ml PFD concentration of MPDA@PFD and MPDA@PFD-FAPI were chosen for the scratch test to measure HFL1 migration. The results showed that both PFD, PFD@MPDA, and PFD@MPDA-FAPI could inhibit the migration of HFL1 treated by TGF-β, and PFD@MPDA-FAPI performed best (**Figures 4A,B**).

The study suggested that PFD@MPDA-FAPI targeting FAP does better than PFD@MPDA on inhibitor the proliferation and migration of activated fibroblast, and had a tiny effect on the normal fibroblast, suggesting that nanoparticle target to FAP is useful in the therapy of pulmonary fibrosis.

3.6 *In Vivo* Biodistribution

Pulmonary fibrosis mice were induced by BLM (2 mg/kg) administered transtracheal *via* a laryngoscope, and after 6 days, micro-CT was performed to confirm the pulmonary fibrosis, then the next day *in vivo* NIR imaging was performed to explore the biodistribution of MPDA and MPDA-FAPI in pulmonary fibrosis mice. The 3D remolding of lungs based on micro-CT showed that, compared to healthy pulmonary, the normal airway structure in fibrosis lungs is reduced (**Figure 5A**). Only MPDA-FAPI has a significant accumulation in the lungs of pulmonary fibrosis mice (**Figure 5B**). After 8 h imaging, the major organs of mice were resected and quantified the radiant efficiency, the lung of the pulmonary fibrosis mouse injected with ICG-MPDA-FAPI also showed a high radiant efficiency, which was consistent with the *in vivo* ICG imaging (**Figures 5C,D**).

The ICG-MPDA and ICG-MPDA-FAPI were first observed in livers because the liver is a typical organ with the endothelial reticular system, in which Kupffer cells uptake nanoparticles. For ICG-MPDA, the accumulation only lasted in the liver; as for ICG-MPDA-FAPI, the nanoparticle gradually accumulates in fibrosis lung, in which FAP is overexpressed. At a later point, ICG-MPDA-FAPI accumulates in the kidneys because the hydrophilic PEG brought by the NH_2-PEG_2-FAPI may change the pharmacokinetic. The NIR imaging indicated the MPDA-FAPI is targeted to the overexpress FAP of fibrosis foci in *in vivo*, MPDA-FAPI is a successful FAP targeted nanodelivery carried out in *in vivo*.

3.7 *In Vivo* Antifibrosis Properties

After the nanodrug treatment, the weight of mice varies mild, which indicates the nanodrug is safe (**Supplementary Figure S6**).

The grades of alveolitis and fibrosis of the mice in the control group were both 0. Compared to the control group, NaCl, MPDA, and PFD@MPDA groups, the PFD@MPDA-FAPI shows the lowest grades of alveolitis and fibrosis (**Figures 6A–C**).

In IHC staining, the control group showed the lowest expression of α-SMA, FAP, and FN. Compared to the control group, the expression of α-SMA, FAP, and FN were increased in NaCl and MPDA groups. The expression of α-SMA, FAP, and FN in PFD, PFD@MPDA, and PFD@MPDA-FAPI groups decreased compared to NaCl and MPDA groups, and the PFD@MPDA-FAPI group manifested the lowest expression (**Figures 7A–D**).

The results of WB were generally consistent with the IHC staining. In WB analyses, the control group showed a low expression of FAP and FN. Compared to the control group, NaCl and MPDA groups show higher expression of FN and FAP. In the PFD@MPDA-FAPI group, the expression of FN and FAP were lower than in the PFD and PFD@MPDA groups, which indicated that the antifibrosis properties of PFD@MPDA-FAPI are the best (**Figures 8A,B**).

In the pathological produce of pulmonary fibrosis, alveolitis comes first, then the fibroblast is activated, expressed FAP, and then activated fibroblast differentiate to myofibroblast, which is a key cell-expressed α-SMA to produce excessive exocellular matrix (Yu and Tang, 2022). The excessive exocellular matrix is comprised of collagen fibers, which can be determined by Masson staining and FN IHC.

Therefore, the WB and IHC results of low FN, FAP, and α-SMA expression in the PFD@MPDA-FAPI group, indicate that PFD@MPDA-FAPI shows good antifibrosis properties *in vivo* and performed better than pure PFD and PFD@MPDA in generally.

We also analyzed the antifibrosis properties of nanodrug after six times treatments. The PFD@MPDA-FAPI also performed the best, which is similar to the result of three times of treatments (**Supplementary Figures S3, S4**). It is considered that the pulmonary fibrosis of mice induced by BLM may change with time, in general, the fibrosis lesion may subside and is close to normal at the end, (Degryse and Lawson, 2011) so it is hard to explain the difference between three times and six times treatment groups, but either three times or six times treatment, we can observe the pleasing antifibrosis properties of PFD@MPDA-FAPI.

4 CONCLUSION

PFD@MPDA-FAPI, a nanoparticle developed based on MPDA, loading PFD, and targeting FAP on activated fibroblast, performs better than pure PFD and MPDA@PFD in inhibiting the proliferation and migration of the activated fibroblast, which is crucial in antifibrosis therapy, and do no harm to normal fibroblast. The nanoparticle is safe for IV administration and can accumulate in the fibrosis lung *in vivo*, also manifesting a good antifibrosis property. PFD@MPDA-FAPI is a promising nanodrug for antifibrosis therapy without the side effects of the stomach caused by PFD orally administrated. In addition, given consideration that FAP is also overexpressed on cancer-associated fibroblast, the MPDA also manifests a photothermal property, so replacing the loading drug with an anticancer drug may also develop a new tumor target nanodrug, which may perform well in cancer therapy combined with chemotherapy and photothermal therapy.

AUTHOR CONTRIBUTIONS

XW designed the study and gave instructions. QF performed the experiment, data analysis, and writing of the original draft. SL, JC, RZ, QH, PH, YL, JL, XZ, and QL helped perform the analysis with constructive discussions.

REFERENCES

Abd Al-Jabbar, S., Atiroğlu, V., Hameed, R. M., Guney Eskiler, G., Atiroğlu, A., Deveci Ozkan, A., et al. (2022). Fabrication of Dopamine Conjugated with Protein @metal Organic Framework for Targeted Drug Delivery: A Biocompatible pH-Responsive Nanocarrier for Gemcitabine Release on MCF-7 Human Breast Cancer Cells. *Bioorg. Chem.* 118, 105467. doi:10.1016/j.bioorg.2021.105467

Acharya, P. S., Zukas, A., Chandan, V., Katzenstein, A.-L. A., and Puré, E. (2006). Fibroblast Activation Protein: a Serine Protease Expressed at the Remodeling Interface in Idiopathic Pulmonary Fibrosis. *Hum. Pathol.* 37 (3), 352 360. doi:10.1016/j.humpath.2005.11.020

Altinoglu, G., and Adali, T. (2020). Alzheimer's Disease Targeted Nano-Based Drug Delivery Systems. *Curr Drug Targets* 21 (7), 628–646. doi:10.2174/1389450120666191118123151

Bergmann, C., Distler, J. H. W., Treutlein, C., Tascilar, K., Müller, A.-T., Atzinger, A., et al. (2021). 68Ga-FAPI-04 PET-CT for Molecular Assessment of Fibroblast Activation and Risk Evaluation in Systemic Sclerosis-Associated Interstitial Lung Disease: a Single-Centre, Pilot Study. *Lancet Rheumatology* 3 (3), e185–e194. doi:10.1016/s2665-9913(20)30421-5

Chen, F., Xing, Y., Wang, Z., Zheng, X., Zhang, J., and Cai, K. (2016). Nanoscale Polydopamine (PDA) Meets π-π Interactions: An Interface-Directed Coassembly Approach for Mesoporous Nanoparticles. *Langmuir* 32 (46), 12119–12128. doi:10.1021/acs.langmuir.6b03294

Degryse, A. L., and Lawson, W. E. (2011). Progress toward Improving Animal Models for Idiopathic Pulmonary Fibrosis. *Am. J. Med. Sci.* 341 (6), 444–449. doi:10.1097/MAJ.0b013e31821aa000

Deng, Z., Fear, M. W., Suk Choi, Y., Wood, F. M., Allahham, A., Mutsaers, S. E., et al. (2020). The Extracellular Matrix and Mechanotransduction in Pulmonary Fibrosis. *Int. J. Biochem. Cell Biol.* 126, 105802. doi:10.1016/j.biocel.2020.105802

Egger, C., Cannet, C., Gérard, C., Suply, T., Ksiazek, I., Jarman, E., et al. (2017). Effects of the Fibroblast Activation Protein Inhibitor, PT100, in a Murine Model of Pulmonary Fibrosis. *Eur. J. Pharmacol.* 809, 64–72. doi:10.1016/j.ejphar.2017.05.022

Fan, M.-H., Zhu, Q., Li, H.-H., Ra, H.-J., Majumdar, S., Gulick, D. L., et al. (2016). Fibroblast Activation Protein (FAP) Accelerates Collagen Degradation and Clearance from Lungs in Mice. *J. Biol. Chem.* 291 (15), 8070–8089. doi:10.1074/jbc.M115.701433

Fernández Pérez, E. R., Daniels, C. E., St. Sauver, J., Hartman, T. E., Bartholmai, B. J., Yi, E. S., et al. (2010). Incidence, Prevalence, and Clinical Course of Idiopathic Pulmonary Fibrosis. *Chest* 137 (1), 129–137. doi:10.1378/chest.09-1002

Garin-Chesa, P., Old, L. J., and Rettig, W. J. (1990). Cell Surface Glycoprotein of Reactive Stromal Fibroblasts as a Potential Antibody Target in Human Epithelial Cancers. *Proc. Natl. Acad. Sci. U.S.A.* 87 (18), 7235–7239. doi:10.1073/pnas.87.18.7235

George, A., Shah, P. A., and Shrivastav, P. S. (2019). Natural Biodegradable

Polymers Based Nano-Formulations for Drug Delivery: A Review. *Int. J. Pharm.* 561, 244–264. doi:10.1016/j.ijpharm.2019.03.011

Keane, F. M., Yao, T.-W., Seelk, S., Gall, M. G., Chowdhury, S., Poplawski, S. E., et al. (2013). Quantitation of Fibroblast Activation Protein (FAP)-specific Protease Activity in Mouse, Baboon and Human Fluids and Organs. *FEBS Open Bio* 4, 43–54. doi:10.1016/j.fob.2013.12.001

King, T. E., Jr., Bradford, W. Z., Castro-Bernardini, S., Fagan, E. A., Glaspole, I., Glassberg, M. K., et al. (2014). A Phase 3 Trial of Pirfenidone in Patients with Idiopathic Pulmonary Fibrosis. *N. Engl. J. Med.* 370 (22), 2083–2092. doi:10.1056/NEJMoa1402582

Lai, Y., Wei, X., Ye, T., Hang, L., Mou, L., and Su, J. (2021). Interrelation between Fibroblasts and T Cells in Fibrosing Interstitial Lung Diseases. *Front. Immunol.* 12, 747335. doi:10.3389/fimmu.2021.747335

Lancaster, L. H., de Andrade, J. A., Zibrak, J. D., Padilla, M. L., Albera, C., Nathan, S. D., et al. (2017). Pirfenidone Safety and Adverse Event Management in Idiopathic Pulmonary Fibrosis. *Eur. Respir. Rev.* 26 (146), 170057. doi:10.1183/16000617.0057-2017

Ley, B., Collard, H. R., and King, T. E., Jr. (2011). Clinical Course and Prediction of Survival in Idiopathic Pulmonary Fibrosis. *Am. J. Respir. Crit. Care Med.* 183 (4), 431–440. doi:10.1164/rccm.201006-0894CI

Lin, K., Gan, Y., Zhu, P., Li, S., Lin, C., Yu, S., et al. (2021). Hollow Mesoporous Polydopamine Nanospheres: Synthesis, Biocompatibility and Drug Delivery. *Nanotechnology* 32 (28), 285602. doi:10.1088/1361-6528/abf4a9

Lin, Y., Ma, Z., Li, Z., Gao, Y., Qin, X., Zhang, Z., et al. (2019). Bioluminescent Probe for Monitoring Endogenous Fibroblast Activation Protein-Alpha. *Anal. Chem.* 91 (23), 14873–14878. doi:10.1021/acs.analchem.9b02117

Liu, B., Yang, W., Che, C., Liu, J., Si, M., Gong, Z., et al. (2021). A Targeted Nano Drug Delivery System of AS1411 Functionalized Graphene Oxide Based Composites. *ChemistryOpen* 10 (4), 408–413. doi:10.1002/open.202000226

Maghsoudi, S., Taghavi Shahraki, B., Rabiee, N., Fatahi, Y., Dinarvand, R., Tavakolizadeh, M., et al. (2020). Burgeoning Polymer Nano Blends for Improved Controlled Drug Release: A Review. *Int. J. Nanomedicine* 15, 4363–4392. doi:10.2147/ijn.S252237

Nathan, S. D., Shlobin, O. A., Weir, N., Ahmad, S., Kaldjob, J. M., Battle, E., et al. (2011). Long-term Course and Prognosis of Idiopathic Pulmonary Fibrosis in the New Millennium. *Chest* 140 (1), 221–229. doi:10.1378/chest.10-2572

Peng, L., Hung, C.-T., Wang, S., Zhang, X., Zhu, X., Zhao, Z., et al. (2019). Versatile Nanoemulsion Assembly Approach to Synthesize Functional Mesoporous Carbon Nanospheres with Tunable Pore Sizes and Architectures. *J. Am. Chem. Soc.* 141 (17), 7073–7080. doi:10.1021/jacs.9b02091

Raghu, G., Collard, H. R., Egan, J. J., Martinez, F. J., Behr, J., Brown, K. K., et al. (2011). An Official ATS/ERS/JRS/ALAT Statement: Idiopathic Pulmonary Fibrosis: Evidence-Based Guidelines for Diagnosis and Management. *Am. J. Respir. Crit. Care Med.* 183 (6), 788–824. doi:10.1164/rccm.2009-040GL

Rockey, D. C., Bell, P. D., and Hill, J. A. (2015). Fibrosis - A Common Pathway to Organ Injury and Failure. *N. Engl. J. Med.* 372 (12), 1138–1149. doi:10.1056/NEJMra1300575

Röhrich, M., Leitz, D., Glatting, F. M., Wefers, A. K., Weinheimer, O., Flechsig, P., et al. (2022). Fibroblast Activation Protein-specific PET/CT Imaging in Fibrotic Interstitial Lung Diseases and Lung Cancer: A Translational Exploratory Study. *J. Nucl. Med.* 63 (1), 127–133. doi:10.2967/jnumed.121.261925

Seth, A., Gholami Derami, H., Gupta, P., Wang, Z., Rathi, P., Gupta, R., et al. (2020). Polydopamine-Mesoporous Silica Core-Shell Nanoparticles for Combined Photothermal Immunotherapy. *ACS Appl. Mat. Interfaces* 12 (38), 42499–42510. doi:10.1021/acsami.0c10781

Sultan, M. H., Moni, S. S., Madkhali, O. A., Bakkari, M. A., Alshahrani, S., Alqahtani, S. S., et al. (2022). Characterization of Cisplatin-Loaded Chitosan Nanoparticles and Rituximab-Linked Surfaces as Target-specific Injectable Nano-Formulations for Combating Cancer. *Sci. Rep.* 12 (1), 468. doi:10.1038/s41598-021-04427-w

Szapiel, S. V., Elson, N. A., Fulmer, J. D., Hunninghake, G. W., and Crystal, R. G. (1979). Bleomycin-induced Interstitial Pulmonary Disease in the Nude, Athymic Mouse. *Am. Rev. Respir. Dis.* 120 (4), 893–899. doi:10.1164/arrd.1979.120.4.893

Wenlong, L., Leilei, Y., Wei, F., Yi, C., Jing, T., Lanzhi, M., et al. (2015). Luciferase Expression Is Driven by the Promoter of Fibroblast Activation Protein-α in Murine Pulmonary Fibrosis. *Biotechnol. Lett.* 37 (9), 1757–1763. doi:10.1007/s10529-015-1855-8

Wu, D., Duan, X., Guan, Q., Liu, J., Yang, X., Zhang, F., et al. (2019). Mesoporous Polydopamine Carrying Manganese Carbonyl Responds to Tumor Microenvironment for Multimodal Imaging-Guided Cancer Therapy. *Adv. Funct. Mat.* 29 (16), 1900095. doi:10.1002/adfm.201900095

Wu, G., Xie, B., Lu, C., Chen, C., Zhou, J., and Deng, Z. (2020). microRNA-30a Attenuates TGF-β1-Induced Activation of Pulmonary Fibroblast Cell by Targeting FAP-α. *J. Cell Mol. Med.* 24 (6), 3745–3750. doi:10.1111/jcmm.15020

Yu, Q. Y., and Tang, X. X. (2022). Irreversibility of Pulmonary Fibrosis. *Aging Dis.* 13 (1), 73–86. doi:10.14336/ad.2021.0730

Zhu, M., Shi, Y., Shan, Y., Guo, J., Song, X., Wu, Y., et al. (2021). Recent Developments in Mesoporous Polydopamine-Derived Nanoplatforms for Cancer Theranostics. *J. Nanobiotechnol* 19 (1), 387. doi:10.1186/s12951-021-01131-9

2

Glycyrrhizic Acid Alleviates Bleomycin-Induced Pulmonary Fibrosis in Rats

Lili Gao[1†], Haiying Tang[1†], Huanyu He[1], Jia Liu[1], Jingwei Mao[2], Hong Ji[3], Hongli Lin[4] and Taihua Wu[1*]*

[1] Department of Respiratory Medicine, The First Affiliated Hospital of Dalian Medical University, Dalian, China, [2] Department of Gastroenterology, The First Affiliated Hospital of Dalian Medical University, Dalian, China, [3] Department of Pediatrics, The First Affiliated Hospital of Dalian Medical University, Dalian, China, [4] Department of Nephrology, The First Affiliated Hospital of Dalian Medical University, Dalian, China

***Correspondence:**
Taihua Wu,
Department of Respiratory Medicine, The First Affiliated Hospital of Dalian Medical University, 222 Zhongshan Road, Dalian 116011, China
wutaihua@sina.com;
Hongli Lin,
Department of Nephrology, The First Affiliated Hospital of Dalian Medical University, 222 Zhongshan Road, Dalian 116011, China
linhongli@vip.163.com

†These authors have contributed equally to this work.

Idiopathic pulmonary fibrosis is a progressive and lethal form of interstitial lung disease that lacks effective therapies at present. Glycyrrhizic acid (GA), a natural compound extracted from a traditional Chinese herbal medicine *Glycyrrhiza glabra*, was recently reported to benefit lung injury and liver fibrosis in animal models, yet whether GA has a therapeutic effect on pulmonary fibrosis is unknown. In this study, we investigated the potential therapeutic effect of GA on pulmonary fibrosis in a rat model with bleomycin (BLM)-induced pulmonary fibrosis. The results indicated that GA treatment remarkably ameliorated BLM-induced pulmonary fibrosis and attenuated BLM-induced inflammation, oxidative stress, epithelial-mesenchymal transition, and activation of transforming growth factor-beta signaling pathway in the lungs. Further, we demonstrated that GA treatment inhibited proliferation of 3T6 fibroblast cells, induced cell cycle arrest and promoted apoptosis *in vitro*, implying that GA-mediated suppression of fibroproliferation may contribute to the anti-fibrotic effect against BLM-induced pulmonary fibrosis. In summary, our study suggests a therapeutic potential of GA in the treatment of pulmonary fibrosis.

Keywords: glycyrrhizic acid, pulmonary fibrosis, bleomycin, transforming growth factor-beta, fibroproliferation

Introduction

Idiopathic pulmonary fibrosis (IPF) is a progressive, usually fatal, form of interstitial lung disease of unknown etiology. IPF is characterized by areas of peripheral fibrosis, interstitial inflammation, failure of alveolar re-epithelialization, persistence of fibroblasts/myofibroblasts, and deposition of extracellular matrix (ECM) molecules in the lung, and it resembles the histopathological pattern of usual interstitial pneumonitis (UIP; White et al., 2003). The progression of IPF may ultimately result in distortion of lung architecture and respiration failure, and the estimated 5-years survival of IPF is approximately 20% (King et al., 2001).

Fibroblasts play a critical role in the repair and regenerative process in almost all human tissues. Following injury, clusters of fibroblasts with an activated myofibroblast phenotype are transiently present in the granulation tissue, namely fibroblast foci, and they represent microscopic zones where fibroblasts migrate, proliferate, and secrete ECM proteins that provide a tissue scaffold for the repair process (Lorena et al., 2002). The activated fibroblasts, or myofibroblasts, are intermediates between fibroblasts and smooth muscle cells, simultaneously producing collagen and expressing α-smooth muscle actin (α-SMA; Hu and Phan, 2013), and they are involved in the physiological wound healing process and in the pathological fibrosis (Lorena et al., 2002; Kramann et al., 2013). Fibroblast foci have long been described in IPF (Katzenstein and Myers, 1998), and fibroblasts/myofibroblasts are recognized to be the key effector cells in fibrogenesis and in the pathogenesis of IPF (White et al., 2003).

The conventional therapeutic strategies for IPF with corticosteroids and immunomodulatory agents are based on the paradigm that chronic inflammation leads to prolonged tissue injury and fibrosis. However, they are largely ineffective and sometimes render prominent adverse effects (Flaherty et al., 2001; Spagnolo et al., 2015). Hence, searching for novel therapeutic agents with high efficacy and low toxicity is critical to manage disease progression and ultimately cure the patients with IPF.

Glycyrrhizic acid (GA), which is extracted from a traditional Chinese herbal medicine *Glycyrrhiza glabra*, is a major active component in *G. glabra* and has been demonstrated by modern scientific approaches to possess a wide spectrum of pharmaceutical properties, such as anti-inflammatory, anti-diabetic, anti-oxidant, anti-tumor, anti-microbial, and anti-viral properties (Ploeger et al., 2001; Ming and Yin, 2013). GA and derivatives have been shown to exert beneficial effects in the lungs against chemical-induced acute lung injury in animal models by modulating the expression and activity of several redox enzymes (Ni et al., 2011; Qamar et al., 2012). Moreover, GA can alleviate asthma in ovalbumin-sensitized mice via the immunoregulatory effects on T cells (Ma et al., 2013). Recently, GA was implicated to inhibit CCl_4-induced liver fibrosis in rats (Guo et al., 2013; Liang et al., 2015), suggesting a protective effect of GA against progressive fibrosis after tissue injury. Yet, whether GA has a protective effect against pulmonary fibrosis remains unclear.

This study aimed to investigate the potential therapeutic effect of GA for IPF using a rat model with bleomycin (BLM)-induced pulmonary fibrosis. The results demonstrated that GA treatment significantly ameliorated BLM-induced pulmonary fibrosis, inflammation, oxidative stress, epithelial-mesenchymal transition (EMT) and activation of transforming growth factor-beta (TGF-β) signaling pathway in the lungs. Furthermore, the *in vitro* study revealed that GA could suppress proliferation, promote apoptosis and inhibit migration of fibroblast cells.

Materials and Methods

Establishment of BLM-induced Pulmonary Fibrosis in Rats and GA Treatment

Forty male 8-weeks-old Sprague-Dawley rats, weighing around 250 g, were used in this study. The rats were hosted in compliance with the international guidelines of laboratory animal care, and the procedures on animals were approved by the Institutional Animal Care and Use Committee of Dalian Medical University. The rats were randomly divided into five groups with eight rats in each group: control, BLM, BLM+GA_{50}, BLM+GA_{100}, and BLM+GA_{200}. Induction of pulmonary fibrosis with BLM was conducted according to a previously described method (Thrall et al., 1979). All rats were anesthetized with 10% hydrate chloride (Sinopharm, Shanghai, China) at 3.5 ml/kg body weight (bw). Following anesthesia, a midline cut of the neck skin was made, and the trachea was exposed by blunt dissection. The needle of 1 ml syringe was inserted into the trachea, and bleomycin (Melonepharma, Dalian, China), dissolved in 100 μl sterile saline, was injected into the rat's lungs at a dose of 5 mg/kg bw, while an equal volume of saline was injected into the rats from the Control group. The rats were rotated immediately after injection to ensure an even distribution of BLM in the lungs, and then the neck skin incision was sewn. Thereafter, the rats from the BLM+GA_{50}, BLM+GA_{100}, and BLM+GA_{200} groups received an intraperitoneal injection of GA at a dose of 50, 100, and 200 mg/kg bw respectively every day for a total of 28 days, and the rest animals received saline. The rats were sacrificed 28 days after BLM induction, the bronchoalveolar lavage fluids (BALFs) were collected by intratracheal instillation and draining of 1.5 ml saline for three times, and then the lungs were excised for further analysis.

Histopathological Examination

The lungs were fixed, paraffin embedded, sectioned at 5 μm and stained with hematoxylin and eosine (H&E; Solarbio, Beijing, China) for microscopic examination of morphological changes. The sections were also subjected to Masson staining to identify collagen fibers. Briefly, the sections were incubated with hematoxylin for 6 min to stain the nuclei and then with Ponceau-Fuchsin acid solution (0.7% w/v ponceau, 0.3% w/v fuchsin acid, 1% v/v glacial acetic acid, all from Sinopharm, Shanghai, China) for 1 min to stain the cytoplasm. After washing with 0.2% glacial acetic acid, the sections were incubated with 1% phosphomolybdic acid for 5 min to destain the connective tissue, and the collagen fibers were stained by aniline blue (2% w/v aniline blue + 2% v/v glacial acetic acid) for 5 min. The sections were dehydrated, mounted, and observed at 200 × magnification.

Lung Index Assay

A fraction of the lung was cut off and weighed prior to and following drying in an incubator at 60°C for 72 h. The pulmonary edema was calculated as the wet/dry (W/D) weight ratio.

Determination of Collagen I and Hydroxyproline Levels in the Lung

To determine the content of collagen I in the lungs, exactly 50 mg lung tissue was physically homogenized in PBS and subjected to freezing-thaw in liquid nitrogen for three times. The level of collagen I in the tissue homogenate was determined with the Collagen Type I Alpha 2 ELISA (enzyme-linked immunosorbent assay) Kit (Cat. No.: SEA571Ra, USCN, Wuhan, China) following the manufacturer's instructions. The tissue homogenates were centrifuged and the supernatant was collected. The protein concentration in the supernatant was determined with the BCA Assay Kit (Beyotime, Haimen, China), and 0.5 mg protein sample was used to measure the content of hydroxyproline using the Hydroxyproline Assay Kit (Cat. No.: A030-1, Jiancheng, Nanjing, China) according to the manufacturer's instructions.

Differential Cell Count in BALF

The BALF was centrifuged at 1,000 *g* for 10 min at 4°C, and the supernatant was stored immediately at −80°C until analysis. The cell pellet was resuspended in 0.5 ml PBS, and 10 μl of the cell suspension was made into the smear on a glass slide. The cell smear was air-dried, fixed in methanol for 15 min, and stained with Giemsa solution (Jiancheng). The total and differential leukocyte counts were determined under 400× magnification.

BALF Biochemical Analysis

The levels of tumor necrosis factor-α (TNF-α), interleukin (IL)-1β, and IL-6 in BALF were determined by ELISA using the commercially available kits (Cat. No.: SEA133Ra, SEA563Ra, and SEA079Ra, USCN) in accordance with the manufacturer's instructions.

Determination of the Level of MDA and the Activity of MPO in the Lung

Lung tissue homogenates were subjected to the assay of myeloperoxidase (MPO) activity using the MPO Assay Kit (Cat. No.: A044, Jiancheng) according to the manufacturer's instructions. The lung homogenates were centrifuged and the supernatant was collected. The protein concentration in the supernatant was determined with the BCA Assay Kit, and the level of malondialdehyde (MDA) was determined with the MDA Assay Kit (Cat. No.: A003-1, Jiancheng) following the manufacturer's instructions.

Immunofluorescence Staining

The lung sections were dewaxed, heated in the antigen retrieval reagent (18 mM citric acid and 82 mM sodium citrate) for 10 min and blocked with goat serum (Solarbio). The sections were incubated with anti-E-cadherin antibody (1:100, Cat. No.: BA0474, Boster, Wuhan, China) overnight at 4°C, followed by incubation with Cy3-conjugated goat anti-rabbit IgG antibody (1:200, Cat. No.: A0516, Beyotime) for 1 h at room temperature. Thereafter, the cell nuclei were briefly stained with DAPI (Biosharp, Korea). The sections were washed, mounted and observed under a BX53 fluorescence microscope (Olympus, Japan).

Immunoblotting

For total protein extraction, lung tissues were physically homogenized and lysed with RIPA lysis buffer containing 1% v/v PMSF (Beyotime), and the cultured cells were lysed with NP-40 lysis buffer (Beyotime). Protein concentration was determined with the BCA Assay Kit. A total of 40 μg proteins from each sample were separated by SDS-PAGE, and then transferred onto PVDF membranes (Millipore, Bedford, MA, USA). The membranes were blocked with 5% non-fat milk and incubated with a specific primary antibody against the protein of interest overnight at 4°C. Anti-TGF-β1 (Cat. No.: sc-146), anti-Cyclin B1 (Cat. No.: sc-245), and anti-P53 (Cat. No.: sc-6243) antibodies were purchased from Santa Cruz (Dallas, TX, USA); anti-Smad2 (Cat. No.: bs-0718R), anti-p-Smad2 (Cat. No.: bs-5618R), anti-Smad3 (Cat. No.: bs-3484R), anti-p-Smad3 (Cat. No.: bs-5459R), and anti-Vimentin (Cat. No.: bs-8533R) antibodies were from Bioss (Beijing, China); anti-E-cadherin (Cat. No.: BA0474), anti-Fibronectin (Cat. No.: BA1772), anti-α-SMA (Cat. No.: BM0002), anti-Cyclin D1 (Cat. No.: BM0771), anti-Cyclin E (Cat. No.: BA0774), anti-P21 (Cat. No.: BA0272), anti-Bcl-2 (Cat. No.: BA0412), anti-MMP-3 (Cat. No.: BA1531), anti-MMP-7 (Cat. No.: PB0071), anti-MMP-8 (Cat. No.: BA2201), and anti-MMP-9 (Cat. No.: BA2202) antibodies were purchased from Boster; anti-cleaved caspase-3 (Cat. No.: ab2302) and anti-PARP (Cat. No.: ab32561) antibodies were from abcam (Cambridge, MA, USA); antibodies against cleaved caspase-8 (WL0153) and cleaved caspase-9 (WL01551) were purchased from Wanleibio (Shenyang, China). After incubation with the primary antibody, the membranes were incubated with horseradish peroxidase (HRP)-conjugated goat anti-mouse or goat anti-rabbit IgG secondary antibody (Beyotime) at room temperature for 45 min, followed by signal visualization using the enhanced chemiluminescence (ECL) system (7Sea Biotech, Shanghai, China). The membranes were stripped with the stripping buffer (Beyotime) and re-probed with anti-β-actin antibody (Cat. No.: sc-47778, Santa Cruz) to verify equal loading and transfer. The blot films were scanned and analyzed with Gel-Pro-Analyzer software to quantify the densitometric values of the target bands.

Cell Culture and Treatment

Murine fibroblast cell line 3T6 was purchased from the Cell Bank of China Academy of Sciences (Shanghai, China). The cells were cultured in DMEM (Gibco, Carlsbad, CA, USA) supplemented with 10% FBS (Hyclone, Logan, UT, USA) at 37°C in a humidified atmosphere of 95% air and 5% CO_2.

GA was dissolved in DMSO to make 180 mM concentrated stocks, which were diluted with PBS to make the 9 mM working solution. 3T6 cells were treated with 5, 10, 25, 50, 100, and 200 μM GA for 24 h, and the cytotoxicity was then analyzed by measuring the activity of lactate dehydrogenase (LDH) in the conditioned culture medium using the LDH Activity Assay Kit (Cat. No.: A020-2, Jiancheng). Low (25 μM), medium (50 μM), and high (100 μM) doses of GA were selected to treat the cells in later experiments.

Proliferation Assay

Cell proliferation was assessed by the 3-(4,5-dimethylthiazol-2-yl)-2,5-diphenyltetrazolium bromide (MTT) assay. 3T6 cells were seeded in 96-well microplates at a density of 3,000 cells per well and cultured at 37°C for 24 h. GA was added into each well to the indicated final concentration (0, 25, 50, or 100 μM). After 24 or 48 h GA treatment, MTT (Sigma-Aldrich, St. Louis, MO, USA) was added into the culture medium to a final concentration of 0.2 mg/ml for 4 h incubation at 37°C. Thereafter, the medium was aspirated and the formazan crystals were dissolved completely in 200 μl DMSO per well. The optical density (OD) at 490 nm was recorded by an ELX-800 microplate reader (BioTek, Winooski, VT, USA). Each assay point was done in five replicates.

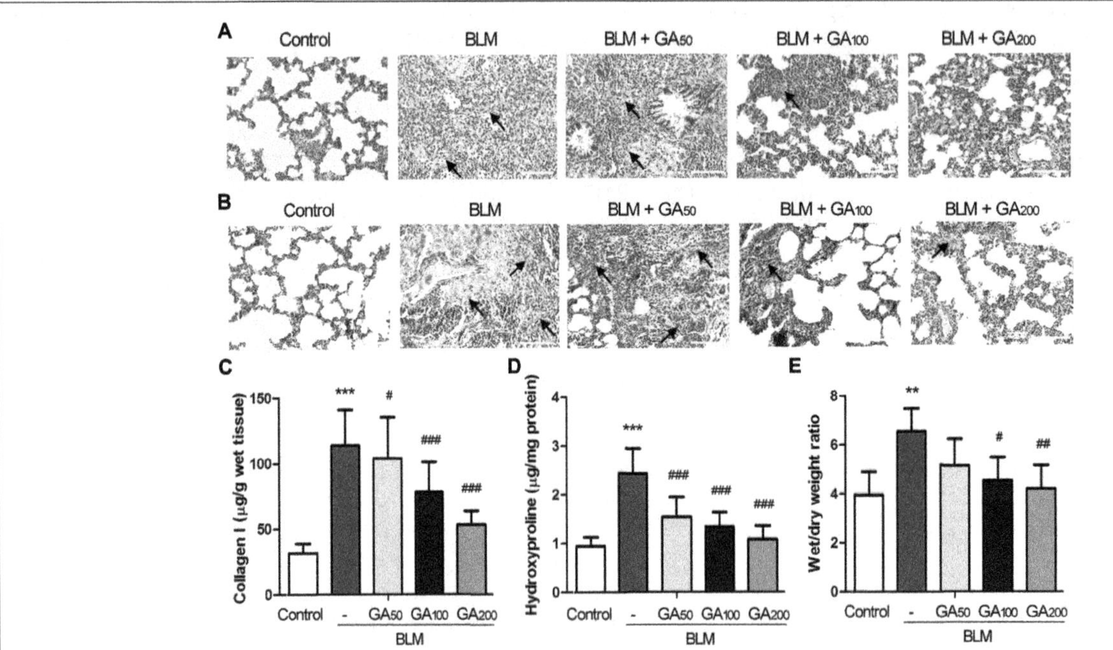

FIGURE 1 | Glycyrrhizic acid (GA) alleviated BLM-induced pulmonary fibrosis in rats. Pulmonary fibrosis was induced by intratracheal instillation of BLM, and the rats received various doses of GA by intraperitoneal injection for 28 days ($n = 8$ per group). **(A)** Histomorphological examination (200 × magnification) of the lung sections following H&E staining. Scale bars = 100 μm. The arrows point at typical areas of fibrosis, manifesting as clusters of cells with protruding cytoplasm, i.e., the fibroblasts. **(B)** Masson's staining of collagen (blue) in the lungs (200 × magnification). Scale bars = 100 μm. The arrows point at typical areas of fibrosis enriched in fibroblasts and collagen fibers. **(C,D)** The levels of collagen I and hydroxyproline in the lungs determined by ELISA. **(E)** Wet/dry weight ratio of the lungs. This figure shows the representative images from each group, and the results are expressed as the mean ± standard deviation. Compared with the control group, $^{**}p < 0.01$, $^{***}p < 0.001$; compared with the BLM group, $^{\#}p < 0.05$, $^{\#\#}p < 0.01$, $^{\#\#\#}p < 0.001$.

TABLE 1 | Effect of GA on BLM-induced changes in total and differential cell counts in the bronchoalveolar lavage fluid of rats.

Group	Total cells (×10^5)	Neutrophils (×10^4)	Macrophages (×10^5)	Lymphocytes (×10^4)
Control	2.55 ± 0.72	4.93 ± 1.66	1.69 ± 0.52	3.69 ± 1.62
BLM	11.0 ± 1.74***	12.2 ± 3.63***	8.84 ± 1.46***	9.82 ± 2.76***
BLM+GA$_{50}$	9.05 ± 2.38	9.4 ± 3.36	7.27 ± 1.87	8.4 ± 3.04
BLM+GA$_{100}$	6.66 ± 1.91##	8.52 ± 2.32	5.16 ± 1.57###	6.5 ± 1.97
BLM+GA$_{200}$	5.42 ± 1.13###	7.13 ± 1.81#	4.16 ± 0.94###	5.45 ± 1.06#

Data are expressed as the mean ± standard deviation ($n = 8$ per group); Compared with the control group, $^{***}p < 0.001$. Compared with the BLM group, $^{\#}p < 0.05$, $^{\#\#}p < 0.01$, $^{\#\#\#}p < 0.001$. GA, glycyrrhizic acid; BLM, bleomycin.

Flow Cytometric Analysis of Cell Cycle and Apoptosis

Following GA treatment for 24 h, the cells were analyzed for cell cycle and apoptosis by flow cytometry. For cell cycle analysis, the cells were harvested, fixed in 70% ethanol at 4°C for 2 h, and incubated with the propidium iodide (PI) solution (Beyotime) for 30 min at 37°C in the dark, followed by analysis in FACSCalibur flow cytometer (BD Biosciences, Franklin Lakes, NJ, USA). Cell apoptosis was assayed with the Annexin V-FITC/PI Apoptosis Detection Kit (Cat. No.: KGA106, KeyGen, Nanjing, China) according to the manufacturer's instructions. Following staining, the apoptotic status of the cells was analyzed by flow cytometry.

Scratch Wound Assay

Cell migration was assessed by the well-established *in vitro* scratch wound assay (Liang et al., 2007). The confluent monolayer of 3T6 cells was incubated with 5 μM mitomycin-C (Sigma-aldrich) for 2 h to inhibit cell proliferation. A scratch was evenly created by horizontally crossing the surface of the cell monolayer with a 200 μl pipette tip. The detached cells were washed off with serum-free medium, and the cells were cultured with serum-free medium containing the indicated concentration of GA for 24 h at 37°C in a 5% CO_2 incubator. The cells were photographed under an inverted microscope at 0, 6, 12, and 24 h post-scratching, and the rate of wound closure was calculated as (original gap distance - gap distance at the indicated time point)/original gap distance × 100%.

Transwell Assay

3T6 cells were pre-treated with 5 μM mitomycin-C for 2 h, and resuspended in culture medium containing the indicated concentration of GA. 2 × 10^4 cells in 200 μl suspension were

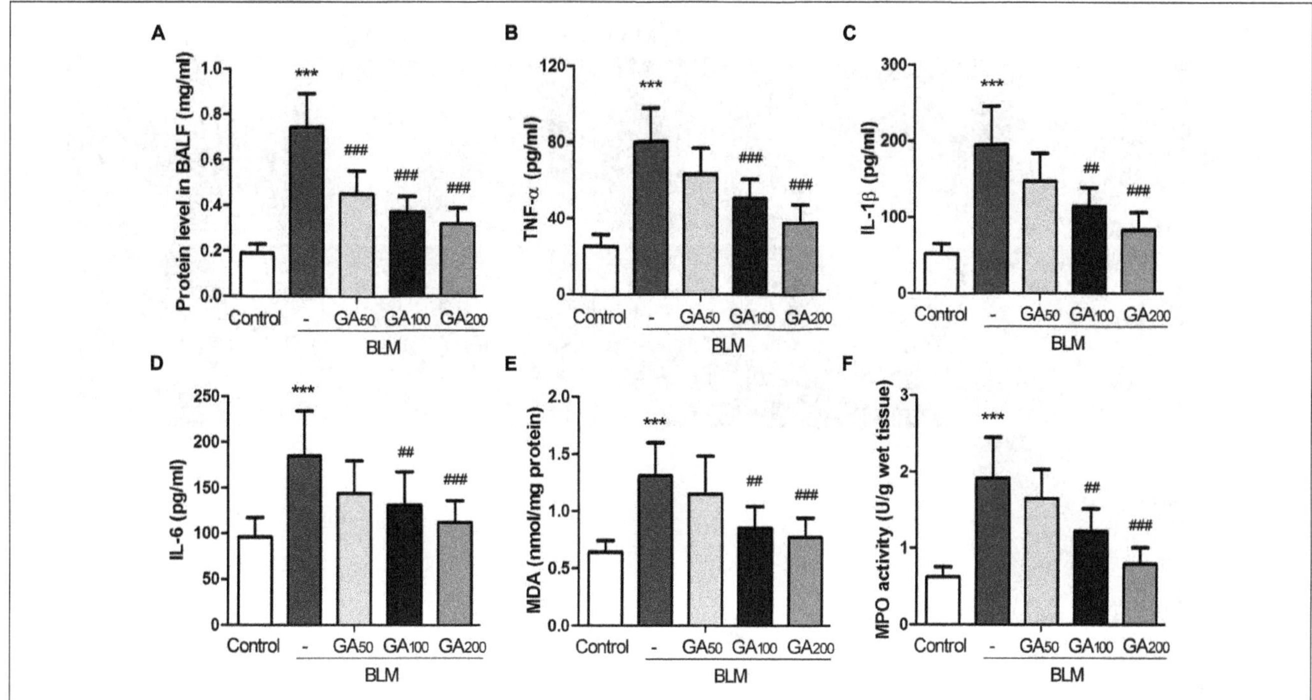

FIGURE 2 | Glycyrrhizic acid reduced BLM-induced elevation of inflammatory cytokines and oxidative stress in the lungs. BALF was collected after the rats were sacrificed. **(A)** The total protein level in the BALF was determined by the BCA assay kit. **(B–D)** The levels of TNF-α, IL-1β and IL-6 in the BALF were assayed by ELISA. **(E)** The MDA content and **(F)** the MPO activity in the lungs were examined by the respective kits. The results are presented as the mean ± standard deviation ($n = 8$ per group). Compared with the control group, $^{***}p < 0.001$; compared with the BLM group, $^{\#\#}p < 0.01$, $^{\#\#\#}p < 0.001$.

plated in one Transwell chamber (Corning) pre-coated with Matrigel (BD Biosciences). The Transwell chamber was then placed into a 24-well plate with each well-containing 800 μl culture medium supplemented with 20% FBS. The cells were cultured for 24 h at 37°C in an atmosphere of 5% CO_2. Thereafter, the cells and the Matrigel on the top surface of the Transwell membrane were wiped off, and the cells on the bottom surface of the membrane were fixed with paraformaldehyde and stained with crystal violet (Amresco, Solon, OH, USA). The cells were observed under a 200 × inverted microscope, and the numbers of the invading cells were counted in five fields on each membrane.

Statistical Analysis

Data were processed with the GraphPad PRISM software (version 5.0; San Diego, CA, USA), and are presented as the mean ± standard deviation (SD). One way analysis of variance (ANOVA) was used to compare differences among multiple groups, followed by Bonferroni *post hoc* test for comparisons between two groups. The differences are considered statistically significant when $p < 0.05$.

Results

GA Attenuated BLM-induced Pulmonary Fibrosis in Rats

Pulmonary fibrosis was primarily assessed by the histomorphological examination following H&E staining of the lung sections. Twenty-eight days after intratracheal instillation of BLM, marked thickening in alveolar septa, collapse of alveolar spaces, loss of alveolar structure, and over-proliferation of fibroblasts were observed in the lungs from the BLM group (**Figure 1A**), indicating a severe pulmonary fibrosis induced by BLM. GA treatment at a dose of 50 mg/kg bw/d (GA_{50}) slightly alleviated BLM-induced pathological changes in the lungs, while higher doses of GA (GA_{100} and GA_{200}) significantly ameliorated BLM-induced pulmonary fibrosis. Local fibrotic lesions were detected in the lungs from the BLM+GA_{100} group, and GA at a dose of 200 mg/kg bw/d (GA_{200}) greatly maintained the alveolar structure after BLM administration with mild thickening of the lung interstitium. In addition to H&E staining, pulmonary fibrosis was verified by Masson's staining of collagen. As shown in **Figure 1B**, the area of collagen deposition spread throughout the entire lung of the rats treated with BLM, whereas GA_{100} and GA_{200} remarkably reduced the areas of collagen deposition after BLM treatment. Moreover, collagen accumulation was quantified by measuring the contents of collagen I and hydroxyproline in the lung (**Figures 1C,D**). BLM treatment resulted in prominent elevation in the levels of collagen I and hydroxyproline in the lungs as compared with the control lungs ($p < 0.001$). Such elevation was significantly reduced by GA treatment in a dose-dependent manner ($p < 0.05$, $p < 0.001$). Since the thickening of the lung interstitum may also due to extra fluid (edema; Dongaonkar et al., 2009), the wet/dry weight ratio of the lung tissues was determined. The results revealed that BLM-induced pulmonary edema was alleviated by GA treatment, and the effect

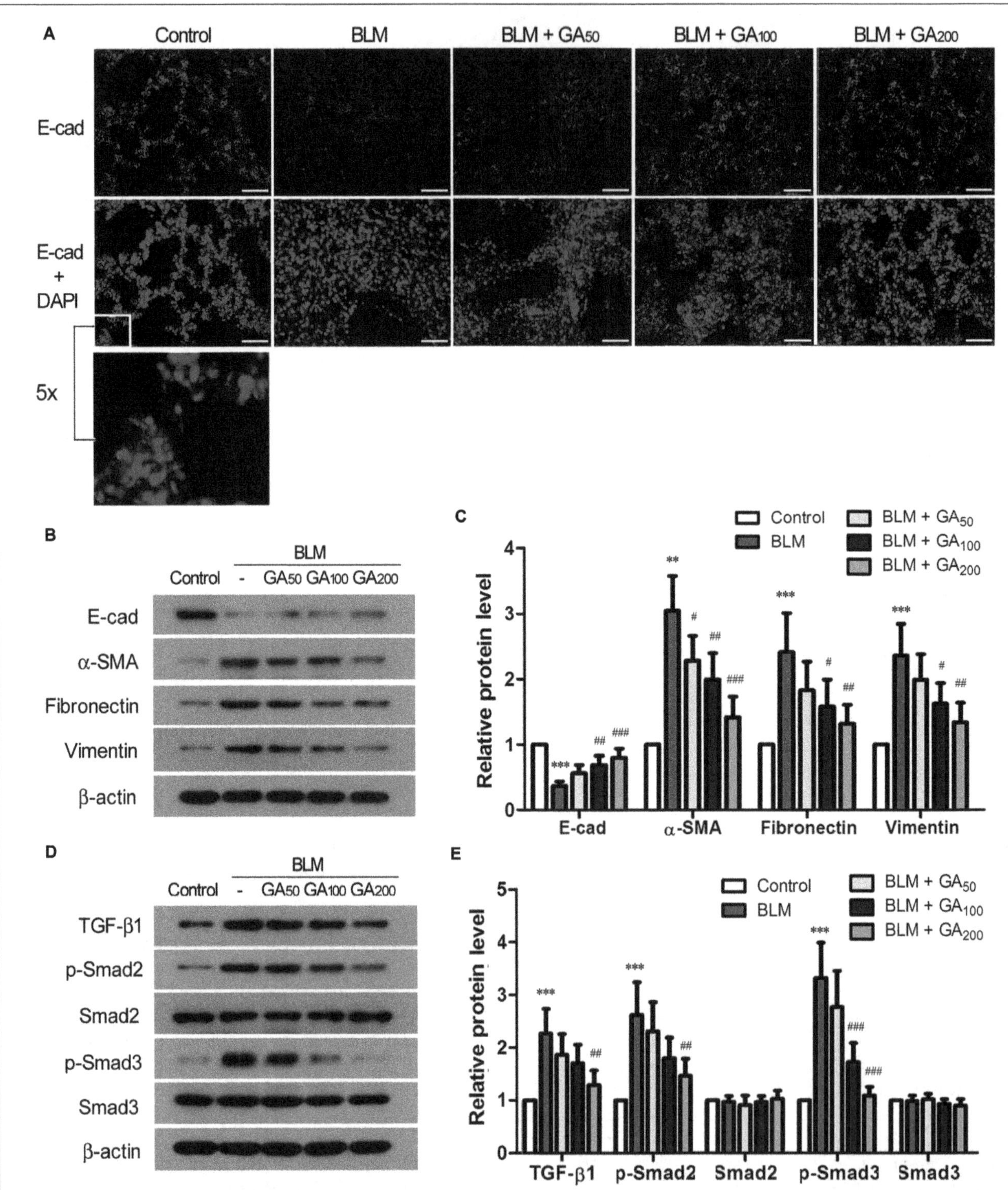

FIGURE 3 | Glycyrrhizic acid inhibited EMT and activation of TGF-β signaling in BLM-induced pulmonary fibrosis. (A) Immunofluorescence staining of E-cadherin (E-cad) in the lungs. The sections were photographed at 400× magnification (scale bars = 50 μm). A small window is enlarged by five times to present the subcellular location of E-cad. **(B)** Immunoblotting for the epithelial marker (E-cad), myofibroblasts maker (α-SMA), and ECM molecules (Fibronectin and Vimenin) in the lung tissues. **(C)** Densitometric analysis of proteins of interest in the immunoblots using β-actin as the internal reference. Values are expressed as the mean ± standard deviation ($n = 8$ per group). Compared with the Control group, $^{**}p < 0.01$, $^{***}p < 0.001$; Compared with the BLM group, $^{\#}p < 0.05$, $^{\#\#}p < 0.01$, $^{\#\#\#}p < 0.001$. **(D)** Immunoblotting for TGF-β1 and its downstream signaling molecules (p-Smad2 and p-Smad3) in the lung tissues. **(E)** Densitometric analysis of target proteins in **(D)** using β-actin as the internal reference. Values are expressed as the mean ± standard deviation ($n = 8$ per group). Compared with the Control group, $^{***}p < 0.001$; Compared with the BLM group, $^{\#\#}p < 0.01$, $^{\#\#\#}p < 0.001$.

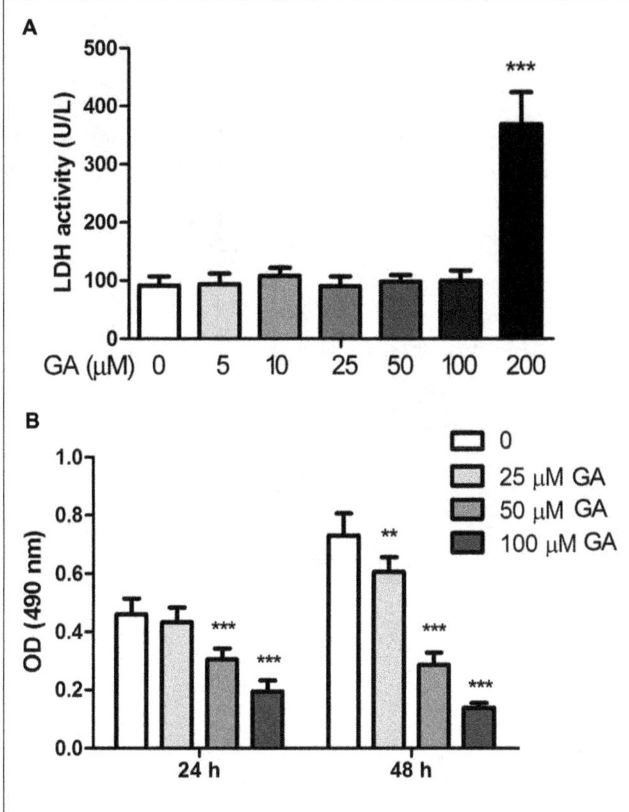

FIGURE 4 | Glycyrrhizic acid suppressed proliferation of 3T6 fibroblast cells. (A) Murine fibroblast cell line 3T6 was treated with various concentrations of GA for 24 h, and the cytotoxicity of GA was detected by the LDH activity in the conditioned culture medium. **(B)** The proliferation of 3T6 cells was assessed by MTT assay after 24 and 48 h GA treatment. The results are presented as the mean ± standard deviation of three independent experiments. Compared with the untreated cells, $^{**}p < 0.01$, $^{***}p < 0.001$.

of GA was dose dependent (**Figure 1E**). Collectively, these results indicated that GA could ameliorate BLM-induced pulmonary fibrosis in a dose-dependent manner.

GA Mitigated Inflammation and Oxidative Stress in BLM-induced Pulmonary Fibrosis

To determine the effect of GA on BLM-induced pulmonary inflammatory responses in rats, the total and differential counts of leukocytes in BALF were firstly determined. Compared with the control rats, a significant influx of inflammatory cells was observed in the BALF from the rats with BLM-induced pulmonary fibrosis, and the numbers of neutrophils, macrophages and lymphocytes were all increased (**Table 1**). Following 28-days GA treatment, BLM-induced increases of inflammatory cell counts were markedly reduced, and such inhibitory effect was dose dependent. In addition, BLM induction resulted in elevated levels of total protein and various inflammatory cytokines in the BALF such as TNF-α, IL-1β and IL-6, which were all reduced by GA treatment in a dose dependent manner (**Figures 2A–D**).

Compared with the control rats, a significant elevation in MDA content, an indicator of lipid peroxidation (Torun et al., 2009), was observed in the lung tissues of the rats exposed to BLM, whereas GA treatment at a dose of 100 and 200 mg/kg bw/d significantly inhibited BLM-induced elevation of MDA in the lungs (**Figure 2E**). Meanwhile, the level of MPO, a marker of neutrophil influx and oxidative stress (Pitanga et al., 2014), was increased in BLM-treated lungs, and such increase was remarkably attenuated by GA treatment in a dose-dependent manner (**Figure 2F**). Thus, these results suggest that GA could combat oxidative stress in BLM-induced pulmonary fibrosis.

GA Inhibited EMT and Activation of TGF-β Signaling Pathway

Epithelial-mesenchymal transition is one of the well-recognized sources of myofibroblasts in pulmonary fibrosis (Willis and Borok, 2007). The epithelial marker E-cadherin, which was expressed in the alveolar septa of normal lungs, was markedly down-regulated in BLM-induced pulmonary fibrosis, while the expression of E-cadherin was resumed in the rats that received medium to high dose of GA (**Figure 3A**). Western blot analysis revealed that α-SMA was upregulated in BLM-treated lungs along with the downregulation of E-cadherin, suggesting an enhanced EMT process in BLM-induced pulmonary fibrosis (**Figures 3B,C**). In contrast, GA treatment inhibited BLM-induced EMT in the lungs by increasing the expression of E-cadherin and simultaneously suppressing the expression of α-SMA after BLM induction. Moreover, GA treatment decreased BLM-induced upregulation of ECM molecules such as Fibronectin and Vimentin, which are normally secreted by myofibroblasts during fibrosis (**Figures 3B,C**).

Transforming growth factor-β signaling is a well-known signaling pathway that plays a critical role in EMT during pulmonary fibrosis (Willis and Borok, 2007). Hence, we examined the activation status of TGF-β signaling pathway in BLM-induced pulmonary fibrosis with and without GA treatment. Compared with the control lungs, the expression of TGF-β1 was significantly upregulated in BLM-induced lungs, accompanied by enhanced phosphorylation of the signaling molecules downstream of TGF-β1, including Smad2 and Smad3 (**Figures 3D,E**). GA treatment of medium and high doses, on the other hand, suppressed BLM-induced upregulation of TGF-β1 as well as decreased the elevation of p-Smad2 and p-Smad3. These results suggest an inhibitory effect of GA on BLM-induced activation of TGF-β signaling in the lungs.

GA Suppressed Growth and Induced Apoptosis of Fibroblasts

Proliferation of fibroblasts takes place at the initial stage of tissue repair in response to injury, and the tightly regulated growth and apoptosis of fibroblasts are critical to restore normal tissue architecture (Lorena et al., 2002). The effect of GA on the proliferation and apoptosis of fibroblasts was investigated *in vitro* by employing a murine fibroblast cell line 3T6. The cytotoxicity of GA on 3T6 cells were examined by incubating the cells with different concentrations of GA ranging from 5 to 200 μM for 24 h, and the LDH activity assay indicated that GA of as high as 100 μM was non-cytotoxic to 3T6 cells (**Figure 4A**). Later on, the effect of GA on the proliferation of

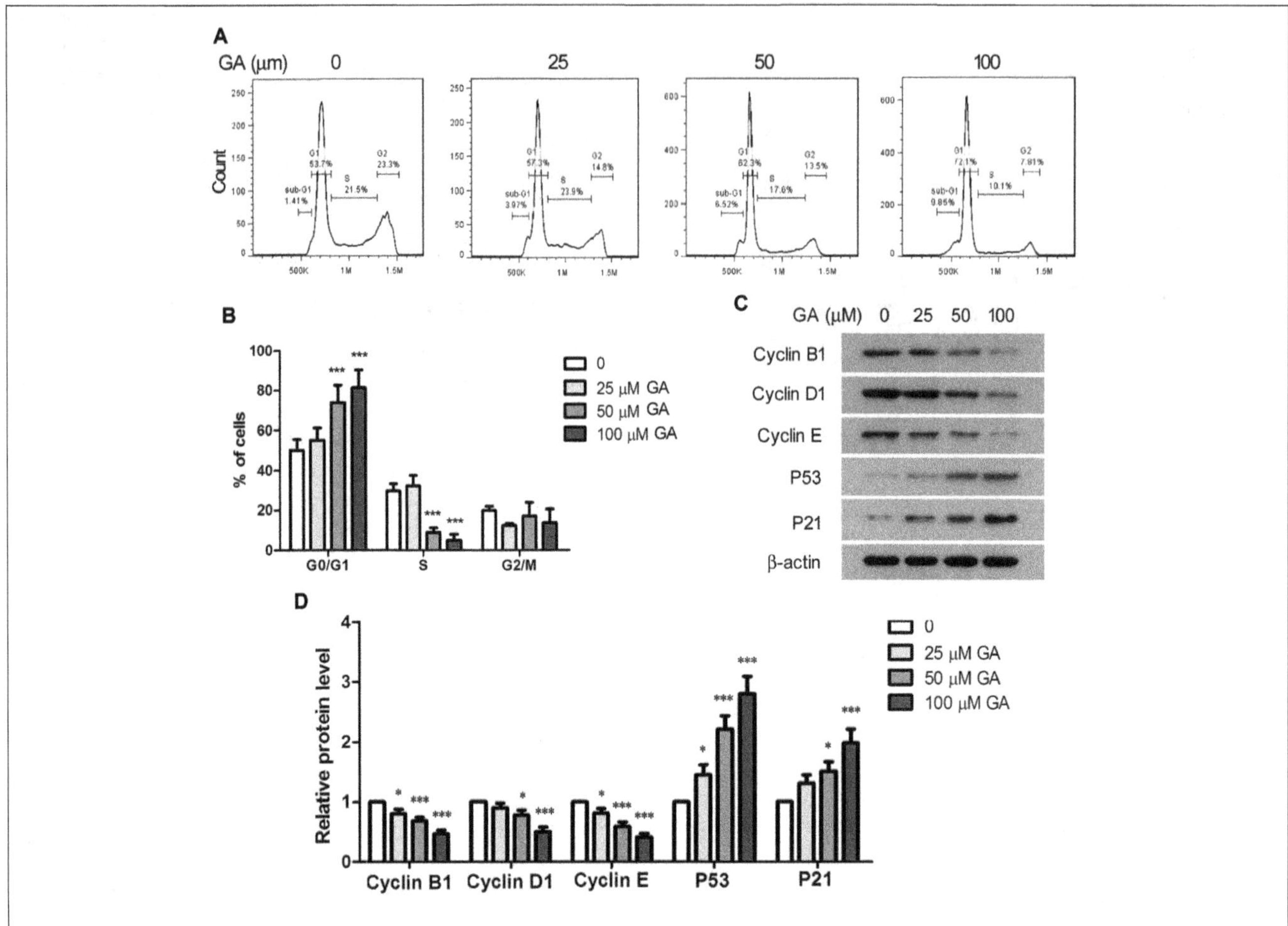

FIGURE 5 | Glycyrrhizic acid induced cell cycle arrest of 3T6 cells. (A) 3T6 cells were treated with the indicated concentration of GA for 24 h. The cells were fixed and stained with PI, followed by flow cytometric analysis. **(B)** The flow cytometric results from three independent experiments were statistically analyzed. **(C)** Western blot analysis of the key cell cycle regulatory proteins in 3T6 cells after 24 h GA treatment. **(D)** Densitometric analysis of proteins of interest in the immunoblots using β-actin as the internal reference. This figure shows the representative images from three independent experiments, and the data are expressed as the mean ± standard deviation. Compared with the untreated cells, *$p < 0.05$, ***$p < 0.001$.

3T6 cells was assessed by MTT assay. It was noted that GA treatment at the doses of 50 and 100 μM led to significant reduction of viable cell numbers after 24 and 48 h incubation as compared to the untreated cells, whereas 25 μM GA displayed the inhibitory effect on cell proliferation only at 48 h (**Figure 4B**). We further examined the cell cycle of 3T6 cells after 24 h treatment with GA. The results revealed that GA of 50 and 100 μM markedly increased the numbers of cells at G_0/G_1 phase and reduced the numbers of cells at S phase (**Figures 5A,B**), indicating that the cell cycle was slowed down by GA treatment. Consistently, GA of 50 and 100 μM led to downregulated expression of a number of cell cycle regulatory proteins such as Cyclin B1, Cyclin D1 and Cyclin E, and upregulated the G1 check-point proteins including P53 and P21 (**Figures 5C,D**). In addition, GA inhibited cell cycle and altered the expression of the cell cycle players in a dose-dependent manner.

Cell apoptosis was analyzed by flow cytometry after 24 h treatment of GA. The ratio of the cells that were stained as Annexin V+ PI- and Annexin V+ PI+, representing early and late apoptotic cells, was statistically analyzed, and the results indicated that GA enhanced apoptosis of 3T6 cells in a dose-dependent manner (**Figures 6A,B**). Further, Western blot results showed that the levels of cleaved caspase-3, cleaved caspase-9 and cleaved PARP, the executors of apoptotic events, were markedly increased by GA, while the level of cleaved caspase-9 was elevated to a less extent (**Figures 6C,D**). Moreover, GA treatment resulted in downregulation of the anti-apoptotic protein Bcl-2 and upregulation of the pro-apoptotic protein Bax (**Figures 6C,D**). Thus, the altered levels of the critical apoptotic players favored the apoptotic phenotype of 3T6 cells after GA treatment.

GA Inhibited Migration and Invasion of 3T6 Cells

In vitro scratch wound assay and Transwell assay were performed to assess the migration and invasion of 3T6 cells after GA treatment. As shown in **Figures 7A,B**, the migration rate of 3T6 cells was significantly reduced by GA at 50 and 100 μM since 6 h of the assay. Notably, the invasiveness of 3T6 cells was

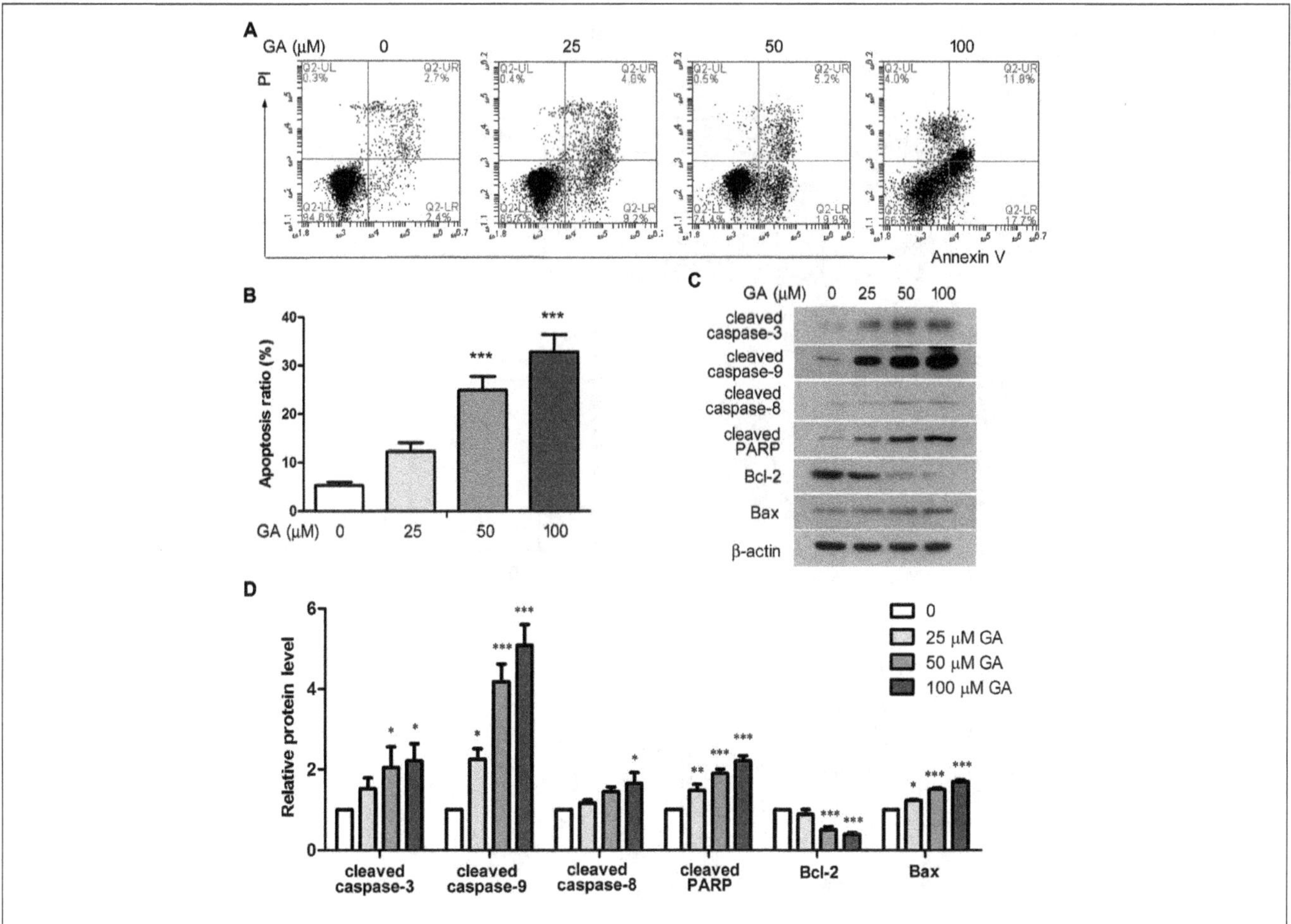

FIGURE 6 | Glycyrrhizic acid promoted apoptosis of 3T6 cell. (A) Following 24 h GA treatment, 3T6 cells were double-stained with Annexin-V-FITC and PI, and then analyzed by flow cytometry. **(B)** The ratio of apoptotic cells (Annexin V+ PI- and Annexin V+ PI+) was statistically analyzed. **(C)** Western blot analysis of several key apoptosis regulatory proteins in 3T6 cells after 24 h GA treatment. **(D)** Densitometric analysis of proteins of interest in **(C)** using β-actin as the internal reference. **(A,C)** Shows the representative images from three independent experiments. The values are expressed as the mean ± standard deviation. Compared with the untreated cells, $^{*}p < 0.05$, $^{**}p < 0.01$, $^{***}p < 0.001$.

strongly inhibited during 24 h incubation with 50 or 100 μM GA (**Figures 7C,D**). Thus, these results demonstrated that GA at the concentration of 50 or 100 μM significantly suppressed migration and invasion of 3T6 cells.

Matrix metalloproteinases (MMPs) are endopeptidases enzymes capable of degrading ECM components during cell invasion, and they have been implicated in the pathology of pulmonary fibrosis (Craig et al., 2015). Here, we show that treatment with GA led to dose-dependent downregulation of MMP-3, MMP-7, MMP-8, and MMP-9 proteins in 3T6 cells (**Figures 7E,F**), suggesting that GA may inhibit cell invasion by interfering with the expression of these MMPs.

Discussion

Intratracheal administration of BLM is one of the most extensively used experimental models in the studies of pulmonary fibrosis at present. BLM is known to stimulate inflammatory responses in the lung tissues with increased infiltration of leukocytes such as macrophages, granulocytes, and lymphocytes. These inflammatory cells stimulate the proliferation of fibroblasts and the activation of myofibroblasts which secrete ECM components into the alveolar interstitial space, gradually resulting in pulmonary fibrosis (Mouratis and Aidinis, 2011). In our study, intratracheal administration of BLM led to the typical phenotypes of BLM-induced pulmonary fibrosis, including marked infiltration of inflammatory cells into the lung tissues, elevation of inflammatory cytokines, excessive proliferation of fibroblasts, massive production of collagen fibers, and deposition of ECM molecules in the lungs. These pathological alterations were all significantly alleviated by intraperitoneal injection of GA at 100 and 200 mg/kg bw/d for 28 days, and the therapeutic effect of GA on pulmonary fibrosis was dose dependent. Hence, our results suggest a potential value of GA in the treatment of IPF.

Idiopathic pulmonary fibrosis is a heterogeneous pulmonary disorder of undefined etiology. Dysregulated fibroproliferation in response to alveolar epithelial injury has drawn extensive attention in recent years, and current understanding of the pathogenesis of IPF is shifting from the conventional concept

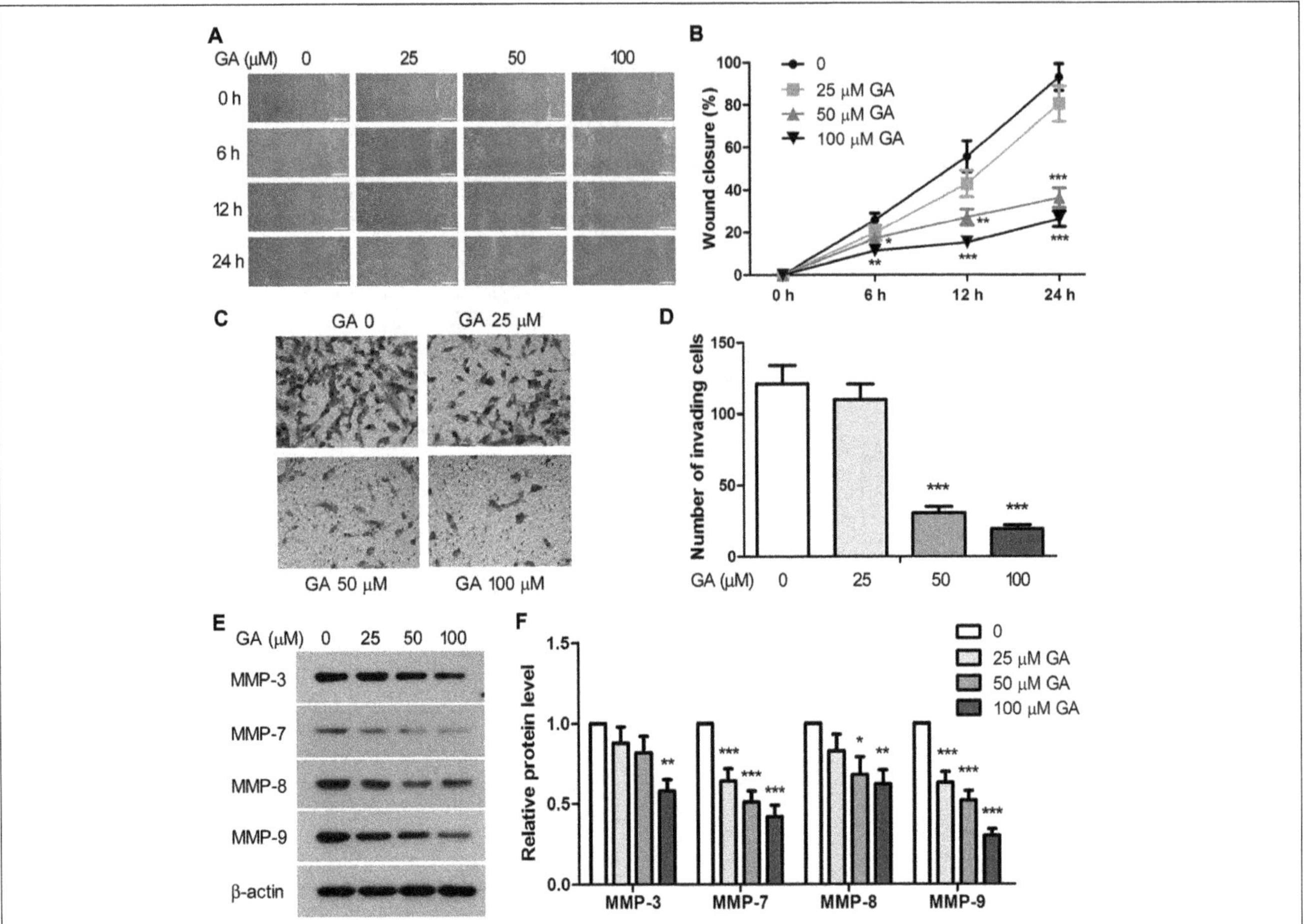

FIGURE 7 | Glycyrrhizic acid inhibited migration and invasion of 3T6 cells. (A) The effect of GA on cell migration was assessed by scratch wound assay. The wound closure was photographed at post-scratching 6, 12, and 24 h. **(B)** The wound closure rate, representing the migration rate, was measured. **(C)** Transwell assay was performed to evaluate the effect of GA on the invasiveness of 3T6 cells. The cells that migrated through the membrane were stained and photographed. **(D)** The number of invading cells in the Transwell assay was statistically analyzed. **(E)** Immunoblotting for the MMP family proteins in 3T6 cells after treatment with various concentrations of GA. **(F)** Densitometric analysis of MMPs in the immunoblots using β-actin as the internal reference. **(A,C,E)** present the representative images from three independent experiments, and the values are expressed as the mean ± standard deviation. Compared with the untreated cells, *$p < 0.05$, **$p < 0.01$, ***$p < 0.001$.

of chronic inflammation toward dysregulated fibroproliferation (Ryu et al., 2014). In this study, we demonstrated that GA inhibited the proliferation of 3T6 fibroblasts by upregulating the cell cycle checkpoint proteins and downregulating several Cyclins. In addition, GA induced apoptosis of 3T6 cells via modulating the levels of a number of key apoptosis regulatory proteins. Particularly, GA treatment augmented the cleavage of caspase-3 and caspase-9 to a much greater extent as compared to GA-induced cleavage of caspase-8, suggesting that GA-stimulated apoptosis is predominantly mediated via the intrinsic apoptotic pathway (Bayir and Kagan, 2008). Apoptosis of fibroblasts is critical at the end of the healing process for restoration of normal tissue architecture (Desmouliere et al., 1995). Thus, it is likely that GA treatment inhibited proliferation and induced apoptosis of fibroblasts during the development of pulmonary fibrosis in BLM-treated rats, thus attenuating BLM-induced fibroproliferation, such as to delay the pathogenesis of pulmonary fibrosis.

TGF-β1 has been implicated in a broad spectrum of activities in the pathogenesis of pulmonary fibrosis such as pulmonary inflammation (Bergeron et al., 2003), differentiation of fibroblasts into active myofibroblasts and inhibition of fibroblast apoptosis (Lee et al., 2006), EMT (Willis and Borok, 2007), as well as synthesis and deposition of collagen and ECM molecules by myofibroblasts (Ignotz and Massague, 1986). Previous studies have demonstrated that TGF-β is the major inducer of EMT in fibrosis via Smad-dependent pathways (Li et al., 2003). In the present study, intratracheal administration of BLM led to increased expression of α-SMA in the lungs, implying an increased number of myofibroblasts, which may be derived from fibroblast transdifferentiation or EMT. GA treatment inhibited BLM-induced upregulation of α-SMA and also reduced BLM-induced upregulation of TGF-β1 and phosphorylation of Smad2/3, suggesting that GA may mitigate BLM-induced pulmonary fibrosis by inhibiting TGF-β signaling pathway.

Previous studies have proposed a therapeutic potential of GA against liver fibrosis (Guo et al., 2013; Liang et al., 2015). Our study demonstrates, for the first time, that GA can ameliorate pulmonary fibrosis in a rat model of BLM-induced pulmonary fibrosis by reducing the infiltration of inflammatory cells, inhibiting the production of inflammatory cytokines, decreasing oxidative stress and suppressing fibroblast proliferation. Since GA is known to possess anti-inflammatory, anti-oxidant and anti-apoptotic properties (Guo et al., 2013; Ming and Yin, 2013; Liang et al., 2015), the therapeutic effect of GA against BLM-induced pulmonary fibrosis might be attributed to these diverse pharmaceutical properties of GA. A previous work by Moro et al. proposed Smad3-mediated transcription of collagen I as the molecular mechanism for the anti-fibrotic effect of GA (Moro et al., 2008). Here, we showed that GA did not only interfere with the activation of Smad3, but also affected the phosphorylation of Smad2 and the expression of TGF-β1. Therefore, our results suggest that GA may exert the anti-fibrotic effect by suppressing the activation of TGF-β signaling pathway, probably through the modulation of TGF-β1 expression.

The levels of most MMP family proteins are elevated in IPF, and several MMPs have been demonstrated to promote pulmonary fibrosis in animal models mainly by upregulating the pro-fibrotic mediators, downregulating the anti-fibrotic mediators, and enhancing cell migration (Craig et al., 2015). MMP-3 and MMP-7, in particular, have been shown to promote the EMT process during the development of pulmonary fibrosis (Zuo et al., 2002; Yamashita et al., 2011). In this study, GA dose-dependently reduced the expression of MMP-3, -7, -8, and -9 in 3T6 cells, suggesting that GA-induced downregulation of MMPs may contribute to the anti-fibrotic action of GA.

In the past few decades, animal models of BLM-induced pulmonary fibrosis have provided important insights in the understanding of IPF pathogenesis. Notably, there are emerging concerns about this model regarding the severe adverse effect of lung injury, which leads to IPF-like phenotypes but only partially recapitulate the disease. Moreover, although a great number of novel compounds were demonstrated to be promising based on this model, most of them fail to show efficacy in clinical trials (Della Latta et al., 2015). Hence, in future studies, alternative models of pulmonary fibrosis may be recruited to confirm the pharmaceutical property of GA, either by chemical induction or using transgenic animals (Wilberding et al., 2001; Moore and Hogaboam, 2008).

Conclusion

Our study demonstrated that GA treatment significantly alleviated BLM-induced pulmonary fibrosis in rats, providing the preliminary evidence for the potential therapeutic value of GA for IPF.

Author Contributions

HL and TW conceived the study. LG and HT carried out the animal model construction and the treatment. LG, HT, HH, and JL performed the examinations of the animal samples. JM and HJ conducted the cell line work. HL and TW reviewed the data and drafted the manuscript.

References

Bayir, H., and Kagan, V. E. (2008). Bench-to-bedside review: mitochondrial injury, oxidative stress and apoptosis–there is nothing more practical than a good theory. *Crit. Care* 12:206. doi: 10.1186/cc6779

Bergeron, A., Soler, P., Kambouchner, M., Loiseau, P., Milleron, B., Valeyre, D., et al. (2003). Cytokine profiles in idiopathic pulmonary fibrosis suggest an important role for TGF-beta and IL-10. *Eur. Respir. J.* 22, 69–76. doi: 10.1183/09031936.03.00014703

Craig, V. J., Zhang, L., Hagood, J. S., and Owen, C. A. (2015). Matrix metalloproteinases as therapeutic targets for idiopathic pulmonary fibrosis. *Am. J. Respir. Cell Mol. Biol.* doi: 10.1165/rcmb.2015-0020TR [Epub ahead of print].

Della Latta, V., Cecchettini, A., Del Ry, S., and Morales, M. A. (2015). Bleomycin in the setting of lung fibrosis induction: from biological mechanisms to counteractions. *Pharmacol. Res.* 97, 122–130. doi: 10.1016/j.phrs.2015.04.012

Desmouliere, A., Redard, M., Darby, I., and Gabbiani, G. (1995). Apoptosis mediates the decrease in cellularity during the transition between granulation tissue and scar. *Am. J. Pathol.* 146, 56–66.

Dongaonkar, R. M., Laine, G. A., Stewart, R. H., and Quick, C. M. (2009). Balance point characterization of interstitial fluid volume regulation. *Am. J. Physiol. Regul. Integr. Comp. Physiol.* 297, R6–R16. doi: 10.1152/ajpregu.00097.2009

Flaherty, K. R., Toews, G. B., Lynch, J. P. III, Kazerooni, E. A., Gross, B. H., Strawderman, R. L., et al. (2001). Steroids in idiopathic pulmonary fibrosis: a prospective assessment of adverse reactions, response to therapy, and survival. *Am. J. Med.* 110, 278–282. doi: 10.1016/S0002-9343(00)00711-7

Guo, X. L., Liang, B., Wang, X. W., Fan, F. G., Jin, J., Lan, R., et al. (2013). Glycyrrhizic acid attenuates CCl(4)-induced hepatocyte apoptosis in rats via a p53-mediated pathway. *World J. Gastroenterol.* 19, 3781–3791. doi: 10.3748/wjg.v19.i24.3781

Hu, B., and Phan, S. H. (2013). Myofibroblasts. *Curr. Opin. Rheumatol.* 25, 71–77. doi: 10.1097/BOR.0b013e32835b1352

Ignotz, R. A., and Massague, J. (1986). Transforming growth factor-beta stimulates the expression of fibronectin and collagen and their incorporation into the extracellular matrix. *J. Biol. Chem.* 261, 4337–4345.

Katzenstein, A. L., and Myers, J. L. (1998). Idiopathic pulmonary fibrosis: clinical relevance of pathologic classification. *Am. J. Respir. Crit. Care Med.* 157, 1301–1315. doi: 10.1164/ajrccm.157.4.9707039

King, T. E. Jr., Tooze, J. A., Schwarz, M. I., Brown, K. R., and Cherniack, R. M. (2001). Predicting survival in idiopathic pulmonary fibrosis: scoring system and survival model. *Am. J. Respir. Crit. Care Med.* 164, 1171–1181. doi: 10.1164/ajrccm.164.7.2003140

Kramann, R., Dirocco, D. P., and Humphreys, B. D. (2013). Understanding the origin, activation and regulation of matrix-producing myofibroblasts for treatment of fibrotic disease. *J. Pathol.* 231, 273–289. doi: 10.1002/path.4253

Lee, C. G., Kang, H. R., Homer, R. J., Chupp, G., and Elias, J. A. (2006). Transgenic modeling of transforming growth factor-beta(1): role of apoptosis in fibrosis and alveolar remodeling. *Proc. Am. Thorac. Soc.* 3, 418–423. doi: 10.1513/pats.200602-017AW

Li, Y., Yang, J., Dai, C., Wu, C., and Liu, Y. (2003). Role for integrin-linked kinase in mediating tubular epithelial to mesenchymal transition and renal interstitial fibrogenesis. *J. Clin. Invest.* 112, 503–516. doi: 10.1172/JCI17913

Liang, B., Guo, X. L., Jin, J., Ma, Y. C., and Feng, Z. Q. (2015). Glycyrrhizic acid inhibits apoptosis and fibrosis in carbon-tetrachloride-induced rat liver injury. *World J. Gastroenterol.* 21, 5271–5280. doi: 10.3748/wjg.v21.i17.5271

Liang, C. C., Park, A. Y., and Guan, J. L. (2007). In vitro scratch assay: a convenient and inexpensive method for analysis of cell migration in vitro. *Nat. Protoc.* 2, 329–333. doi: 10.1038/nprot.2007.30

Lorena, D., Uchio, K., Costa, A. M., and Desmouliere, A. (2002). Normal scarring: importance of myofibroblasts. *Wound Repair Regen.* 10, 86–92. doi: 10.1046/j.1524-475X.2002.00201.x

Ma, C., Ma, Z., Liao, X. L., Liu, J., Fu, Q., and Ma, S. (2013). Immunoregulatory effects of glycyrrhizic acid exerts anti-asthmatic effects via modulation of Th1/Th2 cytokines and enhancement of CD4(+)CD25(+)Foxp3+ regulatory T cells in ovalbumin-sensitized mice. *J. Ethnopharmacol.* 148, 755–762. doi: 10.1016/j.jep.2013.04.021

Ming, L. J., and Yin, A. C. (2013). Therapeutic effects of glycyrrhizic acid. *Nat. Prod. Commun.* 8, 415–418.

Moore, B. B., and Hogaboam, C. M. (2008). Murine models of pulmonary fibrosis. *Am. J. Physiol. Lung. Cell Mol. Physiol.* 294, L152–L160. doi: 10.1152/ajplung.00313.2007

Moro, T., Shimoyama, Y., Kushida, M., Hong, Y. Y., Nakao, S., Higashiyama, R., et al. (2008). Glycyrrhizin and its metabolite inhibit Smad3-mediated type I collagen gene transcription and suppress experimental murine liver fibrosis. *Life Sci.* 83, 531–539. doi: 10.1016/j.lfs.2008.07.023

Mouratis, M. A., and Aidinis, V. (2011). Modeling pulmonary fibrosis with bleomycin. *Curr. Opin. Pulm. Med.* 17, 355–361. doi: 10.1097/MCP.0b013e328349ac2b

Ni, Y. F., Kuai, J. K., Lu, Z. F., Yang, G. D., Fu, H. Y., Wang, J., et al. (2011). Glycyrrhizin treatment is associated with attenuation of lipopolysaccharide-induced acute lung injury by inhibiting cyclooxygenase-2 and inducible nitric oxide synthase expression. *J. Surg. Res.* 165, e29–e35. doi: 10.1016/j.jss.2010.10.004

Pitanga, T. N., De Aragao Franca, L., Rocha, V. C., Meirelles, T., Borges, V. M., Goncalves, M. S., et al. (2014). Neutrophil-derived microparticles induce myeloperoxidase-mediated damage of vascular endothelial cells. *BMC Cell Biol.* 15:21. doi: 10.1186/1471-2121-15-21

Ploeger, B., Mensinga, T., Sips, A., Seinen, W., Meulenbelt, J., and Dejongh, J. (2001). The pharmacokinetics of glycyrrhizic acid evaluated by physiologically based pharmacokinetic modeling. *Drug Metab. Rev.* 33, 125–147. doi: 10.1081/DMR-100104400

Qamar, W., Khan, R., Khan, A. Q., Rehman, M. U., Lateef, A., Tahir, M., et al. (2012). Alleviation of lung injury by glycyrrhizic acid in benzo(a)pyrene exposed rats: probable role of soluble epoxide hydrolase and thioredoxin reductase. *Toxicology* 291, 25–31. doi: 10.1016/j.tox.2011.10.012

Ryu, J. H., Moua, T., Daniels, C. E., Hartman, T. E., Yi, E. S., Utz, J. P., et al. (2014). Idiopathic pulmonary fibrosis: evolving concepts. *Mayo Clin. Proc.* 89, 1130–1142. doi: 10.1016/j.mayocp.2014.03.016

Spagnolo, P., Maher, T. M., and Richeldi, L. (2015). Idiopathic pulmonary fibrosis: recent advances on pharmacological therapy. *Pharmacol. Ther.* 152, 18–27. doi: 10.1016/j.pharmthera.2015.04.005

Thrall, R. S., Mccormick, J. R., Jack, R. M., Mcreynolds, R. A., and Ward, P. A. (1979). Bleomycin-induced pulmonary fibrosis in the rat: inhibition by indomethacin. *Am. J. Pathol.* 95, 117–130.

Torun, A. N., Kulaksizoglu, S., Kulaksizoglu, M., Pamuk, B. O., Isbilen, E., and Tutuncu, N. B. (2009). Serum total antioxidant status and lipid peroxidation marker malondialdehyde levels in overt and subclinical hypothyroidism. *Clin. Endocrinol.* 70, 469–474. doi: 10.1111/j.1365-2265.2008.03348.x

White, E. S., Lazar, M. H., and Thannickal, V. J. (2003). Pathogenetic mechanisms in usual interstitial pneumonia/idiopathic pulmonary fibrosis. *J. Pathol.* 201, 343–354. doi: 10.1002/path.1446

Wilberding, J. A., Ploplis, V. A., Mclennan, L., Liang, Z., Cornelissen, I., Feldman, M., et al. (2001). Development of pulmonary fibrosis in fibrinogen-deficient mice. *Ann. N. Y. Acad. Sci.* 936, 542–548. doi: 10.1111/j.1749-6632.2001.tb03542.x

Willis, B. C., and Borok, Z. (2007). TGF-beta-induced EMT: mechanisms and implications for fibrotic lung disease. *Am. J. Physiol. Lung Cell Mol. Physiol.* 293, L525–L534. doi: 10.1152/ajplung.00163.2007

Yamashita, C. M., Dolgonos, L., Zemans, R. L., Young, S. K., Robertson, J., Briones, N., et al. (2011). Matrix metalloproteinase 3 is a mediator of pulmonary fibrosis. *Am. J. Pathol.* 179, 1733–1745. doi: 10.1016/j.ajpath.2011.06.041

Zuo, F., Kaminski, N., Eugui, E., Allard, J., Yakhini, Z., Ben-Dor, A., et al. (2002). Gene expression analysis reveals matrilysin as a key regulator of pulmonary fibrosis in mice and humans. *Proc. Natl. Acad. Sci. U.S.A.* 99, 6292–6297. doi: 10.1073/pnas.092134099

3

Maimendong Decoction Improves Pulmonary Function in Rats with Idiopathic Pulmonary Fibrosis by Inhibiting Endoplasmic Reticulum Stress in AECIIs

Mengmeng Shen[1], Yanan Nan[2], Lan Zhang[1], Liming Di[1], Shuangshuang He[1], Yu Li[1] and Yadong Li[2*]*

[1] School of Traditional Chinese Medicine, Beijing University of Chinese Medicine, Beijing, China, [2] School of Life Sciences, Beijing University of Chinese Medicine, Beijing, China

***Correspondence:**
Yu Li
liyubeijing1973@163.com
Yadong Li
lydtry@sina.com

This study was designed to investigate the mechanism by which MMDD improves lung function, and observe the effect of MMDD on endoplasmic reticulum stress(ERS) in alveolar type II epithelial cells (AECIIs) of pulmonary fibrosis rats. pulmonary fibrosis animal model was established by intratracheal injection of BLM at a dose of 6mg/kg body weight. Overall, Thirty male SPF Sprague-Dawley rats were randomly divided into control group, BLM group and BLM+MMDD group. BLM+MMDD group rats were fed 24 g/kg over three weeks for twice a day on the fourteenth day after model establishment. MMDD improves pulmonary function of fibrotic rats and reduces the occurrence of endoplasmic reticulum stress in AECIIs. MMDD could significantly improve the forced vital capacity (FVC) of bleomycin-induced pulmonary fibrosis in rats. MMDD reduced the expression of GRP78 and CHOP in AECIIs, increased the secretion of surfactant protein C (SPC) by AECIIs. Moreover, the apoptosis of the fibrosis zone in the lung tissue was remarkably mitigated by administration of MMDD. The finding of this study revealed that MMDD can improve lung function in rats with pulmonary fibrosis by reducing the occurrence of ERS and cell apoptosis of AECIIs. It may provide a new method for the treatment of pulmonary fibrosis.

Keywords: Maimendong decoction, pulmonary function, pulmonary fibrosis, endoplasmic reticulum stress, alveolar type II epithelial cells

INTRODUCTION

IPF is a chronic progressive fibrotic interstitial pneumonia. The lesions caused by IPF are localized in the lungs and occur in middle-aged and elderly men. The symptoms of IPF are mainly manifested by progressively worsened breathing difficulties, with restricted ventilation dysfunction and gas exchange. IPF has a poor prognosis, as it, leads to hypoxemia and respiratory failure. The lung histology and chest high-resolution CT (HRCT) of IPF appear as common interstitial pneumonia (UIP) (Raghu et al., 2015). IPF is a terminal lung disease with pathological manifestations of alveolar structural and its epithelial damage or collapse, and activation and proliferation of lung fibroblasts, and excessive accumulation of extracellular matrix, causing an increased pulmonary interstitial and decreased lung function (Longo et al., 2018). The pathogenesis of pulmonary fibrosis is currently unclear. In recent years, many studies have shown that endoplasmic reticulum stress (ERS) plays an important role in the development of IPF (Korfei et al., 2008; Hsu et al., 2017). These studies have demonstrated that IPF is more sensitive to ERS. ERS can damage AECIIs, and it is more prone to abnormal AECIIs epithelial repairing and processing, which accelerates the development of pulmonary fibrosis (Korfei et al., 2008).

In recent years, with the understanding of pathogenesis of pulmonary fibrosis in Chinese medicine, some progress has been made in the treatment of pulmonary fibrosis with traditional Chinese medicine (Ying et al., 2016; Yunping et al., 2018; Xiaolin et al., 2018). MMDD which consists of the roots consisted of six herbs (Ophiopogonis Radix, Pinelliae Rhizoma Praeparatum Cum Alumine, Ginseng Radix et Rhizoma, Glycyrrhizae Radix et Rhizoma Praeparata Cum Melle, Oryza sativa subsp. japonica S.Kato, Jujubae Fructus) has a variety of pharmacological effects such as regulating the secretion of multi-alveolar surfactant, antitussive, promoting airway purification, and relieving the high sensitivity of the respiratory tract (Wang and Ji, 2016). In addition, MMDD also treats radiation pneumonitis, allergic asthma, chronic bronchitis with lung yin deficiency, and pulmonary fibrosis (Lin et al., 2007; Luo, 2013; Yu, 2015; Kang et al., 2017). Considering the properties of those herbs, and based on the previous research results of our team, this study used MMDD to treat pulmonary fibrosis and observe its effect on ERS. Several active components of MMDD have been shown to be bioactive *in vivo*. Ophiopogonis Radix (Ophiopogon root), which nourishes the yin, has been used in clinical practice to promote fluid secretion and to moisturize the lungs and skin in traditional Chinese Medicine. There are many extractions of *Ophiopogon Radix* also have the anti-inflammatory and anti-apoptotic effects, such as Steroidal saponins, 4′-O-Demethylophiopogonanone E and methylophiopogonanone A (He et al., 2016; Zhao et al., 2017; Wu et al., 2019). Total ginsenosides extract could enhance autophagy flux and induce autophagic cell death through activation of ERS. Emerging evidence demonstrated this process was mediated by the ATF4-CHOP-AKT1-mTOR axis in NSCLC cells (He et al., 2016; Zhao et al., 2019); and Liquiritin had the effects of anti-inflammation, anti-oxidative stress, and anti-cell apoptosis in a rat model (Luo et al., 2019).

In this study, we examined the pulmonary function, pulmonary histomorphology, collagen content, ERS, and cell apoptosis in AECIIs of pulmonary fibrosis rats after administration of MMDD. The purpose of this study was aimed to observe the mechanism by which MMDD improves lung function, and relieves the ERS in AECIIs.

MATERIALS AND METHODS

Reagents

Bleomycin (BLM) was purchased from Nippon Kayaku (Batch number 970592). GRP78/Bip rabbit polyclonal antibody (catalog number:11587-1-AP), GAPDH mouse monoclonal antibody (catalog number: 60004-1-Ig), CHOP/GADD153 mouse monoclonal antibody (catalog number:60304-1-Ig), SFTPC polyclonal antibody (catalog number:10774-1-AP), and CHOP rabbit polyclonal antibody (catalog number:115204-1-AP) were purchased from Proteintech, America.

Sample Preparation and Constituents Identification of MMDD

Ophiopogonis Radix, Pinelliae Rhizoma Praeparatum Cum Alumine, Ginseng Radix et Rhizoma, Glycyrrhizae Radix et Rhizoma Praeparata Cum Melle, Jujubae Fructus were produced by Beijing Tongrentang (Bozhou) Yinpian Co., Ltd. (Anhui, China) and purchased from Guoyi Tang of Beijing University of Chinese Medicine (Beijing, China). Oryza sativa subsp. japonica S.Kato was purchased from Kaiyuan Jefu Trading Company. samples were identified by professor Chunsheng Liu (Voucher numbers: 700003252; 601232835; 501002767; 171103007; 700003080; SC10121128200214). Detailed information of the drug materials and the scan of the vouchers were given in **Supplementary Table 1**. The voucher specimens were deposited in School of Chinese Materia Medica, Beijing University of Chinese Medicine. MMDD derived from *Jinkuiyaolue*, a classic medical book. According to the traditional decoction method of modern Chinese medicine hospital, 42 g of Ophiopogonis Radix, 6 g of Pinelliae Rhizoma Praeparatum Cum Alumine, 1.5 g of Glycyrrhizae Radix et Rhizoma Praeparata Cum Melle, 1.5 g of Ginseng Radix et Rhizoma, 2.5 g of Oryza sativa subsp. japonica S.Kato, 1.8 g of Jujubae Fructus were weighed respectively. all the drugs were mixed together, Soaking in 700 ml deionized water for 30 min, then all the soaked medicine and water were poured into the electric casserole, selected the big fire for 45 min, simmer for 20 min the MMDD decoction were concentrated to 2 g/ml for further use.

LC/MS Conditions

In order to ensure the quality of the drug, the main components of the six herbs of MMDD were analyzed by Ultra Performance Lquid Cromatography/Mss Sctrometry (UPLC/MS). MMDD decoction (100 μl) was taken from the filtrate of the broth, and 1 ml (methanol: water = 1:1) was added, and the mixture was vortexed for 1 h, and centrifuged, and the supernatant was taken for injection. UPLC analysis was performed with a Waters (ThermoFisher, MA, USA) Rapid Separation LC system equipped with a waters UPLC HSS T3 (1.8 um 2.1 mm*100 mm). A gradient elution program was conducted for chromatographic separation with mobile phase A (water 0.1% formic acid) and mobile phase B (acetonitrile) as **Supplementary Table 2**. The flow rate was 0.3 ml/min, the injection volume was 1.0 μl, and the column temperature was 50°C.

The mass spectrometry was performed using a quadrupole orbital ion trap mass spectrometer equipped with a thermoelectric spray ion source. The positive ion source voltages were 3.7 kV, respectively. The capillary heating temperature was 320°C. The plenum pressure is 30 psi and the auxiliary gas pressure is 10 psi.

The volume is heated and evaporated to a temperature of 300°C. Both the updraft and the auxiliary gas are nitrogen. The collision gas was nitrogen and the pressure was 1.5 m Torr. The first-level full scan parameters are: resolution 70000, automatic gain control target of 1×10^6, maximum isolation time of 50ms, and mass-to-charge ratio scanning range of 50–1,500. The liquid quality system is controlled by Xcalibur 2.2 SP1.48 software, and data acquisition and targeted metabolite quantification are performed by the software.

Animals

Male Sprague-Dawley (SD) rats (380 ± 20g) were obtained from Beijing Vital River Laboratory Animal Technology Co., Ltd.(Beijing, China, animal certificate number: SCXK(Beijing) 2016-0006). The animal studies were approved by the Animal Ethics Committee of Beijing University of Traditional Chinese Medicine(BUCM-4-2017101301-402). The laboratory temperature was maintained at 22.9 degrees Celsius (°C), and relative humidity at 46.4%, and 12 h dark-light cycle. All rats were fed with standard food and water ad libitum in the laboratory for 14 days before experiment.

Model Preparation and Administrations

After 14 days of adoption, all rats were randomly divided into control group (n=10), BLM group (n=10), BLM+MMDD group (n=10). To establish the pulmonary fibrosis model, the control group treated with nothing, the other groups rats were intratracheally injected with bleomycin (6 mg/kg) dissolved in saline. The control group and BLM group rats were tread by saline, and the BLM+MMDD group rats were given MMDD was administered at a dose of 2.4 g/100 g body weight via oral gavage administration for 21 days. All the treatments were initiated 14 days after bleomycin established a pulmonary fibrosis model, twice a day for 21 days. All the rats were sacrificed on day 35.

The rats were anesthetized with 1% sodium pentobarbital, lung function test was performed first, and then left and right lung tissues of the rats were taken. The rats were anesthetized with 1% sodium pentobarbital, lung function tests were performed first, and then left and right lung tissues of the rats were taken. The left lung is centered on the hilum and divided into three parts. The lower 1/3 of the left lung, which was fixed with 10% neutral formalin solution, was treated with HE staining, MASSON staining, immunohistochemical staining, immunofluorescent staining, and TUNEL staining. The middle 1/3 and upper 1/3 of the left lung were stored at -80°C, which were used for WB analysis and HYP content determination, respectively.

Pulmonary Function Test

1% sodium pentobarbital (70 mg/kg) was anesthetized by intraperitoneal injection. The tracheal intubation was performed after tracheotomy, and the intubation was fixed with the trachea. The rat was placed supine in a medium-sized body drawing box, connected to a breathing machine, and set a breathing ratio of 20:10 and a respiratory rate of 65 times/min. The forced vital capacity (FVC) and dynamic pulmonary compliance (Cdyn) were measured by a 30 cm H_2O pressure. FVC was tested by ventilator (Bestlab, Beijing).

Hydroxyproline Assay in Lung Tissue

HYP contents were measured according to the manufacture's instruction of the kit (Jiancheng, Nanjing, China). Lung tissues (100 mg) were hydrolyzed with 750 ul akaline hydrolysate and high pressure at 120°C for 60 min and then centrifuged at 5,000 rpm for 10 min at 4°C. The supernatant was obtained, and hydroxyproline content was measured on an ultraviolet spectrophotometer (Thermo, US). Results were expressed in microgram per gram tissue (ug/g tissue).

Histomorphology and Immunohistochemical Analysis

The lower 1/3 of the left lung was fixed with 10% neutral formalin solution, paraffin-embedded, coronal section, standard hematoxylin and eosin (HE) solution (Solarbio, Beijing, China) and Masson's trichrome staining kit (Solarbio, Beijing, China) and immunohistochemical staining (Boster, Beijing, China) was carried out to observe and photograph. Immunohistochemical staining was performed strictly according to the instructions of the ready-to-use immunohistochemistry kit. Conventional baking, dewaxing, antigen inactivation, heat repair of antigen, and blocking endogenous peroxides. Primary antibody: rabbit-derived GRP78(1:1,000), CHOP antibody (1:200) and SPC antibody (1:300) were incubated overnight at 4°C; After washing the slides thrice with PBS, the sections were then incubated with secondary antibody for 20 min at 35°C. Sections were then washed with PBS and incubated with DAB for 10 min. Nuclei were counterstained with hematoxylin. Positive staining for GRP78, CHOP and SPC were brown. Expression of GRP78, CHOP, and SPC was compared between groups by calculating the ratio of positive staining area.

Immunofluorescence Staining

The paraffin sections were baked in a constant temperature oven at 60°C for 2 h, gradient dewaxing with xylene and alcohol. Endogenous performed activity was blocked in a solution of 3% hydrogen peroxide. Antigen retrieval by microwave heating with 0.1 M sodium citrate buffer (pH 6.0), 0.3% Titron X solution diluted with 0.1 M PBS was added to the sections and placed in a wet box, and allowed to stand at room temperature for 30 min; 5% normal goat serum was added dropwise, and the mixture was sealed at room temperature for 30 min to remove excess liquid, and the primary antibodies of GRP78 (1:100) and SPC (1:100) were incubated overnight at 4°C. After washing the slides three times with PBS, the sections were then incubated with secondary antibody for 20 min at room temperature, the fluorescently labeled secondary antibody (1:100) was added dropwise and incubated for 1 h at room temperature, then nuclei were counterstained with DAPI (1 ug/ml). The sections were sealed with anti-fluorescence quencher.

Western Blotting Analysis

100 mg left lung upper lobe tissue was placed in a glass grinder, 200 µl RIPA lysate and 2 µl PMSF were added per 20 mg, and the tissue homogenate was repeatedly ground on ice. After centrifugation (12,000 r/min, 10 min at 4°C), the supernatant

was collected, packed, and stored in -80°C. Just before using, the loading buffer was mixed into the supernatant at a ratio of 1:4 and cooked in boiling water for 10 min. Proteins in the supernatant were separated by SDS-PAGE on a 10% SDS polyacrylamide gel, 20 μg protein sample per well was loaded, and then transferred to polyvinylidene fluoride (PVDF) membranes. The blotted membranes were blocked with 5% non-fat dairy milk (w/v). Blotted membranes were washed by 0.1% Tween-TBS (TBST) three times (10 min per time) after 2 h. Then blotted membranes were incubated at 4°C overnight with primary anti-GRP78 antibodies (1:1,500, Proteintech, Chicago, USA), anti-chop antibodies (1:300, Proteintech, Chicago, USA) and with secondary antibodies at room temperature for 1 h. After being washed with TBST three times (10 min per time), the blots were visualized with ECL reagent (MilliPore, Massachusetts, USA). Protein levels were analyzed using Image Lab software. Gray-scale analysis of the target strip was performed using Image J software to calculate the relative integrated optical density value.

TUNEL Staining

Apoptotic cells were visualized by terminal deoxynucleo-tidyl transferase-mediated dUTP nick end labeling (TUNEL) staining according to the manufacturer's instructions (Key Gen biological Technology, Nanjing, China). The paraffin sections were baked in a constant temperature oven at 60°C for 2 h, gradient dewaxing with xylene and alcohol; the sections were digested with proteinase K and washed three times with 1× PBS. After that, the sections were incubated with 50 μl terminal deoxynucleotidyl transferase (TdT) enzyme at 37°C for 60 min in a wet box. At last, streptavidin-labeled horseradish peroxidase (HPR) were added in a wet box at 37°C for 60 min, then the nuclei were counterstained with DAPI (1 ug/ml). Sealing was with anti-fluorescence quencher.

Statistical Analysis

All the data were statistically analyzed using SPSS20.0 software (IBM, NY, USA), and the normal measurement data conforming to the normal distribution was expressed by the mean ± SEM, Kruskal-Wallis *H* test was used if the data do not comply with the normal distribution; if the data comply with the normal distribution, one-way analysis of variance followed by SNK or Dunnett's T3 *post hoc* test was used for multiple comparisons. Differences were considered to be significant at *P* values < 0.05.

RESULTS

The Result of LC/MS

LC/MS was used to analyze the main components of MMDD. Five major components, including ophiopogonin D, Succinate, ginsenoside Rg1, ginsenoside Re, Ginsenoside Rb1, Ammonium glycyrrhizinate, Liquiritin were identified in MMDD (**Figure 1**).

MMDD Ameliorated Pulmonary Function in Rats

As we know, progressive aggravation of pulmonary function is a feature of IPF. To elucidate the effects of MMDD on BLM-induced pulmonary dysfunction, pulmonary function test was tested dynamically. We observed that compared with control group, FVC, FVC/weight and Cdyn of the BLM group were

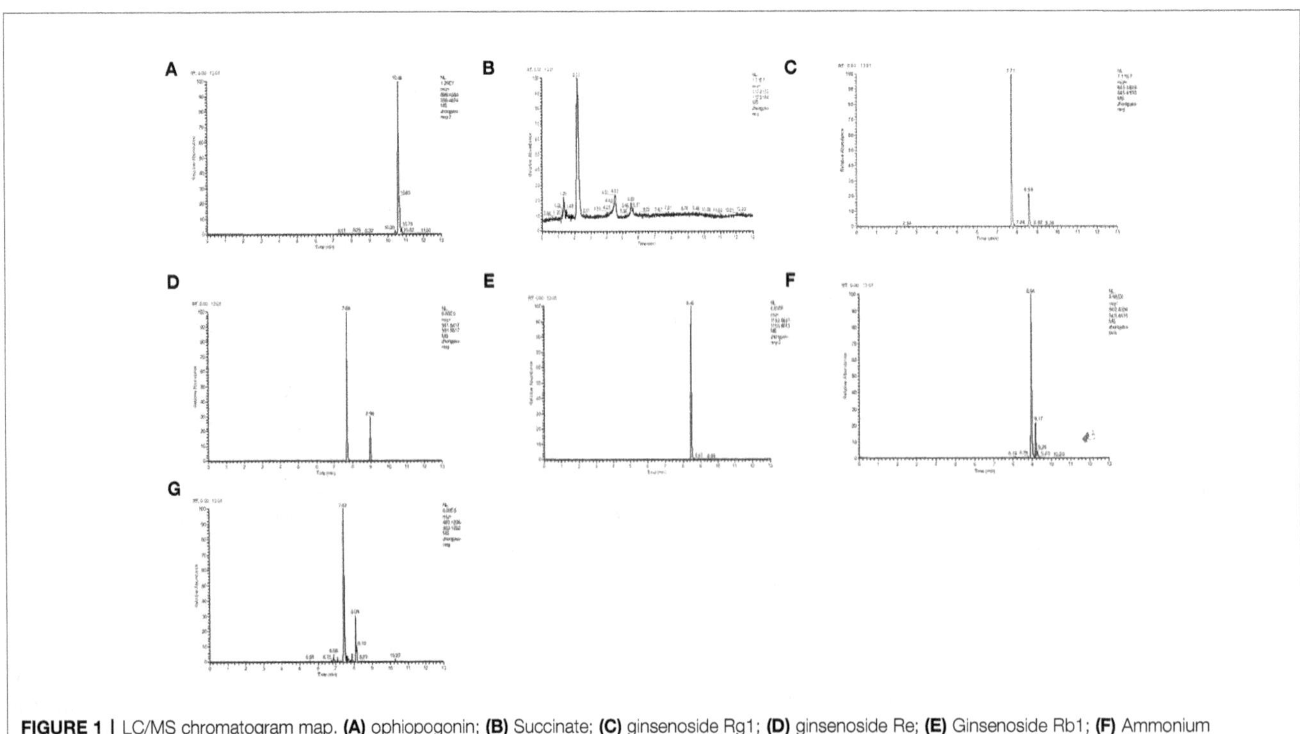

FIGURE 1 | LC/MS chromatogram map. **(A)** ophiopogonin; **(B)** Succinate; **(C)** ginsenoside Rg1; **(D)** ginsenoside Re; **(E)** Ginsenoside Rb1; **(F)** Ammonium glycyrrhizinate; **(G)** Liquiritin.

significantly decreased (**Figures 2B–D**). After using MMDD, FVC, lung coefficient, and lung compliance were increased significantly in comparison with the BLM group rats. These data indicated that MMDD improved the lung function induced by BLM in fibrotic rats.

MMDD Alleviated Pulmonary Injuries in Rats

o identify the degree of lung injury after treatment, sections of lung tissue were stained with H&E and Masson trichrome. The infiltration of numerous inflammatory cells was observed in the alveolar and interstitial space of the lung by HE staining, with the lung tissue of the BLM group was extensively transformed, the alveolar structure was disordered or collapsed, and the alveolar septum was relatively thicker (**Figure 2A**). In the BLM+MMDD group, apparent alleviation of pulmonary alveolitis was observed. Pulmonary fibrosis zone was reduced largely, the alveolar structure was gradually healed, the alveolar septum was thinner, and the number of interstitial inflammatory cells was significantly reduced. Additionally, the Masson staining showed that blue-stained collagen was massively increased in the BLM group. The collagen deposit of BLM+MMDD group was alleviated significantly according to the result of the Masson staining.

MMDD Reduced Collagen Content in Lung Tissue of Fibrotic Rats

Pulmonary fibrosis was characterized by collagen accumulation. HYP was an index of collagen contents. Analyses of HYP contents were conducted to evaluate the effect of MMDD formula (**Figure 3A**). Compared with the BLM group, The contents of HYP were significantly decreased. in the BLM+MMDD group (*P*<0.05). The expression of α-SMA was tested by Western blot analysis (**Figure 3B**). After modeling, the level of α-SMA was significantly increased compared with control group. In the BLM+MMDD group, the expression of the level of α-SMA was much lower than the BLM groups (**Figure 3C**).

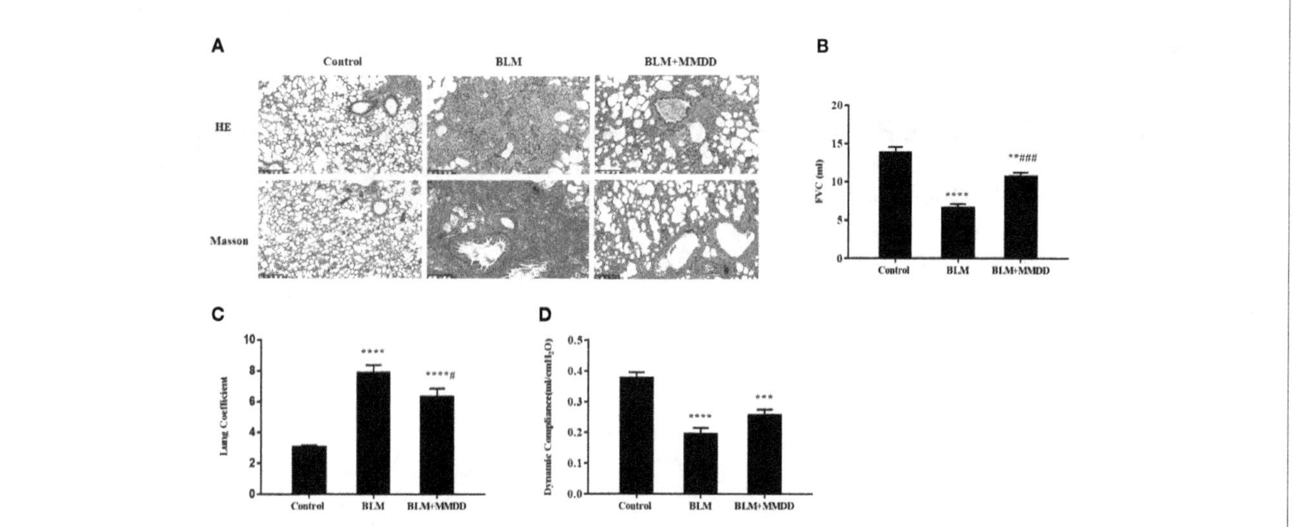

FIGURE 2 | Effect of MMDD on histopathologic changes and Pulmonary Function in BLM-induced pulmonary fibrosis rats. **(A)** All sections were stained with HE and representative sections are shown at the same magnification. All sections were stained with HE and representative sections were shown at the same magnification. Bars: 50 μm. **(B)** FVC; **(C)** Lung coefficient; **(D)** Dynamic compliance. Data were analyzed by one way ANOVA (Mean ± SEM). **P < 0.01, ***P < 0.001, ****P < 0.0001, compared with the control group. #P < 0.05, ###P < 0.001, compared with the BLM group.

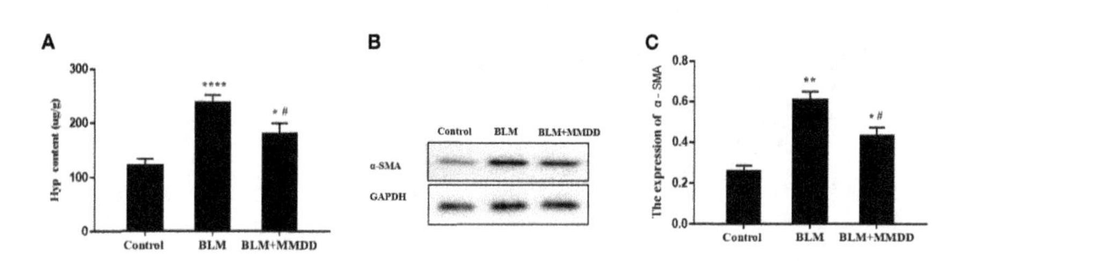

FIGURE 3 | MMDD reduced collagen content in lung tissue of Fibrotic rats. Data were analyzed by one way ANOVA (Mean ± SEM). **(A)** HYP content in lung tissue of rats in each group; **(B)** The expression level of the α-SMA was detected by Western blot analysis; **(C)** The quantitative result of the α-SMA expression. *P < 0.05, **P < 0.01, ****P < 0.0001, compared with the control group. #P < 0.05, compared with the BLM group.

Results of Immunohistochemistry Staining for GRP78, CHOP, and SPC

In **Figures 4A, B**, compared with the control group, the expression of GRP78 and CHOP was markedly increased in the BLM group, and Positive cells are stained brownish yellow. When compared with BLM group, the expression of GRP78 and CHOP could be inhibited in groups that were treated with MMDD by immunohistochemistry testing. The SPC synthesized and secreted by AECIIs in rat normal lung tissue was evenly distributed on the alveolar surface. In lung tissue, only AECIIs secreted SP-C. As shown in **Figure 4C**, the SPC immunohistochemical staining was light brown. Compared with the control group, the SPC was observed in the fibrosis zone of the lung tissue of the BLM group. The brown color was strongly positively expressed, and its distribution was mainly confined to AECIIs. At the same time, the cytoplasm of AECIIs was significantly vacuolated. Compared with the BLM group, SPC retained in AECIIs of BLM + MMDD group was decreased, and SPC secreted to the alveolar surface was increased. The Positive expression of GRP78 and CHOP indicated that ERS occurred in pulmonary fibrosis caused by bleomycin. AECIIs secreted more SPC to the surface of the alveoli, which contributed to the alveolar contraction and stability.

Expression of GRP78, CHOP, and SPC in Lung Tissues

The expression levels of GRP78, CHOP and SPC were tested by Western blot analysis (**Figure 5**). After modeling, when compared to the control group, the expression levels of GRP78 and CHOP were obviously increased, while the expression of SPC was significantly decreased. Compared with the BLM group, the expression levels of GRP78 and CHOP of the BLM+MMDD group were significantly decreased ($P<0.05$). In contrast, the expression of SPC was increased. These findings revealed that ERS was increased and the secretion of SPC was significantly reduced in the model of bleomycin-induced pulmonary fibrosis. After treatment with MMDD, endoplasmic reticulum stress was relieved, and the secretion of SPC in AECIIs was enhanced.

Results of Immunohistochemistry Staining for GRP78, CHOP, and SPC

From the results of immunohistochemistry, we found that GRP78, CHOP and SPC were expressed in the cytoplasm of the cells, so we used co-localization detection of GRP78/SPC and CHOP/SPC by immunofluorescence double staining. we observed that GRP78 and SPC were expressed in the same cell. Since SPC is expressed only by AECIIs in lung tissue (**Figure 6A**), it can be confirmed that GRP78 and SPC are co-expressed in AECIIs. In addition, we also found that GRP78 was not only expressed in the cytoplasm of AECIIs, but also expressed in the cytoplasm of other cells, which cell is subject to further study. Similarly, we found that in the double staining of CHOP and SPC (**Figure 6B**), CHOP and SPC fluid were co-expressed in the AECIIs.

Apoptosis of TUNEL Staining

There was almost no apoptosis in the lung tissue of the control group. Compared with the control group, the apoptotic cells in the fibrosis zone in the lung tissue of the model group increased. Compared with the BLM group, the number of apoptotic cells in the AECIIs of the BLM+MMDD group was significantly decreased (**Figure 7**).

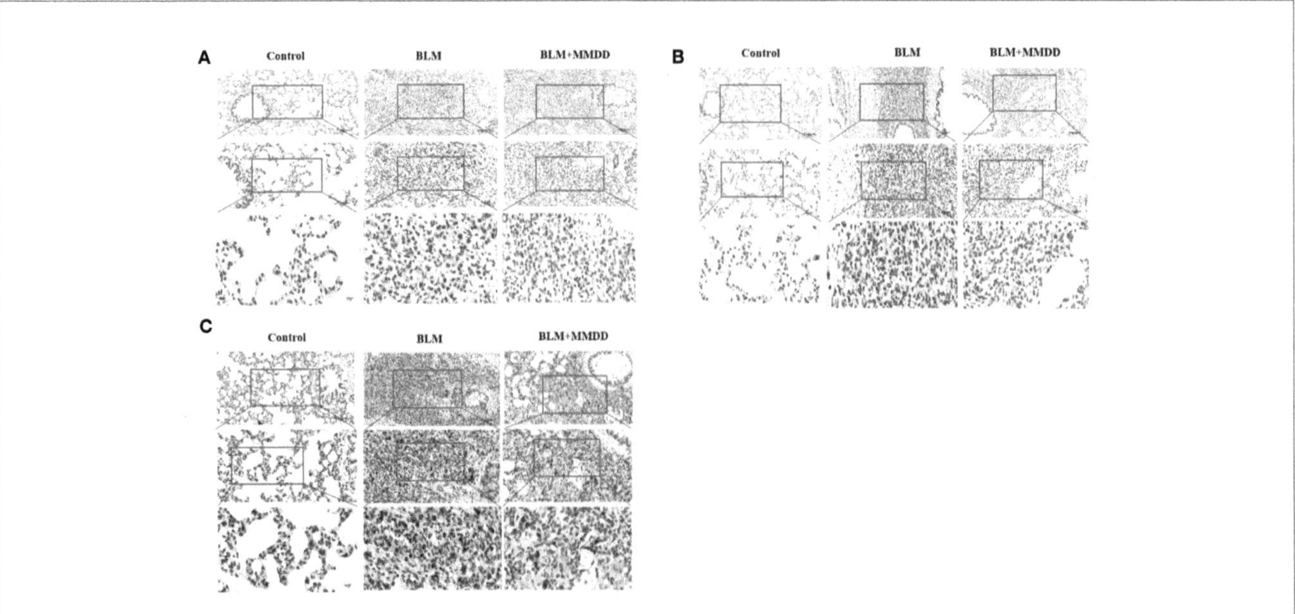

FIGURE 4 | Effect of MMDD on the expression of GRP78, CHOP, and surface active protein C (SPC) in the lung tissue of BLM-induced pulmonary fibrosis rat by immunohistochemical analysis. **(A)** The expression of GRP78 in each groups; **(B)** The expression of CHOP in each groups; **(C)** The expression of SPC in each groups. All the sections were detected by immunohistochemical analysis. Bars: (upper panels: 100 μm; middle panels: 50 μm; lower panels: 10 μm.)

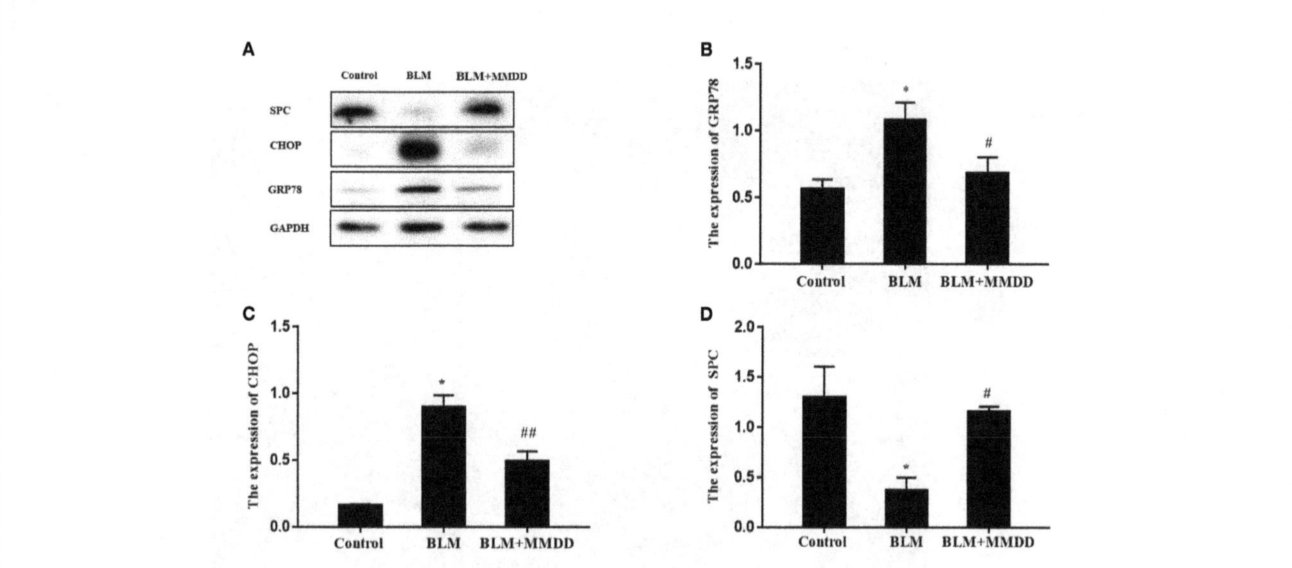

FIGURE 5 | Effect of MMDD on the expression of GRP78 and CHOP in the lung tissues of BLM-induced pulmonary fibrosis rat by Western blot analysis. **(A)** The expression of GRP78, CHOP and surface active protein C (SPC) in the lung tissues were detected by Western blot analysis; **(B)** The quantitative result of the GRP78 expression; **(C)** The quantitative result of the CHOP expression; **(D)** The quantitative result of the SPC expression. Data analyzed by one way ANOVA (Mean ± SEM). *P < 0.05, compared with the control group. #P < 0.05, ##P < 0.01,compared with the BLM group.

DISCUSSION

In animal experimental research, BLM-induced pulmonary fibrosis rat or mouse models are generally used to study the pathogenesis and corresponding treatment methods (Moore and Hogaboam, 2008). Bleomycin has been used as an anti-tumor drug, but it is now thought to cause dose-dependent interstitial pulmonary fibrosis (Chen and Stubbe, 2005). Chen J has reported that BLM can activate endoplasmic reticulum stress-related proteins including GRP78, CHOP and ATF-4 *in vivo* and *in vitro*. When ERS inhibitors or Pakt inhibitors are used, lung fibroblasts are reduced and can effectively improve lung function (Zhang et al., 2017).

In the present study, our finding showed that MMDD not only delayed the pathological process of BLM-induced fibrotic rats, but also ameliorated the lung function of fibrotic rats. Those might be through reducing the inflammatory infiltration of the lung tissue of fibrotic rats, reducing the content of extracellular matrix collagen, and increasing the amount of active SPC secreted by AECIIs to the surface of the alveoli. Our previous studies have also shown that MMDD attenuated BLM-induced rat IPF by improving lung function and alleviating chronic inflammatory responses in fibrotic lung tissue (Kang et al., 2017).

Extensive extracellular matrix deposition in the lung septum is an important pathological feature of pulmonary fibrosis. Collagen is the main component of the extracellular matrix. HYP is a unique amino acid that makes up the body's collagen. Except that elastin contains a small amount of HYP (about 1%), almost all HYP is present as collagen. Therefore, the HYP content in the tissue can directly reflect the degree of organ fibrosis. The direct source of collagen in the lung septum is

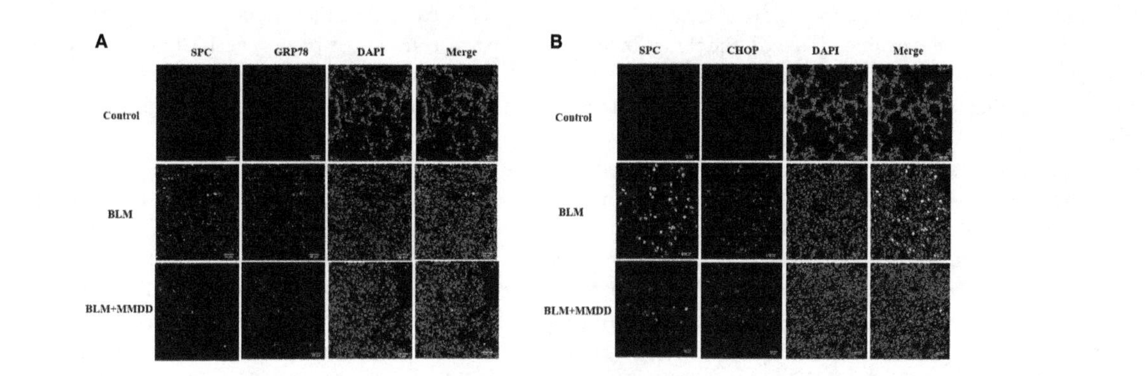

FIGURE 6 | Effect of MMDD on the expression of GRP78, CHOP, and surface active protein C (SPC) in the lung tissue of BLM-induced pulmonary fibrosis rat by Immunofluorescence double staining. **(A)** Immunofluorescence staining images for detection of CY3 (red), FITC (green) expression. **(B)** Immunofluorescence staining images for detection of CY3 (red), FITC (green) expression. DAPI (blue) was used for staining of nuclei. Bars: 50μm.

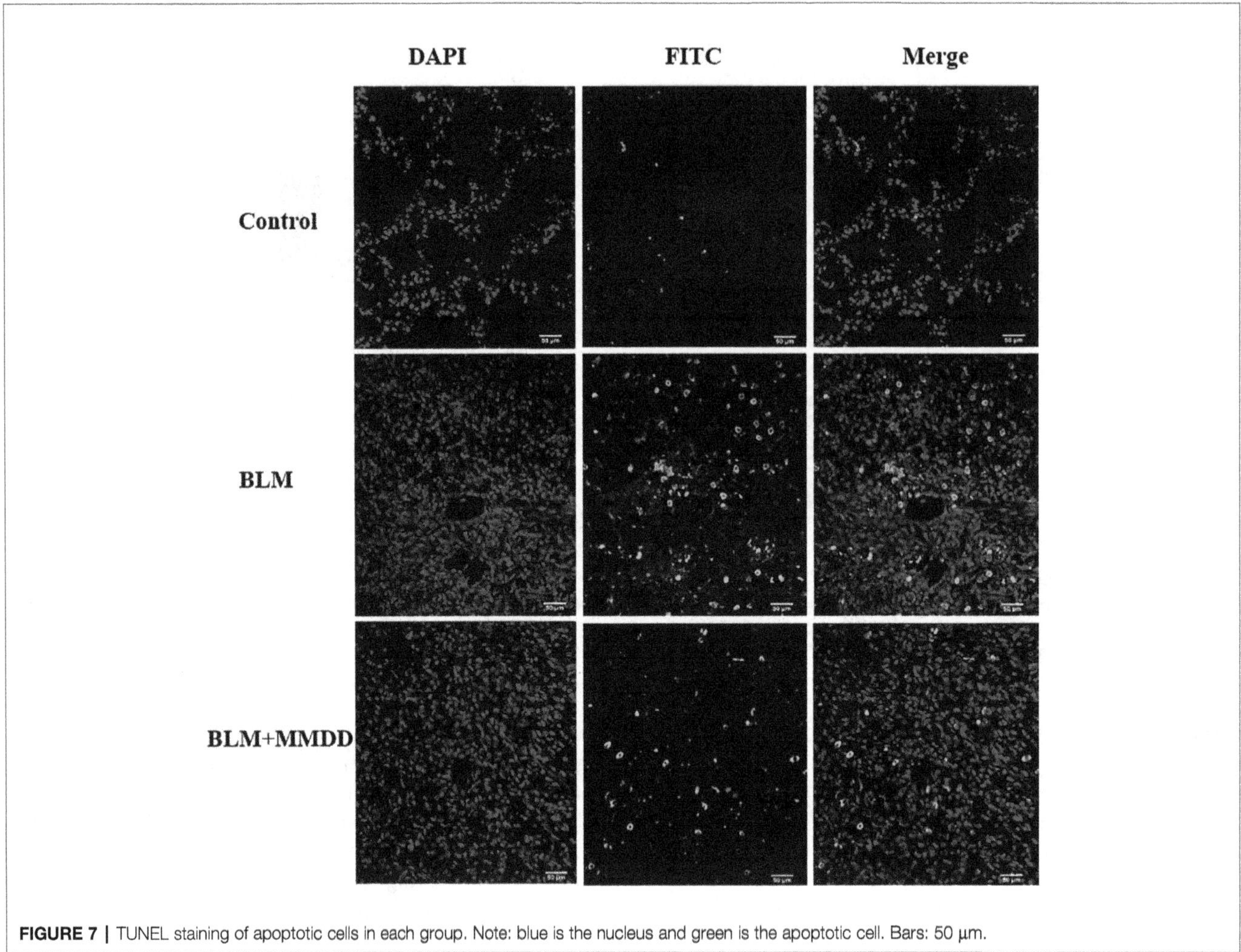

FIGURE 7 | TUNEL staining of apoptotic cells in each group. Note: blue is the nucleus and green is the apoptotic cell. Bars: 50 μm.

secreted by activated myofibroblasts, while α-SMA is a special marker protein for myofibroblasts (Waisberg et al., 2012). Therefore, α-SMA is an indirect indicator of collagen content. So we used HYP and α-SMA as indicator to measure the degree of fibrosis in our research. Our experimental results showed that MMDD remarkably reduced the content of HYP and the expression of α-SMA in lung tissue of rats with BLM-induced pulmonary fibrosis. This might be one reason for the improvement of pulmonary function in fibrotic rats.

The alveoli are the terminal part of the lung bronchial bundle and the place where gas exchange takes place. It is the main structure that constitutes the lung. Alveolar epithelium is classified into AECIs and AECIIs according to their morphological structure and function (Dobbs et al., 1998). AECIIs are sites for the synthesis, storage and secretion of pulmonary surfactants (Fehrenbach, 2001; Schmitz and Müller, 1991). Alveolar surfactant is a secreted lipoprotein composed mainly of four related proteins, SP-A, SP-B, SP-C, and SP-D. Only AECIIs secrete SP-C. They have the function of reducing the surface tension of the alveoli, increasing the compliance of the lungs, maintaining the stability of the alveolar size, preventing atelectasis and preventing pulmonary edema. In addition, AECIIs also have the beneficial functions in alveolar fluid balance, cellular (epithelial) repair, removal of dead or apoptotic cells, immune regulation and host defense. William E et al. developed a transgenic mouse model by using the Tet-On system, in which the expression of the mutant L188Q SFTPC was induced. AECIIs are more susceptible to apoptosis after BLM treatment, and the presence of ERS in AECIIs enhances bleomycin-induced pulmonary fibrosis in mice (Lawson et al., 2011). In patients with sporadic IPF, Martina Korfei et al. observed that in patients with IPPD, severe ERS occurred in AECIIs in lung tissue of patients with IPF, and ERS participates in the pathogenesis of pulmonary fibrosis by inducing apoptosis of alveolar epithelial cells in patients with IPF (Korfei et al., 2008). In our study, our results show that the active SPC secreted by AECIIs was reduced in the rat model of pulmonary fibrosis, and most of the SPC was accumulated and existed in AECIIs in an inactive form. After treatment with MMDD, the active SPC secretion was increased. This may be another reason for the improvement of pulmonary function in fibrotic rats.

Furthermore, MMDD can reduce the occurrence of endoplasmic reticulum stress and apoptosis in AECIIs. Endoplasmic reticulum (ER) is an organelle responsible for the correct folding of membranes and secreted proteins, lipid biosynthesis, glycogen production and storage, and intracellular calcium homeostasis (Sevier and Kaiser, 2002; Tu, 2004). Under physiological conditions, the normal function of nascent proteins needs to undergo correct folding based on chaperone proteins and post-translational modifications are mainly aided by chaperone proteins such as the Hsp70 family members GRP78, calnexin and calreticulin (Ron and Walter, 2007; Saibil, 2013). However, under the action of various conditions that impair ER function, the accumulation of unfolded or misfolded proteins in the ER leads to the unfolded protein response (UPR) (Brown, 1996; Schröder et al., 2005). GRP78 is a molecular chaperone widely distributed in the endoplasmic reticulum, which is the main UPR regulator and promotes protein folding and prevents protein aggregation in ER, stabilizes protein conformation and improves ER folding, and serves as a quality control system for identifying, retaining, and ultimately eliminating targets (Welch and Brown, 1996). Normally, proteins involved in transmembrane are inactive with GRP78 in combination with protein kinase RNA-like endoplasmic reticulum kinase (PERK), activated transcription factor 6 (ATF-6), and inositol 1 (IRE-1). When UPR is activated, PERK, ATF-6, and IRE-1 are separated from GRP78, isolated GRP78 is involved in the correct folding of unfolded or misfolded proteins to reduce their accumulation in the endoplasmic reticulum cavity and reduce endoplasmic reticulum stress. If UPR does not rescue cells, the cells eventually undergo apoptosis through increased expression of CHOP or activation of ER-specific caspase, thus GRP78 or induction of CHOP is widely used as a marker for ER stress (**Figure 8**).

GRP78 immunoreactivity was observed in mouse AT2 cells after bleomycin injury, while overexpression of SPC - BRICHOS mutant SP-CDExon4 in A549 cells increased GRP78 (Zhong et al., 2011). After bleomycin was modeled, the expression of GRP78 was increased in rat lung tissue. These observations suggest that endoplasmic reticulum stress does occur in a bleomycin-induced rat fibrosis model. After treatment with MMDD, ERS in fibrotic rats was suppressed. CHOP is thought to represent a key regulator of pro-apoptotic responses under ER stress. Chop deficiency protects mice from BLM-induced lung injury and fibrosis (Yao et al., 2016). Our study found that the content of CHOP protein in lung tissue was significantly reduced after treatment with MMDD, indicating that MMDD can inhibit the development of pulmonary fibrosis through apoptosis of related cells. To determine whether ERS and apoptosis occurred in AECIIs, we used confocal immunofluorescent

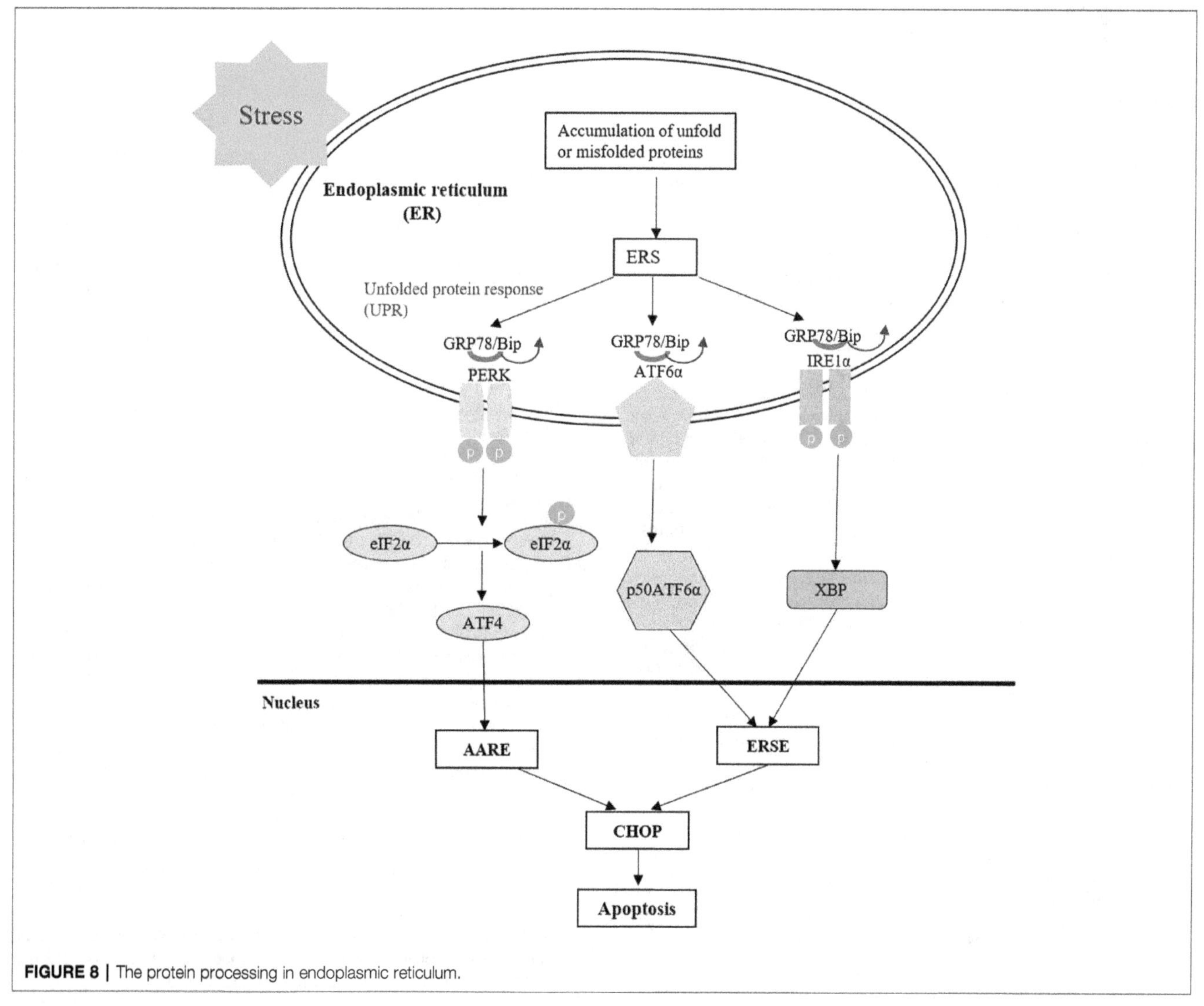

FIGURE 8 | The protein processing in endoplasmic reticulum.

microscopy. Double-staining for GRP78 and SPC, CHOP, and SPC confirmed the increased ERS and apoptosis in AECIIs. In addition, TUNEL staining showed that MMDD can reduce the apoptosis of lung tissue cells in rats with pulmonary fibrosis lesions. Moreover, MMDD effectively inhibited the occurrence of ERS in AECIIs and the apoptosis of AECIIs.

There are three apoptotic pathways due to CHOP-mediated apoptosis. Therefore, the inhibition of apoptotic pathway and signaling pathway in fibrotic lung tissue by MMDD remain to be further studied. This study provides a basis for the study of traditional Chinese medicine compound, presents a new method for the treatment of pulmonary fibrosis, and established an experimental basis for exploring new targets for the treatment of pulmonary fibrosis.

CONCLUSIONS

MMDD can mitigate the pathological development of pulmonary fibrosis. MMDD improved lung function by inhibiting the occurrence of ERS in AECIIs, reducing the apoptosis of AECIIs, and increasing the secretion of active SPC in AECIIs in lung tissue of fibrotic lesions. It may become a novel method for treating IPF.

AUTHOR CONTRIBUTIONS

YaL and YuL designed this research. MS performed the animal experiments. LT and YN conducted the pulmonary function test. LZ, LD, and SH conducted LC/MS. MS conducted the biochemical experiments and analyzed the data. MS wrote the manuscript. All authors contributed to the article and approved the submitted version.

ACKNOWLEDGMENTS

We thank National Center for Protein Science at Peking University in Beijing, china, for assistance with Peking University School of Life Sciences Public Instrument Center and Mz. Liqin Fu for help with data collection. This work was financially supported by the National Natural Science Foundational of China (NSFC) (81573716), Ministry of Education Research Innovation Team Project (IRT-17R11), Beijing University of Traditional Chinese Medicine School Research Project (2017-JYB-JS-175), National Natural Science Foundational of China (NSFC) (81202787), Innovation Team of the Beijing University of Chinese Medicine (2019-JYB-TD-006).

REFERENCES

Brown, W. J. W. R. (1996). Influence of molecular and chemical chaperones on protein folding. *Cell Stress Chaperones* 1 (2), 109–115. doi: 10.2307/1601909

Chen, J., and Stubbe, J. A. (2005). Bleomycins: towards better therapeutics. *Nat. Rev. Cancer* 5 (2), 102–112. doi: 10.1038/nrc1547

Dobbs, L. G., Gonzalez, R., Matthay, M. A., Carter, E. P., Allen, L., and Verkman, A. S. (1998). Highly water-permeable type i alveolar epithelial cells confer high water permeability between the airspace and vasculature in rat lung. *Proc. Natl. Acad. Sci.* 95 (6), 2991–2996. doi: 10.1073/pnas.95.6.2991

Fehrenbach, H. (2001). Alveolar epithelial type ii cell: defender of the alveolus revisited. *Respir. Res.* 2 (1), 33. doi: 10.1186/rr36

He, F., Xu, B. L., Chen, C., Jia, H. J., Wu, J. X., Wang, X. C., et al. (2016). Methylophiopogonanone A suppresses ischemia/ reperfusion-induced myocardial apoptosis in mice via activating PI3K/Akt/eNOS signaling pathway. *Acta Pharmacol. Sin.* 037 (006), 763–771. doi: 10.1038/aps.2016.14

Hsu, H. S., Liu, C. C., Lin, J. H., Hsu, T. W., Hsu, J. W., Su, K., et al. (2017). Involvement of er stress, pi3k/akt activation, and lung fibroblast proliferation in bleomycin-induced pulmonary fibrosis. *Sci. Rep.* 7 (1), 14272. doi: 10.1038/s41598-017-14612-5

Kang, D., Li, Y., Zhu, M., Tang, L., Shen, M. M., Chang, L. G., et al. (2017). Experimental study on lung function of pulmonary fibrosis rat under lung withered theory. *World Chin. Med.* 12 (2), 390–393. doi: 10.3969/j.issn.1673-7202.2017.02.038

Kang, D. (2017). *Experimental study on treatment of pulmonary fibrosis with fei wei. [master"s thesis]* (Beijing: Beijing university of Traditional Chinese Medicine).

Korfei, M., Ruppert, C., Mahavadi, P., Henneke, I., Markart, P., Koch, M., et al. (2008). Epithelial endoplasmic reticulum stress and apoptosis in sporadic idiopathic pulmonary fibrosis. *Am. J. Respir. Crit. Care Med.* 178 (8), 838–846. doi: 10.1164/rccm.200802-313oc

Lawson, W. E., Cheng, D. S., Degryse, A. L., Tanjore, H., Polosukhin, V. V., Xu, X. C., et al. (2011). Endoplasmic reticulum stress enhances fibrotic remodeling in the lungs. Proc. *Natl. Acad. Sci.* 108 (26), 10562–10567. doi: 10.1073/pnas.1107559108

Lin, J. H., Walter, P., and Yen, T. S. B. (2007). Endoplasmic reticulum stress in disease pathogenesis. *Annu. Rev. Pathol.* 3 (1), 399–425. doi: 10.1146/annurev.pathol.3.121806.151434

Longo, D. L., Lederer, D. J., and Martinez, F. J. (2018). Idiopathic pulmonary fibrosis. *N. Engl. J. Med.* 378 (19), 1811–1823. doi: 10.1056/NEJMra1705751

Luo, Y. S., Chen, S. H., Li, T., Guan, Y. L., Liu, Y. M., and Ma, B. X. (2019). Liquiritin alleviates spinal cord injury through suppression of inflammation, oxidative stress, and cell apoptosis in a rat model. *Trop. J. Pharm. Res.* 18, 1683–1689. doi: 10.4314/tjpr.v18i8.17

Luo, M. (2013). Clinical Observation on 38 Cases of Chronic Bronchitis with Clinical Relief of Lung and Yin Deficiency Treated with Maimendong formula. *Guiding J. Tradit. Chin. Med. Pharm.* 19 (11), 107–108.

Moore, B. B., and Hogaboam, C. M. (2008). Murine models of pulmonary fibrosis. *Am. J. Physiol. Lung Cell Mol. Physiol.* 294 (2), 152–160. doi: 10.1152/ajplung.00313.2007

Raghu, G., Rochwerg, B., Zhang, Y., Garcia, C. A. C., Azuma, A., Behr, J., et al. (2015). An official ats/ers/jrs/alat clinical practice guideline: treatment of idiopathic pulmonary fibrosis: an update of the 2011 clinical practice guideline. *Am. J. Respir. Crit. Care Med.* 192 (5), e3. doi: 10.1164/rccm.1925erratum

Ron, D., and Walter, P. (2007). Signal integration in the endoplasmic reticulum unfolded protein response. *Nat. Rev. Mol. Cell Biol.* 8 (7), 519–529. doi: 10.1038/nrm2199

Saibil, H. R. (2013). Chaperone machines for protein folding, unfolding and disaggregation. *Nat. Rev. Mol. Cell Biol.* 14 (10), 630–642. doi: 10.1038/nrm3658

Schmitz, G., and Müller, G. (1991). Structure and function of lamellar bodies, lipid-Protein complexes involved in storage and secretion of cellular lipids. *J. Lipid Res.* 32 (10), 1539–1570.

Schröder, M., and Kaufman, R. J. (2005). The mammalian unfolded protein response. *Annu. Rev. Biochem.* 74 (1), 739–789. doi: 10.1146/annurev.biochem.73.011303.074134

Sevier, C. S., and Kaiser, C. A. (2002). Formation and transfer of disulphide bonds in living cells. *Nat. Rev. Mol. Cell Biol.* 3 (11), 836. doi: 10.1038/nrm954

Tu, B. P. (2004). Oxidative protein folding in eukaryotes: mechanisms and consequences. *J. Cell Biol.* 164 (3), 341–346. doi: 10.1083/jcb.200311055

Waisberg, D. R., Parra, E. R., Barbas-Filho, JoãoV., Fernezlian, S., and Capelozzi, V. L. (2012). Increased fibroblast telomerase expression precedes myofibroblast α-smooth muscle actin expression in idiopathic pulmonary fibrosis. *Clinics (São Paulo Brazil).* 67 (9), 1039–1046. doi: 10.6061/clinics/2012(09)10

Wang, Y. W., and Ji, J. (2016). Therapeutic effect of Maimendong formula on the treatment of cough with qi and yin deficiency in patients with advanced lung cancer. *Jiangxi J. Tradit. Chin. Med.* 47 (07), 47–49.

Welch, W. J., and Brown, C. R. (1996). Influence of molecular and chemical chaperones on protein folding. *Cell Stress Chaperones.* 1 (2), 109 –115 doi: 10.1379/1466-1268(1996)001<0109:IOMACC>2.3.CO;2

Wu, Z., Zhao, X., Miyamoto, A., Zhao, S. J., Liu, C. Q., Zheng, W. M., et al. (2019). Effects of steroidal saponins extract from Ophiopogon japonicus root ameliorates doxorubicin-induced chronic heart failure by inhibiting oxidative stress and inflammatory response. *Pharm. Biol.* 57 (1), 176–183. doi: 10.1080/13880209.2019.1577467

Xiaolin, Y., Yanxia, Z., Xiaohua, Y., Xiaomei, Z., Xinxiang, W., Xuemei, L., et al. (2018). The influence of buqihuoxuetongluo formula on histopathology and pulmonary function test in bleomycin-induced idiopathic pulmonary fibrosis in rats. *J. Evidence-Based Complement. Altern Med.* 2018, 1–13. doi: 10.1155/2018/8903021

Yao, Y., Wang, Y., Zhang, Z., He, L., Zhu, J., Zhang, M., et al. (2016). Chop deficiency protects mice against bleomycin-induced pulmonary fibrosis by attenuating m2 macrophage production. *Mol. Ther.* 24 (5), 915–925. doi: 10.1038/mt.2016.36

Ying, G., Li-Fu, Y., Yang, Z., Li-Man, W., Peng, G., Meng, Y., et al. (2016). The chinese herbal medicine formula mkg suppresses pulmonary fibrosis of mice induced by bleomycin. *Int. J. Mol. Sci.* 17 (2), 238–. doi: 10.3390/ijms17020238

Yu, L. (2015). Treatment of 30 cases of idiopathic pulmonary fibrosis with Maimendong formula. *Chin. Med. Modern Distance Educ. China* 13 (06), 55–56. doi: 10.3969/j.issn.1672-2779.2015.06.028

Yunping, B., Jiansheng, L., Peng, Z., Ya, L., Meng, L., Suxiang, F., et al. (2018). A chinese herbal formula ameliorates pulmonary fibrosis by inhibiting oxidative stress via upregulating nrf2. *Front. Pharmacol.* 9, 628. doi: 10.3389/fphar.2018.00628

Zhang, L., Wang, Y., Wu, G., Xiang, X., Gong, Q., Xiong, W., et al. (2017). Endoplasmic reticulum stress, a new wrestler, in the pathogenesis of idiopathic pulmonary fibrosis. *Am. J. Transl. Res.* 9 (2), 722. eCollection 2017

Zhao, J. W., Chen, D. S., Deng, C. S., Wang, Q., Zhu, W., and Lin, L. (2017). Evaluation of anti-inflammatory activity of compounds isolated from the rhizome of ophiopogon japonicas. *BMC Complement. Altern Med.* 17 (1), 7. doi: 10.1186/s12906-016-1539-5

Zhao, M., Chen, Q. F., Xu, W. F., Wang, H., Che, Y., Wu, M. Q., et al. (2019). Total ginsenosides extract induce autophagic cell death in NSCLC cells through activation of endoplasmic reticulum stress. *J. Ethnopharmacol.* 243. doi: 10.1016/j.jep.2019.112093

Zhong, Q., Zhou, B., Ann, D. K., Minoo, P., Liu, Y., Banfalvi, A., et al. (2011). Role of endoplasmic reticulum stress in epithelial–mesenchymal transition of alveolar epithelial cells. *Am. J. Respir. Cell Mol. Biol.* 45 (3), 498–509. doi: 10.1165/rcmb.2010-0347oc

4

Protective Effect of Arbidol against Pulmonary Fibrosis and Sepsis in Mice

Hailong Li[1,2], *Rui Liu*[1,2], *Ruotong Zhang*[1,2], *Shanshan Zhang*[1], *Yiying Wei*[1,2], *Liang Zhang*[3], *Honggang Zhou*[1,2]* *and Cheng Yang*[1,2]*

[1] *The State Key Laboratory of Medicinal Chemical Biology, College of Pharmacy and Key Laboratory of Molecular Drug Research, Nankai University, Tianjin, China,* [2] *High-Throughput Molecular Drug Screening Centre, Tianjin International Joint Academy of Biomedicine, Tianjin, China,* [3] *Department of Thoracic Surgery, Tian Jin First Central Hospital, Tianjin, China*

***Correspondence:**
Honggang Zhou
honggang.zhou@nankai.edu.cn
Cheng Yang
yangcheng@nankai.edu.cn

From the perspective of epidemiology, viral immunology and current clinical research, pulmonary fibrosis may become one of the complications of patients with Coronavirus Disease 2019 (COVID-19). Cytokine storm is a major cause of new coronavirus death. The purpose of this study was to explore the effects of antiviral drug arbidol on cytokine storm and pulmonary fibrosis. Here, we use a mouse model of bleomycin-induced pulmonary fibrosis and a mouse model of fecal dilution-induced sepsis to evaluate the effects of arbidol on pulmonary fibrosis and cytokine storm. The results showed that arbidol significantly reduced the area of pulmonary fibrosis and improved lung function (reduced inspiratory resistance, lung dynamic compliance and forced vital capacity increased). Treatment with arbidol promoted reduced sepsis severity 48 h after sepsis induction, based on weight, murine sepsis score and survival rate. Arbidol observably alleviates inflammatory infiltrates and injury in the lungs and liver. Finally, we also found that arbidol reduced serum levels of pro-inflammatory factors such as TNF-α and IL-6 induced by fecal dilution. In conclusion, our results indicate that arbidol can alleviate the severity of pulmonary fibrosis and sepsis, and provide some reference for the treatment of cytokine storm and sequelae of pulmonary fibrosis in patients with COVID-19.

Keywords: arbidol, COVID-19, pulmonary fibrosis, cytokine storm, sepsis

INTRODUCTION

On December 30, 2019, 27 pneumonia cases linked to a seafood wholesale market were found in Wuhan, China, and promptly reported to the National Health Commission of China (Lake, 2020). A new type of coronavirus (HCoV), severe acute respiratory syndrome coronavirus-2 (SARS-CoV-2), was discovered through deep sequencing and analysis of lower respiratory tract samples (Gorbalenya et al., 2020; Zhu et al., 2020a). SARS-COV-2 is similar to SARS-COV and has sequence homology, but it spreads faster (Gorbalenya et al., 2020). As of November 30, SARS-COV-2 is still raging around the world, with a total of 63 million confirmed cases worldwide (Data comes from the World Health Organization, official notifications and authoritative media reports), but there are still no effective treatment drugs and methods.

Many critically ill patients and deceased patients have no serious clinical manifestations in the early stage of the virus infection, and only show mild fever, cough and other physical discomfort, but their bodily condition suddenly deteriorated during the treatment and turned into severe patients. Numerous severe COVID-19 patients will develop acute respiratory distress syndrome (ARDS) and multiple organ failure, which will eventually lead to death (Azkur et al., 2020; Yang et al., 2020). Dina Ragab and Harapan et al. (Harapan et al., 2020; Ragab et al., 2020) suggest that mortality in COVID-19 patients is related to the "cytokine storm" caused by the virus. Excessive production of proinflammatory cytokines lead to ARDS aggravation and extensive tissue damage, leading to multiple organ failure and death. In the case of COVID-19, clinical studies have concluded that the rapid deterioration of COVID-19 patients is closely related to the outbreak of cytokine storms in the body. Cytokine storm is an important cause of death. In addition, cytokine storms are a major cause of death in patients with SARS, MERS, and influenza (Liu et al., 2016; Channappanavar and Perlman, 2017; Rat et al., 2020). Therefore, inhibiting cytokine storms can effectively prevent death in COVID-19 patients. Sepsis refers to systemic inflammatory response syndrome (SIRS) caused by infection (Butler, 2015; Schlapbach et al., 2015). Sepsis, with its rapid development and high fatality rate, has always been one of the major difficulties in the study of acute illness (Li et al., 2015). The severity of sepsis infection is caused by a cascade reaction, which makes the automatic amplification of cytokines, and finally leads to a cytokine storm (Chousterman et al., 2017). Mouse models of sepsis are usually study cytokine storms. Song et al. (Qiu et al., 2019) found that regulatory T cells lacking Gpr174 reduced cytokine storms in septic mice. Tang et al. (Yao et al., 2017) revealed that α-lactose can reduce the cytokine storm by preventing TIM-3 signal transduction, thereby improving the survival rate of septic mice. Therefore, exploring the cytokine storm in sepsis mice has partial reference significance for the clinical cytokine storm.

Although the spread of the epidemic is still not ended, the sequelae of the epidemic are gradually emerging, and we need to explore in depth. At present, the familiar coronaviruses include SARS coronavirus, MERS and Novel Coronavirus. The study found that idiopathic pulmonary fibrosis (PF) was the most important cause of high mortality and low quality of life in patients infected with SARS coronavirus (Venkataraman and Frieman, 2017). Recently, through retrospective analysis of lung computed tomography imaging of 50 patients with COVID-19 pneumonia. It was found that the formation of fibrous streaks during rehabilitation (Xu et al., 2020). A meta-analysis found that viral infections increase the risk of idiopathic pulmonary fibrosis, and COVID-19 patients in the recovery period may cause additional complications due to PF (Sheng et al., 2020; Taz et al., 2020). Therefore, pulmonary fibrosis is likely to be one of the major complications in COVID-19 patients. The U.S. Food and Drug Administration (FDA) approved nintedanib and pirfenidone to inhibit the progression of PF (Raghu et al., 2015). They can only alleviate the decline in lung function and cannot reverse the fibrosis that has formed (Holtze et al., 2020). Therefore, it is very necessary to develop novel therapies for the treatment of PF and pay attention to the sequelae of SARS-COV-2 pulmonary fibrosis.

Arbidol (ethyl-6-bromo-4-[(dimethylamino) methyl]-5-hydroxy-1-methyl-2-[(phenylthio) methyl]-indole-3 carboxylate hydrochloride monohydrate, also known as UMifenovir), a broad-spectrum antiviral compound synthesized by the Russian Institute of Chemistry and Medicine in 1988, has been approved for the prevention and treatment of influenza A and B infections and post-influenza complications in China and Russia (Haviernik et al., 2018). Previous studies have shown that arbidol has an inhibitory effect on many global viruses with significant morbidity and mortality (Pécheur et al., 2016). Arbidol, oseltamivir, ribavirin and lopinavir (individualized or combined medication) are widely used in Chinese patients with COVID-19, but none of them have obvious effects. However, a retrospective study in a clinical trial found that in 220 non-emergency COVID 19 patients in Wuhan Dongxihu Hospital, China, arbidol could accelerate the fever recovery and virus clearance of respiratory specimens, especially in men, and also help shorten the length of hospital stay, And no obvious adverse reactions (Gao et al., 2020). However, the effect of arbidol on the cytokine storm and PF produced in patients with COVID-19 has not been reported.

Since our laboratory is not qualified for virus testing, in this study we used a fecal diluent-induced sepsis mouse model and a bleomycin-induced IPF mouse model to evaluate the effect of arbidol on cytokine storm and IPF, in order to provide reference for the clinical treatment and sequelae prevention of COVID-19.

MATERIALS AND METHODS

Materials

Nintedanib (>99%) was purchased from HWRK Chem Co., Ltd. (Beijing, China). BLM was purchased from HANHUI Pharmaceuticals Co., Ltd (Shanghai, China). Cefpirome sulfate was obtained from Yuanye Bio-Technology Co., Ltd. (Shanghai, China). Arbidol (>98%) was purchased from Bidepharm (Shanghai, China).

Experimental Animals

Male C57BL/6 mice of about 6–8 weeks and weighed (18 ± 4) g were provided by Beijing Academy of Military Sciences (Beijing, China). Mice had free access to food and water and housed in a room at a temperature of 20°–26°C and a humidity between 50 and 55%, with 12 h light/dark cycle. All experimental protocols were approved by the Animal Experiment Committee of Tianjin International Joint Academy of Biomedicine (approval no. SYXK (JIN) 2017-0003).

Modeling and Animal Grouping

In bleomycin (BLM)-induced pulmonary fibrosis model, the mice were randomly divided into five groups (n = 8): Saline group, BLM only group (2 mg·kg^{-1}), BLM with nintedanib group (100 mg·kg^{-1}) and BLM with arbidol (100 and 200 mg·kg^{-1}) treatment groups. At day 0, C57BL/6 mice were anesthetized by intraperitoneal injection of 10% chloral hydrate (5·ml/kg), and then intratracheal injection of 2 mg/kg BLM (Nippon Kayaku Co., Ltd. Tokyo, Japan). Saline group received normal saline by the same procedure. Normal saline, nintedanib and arbidol were applied intragastrically from day 7 to day 13.

In fecal dilution-induced sepsis model, the mice were randomly divided into five groups (n = 8): Saline group, 10% fecal dilution only group, fecal dilution with cefpirome sulfate (CS) group (100 mg·kg^{-1}) and fecal dilution with arbidol (100 and 200 mg·kg^{-1}) treatment groups. At day 0, Intraperitoneal injection of 10% fecal dilution was given to model group and treatment group to establish the sepsis models. For the treatment group, intraperitoneal injection of cefpirome sulfate

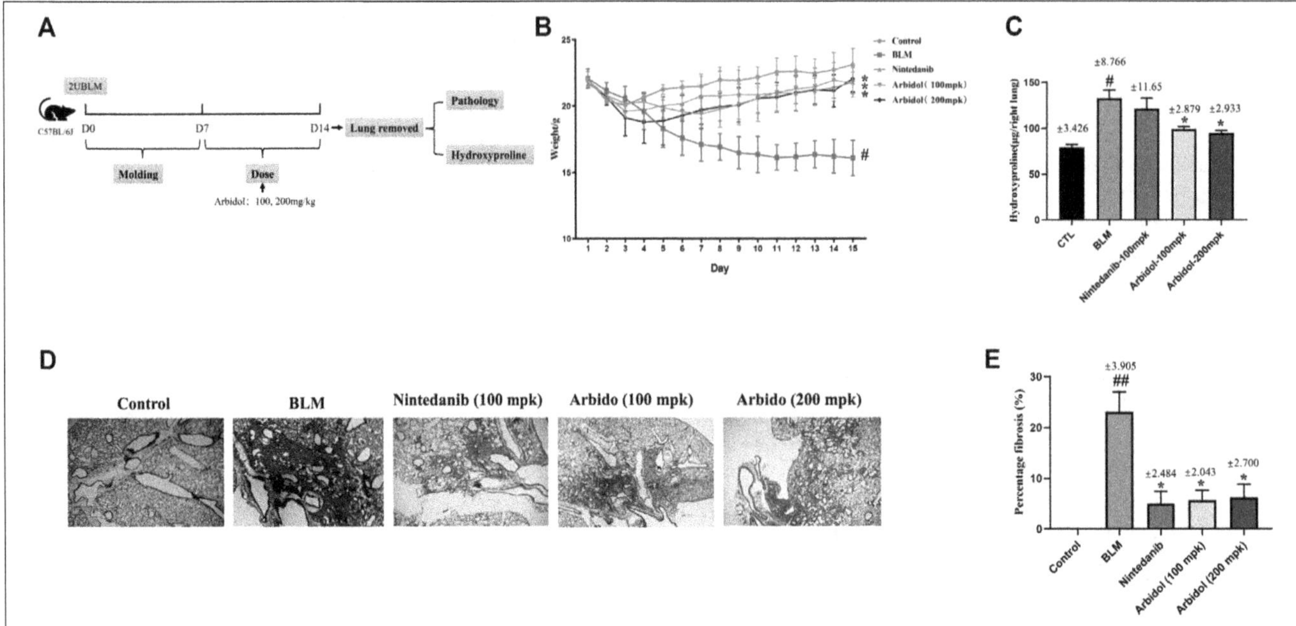

FIGURE 1 | Effect of arbidol on BLM-induced pulmonary fibrosis in mice. **(A)** Experimental protocol of BLM-induced IPF in mice. **(B)** Arbidol significantly inhibited BLM-induced weight loss in mice. **(C)** Arbidol significantly inhibited the levels of hydroxyproline in the lung tissue of mice **(D)** HE staining was used to evaluate the effect of arbidol on BLM-induced pathological changes (20x magnification). **(E)** Percentage of fibrosis was quantified by Ashcroft score system. Values are presented as the mean ± SEM (n = 5), $^{\#}p < 0.05$, significantly different from control group; $^{*}p < 0.05$ significantly different from model groups.

(100 mg·kg^{-1}) and arbidol (100 and 200 mg·kg^{-1}) were given 2 h before fecal dilution injection. Saline group received normal saline by the same procedure.

Histological

The heart, liver, spleen, lung and kidney tissues were fixed in 4% paraformaldehyde, embedded in paraffin and sectioned into 5 μm slices. Put the prepared slices in a 60°C oven for drying, and then dewax them as usual. Hematoxylin staining for 5–10 min, hydrochloric ethanol separation for 10–20 s. Then rinse with ultra-pure water for 15–20 min and dye with eosin for 3 min (H&E; Solarbio). After dehydration and transparency, add neutral gum to seal the slice. The histologic severity was quantified by Ashcroft scoring system (Ashcroft et al., 1988).

Hydroxyproline Determination

The improved method of Dong et al. (Dong et al., 2015). was used to isolate the right lung tissue of mice with bleomycin pulmonary fibrosis and determine the level of Hydroxyproline.

Pulmonary Function Test

The mice were kept supine and fixed on the operating table after anesthesia. When the trachea is exposed, insert the tube into the trachea and secure it with cotton thread. The pulmonary dynamic compliance (Cldyn) and forced vital capacity (FVC), expiratory resistance (Re) and inspiratory resistance (Ri) mice was measured after the mice were transferred to the body description platform.

ELISA for the Detection of Inflammatory Factors

The levels of IL-6 and TNF-α in serum of fecal dilution-induced sepsis mice were determined by enzyme-linked immunosorbent assay (ELISA) kit. The experimental process strictly followed the instructions of the ELISA kit (Proteintech, United States).

Statistical Analysis

All the data were analyzed using Graph Pad Prism 8.1 (Graph Pad Software, Inc., San Diego, CA) and expressed as mean ± SEM. All the data were statistically evaluated using one-way ANOVA for post-mortem multiple group comparisons. $p < 0.05$ was considered to be statistically significant.

RESULTS

Arbidol Attenuates BLM-Induced Pulmonary Fibrosis in Mice

We first evaluated the effects of arbidol treatment on BLM-induced pulmonary fibrosis, and the experimental program is shown in **Figure 1A**. The change of body weight was displayed in **Figure 1B**. The body weight was decreased apparently with the treatment of BLM. As showed in **Figure 1C**, compared with saline group, the content of hydroxyproline in the right lung of mice in bleomycin group was significantly increased. In BLM with arbidol treatment groups, the hydroxyproline content decreased, indicating that arbidol inhibited ECM deposition. Histological changes of the lung were shown in **Figures 1D,E**, in the saline

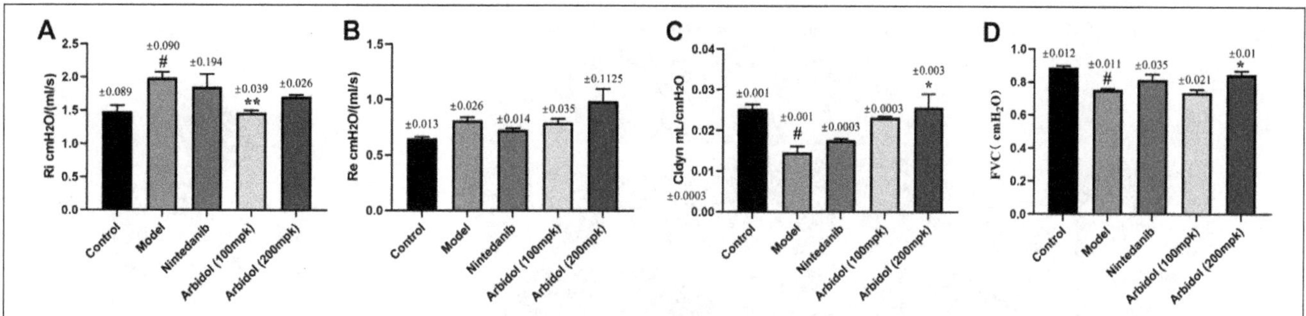

FIGURE 2 | Effect of arbidol on BLM-induced pulmonary function impairment in mice. Lung function **(A)** (inspiratory resistance, RI) **(B)** (expiratory resistance, Re) **(C)** (dynamic lung compliance, Cldyn) and **(D)** (forced vital capacity, FVC) of the mice in the different groups described above were measured by pulmonary function apparatus. Values are presented as the mean ± SEM (n = 5), $^{\#}p < 0.05$, significantly different from control group; $^{*}p < 0.05$, $^{**}p < 0.01$ significantly different from model groups.

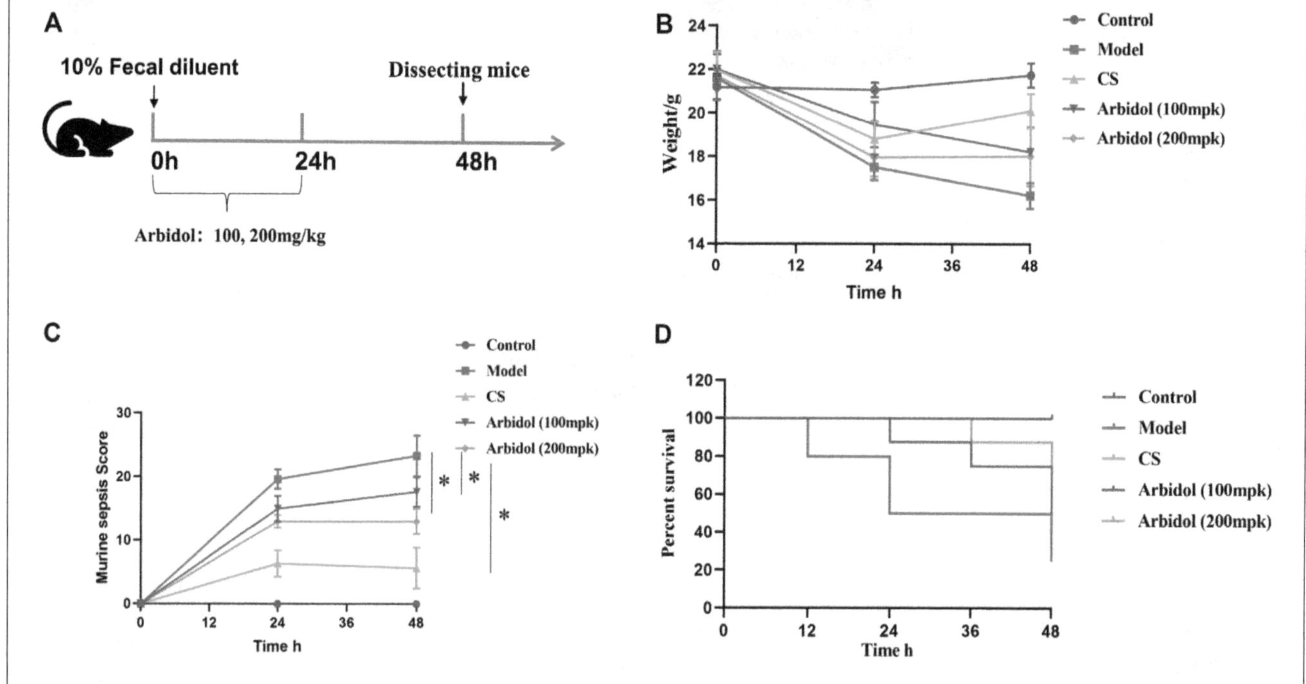

FIGURE 3 | Effect of arbidol on fecal dilution -induced sepsis in mice **(A)** Experimental scheme of mice sepsis induced by fecal diluent **(B)** Changes in body weight in different groups of mice (Control, Model, cefpirome sulfate or CS, 100 and 200 mpk arbidol) **(C)** The effect of arbidol on murine sepsis score (MSS) of the different groups of mice described above **(D)** The effect of arbidol on the survival time of the different groups of mice described above. Values are presented as the mean ± SEM (n = 5), $^{\#}p < 0.05$, significantly different from control group; $^{*}p < 0.05$, significantly different from model groups.

group, the lung tissue structure was normal without obvious inflammatory cell infiltration. After injection of bleomycin, the lung tissues of mice showed significant alveolar inflammation, and some alveolar changes and fibrosis occurred. After arbidol treatment, the tissue lesions were alleviated and the percentage fibrosis was observably reduced.

Arbidol Alleviated BLM-Induced Pulmonary Function Impairment in Mice

Pulmonary function determination is an important clinical examination of lung diseases and respiratory physiology. It is helpful for early detection of lung and airway lesions, assessing the severity and prognosis of the disease, and can also be used to evaluate the efficacy of drugs or other treatment methods. We have evaluated the effect of arbidol on BLM-induced pulmonary function impairment in mice. As showed in **Figures 2A,B**, compared with model group, arbidol significantly decreased Ri, but have no effect of Re. The results suggested that arbidol could reduce the airway resistance induced by BLM in mice, and thus alleviate the pulmonary function impairment caused by pulmonary fibrosis in mice. Cldyn is often used to detect the elastic resilience of lung tissue and determine the severity of obstructive lung disease. The decline in FVC is an alternative

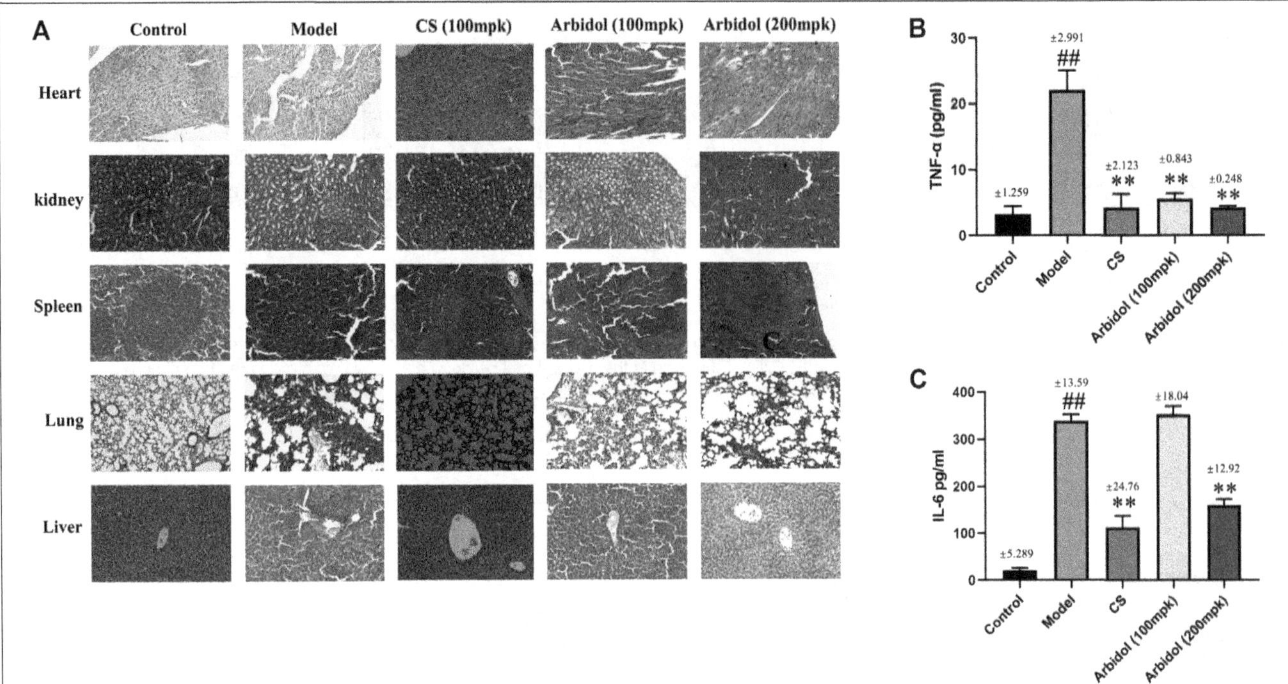

FIGURE 4 | Effect of arbidol on serum proinflammatory cytokine expression. **(A)** HE staining was used to evaluate the effect of arbidol on fecal dilution -induced pathological changes (20× magnification). **(B,C)** Serum TNF-α and IL-6 were detected by ELISA. Arbidol significantly inhibits the levels of TNF-α and IL-6 in mouse serum. Values are presented as the mean ± SEM (n = 5), $^{##}p < 0.01$, significantly different from control group; $^{**}p < 0.01$, significantly different from model groups.

endpoint for death in IPF studies, and new drug development needs to demonstrate its efficacy against FVC under current treatment standards. As showed in **Figures 2C,D**, compared with the model group, arbidol significantly increased Cldyn and FVC. In conclusion, these data suggested arbidol could restore some lung function impairment indicators in pulmonary fibrosis mice.

Arbidol Attenuates Fecal Dilution -Induced Sepsis in Mice

The experimental program is shown in **Figure 3A**. The change of body weight was displayed in **Figure 3B**. Sepsis-induced a decrease in body weights compared with the Control group, the body weight in mice treated with arbidol was higher than model group. The murine sepsis score (MSS) was tested according to the introduction of reference (Shrum et al., 2014). MSS values increased 24 and 48 h after induction of fecal diluent. However, the severity of sepsis evaluated by MSS was lower 24 and 48 h after sepsis induction in mice treated with arbidol (**Figure 3C**). A total of 40 mice were used in the survival experiments that were conducted independently over a period of 48 hour. As showed in **Figure 3D**, compared with the sepsis group, survival was improved in the arbidol treatment groups. The survival rate of the model group was 50% after 48 h induction of fecal diluent, whereas, during the same time period, the survival rates of arbidol group (100 and 200 mg·kg^{-1}) were 80 and 90%, respectively.

Arbidol Inhibits the Release of Pro-inflammatory Cytokines in Serum

We also evaluated the effect of arbidol on sepsis induced tissue damage in mice. The histological changes are shown in **Figure 4A**. In the spleen of model group, the white pulp is significantly enlarged. In the lung of model group, mild alveolar space edema and leukocyte accumulation around pulmonary arterioles. In the liver and kidney of mice with fecal diluent, the tissue exhibited numerous inflammatory infiltrates. In the heart of model group, the cardiomyocytes are disorganized and loose. After arbidol intervention, the above lesions were alleviated.

As showed in **Figures 4B,C**, compared with the control group, content of inflammatory factors IL-6 and TNF-a in serum significantly increased after the injection of fecal diluent, while the content markedly decreased after the treatment of arbidol. These data suggested that arbidol could inhibit the elevation of serum inflammatory cytokines induced by sepsis.

DISCUSSION

Arbidol can inhibit the fusion of the viral lipid membrane and the cell body membrane under physiological conditions in the cell, and prevent the release of viral genetic material. At the same time, arbidol can enter the cell nucleus in its original form, change the permeability of the cell membrane, activate 2, 5-A synthetase, and induce the synthesis of 2, 5-oligoadenine nucleotides, which is an interferon-like effect, which leads to Disruption of cell metabolism, inhibit virus growth and cell proliferation (Boriskin et al., 2008). As a broad-spectrum antiviral, arbidol inhibits a variety of viruses, including parainfluenza, Lassa, Ebola, hepatitis B and C viruses (Blaising et al., 2014; Hulseberg et al., 2019). With regard to COVID-19, Xue et al. (Zhu et al., 2020b) showed that the duration of viral loss and hospital stay was significantly shorter in patients treated with arbidol, Lopinavir/Ritonavir, and recombinant interferon alpha-2B triple antiviral therapy compared to those treated without arbidol. Li et al. (Gao et al., 2020) analyzed the efficacy of arbidol and found that it accelerated fever recovery and virus clearance in respiratory tract samples. However, the effect of arbidol on sudden cytokine storms and pulmonary fibrosis in COVID-19 patients remains unknown. In this study, we used fecal diluent-induced septic mice and bleomycin-induced pulmonary fibrosis mice to partially simulate the symptoms of COVID-19 patients, including cytokine storm and sequelae of pulmonary fibrosis. The experimental results demonstrated that arbidol could significantly inhibit PF and sepsis in mice.

A single tracheal instillation of bleomycin in rodents is a widely used model for studying the occurrence of pulmonary fibrosis and evaluating the effects of anti-fibrosis treatments (Kolb et al., 2020). Bleomycin-induced pulmonary fibrosis model was in the early inflammatory stage from 0 to 7 days, and changed to fibrosis after 7 days (Plantier et al., 2018). This induction mode makes the timing of anti-pulmonary fibrosis treatment very important. Therefore, in order to accurately evaluate the anti-fibrosis effect of the drug, the intervention should be after 7 days without affecting the early inflammation. In this study, seven days after bleomycin-induced mice, arbidol treatment was started. Hydroxyproline (HYP) is mainly found in animal collagen and can enhance the elasticity of connective tissue. The content of hydroxyproline in the tissue reflects the catabolism of collagen. Therefore, accurate determination of the content of hydroxyproline in lung tissue can be directly and effectively determine the degree of development of pulmonary fibrosis (Srivastava et al., 2016). The results showed that arbidol could significantly reduce the area of fibrosis and the level of hydroxyproline in mouse lung tissue. Many types of lung function decline can affect the lower respiratory system, from the conducting trachea to the pulmonary vascular system. The clinical expression of pulmonary fibrosis is directly related to changes in lung function (Plantier et al., 2018). By testing the lung function of mice, it was found that arbidol could reduce the Ri of mice and increase Cldyn and FVC, but had no obvious effect on Re. Of course, we will continue to conduct in-depth research on the efficacy and mechanism of arbidol against pulmonary fibrosis.

Harapan et al. pointed out that SARS-CoV-2 infection induces an extremely active inflammatory response called cytokine storm, which subsequently leads to uncontrolled lung inflammation (Harapan et al., 2020). Another study also pointed out that COVID-19 infection is accompanied by an aggressive inflammatory response that releases a large amount of pro-inflammatory cytokines. This event is called a "cytokine storm" and is closely related to the mortality of patients with COVID-19 (Ragab et al., 2020). Sepsis, a complex disease, characterized by a host's dysfunctional response to infection that leads to life-threatening multiorgan dysfunction (Dugar et al., 2020). Studies have found that the release of inflammatory cytokines, such as tumor necrosis factor (TNF-α) and interleukins (IL-1β and IL-6) increases, and promotes many immunopathological processes in sepsis, which are often referred to as "cytokines storm" (Ono et al., 2018; Hwang et al., 2020). As the most common source of infection in patients with sepsis comes from the abdominal cavity, in recent years, the abdominal infection model has been gradually used as a commonly used animal model of sepsis. Animal models of fecal peritonitis have been widely used in sepsis research (Dyson et al., 2011; Rudiger et al., 2013; Jeger et al., 2017; Sulzbacher et al., 2020). Since our laboratory cannot perform virus tests, in this study, we used fecal diluent-induced sepsis mice to simulate the cytokine storm symptoms of COVID-19 to a certain extent. The result revealed that arbidol notably attenuates fecal dilution -induced sepsis in mice. ELISA assay revealed that arbidol inhibits the release of pro-inflammatory cytokines (TNF-α and IL-6) in serum. Taken together, these data indicated that arbidol could inhibit the cytokine storm induced by fecal diluent in septic mice, and we hypothesized that arbidol may have a better inhibitory effect on cytokine storm in COVID-19 patients.

CONCLUSION

In summary, our study found that arbidol can relieve PF and sepsis in mice. This study proves to a certain extent that arbidol may have a certain therapeutic effect in the cytokine storm that appears in the clinic of COVID-19 patients and the PF that appears during the rehabilitation period. Of course, the mechanism of action of arbidol on PF and sepsis needs to be further analyzed.

AUTHOR CONTRIBUTIONS

All authors listed have made a substantial, direct, and intellectual contribution to the work and approved it for publication.

REFERENCES

Ashcroft, T., Simpson, J. M., and Timbrell, V. (1988). Simple method of estimating severity of pulmonary fibrosis on a numerical scale. *J. Clin. Pathol.* 41, 467–470. doi:10.1136/jcp.41.4.467

Azkur, A. K., Akdis, M., Azkur, D., Sokolowska, M., Van De Veen, W., Brüggen, M. C., et al. (2020). Immune response to SARS-CoV-2 and mechanisms of immunopathological changes in COVID-19. *Allergy* 75, 1564–1581. doi:10.1111/all.14364

Blaising, J., Polyak, S. J., and Pécheur, E. I. (2014). Arbidol as a broad-spectrum antiviral: an update. *Antivir. Res.* 107, 84–94. doi:10.1016/j.antiviral.2014.04.006

Boriskin, Y. S., Leneva, I. A., Pécheur, E. I., and Polyak, S. J. (2008). Arbidol: a broad-spectrum antiviral compound that blocks viral fusion. *Curr. Med. Chem.* 15, 997–1005. doi:10.2174/092986708784049658

Butler, T. (2015). *Capnocytophaga canimorsus*: an emerging cause of sepsis, meningitis, and post-splenectomy infection after dog bites. *Eur. J. Clin. Microbiol. Infect. Dis.* 34, 1271–1280. doi:10.1007/s10096-015-2360-7

Channappanavar, R., and Perlman, S. (2017). Pathogenic human coronavirus infections: causes and consequences of cytokine storm and immunopathology. *Semin. Immunopathol.* 39, 529–539. doi:10.1007/s00281-017-0629-x

Chousterman, B. G., Swirski, F. K., and Weber, G. F. (2017). Cytokine storm and sepsis disease pathogenesis. *Semin. Immunopathol.* 39, 517–528. doi:10.1007/s00281-017-0639-8

Dong, Y., Geng, Y., Li, L., Li, X., Yan, X., Fang, Y., et al. (2015). Blocking follistatin-like 1 attenuates bleomycin-induced pulmonary fibrosis in mice. *J. Exp. Med.* 212: 235–252. doi:10.1084/jem.20121878

Dugar, S., Choudhary, C., and Duggal, A. (2020). Sepsis and septic shock: guideline-based management. *Cleve. Clin. J. Med.* 87, 53–64. doi:10.3949/ccjm.87a.18143

Dyson, A., Rudiger, A., and Singer, M. (2011). Temporal changes in tissue cardiorespiratory function during faecal peritonitis. *Intensive Care Med.* 37, 1192–1200. doi:10.1007/s00134-011-2227-z

Gao, W., Chen, S., Wang, K., Chen, R., Guo, Q., Lu, J., et al. (2020). Clinical features and efficacy of antiviral drug, Arbidol in 220 nonemergency COVID-19 patients from East-West-Lake Shelter Hospital in Wuhan: a retrospective case series. *Virol. J.* 17, 162. doi:10.1186/s12985-020-01428-5

Gorbalenya, A. E., Baker, S., Baric, R., De Groot, R. J., Drosten, C., Perlman, S., et al. (2020). The species Severe acute respiratory syndrome-related coronavirus: classifying 2019-nCoV and naming it SARS-CoV-2. *Nat. Microbiol.* 5, 536–544. doi:10.1038/s41564-020-0695-z

Harapan, H., Ryan, M., Yohan, B., Abidin, R. S., Nainu, F., Rakib, A., et al. (2020). Covid-19 and dengue: double punches for dengue-endemic countries in Asia. *Rev. Med. Virol.* E2161. doi:10.1002/rmv.2161

Haviernik, J., Štefánik, M., Fojtíková, M., Kali, S., Tordo, N., Rudolf, I., et al. (2018). Arbidol (umifenovir): a broad-spectrum antiviral drug that inhibits medically important arthropod-borne flaviviruses. *Viruses* 10 (4), 184. doi:10.3390/v10040184

Holtze, C. H., Freiheit, E. A., Limb, S. L., Stauffer, J. L., Raimundo, K., Pan, W. T., et al. (2020). Patient and site characteristics associated with pirfenidone and nintedanib use in the United States; an analysis of idiopathic pulmonary fibrosis patients enrolled in the pulmonary fibrosis foundation patient registry. *Respir. Res.* 21, 48. doi:10.1186/s12931-020-1315-4

Hulseberg, C. E., Fénéant, L., Szymańska-de Wijs, K. M., Kessler, N. P., Nelson, E. A., Shoemaker, C. J., et al. (2019). Arbidol and other low-molecular-weight drugs that inhibit lassa and ebola viruses. *J. Virol.* 93, e02185–e02218. doi:10.1128/JVI.02185-18

Hwang, M. I., Bond, W. F., and Powell, E. S. (2020). Sepsis alerts in emergency departments: a systematic review of accuracy and quality measure impact. *West. J. Emerg. Med.* 21, 1201–1210. doi:10.5811/westjem.2020.5.46010

Jeger, V., Arrigo, M., Hildenbrand, F. F., Müller, D., Jirkof, P., Hauffe, T., et al. (2017). Improving animal welfare using continuous nalbuphine infusion in a long-term rat model of sepsis. *Intensive Care Med. Exp.* 5, 23. doi:10.1186/s40635-017-0137-2

Kolb, P., Upagupta, C., Vierhout, M., Ayaub, E., Bellaye, P. S., Gauldie, J., et al. (2020). The importance of interventional timing in the bleomycin model of pulmonary fibrosis. *Eur. Respir. J.* 55, 1901105. doi:10.1183/13993003.01105-2019

Lake, M. A. (2020). What we know so far: COVID-19 current clinical knowledge and research. *Clin. Med.* 20, 124–127, doi:10.7861/clinmed.2019-coron

Li, J., Li, M., Su, L., Wang, H., Xiao, K., Deng, J., et al. (2015). Alterations of T helper lymphocyte subpopulations in sepsis, severe sepsis, and septic shock: a prospective observational study. *Inflammation* 38, 995–1002. doi:10.1007/s10753-014-0063-3

Liu, Q., Zhou, Y. H., and Yang, Z. Q. (2016). The cytokine storm of severe influenza and development of immunomodulatory therapy. *Cell. Mol. Immunol.* 13, 3–10. doi:10.1038/cmi.2015.74

Ono, S., Tsujimoto, H., Hiraki, S., and Aosasa, S. (2018). Mechanisms of sepsis-induced immunosuppression and immunological modification therapies for sepsis. *Ann. Gastroenterol. Surg.* 2, 351–358. doi:10.1002/ags3.12194

Pécheur, E. I., Borisevich, V., Halfmann, P., Morrey, J. D., Smee, D. F., Prichard, M., et al. (2016). The synthetic antiviral drug arbidol inhibits globally prevalent pathogenic viruses. *J. Virol.* 90, 3086–3092. doi:10.1128/JVI.02077-15

Plantier, L., Cazes, A., Dinh-Xuan, A. T., Bancal, C., Marchand-Adam, S., and Crestani, B. (2018). Physiology of the lung in idiopathic pulmonary fibrosis. *Eur. Respir. Rev.* 27, 170062. doi:10.1183/16000617.0062-2017

Qiu, D., Chu, X., Hua, L., Yang, Y., Li, K., Han, Y., et al. (2019). Gpr174-deficient regulatory T cells decrease cytokine storm in septic mice. *Cell Death Dis.* 10, 233. doi:10.1038/s41419-019-1462-z

Ragab, D., Salah Eldin, H., Taeimah, M., Khattab, R., and Salem, R. (2020). The COVID-19 cytokine storm; what we know so far. *Front. Immunol.* 11, 1446. doi:10.3389/fimmu.2020.01446

Raghu, G., Rochwerg, B., Zhang, Y., Garcia, C. A., Azuma, A., Behr, J., et al. (2015). An official ATS/ERS/JRS/ALAT clinical practice guideline: treatment of idiopathic pulmonary fibrosis. an update of the 2011 clinical practice guideline. *Am. J. Respir. Crit. Care Med.* 192, e3–e19. doi:10.1164/rccm.201506-1063ST

Rat, P., Olivier, E., and Dutot, M. (2020). SARS-CoV-2 vs. SARS-CoV-1 management: antibiotics and inflammasome modulators potential. *Eur. Rev. Med. Pharmacol. Sci.* 24, 7880–7885. doi:10.26355/eurrev_202007_22293

Rudiger, A., Dyson, A., Felsmann, K., Carré, J. E., Taylor, V., Hughes, S., et al. (2013). Early functional and transcriptomic changes in the myocardium predict outcome in a long-term rat model of sepsis. *Clin. Sci.* 124, 391–401. doi:10.1042/CS20120334

Schlapbach, L. J., Straney, L., Alexander, J., MacLaren, G., Festa, M., Schibler, A., et al. (2015). Mortality related to invasive infections, sepsis, and septic shock in critically ill children in Australia and New Zealand, 2002–13: a multicentre retrospective cohort study. *Lancet Infect. Dis.* 15, 46–54. doi:10.1016/S1473-3099(14)71003-5

Sheng, G., Chen, P., Wei, Y., Yue, H., Chu, J., Zhao, J., et al. (2020). Viral infection increases the risk of idiopathic pulmonary fibrosis: a meta-analysis. *Chest* 157, 1175–1187. doi:10.1016/j.chest.2019.10.032

Shrum, B., Anantha, R. V., Xu, S. X., Donnelly, M., Haeryfar, S. M., McCormick, J. K., et al. (2014). A robust scoring system to evaluate sepsis severity in an animal model. *BMC Res. Notes* 7, 233. doi:10.1186/1756-0500-7-233

Srivastava, A. K., Khare, P., Nagar, H. K., Raghuwanshi, N., and Srivastava, R. (2016). Hydroxyproline: a potential biochemical marker and its role in the pathogenesis of different diseases. *Curr. Protein Pept. Sci.* 17, 596–602. doi:10.2174/1389203717666151201192247

Sulzbacher, M. M., Sulzbacher, L. M., Passos, F. R., Bilibio, B. L. E., Althaus, W. F., Weizenmann, L., et al. (2020). A single dose of eHSP72 attenuates sepsis severity in mice. *Sci. Rep.* 10, 9198. doi:10.1038/s41598-020-66011-y

Taz, T. A., Ahmed, K., Paul, B. K., Kawsar, M., Aktar, N., Mahmud, S. M. H., et al. (2020). Network-based identification genetic effect of SARS-CoV-2 infections to idiopathic pulmonary fibrosis (IPF) patients. *Brief Bioinform.* bbaa235, 1–13. doi:10.1093/bib/bbaa235

Venkataraman, T., and Frieman, M. B. (2017). The role of epidermal growth factor receptor (EGFR) signaling in SARS coronavirus-induced pulmonary fibrosis. *Antivir. Res.* 143, 142–150. doi:10.1016/j.antiviral.2017.03.022

Xu, Y. H., Dong, J. H., An, W. M., Lv, X. Y., Yin, X. P., Zhang, J. Z., et al. (2020). Clinical and computed tomographic imaging features of novel coronavirus pneumonia caused by SARS-CoV-2. *J. Infect.* 80, 394–400. doi:10.1016/j.jinf.2020.02.017

Yang, X., Yu, Y., Xu, J., Shu, H., Xia, J., Liu, H., et al. (2020). Clinical course and outcomes of critically ill patients with SARS-CoV-2 pneumonia in Wuhan, China: a single-centered, retrospective, observational study. *Lancet Respir. Med.* 8, 475–481. doi:10.1016/S2213-2600(20)30079-5

Yao, Y., Deng, H., Li, P., Zhang, J., Zhang, J., Wang, D., et al. (2017). α-lactose improves the survival of septic mice by blockade of TIM-3 signaling to prevent NKT cell apoptosis and attenuate cytokine storm. *Shock* 47, 337–345. doi:10.1097/SHK.0000000000000717

Zhu, N., Zhang, D., Wang, W., Li, X., Yang, B., Song, J., et al. (2020a). A novel coronavirus from patients with pneumonia in China, 2019. *N. Engl. J. Med.* 382, 727–733. doi:10.1056/NEJMoa2001017

5

Extracellular HSP90α Interacts with ER Stress to Promote Fibroblasts Activation through PI3K/AKT Pathway in Pulmonary Fibrosis

Jinming Zhang[1†], Wenshan Zhong[1†], Yuanyuan Liu[1†], Weimou Chen[1], Ye Lu[1], Zhaojin Zeng[1], Yujie Qiao[1], Haohua Huang[1], Xuan Wan[1], Wei Li[2], Xiaojing Meng[3], Fei Zou[3], Shaoxi Cai[1] and Hangming Dong[1]**

[1]*Chronic Airways Diseases Laboratory, Department of Respiratory and Critical Care Medicine, Nanfang Hospital, Southern Medical University, Guangzhou, China,* [2]*Department of Dermatology and The Norris Comprehensive Cancer Centre, University of Southern California Keck Medical Centre, Los Angeles, CA, United States,* [3]*School of Public Health, Southern Medical University, Guangzhou, China*

***Correspondence:**
Hangming Dong
dhm@smu.edu.cn
Shaoxi Cai
hxkc@smu.edu.cn

[†]*These authors contributed equally to this work*

Pulmonary fibrosis is characterized by alveolar epithelial cell injury, lung fibroblast proliferation, differentiation, and extracellular matrix (ECM) deposition. Our previous study indicated that extracellular HSP90α (eHSP90α) promotes pulmonary fibrosis by activating the MAPK signaling pathway. Thus, treatment with 1G6-D7 (a selective HSP90α monoclonal antibody) to antagonize eHSP90α could effectively ameliorate fibrosis. This study aimed to elucidate the mechanism underlying the effects of eHSP90α in pulmonary fibrosis by focusing on its link with endoplasmic reticulum (ER) stress. Our results showed that eHSP90α promoted lung fibroblast differentiation by activating ER stress. Treatment with the ER stress inhibitor tauroursodeoxycholate (TUDCA) or glucose-regulated protein 78 kDa (GRP78) depletion significantly abrogated the effect of eHSP90α on ER stress and fibroblast activation. In addition, eHSP90α induced ER stress in fibroblasts *via* the phosphoinositide-4,5-bisphosphate 3-kinase (PI3K)-protein kinase B (AKT) signaling pathway, which could be blocked by the PI3K/AKT inhibitor LY294002, and blockade of eHSP90α by 1G6-D7 markedly inhibited ER stress in the model, indicating preventive and therapeutic applications. Intriguingly, we observed that TUDCA effectively reduced the secretion of eHSP90α *in vitro* and *in vivo*. In conclusion, this study shows that the interaction between eHSP90α and ER stress plays a crucial role in pulmonary fibrosis, indicating a positive feedback in lung fibroblasts. Targeting eHSP90α and alleviating fibroblast ER stress may be promising therapeutic approaches for pulmonary fibrosis.

Keywords: extracellular Hsp90α, er stress, fibroblasts activation, PI3K/AKT, pulmonary fibrosis

INTRODUCTION

Pulmonary fibrosis is a chronic, progressive, fibrotic interstitial pulmonary disease of unknown origin that results in reduced exchange and impaired pulmonary function. To our knowledge, pulmonary fibrosis is one of the most forms of common interstitial pneumonia, presenting with a high morbidity rate and lacking effective therapies to improve the survival rate. Pirfenidone and nintedanib have been recently shown to have a moderate effect on disease progression. However, neither agent stops pulmonary fibrosis progression (Martinez et al., 2017; Richeldi et al., 2017). Therefore, it is essential to develop alternative therapeutic strategies for patients with PF. The pathological characteristics of pulmonary fibrosis include alveolar epithelial injury, aberrant fibroblast differentiation and proliferation, and excessive pro-fibrotic cytokine secretion (Wolters et al., 2014). Notably, with the stimulation of multiple pro-fibrotic cytokines, lung fibroblasts differentiate into myofibroblasts, leading to massive ECM accumulation and accelerated fibrosis progression (Kwon et al., 2018; Duan et al., 2019; Li et al., 2019). Therefore, fibroblasts/myofibroblasts play a central role in fibrosis formation, and suppression of fibroblast differentiation could be an important strategy to alleviate pulmonary fibrosis.

The endoplasmic reticulum (ER) plays a key role in cellular homeostasis and is extremely sensitive to various changes. Failure of the ER to fold and assemble proper protein architecture leads to accumulation of misfolded/unfolded proteins in the ER lumen, disturbing ER homeostasis and provoking ER stress. ER stress-associated proteins mainly include GRP78, activating transcription factor-6 (ATF6), and inositol-requiring enzyme-1α (IREα). The main function of these proteins is to expand the ER protein-folding capacity and reduce ER load. ER stress has been recently noted in various diseases, including cancer, asthma, and diabetes (Cubillos-Ruiz et al., 2017; Bhakta et al., 2018; Crookshank et al., 2018). For instance, multiple cancers have a sustained and abnormally high expression of ER-related proteins (Fernandez et al., 2000; Shuda et al., 2003; Carrasco et al., 2007). In addition, ER stress is also involved in lung fibrosis by regulating fibroblast proliferation, differentiation, and alveolar epithelial injury (Lee et al., 2020a; Borok et al., 2020). Treatment with the ER stress inhibitor 4-phenylbutyrate (4-PBA) or TUDCA could effectively attenuate pulmonary fibrosis (Hsu et al., 2017; Lee et al., 2020b). Therefore, further investigation of the molecular mechanisms underlying ER stress in pulmonary fibrosis is highly appreciated.

The levels of heat shock protein 90 (HSP90), one of the most abundant HSPs, have been reported to be elevated in IPF patients and experimental pulmonary fibrosis. Furthermore, HSP90 inhibition with 17-AAG or AUY-922 could help alleviate pulmonary fibrosis by blocking the transforming growth factor-β (TGF-β) signaling pathway (Colunga et al., 2020). Notably, HSP90 has been confirmed to be secreted from cells following multiple stresses such as hypoxia, reactive oxygen species and heat, and this secreted form is called eHSP90α. Emerging evidence indicates that eHSP90α is associated with tumor progression and wound healing (Li et al., 2012; Fan et al., 2019). In addition, we previously confirmed that eHSP90α promotes pulmonary fibrosis by activating the MAPK signaling pathway, and the use of the monoclonal antibody 1G6-D7 could effectively attenuate pulmonary fibrosis (Dong et al., 2017). As mentioned above, ER stress has a positive effect on the activation of lung fibroblasts in pulmonary fibrosis. However, the relationship between eHSP90α and ER stress in pulmonary fibrosis has not yet been completely clarified.

In this study, we examined the crosstalk between eHSP90α and ER stress in lung fibroblasts. The role of eHSP90α in the regulation of ER stress depends on activating the PI3K/AKT signaling pathway. We also confirmed ER stress mediated eHSP90α released in the pulmonary fibrosis.

MATERIALS AND METHODS

Cell Culture

IMR90 cells were purchased from ATCC and cultured in EMEM medium supplemented with 10% fetal bovine serum (PAN, German) in an atmosphere of 5% CO2. When the cells were 80–90% confluent, they were stimulated with recombinant TGF-β1 (R&D Systems, United States) with or without TUDCA (MCE, United States) for another 24 h. Before stimulation with human recombinant Hsp90α (hrHsp90α; Stress Marq Biosciences, British Columbia), the cells were pretreated with LY294002 (MCE, United States) for 2 h.

Animal Study

120 Female C57BL/6J mice (6–8 weeks of age) were obtained from Southern Medical University Animal Centre (Guangzhou, China) and maintained in a specific pathogen-free environment. All experiments were performed according to the guidelines for experimental animals and approved by the Institutional Animal Care and Use Committee of the Institute of Biophysics, Chinese Academy of Sciences. The mice were intratracheally administered with either bleomycin (BLM, 3 mg/kg) or vehicle on Day 0. In the TUDCA prevention model, mice were first randomly assigned into four groups (n = 10 for each group): vehicle, TUDCA, BLM and BLM + TUDCA. TUDCA (50 mg/kg) was intraperitoneal injected at an interval of 1 day from Day1. Mice were sacrificed 3 weeks after TUDCA treatment. For the 1G6-D7 treatment model, 7 days after delivery of BLM, 3 weeks after 1G6-D7 nasal inhalation treatment, the mice were sacrificed and lungs were collected. The protocol of 1G6-D7 prevention model was reported previously (Dong et al., 2017). Lung microsections (5 μm) were stained with Masson's trichrome and hematoxylin and eosin (H&E) to visualize fibrotic lesions.

Cell Counting Kit-8 Assay

The cells were seeded in a 96-well plate, and then treated with different concentrations of rHSP90α to evaluate cell viability at different time points. Cell proliferation was detected by CCK8 (Dojindo, Japan) following the manufacturer's protocol.

EdU Assay

EdU assay was performed according to the manufacturer's instructions of the EdU kit (Beyotime, China). The EdU reagent was diluted to 20 μM in serum-free medium, added to the cells and incubated for 4 h. After PBS washing, cells were fixed in 4% paraformaldehyde for 30 min and permeabilized with 0.3% Triton X-100 for 15 min. Dye these cells with Click Additive Solution according to the instructions. DAPI was added to stain the nucleus for 10 min. Finally, positive cells were counted by fluorescence microscope.

Wound Healing Assay

IMR90 cells were seeded in six-well plates. When cells were grown to about 90% confluency and then scratched with a sterile 100 μl pipette tip. The cells were washed with PBS three

TABLE 1 | Antibody information.

Antibody	CAS No	Company
CollagenI	AF7001	Affinity
α-SMA	Ab5694	Abcam
GRP78	Sc-376768	Santa cruz
ATF6	Sc-1666659	Santa cruz
IRE1A	Sc-390960	Santa cruz
HSP90α	Ab59459	Abcam
β-actin	6008-1-Ig	Proteintech
AKT	4685s	CST
p-AKT (Ser473)	4060s	CST
p-AKT (Thr308)	2965s	CST
Alexa Fluor 488	A32723	ThermoFisher

times. Images of the wounded area were created at indicated time points with the same microscopic cross point by light microscopy.

Immunofluorescence Staining

IMR90 cells were fixed in 4% paraformaldehyde for 30 min, permeabilized with 0.1% Triton X-100 for 20 min and then blocked with 1% BSA for 30 min. Cells were incubated with α-SMA and Collagen I were visualized with an overnight with specific fluorochrome primary antibodies including α-SMA (Abcam, United States), Collagen I (Affinity, China) at a concentration of 1:100. After extensive washing with PBS, cells were incubated with goat Alexa Fluor 488-labeled secondary antibody (Life Technologies, United States) for 1 h at room temperature and nuclei were stained with DAPI. The images were obtained by using Olympus FluoView® FV1200 confocal laser scanning microscope (Olympus Corporation, Center Valley, PA).

Western Blot Analysis

Lung tissues and cultured cells were extracted with RIPA buffer and then centrifuged at 15,000 rpm, 4°C for 15 min, the supernatant was collected. Protein concentration was quantified using a Bradford protein assay Kit (Beyotime Biotechnology, Shanghai, China). Equal amounts of protein were separated on SDS-PAGE, transferred onto PVDF membranes and then incubated with primary antibodies (**Table 1**). After being washed with TBST three times, membranes were then incubated with IRDye® 800CW- or 680RD- conjugated secondary antibodies and visualized using a LI-COR Odyssey Imaging System (LI-COR Biosciences, Lincoln, NE, United States).

RNA-Seq

RNA was isolated from three biological replicates in both untreated and rHSP90α-treated group according to the manufacturer's instructions. The cDNA fragments were purified and enriched by PCR to construct the cDNA library. Finally, the cDNA library was sequenced on the Illumina sequencing platform (Illumina HiSeq ™ 4000). The threshold of the *p*-value in multiple tests was determined by the false discovery rate (FDR). A threshold of the FDR ≤0.05 was used to judge the significance of gene expression differences. The RNA-seq data was uploaded to SRA database. Accession to cite for these SRA data: PRJNA716070.

TABLE 2 | The sequences of siRNA.

GRP78 siRNA-1	GAGGCUUAUUUGGGAAAGATT (5′ to 3′) UCUUUCCCAAAUAAGCCUCTT (5′ to 3′)
GRP78 siRNA-2	GGGCAAAGAUGUCAGGAAATT (5′ to 3′) UUUCCUGACAUCUUUGCCCTT (5′ to 3′)
GRP78 siRNA-3	GAGGUGUCAUGACCAAACUTT (5′ to 3′) AGUUUGGUCAUGACACCUCTT (5′ to 3′)
Negative control	UUCUCCGAACGUGUCACGUTT (5′ to 3′) ACGUGACACGUUCGGAGAATT (5′ to 3′)

RNAi and Transfection

siRNAs were synthesized by GenePharma (Shanghai, China). The sequences used are show in **Table 2**. IMR90 cells transfections were conducted using Lipo3000 (Thermo Fisher Scientific) following the manufacturer's protocol.

Immunohistochemistry

The expressions of α-SMA, GRP78 and HSP90α were characterized by immunohistochemistry using specific antibodies. Briefly, lung slices were dewaxed in xylene, followed by antigen retrieval with citrate buffer (pH 6.0) and incubated overnight with antibodies against α-SMA (Abcam, 1:400), GRP78 (Santa Cruz, 1:50) and HSP90α (Abcam, 1:200). Then, lung slices were incubated with secondary antibody for 30 min and visualized with a DAB substrate kit (Zhong Shan Jin Qiao, Beijing, China).

ER-Tracker

ER-Tracker was performed to detect ER activity according to the instruction of the ER-Tracker kit (C1041, Beyotime, China). Briefly, cells were incubated with ER-Tracker working fluid for 20 min, followed by image acquisition.

Quantitative RT-PCR

Lung fibroblasts were transfected with siRNA for 24 h and extracted the RNA with Trizol reagent (Takara, Japan). The SYBR Premix Ex Taq II Kit (Takara, Japna) was used to detect the expression of GRP78, normalized to the expression of the endogenous control GAPDH. The primer sequences were GRP78: 5′-ACCTCCAACCCCGAGAACA-3′ (forward), 5′-TTCAACCACCTTGAACGGC-3′ (reverse); GAPDH:5′-AATTCCATGGCACCGTCAAG-3′ (forward), 5′-GGTGAA GACGCCAGTGGACT-3′ (reverse).

Enzyme-Linked Immunosorbent Assay

Bronchoalveolar lavage fluid (BALF) and serum samples were collected as described previously (Yao et al., 2016). All the samples were centrifuged and the supernatant was collected and stored at −80°C until further analysis. The HSP90α (Cloud-Clone, Buckingham, United Kingdom) ELISA kit was used according to the manufacturer's instruction.

Preparation of Conditioned Media

The conditioned media was collected as previously described (Li et al., 2007) and then utilized to evaluate secretion of HSP90α.

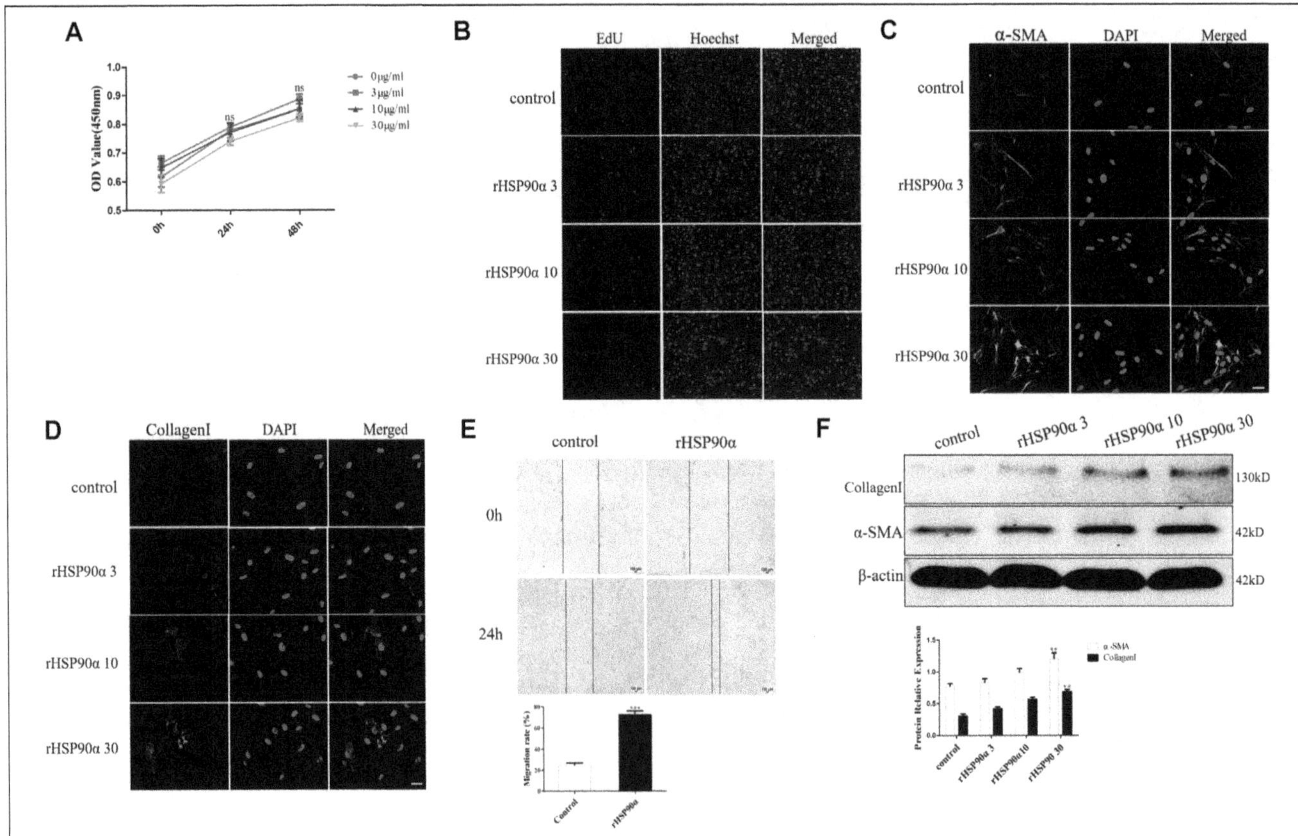

FIGURE 1 | Extracellular HSP90α promotes lung fibroblasts activation but has no influence on proliferation. **(A)**. Cell proliferation was assessed *via* the CCK8 assay after stimulation with 0, 3, 10 and 30 ug/ml rHSP90α for indicated times (24 and 48 h) in the IMR90 cells. **(B)**. Proliferative capacity was analyzed using an EdU assay after treatment with 0, 3, 10 and 30 ug/ml rHSP90α in the IMR90 cells for 24 h. Lung fibroblasts activation was assessed by immunofluorescence staining for α-SMA and CollagenI **(C,D)**, representative staining images of α-SMA–positive stress fibers (green), CollagenI-positive collagen deposition (green) and DAPI (blue) showing nuclei under confocal laser scanning microscopy (scale bar = 50 μm). **(E)**. Fibroblasts migration were performed by wound-healing assays. **(F)**. The protein expression of CollagenI and α-SMA were determined by western blot after stimulation of different concentrations of rHSP90α for 24 h, β-actin was used as an internal control. **ns** = no significance, $^{*}p < 0.05$, $^{**}p < 0.01$.

Statistical Analysis

All the experiments were conducted at least in triplicate. The data were presented as the means ± SEM or means ± SD. Data were analyzed with the use of an unpaired *t* test for comparisons between two conditions or ANOVA with the Tukey post test to determine the differences among all groups. The data of *in vivo* experiments were analyzed with the one-way ANOVA. The significance level was set at $p < 0.05$. Statistical analysis was performed using GraphPad Prism software (GraphPad Software, United States).

RESULTS

Extracellular HSP90α Promotes Lung Fibroblasts Activation But Have No Influence on Proliferation

Pulmonary fibrosis is characterized by the proliferation and differentiation of lung fibroblasts (Penke et al., 2018). To evaluate the role of eHSP90α in the pulmonary fibrosis, the effect of eHSP90α on fibroblasts proliferation and differentiation was measured first. Lung fibroblasts were treated with different concentrations of eHSP90α for the indicated times. Proliferation ability was determined by the CCK8 assay. As shown in **Figure 1A**, there was no significant difference between the rHSP90α-treated and untreated groups. In addition, the EdU assay was performed, and the EdU-positive cells in the rHSP90α-treated groups showed no obvious differences in comparison with the control group (**Figure 1B**). The differentiation of fibroblasts to myofibroblasts is accompanied by an increase in α-SMA and collagen I expression and migration (Chen et al., 2019). Next, to test the expression of eHSP90α on myofibroblast markers, lung fibroblasts were treated with different concentrations of rHSP90α for 24 h and evaluated by immunofluorescence staining. The results showed that α-SMA and collagen I expression increased in a concentration-dependent manner in comparison with the control group (**Figures 1C,D**). Next, to investigate whether eHSP90α affects lung fibroblast migration, a wound-healing assay was performed. As shown in **Figure 1E**, rHSP90α significantly promoted the migration of lung fibroblasts. Consistently, western blotting analysis confirmed that the

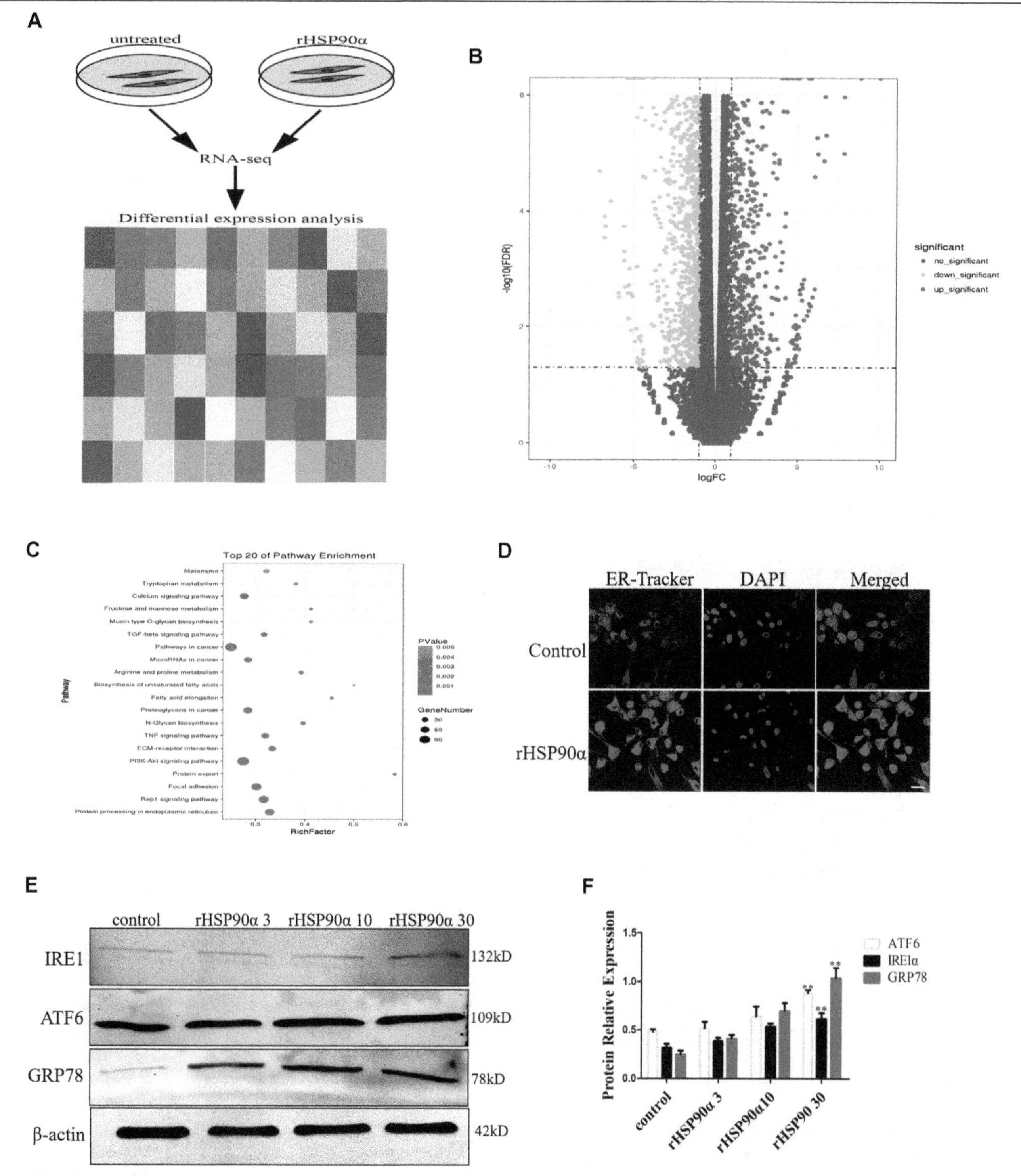

FIGURE 2 | Extracellular HSP90α induces ER Stress in lung fibroblasts. **(A).** Schematic diagram of RNA-seq with or without rHSP90α treatment. **(B).** Volcano plot displays the overall genes identified with a $p < 0.05$ and |log2FC|>1.0 a cutoff. **(C).** KEGG pathway analysis of pathway enrichment. The vertical axis represents the pathway category and the horizontal axis represents the enrichment score [–log (*p*-value)] of the pathway. Significantly enriched KEGG pathways ($p < 0.05$) are presented. The data were analyzed by DAVID bioinformatics tools. **(D).** Endoplasmic reticulum (ER) activity was assessed by immunofluorescence staining ER-Tracker. Representative staining images of ER-positive cells and DAPI (blue) showing nuclei under confocal laser scanning microscopy (scale bar = 50 μm). **(E,F).** Western blot analysis of expression of ATF6, IRE1α and GRP78 after different concentrations of rHSP90α treatment for 24 h, β-actin was used as an internal control. *$p < 0.05$, **$p < 0.01$.

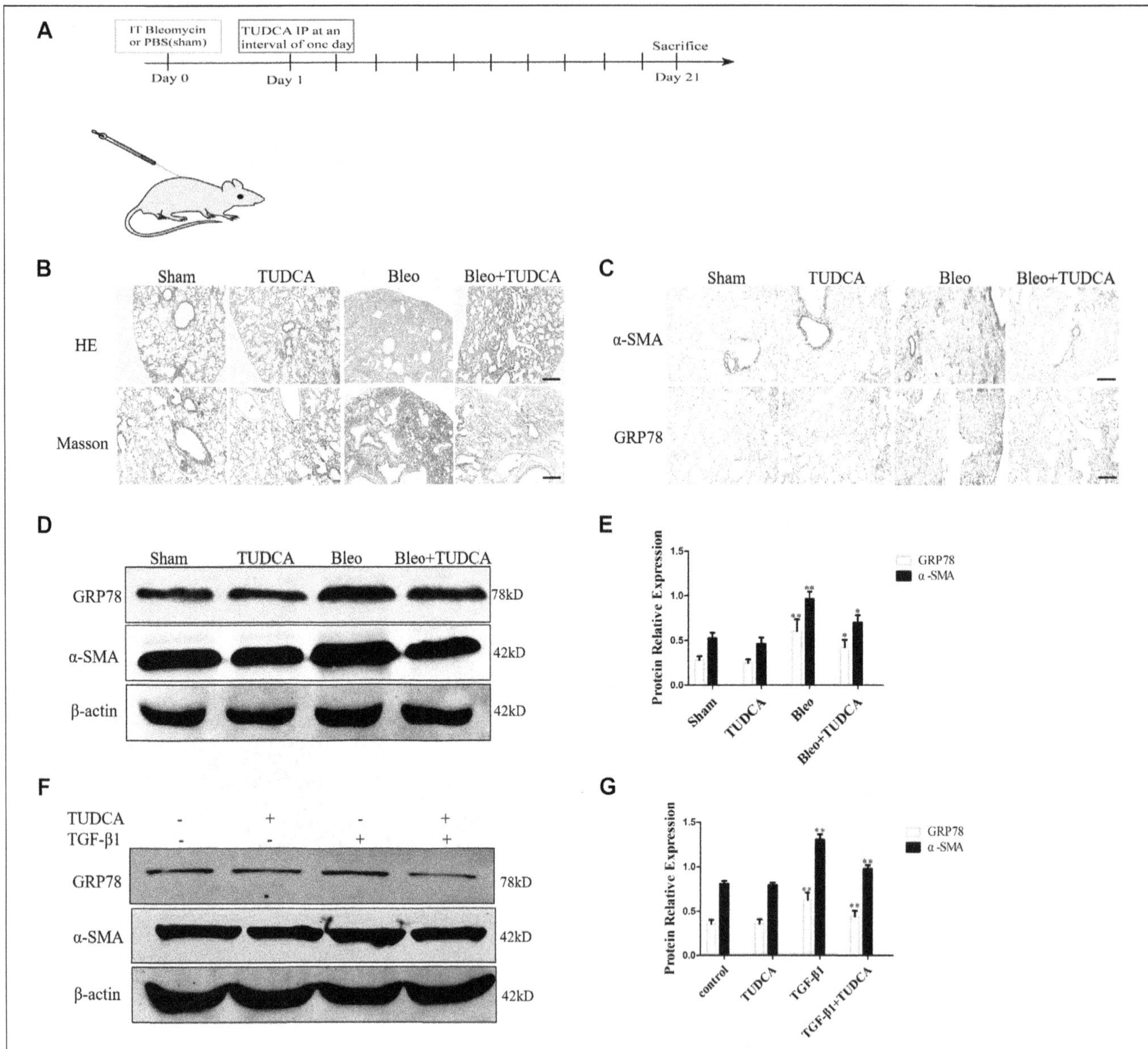

FIGURE 3 | ER stress in the lung fibroblasts is critical for pulmonary fibrosis progression. **(A)**. Experimental scheme of the mouse model of bleomycin-induced pulmonary fibrosis. Mice were intratracheally injected with saline or bleomycin (3 mg/kg) at day 0. On day 1, mice were administrated with TUDCA (50 mg/kg) or DMSO by intraperitoneal injection every 2 days. Mice were sacrificed on day 21 (n = 10 for each group). **(B)**. Histological images and collagen deposition of the lung tissue was detected by H&E and Masson staining. Scale bar = 100 μm. **(C)**. Representative images showing GRP78 and α-SMA staining of lung tissues of mice treated with saline, bleomycin without or with TUDCA. Scale bar = 100 μm. **(D,E)**, Western blot analysis of expression of GRP78 and α -SMA. **(F,G)**, IMR90 were pre-treated with TUDCA (100 μM) for 2 h and followed by TGF-β1 (10 ng/ml) for 24 h. The expression levels of GRP78 and α-SMA was measured by western blot. β-actin was used as an internal control. $^{*}p < 0.05$, $^{**}p < 0.01$.

expression of α-SMA and collagen I increased with increasing concentrations of eHSP90α (**Figure 1F**). Taken together, these results showed that eHSP90α could activate lung fibroblasts but had no obvious influence on proliferation.

Extracellular HSP90α Induces ER Stress in Lung Fibroblasts

To further explore the potential mechanisms by which eHSP90α promotes fibroblast activation, RNA-seq was performed in lung fibroblasts with or without rHSP90α treatment (**Figure 2A**). According to the cut-off criteria of $p < 0.05$ and |log2FC|>1.0, 4905 dysregulated genes were identified (**Figure 2B**). KEGG pathway enrichment analysis showed that these genes were principally categorized into regulation of protein processing in the ER, focal adhesion, and PI3K-AKT pathway. To validate ER activity in rHSP90α-treated fibroblasts, ER-Tracker staining was performed. As shown in **Figure 2D**, treatment of lung fibroblasts with rHSP90α for 24 h significantly increased the ER-Tracker staining intensity. In addition, we stimulated lung fibroblasts with

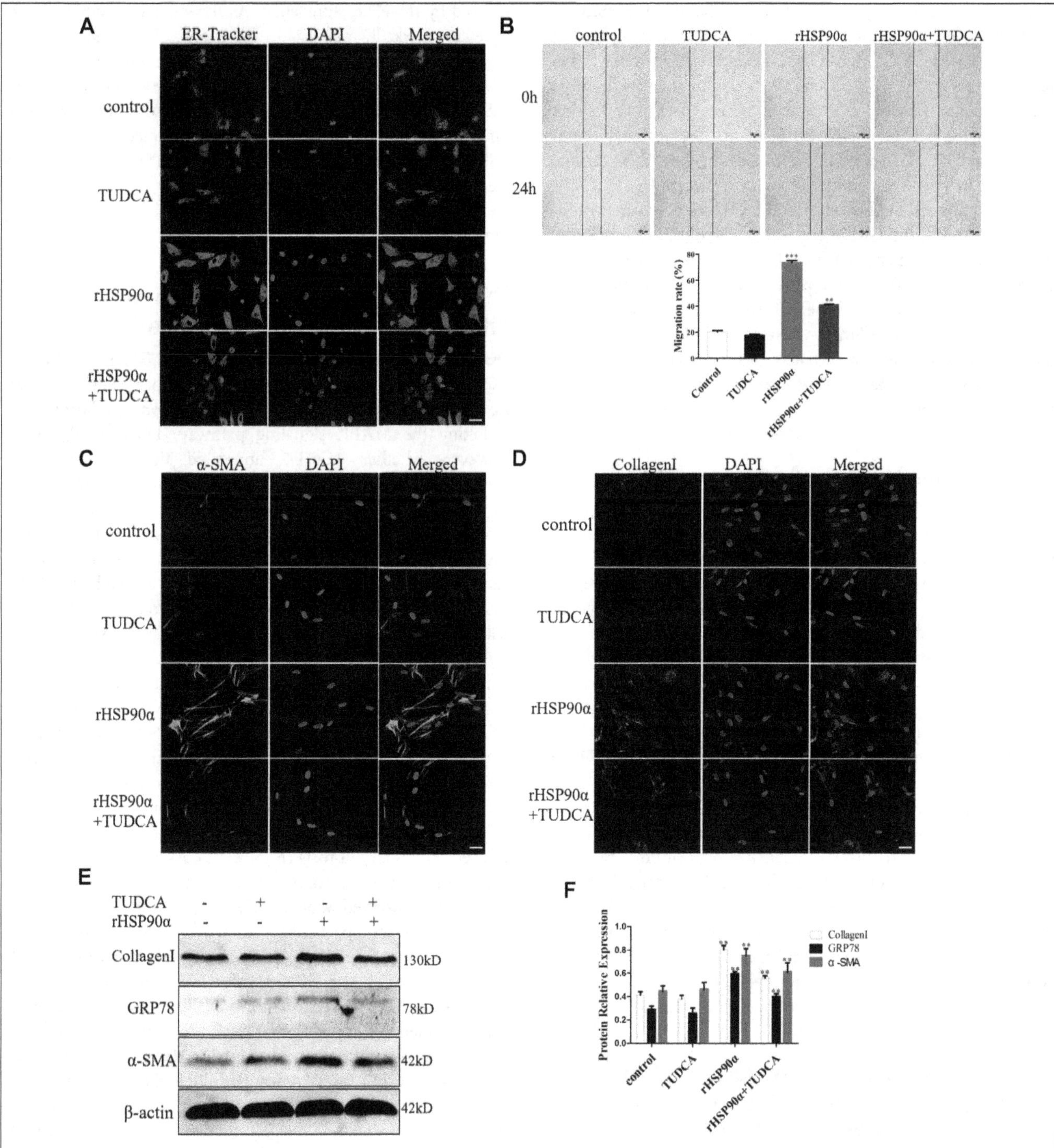

FIGURE 4 | Extracellular HSP90α activates lung fibroblasts *via* ER Stress. **(A)**. Representative images showing ER-Tracker staining of IMR90 cells pre-treated with or without TUDCA (100 μM) and followed by rHSP90α for 24 h, scale bar = 50 μm. **(B)**. Cell migration was examined in IMR90 cells by a wound healing assay. **(C,D)**. Representative images showing immunofluorescence staining of α-SMA and CollagenI in IMR90 cells. **(E,F)**. Western blot analysis of the expression of CollagenI, GRP78 and α-SMA. β-actin was used as an internal control. $^*p < 0.05$, $^{**}p < 0.01$.

different concentrations of rHSP90α for 24 h and found that the ER stress markers GRP78, ATF6, IRE1α upregulated effectively (**Figures 2E,F**). These data suggested that eHSP90α could induce the ER stress in the lung fibroblasts.

ER Stress Mediated Lung Fibroblasts Activation in Pulmonary Fibrosis

To determine whether ER stress is involved in lung fibroblast activation in pulmonary fibrosis, we established a mouse model of lung fibrosis induced by intratracheal instillation of bleomycin. TUDCA, an ER stress inhibitor, was intraperitoneally injected at 1 d intervals from Day 1 (**Figure 3A**). As expected, H&E and Masson staining revealed that TUDCA effectively ameliorated the distorted alveolar structure, thickened alveolar walls and collagen deposition induced by BLM (**Figure 3B**). In addition, IHC staining results showed that TUDCA significantly decreased the GRP78 expression, particularly in the α-SMA positive fibrotic foci (**Figure 3C**). Similarly, western blotting results showed that TUDCA downregulated BLM-stimulated α-SMA and GRP78 expression (**Figures 3D,E**). We used TGF-β1 to treat human lung fibroblasts as an *in vitro* model. As shown in **Figures 3F,G**, TGF-β1 treatment in lung fibroblasts increased the expression of the ER stress marker GRP78 and myofibroblast marker α-SMA, whereas the expression of these markers was attenuated by TUDCA treatment (100 μM). Taken together, these data suggest that ER stress plays a crucial role in lung fibroblast activation.

Extracellular HSP90α Activates Lung Fibroblasts *via* ER Stress

The above data showed that the most significant pathway enrichment between the untreated group and the rHSP90α-treated group was protein processing in the ER. Therefore, we speculated that eHSP90α activated fibroblasts and promoted fibrosis by inducing ER stress. To test this assumption, we first used ER-Tracker to detect the ER activity. As shown in **Figure 4A**, we found that TUDCA effectively abrogated the staining intensity of ER-Tracker, which was increased by eHSP90α. In addition, wound healing results showed that lung fibroblast migration was markedly increased by eHSP90α stimulation, while TUDCA alleviated this effect (**Figure 4B**). We further used immunofluorescence staining to examine α-SMA and collagen I expression and observed lower α-SMA positive cells and less collagen deposition in the rHSP90α+TUDCA group than in the rHSP90α group (**Figures 4C,D**). Consistent with these observations, western blotting analysis indicated that TUDCA significantly reduced rHSP90α-induced α-SMA and collagen I expression (**Figures 4E,F**). Taken together, these results suggest that eHSP90α promotes lung fibroblast differentiation by activating ER stress.

Knockdown of GRP78 Abrogates Lung Fibroblast Activation Induced by eHSP90α

GRP78 is a crucial modulator of the ER that responds to UPR and maintains cellular homeostasis, contributing to proliferation and differentiation (Aran et al., 2018; van Lidth et al., 2018; Du T et al., 2019; Merkel et al., 2019). Thus, we hypothesized that eHSP90α induces ER stress to further activate fibroblasts by upregulating GRP78 expression. To confirm our assumption, we designed three siRNAs and transfected them into lung fibroblasts to knock down GRP78. The interference efficiency was verified using western blotting and qRT-PCR. As shown in **Figure 5A,C**, the results revealed that the relative level of GRP78 was significantly decreased by the siRNAs. Thus, si-3 was selected as the target siRNA for GRP78. Next, GRP78 was knocked down in lung fibroblasts with siRNA, followed by rHSP90α stimulation. As shown in **Figure 5D**, GRP78 depletion markedly abrogated the effects of eHSP90α on cell migration. In addition, knockdown GRP78 significantly reduced α-SMA staining intensity and collagen deposition induced by eHSP90α in fibroblasts (**Figures 5E,F**). Consistent with the immunofluorescence staining results, the protein expression of α-SMA and collagen I upregulated by eHSP90α was effectively attenuated by depletion of GRP78 (**Figures 5G,H**). These data strongly suggest that GRP78 is essential for eHSP90α-induced lung fibroblast activation and ECM production.

The Monoclonal Antibody 1G6-D7 Attenuates Pulmonary Fibrosis by Decreasing ER Stress *in vitro* and *in vivo*

1G6-D7, a selective anti-HSP90α monoclonal antibody, was previously reported to attenuate pulmonary fibrosis by inhibiting the MAPK signaling pathway (Dong et al., 2017). However, whether 1G6-D7 abrogated the ER stress and fibroblast activation induced by eHSP90α remains unclear. First, lung fibroblasts were pre-treated with 1G6-D7 and followed by rHSP90α for 24h, and ER-Tracker staining was used to examine the role of 1G6-D7 on ER activity. As shown in **Figure 6A**, 1G6-D7 significantly decreased the staining intensity induced by rHSP90α. Next, a wound-healing assay was performed to detect the effect of 1G6-D7 on the migration of lung fibroblasts. As shown in **Figure 6B**, 1G6-D7 remarkably inhibited the migration stimulated by rHSP90α. We further found that treatment with 1G6-D7 inhibited the effects of fibroblast activation by preventing α-SMA and collagen upregulation (**Figures 6C,D**). Consistently, western blot results showed that 1G6-D7 effectively downregulated the expression of GRP78, collagen I and α-SMA induced by rHSP90α. *In vivo*, we established prophylactical and therapeutical models to confirm the effect of 1G6-D7 on BLM-induced pulmonary fibrosis (**Figure 7A**). As shown in **Figure 7B**, IHC was performed to examine GRP78 and α-SMA in the cortical model. We observed that 1G6-D7 significantly decreased the GRP78 expression, particularly in the α-SMA positive fibrotic foci. In the therapeutical model, blocking HSP90α with 1G6-D7 similarly decreased the GRP78 and α-SMA expression through IHC (**Figure 7C**). Western blotting results showed that 1G6-D7 downregulated the expression of GRP78 and α-SMA induced by BLM in the prevention model (**Figures 7D,E**). Consistently, we found that 1G6-D7 also significantly inhibited the upregulation of GRP78 and α-SMA upon the BLM treatment in the treatment model (**Figures 7F,G**). These results demonstrates that 1G6-D7 attenuates the pulmonary fibrosis by inhibiting ER stress and that 1G6-D7 might be a potential therapeutic agent for pulmonary fibrosis patients.

Extracellular HSP90α Facilitates ER Stress Through the PI3K/AKT Pathway

Several studies have revealed that the PI3K/AKT signaling pathway is involved in regulating ER stress (Hsu et al., 2017). However, whether eHSP90α induces ER stress through PI3K/AKT signaling pathway has not been clarified. Based on the

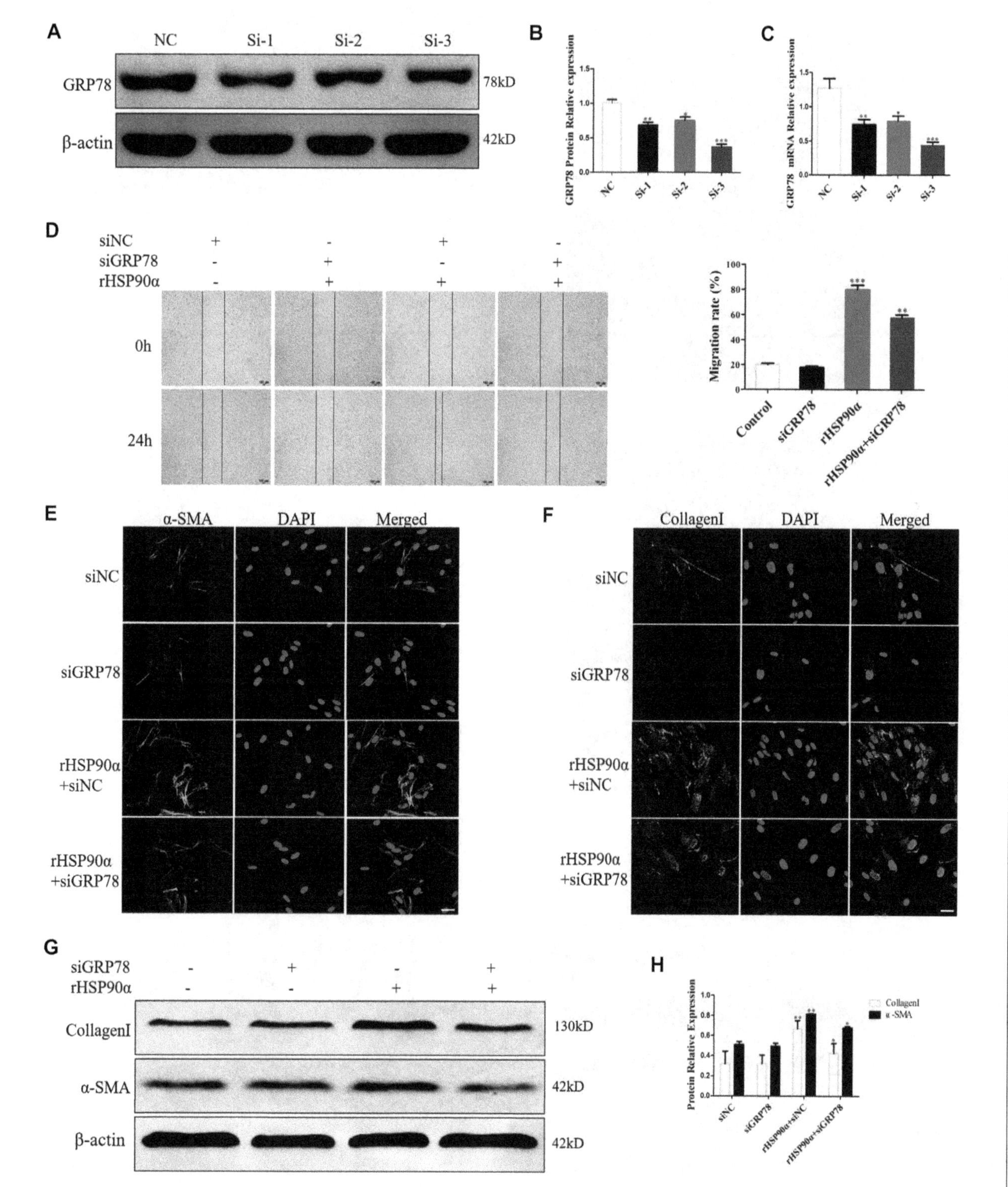

FIGURE 5 | GRP78 is essential for lung fibroblast activation induced by eHSP90α. IMR90 cells were transfected with siGRP78 or siNC and the efficiency was assessed by western blot **(A,B)** and qPCR **(C)**. Cell migration was examined in IMR90 cells by a wound healing assay **(D)**. Lung fibroblasts activation was assessed by immunofluorescence staining for α-SMA and CollagenI **(E,F)**, representative staining images of α-SMA–positive stress fibers (green), CollagenI-positive collagen deposition (green) and DAPI (blue) showing nuclei under confocal laser scanning microscopy (scale bar = 50 μm). **(G,H)**. The expression of CollagenI and α-SMA were measured by western blot. β-actin was used as an internal control. $^{*}p < 0.05$, $^{**}p < 0.01$.

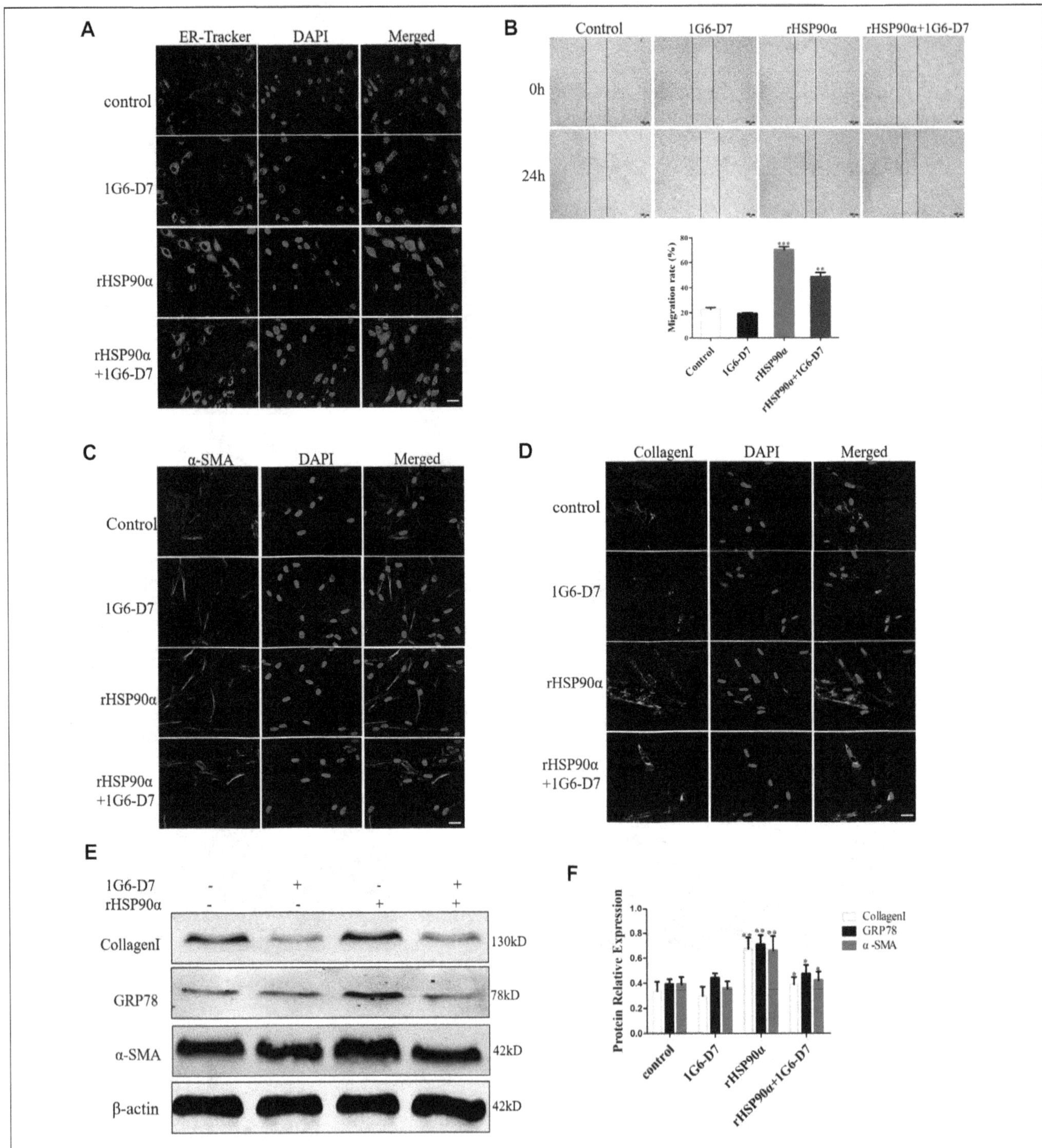

FIGURE 6 | Monoclonal antibody 1G6-D7 inhibits ER stress induced by eHSP90α ***in vitro*. (A)**. Representative images showing ER-Tracker staining of IMR90 cells pre-treated with or without 1G6-D7 (10 μg/ml) and followed by rHSP90α for 24 h, scale bar = 50 μm. **(B)** Cell migration was examined in IMR90 cells by a wound healing assay. **(C,D)**. Representative images showing immunofluorescence staining of α -SMA and CollagenI in IMR90 cells. **(E,F)**. Western blot analysis of the expression of CollagenI, GRP78 and α-SMA. β-actin was used as an internal control. $^{*}p < 0.05$, $^{**}p < 0.01$.

KEGG pathway enrichment analysis, PI3K/AKT signaling pathway was found to be significantly enriched among differentially expressed genes between the rHSP90α-treated group and the untreated group. We first examined the phosphorylation of AKT *in vivo* by using western blot. As shown in **Figures 8A,B**, phosphorylation of AKT were upregulated by BLM, but was significantly attenuated by the monoclonal antibody 1G6-D7 in the prevention model. In

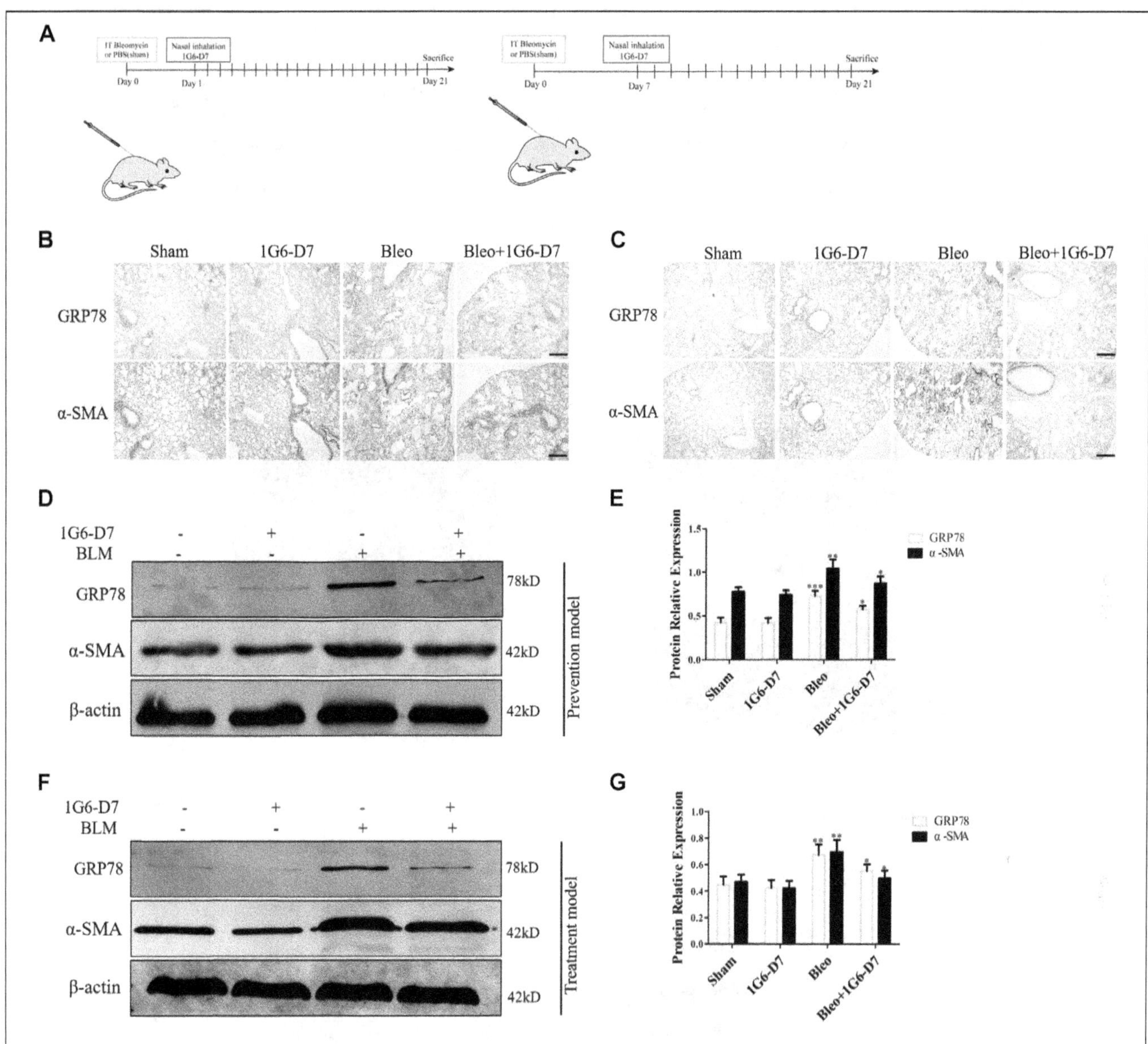

FIGURE 7 | Monoclonal antibody 1G6-D7 inhibits ER stress in the bleomycin-induced pulmonary fibrosis model. **(A)**. Schematic diagram of mouse model establishment ($n = 10$ for each group). **(B)**. Representative images showing GRP78 and α-SMA staining of lung tissues of mice in the prophylactical model. Scale bar = 100 μm. **(C)**. Representative images showing GRP78 and α-SMA staining of lung tissues of mice in the therapeutical model. Scale bar = 100 μm. Western blot analysis of the expression of GRP78 and α-SMA in the prophylactical model **(D,E)** and therapeutical model **(F,G)**. β-actin was used as an internal control. $^{*}p < 0.05$, $^{**}p < 0.01$.

the treatment model, 1G6-D7 effectively reduced the phosphorylation of AKT (**Figures 8C,D**). In addition, immunofluorescence staining results showed that the PI3K/AKT inhibitor (LY294002) largely abolished the effect of rHSP90α on increasing the α-SMA and collagen I expression (**Figures 8E,F**). We further examined the effect of LY294002 on ER stress and fibroblast activation induced by rHSP90α. As shown in **Figures 8G,H**, pre-treatment with LY294002 effectively reduced the ER stress marker GRP78 and the increased phosphorylation of Akt induced by rHSP90α. Western blotting analysis also showed that pre-treatment with LY294002 significantly downregulated the expression of α-SMA and collagen I following treatment with rHSP90α. Collectively, these data suggest that eHSP90α induces ER stress, promotes fibroblast activation *via* the PI3K/AKT pathway, and inhibited PI3K/AKT, with LY294002 significantly attenuates the ER stress and fibroblasts activation induced by eHSP90α.

ER Stress Inhibitor TUDCA Suppress Extracellular HSP90α Secretion

Some studies have reported that ER stress could regulate cellular homeostasis and stimulate extracellular vesicle secretion, and eHSP90α was also reported to be secreted through exosomes (Kakazu et al., 2016a; Guo et al., 2017; Zhang et al., 2017; Liu et al., 2019). In addition, previous studies demonstrated that TGF-β1 or

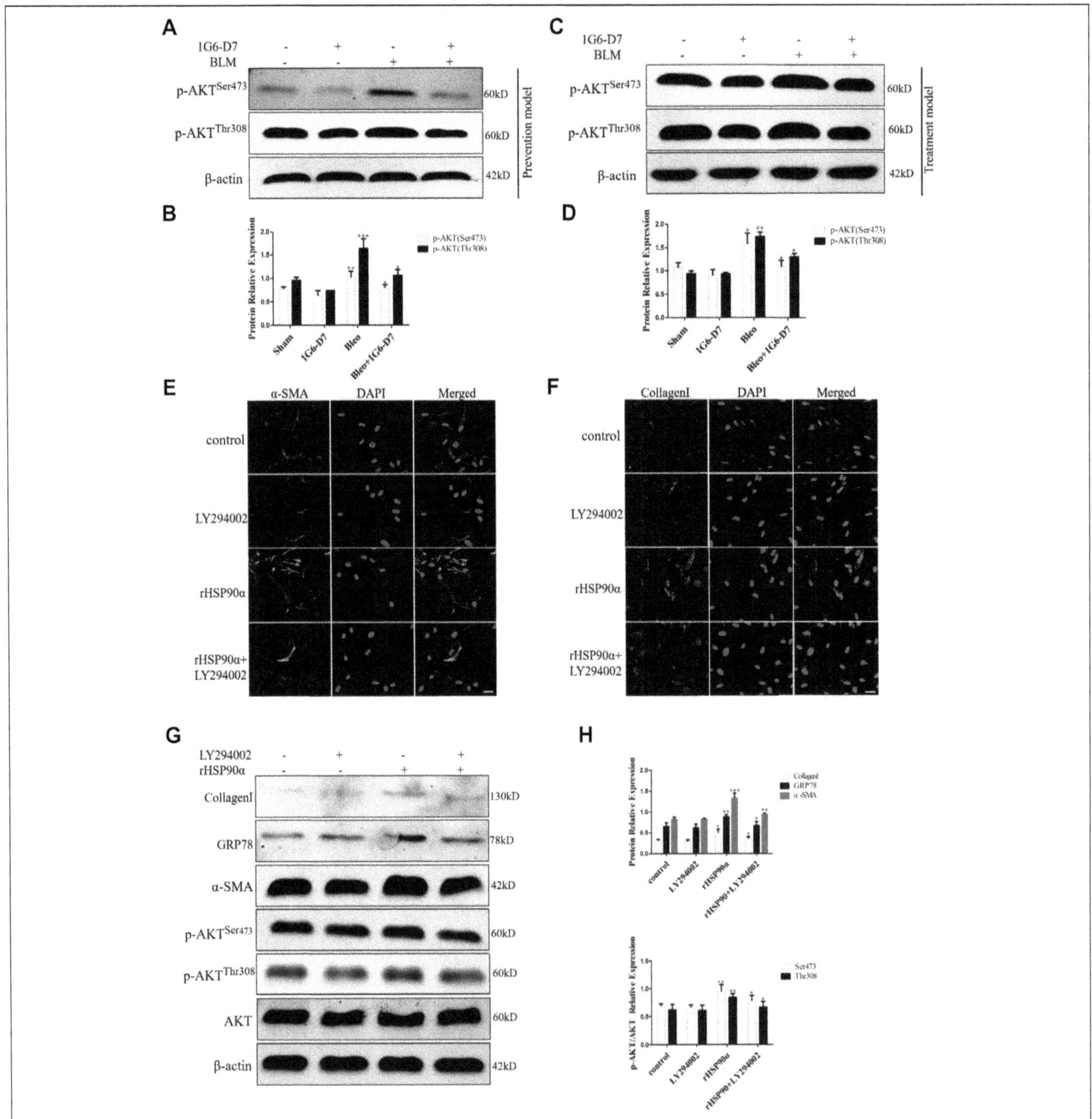

FIGURE 8 | PI3K/AKT signaling pathway is involved in ER stress induced by eHSP90α. The expression of *p*-AKT^{Ser473} and *p*-AKT^{Thr308} was measured by western blot in the prophylactical model **(A,B)** and in the therapeutical model **(C,D)**. Immunofluorescence staining showed that α -SMA and CollagenI in IMR90 cells pre-treated with or without LY294002 (10 μM) followed by rHSP90α stimuli **(E,F)**. Scale bar = 50 μm. **(G,H)**. Western blot analysis of the expression of CollagenI, GRP78, α-SMA, *p*-AKT^{Ser473}, *p*-AKT^{Thr308} and AKT. β-actin was used as an internal control. $^{*}p < 0.05$, $^{**}p < 0.01$, $^{***}p < 0.001$.

BLM increased the secretion of eHSP90α in a pulmonary fibrosis model (Dong et al., 2017). Therefore, we hypothesized that eHSP90α secretion may respond to ER stress in pulmonary fibrosis. We first detected the expression of HSP90α by using IHC. As shown in **Figure 9A**, BLM significantly increased the expression of HSP90α and was abrogated by TUDCA. Similarly, western blotting results showed that TUDCA markedly decreased the BLM-induced expression of HSP90α (**Figures 9B,C**). Furthermore, eHSP90α levels were examined using ELISA, and TUDCA was found to effectively decrease BLM-induced eHSP90α content in both BALF and serum (**Figures 9D,E**). Moreover, to elucidate whether TUDCA can inhibit eHSP90α secretion *in vitro*, we pre-treated the lung fibroblasts with TUDCA, followed by TGF-β1. As shown in **Figures 9F,G,**

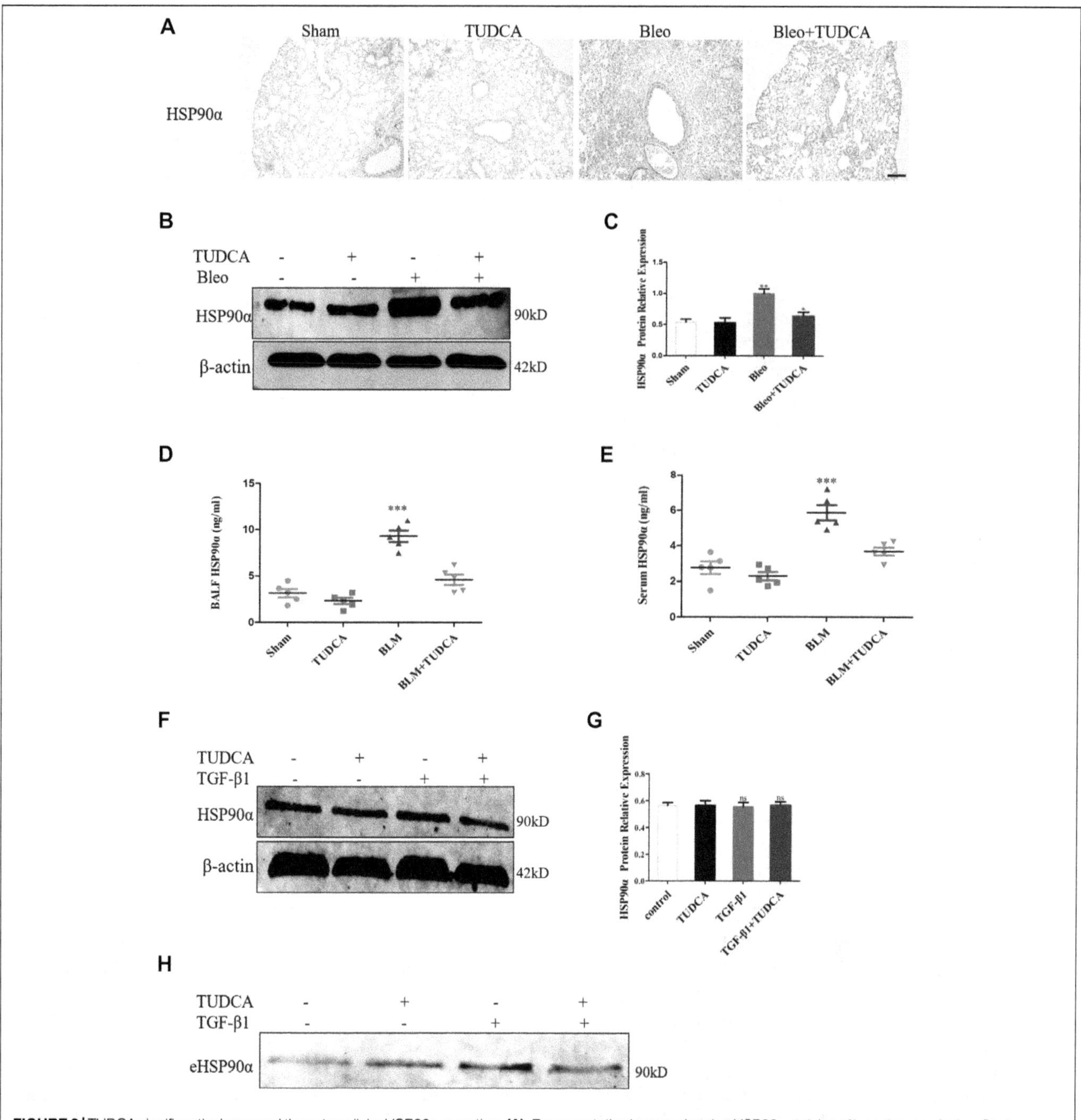

FIGURE 9 | TUDCA significantly decreased the extracellular HSP90α secretion. **(A)**. Representative images showing HSP90α staining of lung tissues of mice. Scale bar = 100 μm. **(B,C)**. The expression of HSP90α was assessed by western blot. The content of HSP90α in BALF **(D)** and in serum **(E)** samples in the mice were measured by ELISA (n = 5 for each group). **(F,G)**. Western blot analysis of the expression of HSP90α in IMR90 cells pre-treated with TUDCA (100 μM) followed by TGF-β1 stimuli. β-actin was used as an internal control. **(H)**. Secretion of HSP90α in IMR90 cells pre-treated with TUDCA followed by TGF-β1 treatment was detected by western blot. **ns** = no significance, *$p < 0.05$, **$p < 0.01$, ***$p < 0.001$.

cellular HSP90α expression was not significantly different between the TGF-β1 and the TUDCA + TGF-β1 groups. However, we were surprised to find that TUDCA remarkably inhibited the secretion of eHSP90α (**Figure 9H**). These results suggest that eHSP90α secretion is associated with ER stress, and that inhibition of ER stress by TUDCA can effectively reduce eHSP90α in the pulmonary fibrosis.

DISCUSSION

Pulmonary fibrosis is mainly characterized by alveolar injury, fibroblast activation, proliferation, and ECM accumulation. Fibroblasts/myofibroblasts play an essential role in the progression of pulmonary fibrosis. As a member of the heat shock protein family, the role of HSP90α in cancer progression, fibrosis, and diabetes has

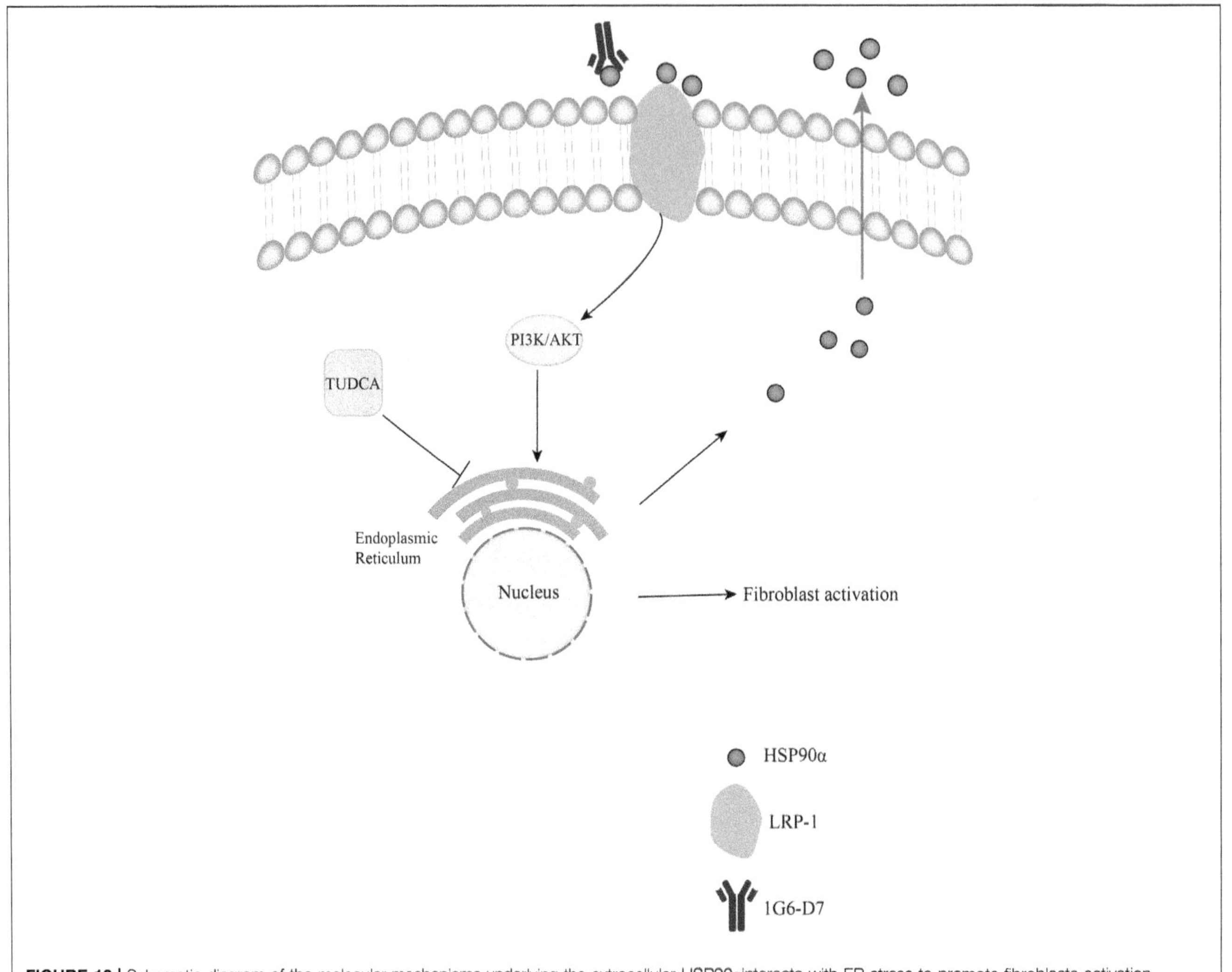

FIGURE 10 | Schematic diagram of the molecular mechanisms underlying the extracellular HSP90αinteracts with ER stress to promote fibroblasts activation through PI3K/AKT pathway in pulmonary fibrosis.

been widely investigated (Cheng et al., 2011; Bonniaud et al., 2018; Zhou et al., 2019). The main function of HSP90α is to regulate cell proliferation, differentiation, and epithelial mesenchymal transition (As et al., 2004). Notably, HSP90α can be secreted into the extracellular space to exert its function by interacting with LDL Receptor–Related Protein 1 (LRP-1) (Chen et al., 2010). We previously reported that eHSP90α promotes pulmonary fibrosis by activating the MAPK signaling pathway (Dong et al., 2017). In addition, Bellaye et al. also found that eHSP90α was strongly associated with disease severity in pulmonary fibrosis and promoted pulmonary fibrosis *via* LRP-1 (Bellaye et al., 2018). Thus, eHSP90α may play a crucial role in pulmonary fibrosis. Our study aimed to explore the molecular mechanisms underlying the effects of eHSP90α in pulmonary fibrosis. In this study, we demonstrated that eHSP90α promoted fibroblast activation by inducing ER stress *via* the PI3K/AKT signaling pathway. We also examined the relationship between eHSP90α secretion and ER stress and observed that eHSP90α secretion could be regulated by ER stress (**Figure 10**).

ER stress can be induced by several pathological stimuli, including glucose starvation, hypoxia and oxidative stress (Yoshida, 2007; Cao and Kaufman, 2014). Emerging evidence has demonstrated that ER stress can regulate cell differentiation, including the differentiation of lung fibroblasts (Matsuzaki et al., 2015; Tanimura et al., 2018; Peñaranda-Fajardo et al., 2019). However, whether ER stress is involved in the effect of eHSP90α on pulmonary fibrosis has not been fully clarified. In this study, we found that the expression of ER stress-related proteins GRP78, IRE1α and ATF6 was significantly higher in rHSP90α-treated IMR90 cells compared to untreated IMR90 cells. GRP78 is a key modulator that assists in the correct folding of newly synthesized proteins. Our results showed that GRP78 was upregulated in activated fibroblasts both *in vitro* or *in vivo*. Depletion of GRP78 strikingly inhibited eHSP90α-induced fibroblast differentiation and ECM deposition. Consistently, a recent study confirmed that cigarette smoke extract could promote human lung myofibroblast differentiation through GRP78 upregulation (Song et al., 2019a).Interestingly, GRP78 was contradictorily downregulated in the type II alveolar epithelial cells of patients with IPF (Borok et al., 2020). By combining these two results, we speculated that GRP78 might play distinct roles in different cells, and we would attempt to explore its mechanism. Furthermore, inhibiting ER stress with TUDCA remarkedly attenuated fibroblast activation and pulmonary fibrosis progression *in vitro* and *in vivo*. These findings elucidated the mechanism by which eHSP90α contributes to the development of pulmonary fibrosis by inducing ER stress in lung fibroblasts.

HSP90 inhibitors have been reported to be potential treatments for multiple cancers and pulmonary fibrosis (Trepel et al., 2010; Colunga et al., 2020). However, almost all the clinical trials have failed because of the pan-inhibitory activity of HSP90 inhibitors (Sanchez et al., 2020). Therefore, a selectively HSP90α-inhibiting agent is more suitable for pulmonary fibrosis treatment. We previously utilized monoclonal antibody 1G6-D7 to antagonize HSP90α to evaluate the effect of eHSP90α on pulmonary fibrosis in a prophylactical model. Although we observed that 1G6-D7 could protect against BLM-induced pulmonary fibrosis, whether 1G6-D7 played a similar role in the therapeutical model was not fully understood. In this study, we confirmed that administration of 1G6-D7 from Day7 to Day 21 after intratracheal BLM injection also effectively attenuated pulmonary fibrosis. We further demonstrated that 1G6-D7 decreased the expression of ER stress marker GRP78 in our model both prophylactically and therapeutically. Consistently, the effect of extracellular HSP90α on lung fibroblasts could be hampered by 1G6-D7 *in vitro*. Our findings suggest that antagonism with 1G6-D7 might have a potential antifibrotic effect on pulmonary fibrosis through inhibiting ER stress.

The PI3K/AKT pathway is the most commonly signaling pathway in pulmonary diseases, including pulmonary fibrosis (Hsu et al., 2017; Wang et al., 2018; Shi et al., 2019; Wan et al., 2019). Several studies have suggested that the PI3K/AKT signaling pathway is particularly important in mediating ER stress in various diseases (Hsu et al., 2017; Song et al., 2019b; Wang et al., 2020). However, the mechanisms of the PI3K/AKT signaling pathway underlying the effect of eHSP90α on pulmonary fibrosis remain poorly understood. Our RNA-seq data showed that treatment of lung fibroblasts with rHSP90α activated the PI3K/AKT signaling pathway in comparison with the untreated group. Notably, by using a selective PI3K/AKT inhibitor (LY294002), we verified that the PI3K/AKT signaling pathway is essential for eHSP90α-induced fibroblast activation and ER stress. Similarly, a recent study indicated that ultrafine silicon dioxide nanoparticle could cause lung epithelial cells ER stress *via* the PI3K/AKT signaling pathway. Treatment with the ROS inhibitor N-acetyl-l-cysteine (NAC) and LY294002 reversed the signals induced by ultrafine silicon dioxide nanoparticle (Lee et al., 2020). Collectively, these findings suggest that eHSP90α activates ER stress and fibroblasts *via* the PI3K/AKT signaling pathway.

Some studies have demonstrated that ER stress could stimulate extracellular vesicle secretion to further promote cancer immune escape and inflammation (Dasgupta et al., 2020; Yao et al., 2020). We previously observed that eHSP90α secretion was increased whether in the lung fibroblasts stimulated by TGF-β1 or BALF/serum induced by BLM (Dong et al., 2017). TGF-β1 has been to induce ER stress in lung fibroblasts (Hsu et al., 2017). Thus, we speculated that the eHSP90α production might be regulated by ER stress. In our study, we discovered that treatment with TUDCA significantly decreased HSP90α levels in the BALF and serum. Intriguingly, TUDCA did not alter HSP90α expression at the intracellular level, but markedly reduced the eHSP90α content. Thus, these findings suggest that eHSP90α production is involved in ER stress in the pulmonary fibrosis.

However, one of the limitations of this study is that we were unable to demonstrate that the direct molecular mechanism by which ER stress regulates the eHSP90α secretion in pulmonary fibrosis. Several studies reported that exosome induced by ER stress was highly associated with IRE1α (Kakazu et al., 2016b; Hosoi et al., 2018; Xu et al., 2019). Future research will focus on whether eHSP90α secretion is IRE1α-dependent. This future direction may be important to better understand how eHSP90α regulates pulmonary fibrosis.

In summary, the present study demonstrated that eHSP90α promoted lung fibroblast activation in the pulmonary fibrosis by inducing ER stress *in vitro* and *in vivo*. The role of eHSP90α in ER stress is, at least partially, mediated by activation of the PI3K/Akt signaling pathway. The production of eHSP90α in the pulmonary fibrosis is mediated by ER stress activation. These observations strengthen our notion that eHSP90α interacts with ER stress to promote lung fibroblast activation in pulmonary fibrosis and provide a potential therapeutic strategy for pulmonary fibrosis.

AUTHOR CONTRIBUTIONS

ZJM, DHM and CSX designed research experiments; ZJM, ZWS and LYY performed experiments; ZJM, ZWS, CWM, LYY, LY, WX, ZJZ, QYJ, LY, and ZF collected and analyzed data; ZJM, DHM and CSX prepared and edited the manuscript. All authors have given approval to the final version of the manuscript.

REFERENCES

Aran, G., Sanjurjo, L., Bárcena, C., Simon-Coma, M., Téllez, É., Vázquez-Vitali, M., et al. (2018). CD5L Is Upregulated in Hepatocellular Carcinoma and Promotes Liver Cancer Cell Proliferation and Antiapoptotic Responses by Binding to HSPA5 (GRP78). *FASEB J.* 32 (7), 3878–3891. doi:10.1096/fj.201700941RR

As, S., Kalmár, E., Csermely, P., and Yf, S. (2004). Hsp90 Isoforms: Functions, Expression and Clinical Importance. *FEBS Lett.* 562, 11–15. doi:10.1016/s0014-5793(04)00229-710.1002/feb2.2004.562.issue-1-3

Bellaye, P. S., Shimbori, C., Yanagihara, T., Carlson, D. A., Hughes, P., Upagupta, C., et al. (2018). Synergistic Role of HSP90α and HSP90β to Promote Myofibroblast Persistence in Lung Fibrosis. *Eur. Respir. J.* 51 (2). doi:10.1183/13993003.00386-2017

Bhakta, N. R., Christenson, S. A., Nerella, S., Solberg, O. D., Nguyen, C. P., Choy, D. F., et al. (2018). IFN-stimulated Gene Expression, Type 2 Inflammation, and Endoplasmic Reticulum Stress in Asthma. *Am. J. Respir. Crit. Care Med.* 197 (3), 313–324. doi:10.1164/rccm.201706-1070OC

Bonniaud, P., Burgy, O., and Garrido, C. (2018). Heat Shock Protein-90 toward Theranostics: a Breath of Fresh Air in Idiopathic Pulmonary Fibrosis. *Eur. Respir. J.* 51 (2). doi:10.1183/13993003.02612-2017

Borok, Z., Horie, M., Flodby, P., Wang, H., Liu, Y., Ganesh, S., et al. (2020). Grp78 Loss in Epithelial Progenitors Reveals an Age-Linked Role for Endoplasmic Reticulum Stress in Pulmonary Fibrosis. *Am. J. Respir. Crit. Care Med.* 201 (2), 198–211. doi:10.1164/rccm.201902-0451OC

Cao, S. S., and Kaufman, R. J. (2014). Endoplasmic Reticulum Stress and Oxidative Stress in Cell Fate Decision and Human Disease. *Antioxid. Redox Signal.* 21 (3), 396–413. doi:10.1089/ars.2014.5851

Carrasco, D. R., Sukhdeo, K., Protopopova, M., Sinha, R., Enos, M., Carrasco, D. E., et al. (2007). The Differentiation and Stress Response Factor XBP-1 Drives Multiple Myeloma Pathogenesis. *Cancer Cell* 11 (4), 349–360. doi:10.1016/j.ccr.2007.02.015

Chen, J. S., Hsu, Y. M., Chen, C. C., Chen, L. L., Lee, C. C., and Huang, T. S. (2010). Secreted Heat Shock Protein 90alpha Induces Colorectal Cancer Cell Invasion through CD91/LRP-1 and NF-kappaB-Mediated Integrin alphaV Expression. *J. Biol. Chem.* 285 (33), 25458–25466. doi:10.1074/jbc.M110.139345

Chen, Y., Zhao, X., Sun, J., Su, W., Zhang, L., Li, Y., et al. (2019). YAP1/Twist Promotes Fibroblast Activation and Lung Fibrosis that Conferred by miR-15a Loss in IPF. *Cell Death Differ* 26 (9), 1832–1844. doi:10.1038/s41418-018-0250-0

Cheng, C. F., Sahu, D., Tsen, F., Zhao, Z., Fan, J., Kim, R., et al. (2011). A Fragment of Secreted Hsp90α Carries Properties that Enable it to Accelerate Effectively Both Acute and Diabetic Wound Healing in Mice. *J. Clin. Invest.* 121 (11), 4348–61. doi:10.1172/JCI46475

Colunga Biancatelli, R. M. L., Solopov, P., Gregory, B., and Catravas, J. D. (2020). HSP90 Inhibition and Modulation of the Proteome: Therapeutical Implications for Idiopathic Pulmonary Fibrosis (IPF). *Int. J. Mol. Sci.* 21 (15). doi:10.3390/ijms21155286

Crookshank, J. A., Serrano, D., Wang, G. S., Patrick, C., Morgan, B. S., Paré, M. F., et al. (2018). Changes in Insulin, Glucagon and ER Stress Precede Immune Activation in Type 1 Diabetes. *J. Endocrinol.* 239 (2), 181–195. doi:10.1530/JOE-18-0328

Cubillos-Ruiz, J. R., Bettigole, S. E., and Glimcher, L. H. (2017). Tumorigenic and Immunosuppressive Effects of Endoplasmic Reticulum Stress in Cancer. *Cell* 168 (4), 692–706. doi:10.1016/j.cell.2016.12.004

Dasgupta, D., Nakao, Y., Mauer, A. S., Thompson, J. M., Sehrawat, T. S., Liao, C. Y., et al. (2020). IRE1A Stimulates Hepatocyte-Derived Extracellular Vesicles that Promote Inflammation in Mice with Steatohepatitis. *Gastroenterology* 159 (4), 1487–e17. e17. doi:10.1053/j.gastro.2020.06.031

Dong, H., Luo, L., Zou, M., Huang, C., Wan, X., Hu, Y., et al. (2017). Blockade of Extracellular Heat Shock Protein 90α by 1G6-D7 Attenuates Pulmonary Fibrosis through Inhibiting ERK Signaling. *Am. J. Physiol. Lung. Cel. Mol. Physiol.* 313 (6), L1006–L1015. doi:10.1152/ajplung.00489.2016

Du, T., Li, H., Fan, Y., Yuan, L., Guo, X., Zhu, Q., et al. (2019). The Deubiquitylase OTUD3 Stabilizes GRP78 and Promotes Lung Tumorigenesis. *Nat. Commun.* 10 (1), 2914. doi:10.1038/s41467-019-10824-7

Duan, F. F., Barron, G., Meliton, A., Mutlu, G. M., Dulin, N. O., and Schuger, L. (2019). P311 Promotes Lung Fibrosis via Stimulation of Transforming Growth Factor-B1, -β2, and -β3 Translation. *Am. J. Respir. Cel Mol. Biol.* 60 (2), 221–231. doi:10.1165/rcmb.2018-0028OC

Fan, C. S., Chen, L. L., Hsu, T. A., Chen, C. C., Chua, K. V., Li, C. P., et al. (2019). Endothelial-mesenchymal Transition Harnesses HSP90α-Secreting M2-Macrophages to Exacerbate Pancreatic Ductal Adenocarcinoma. *J. Hematol. Oncol.* 12 (1), 138. doi:10.1186/s13045-019-0826-2

Fernandez, P. M., Tabbara, S. O., Jacobs, L. K., Manning, F. C., Tsangaris, T. N., Schwartz, A. M., et al. (2000). Overexpression of the Glucose-Regulated Stress Gene GRP78 in Malignant but Not Benign Human Breast Lesions. *Breast Cancer Res. Treat.* 59 (1), 15–26. doi:10.1023/a:1006332011207

Guo, J., Chang, C., and Li, W. (2017). The Role of Secreted Heat Shock Protein-90 (Hsp90) in Wound Healing - How Could it Shape Future Therapeutics?. *Expert Rev. Proteomics* 14 (8), 665–675. doi:10.1080/14789450.2017.1355244

Hosoi, T., Nakashima, M., and Ozawa, K. (2018). Incorporation of the Endoplasmic Reticulum Stress-Induced Spliced Form of XBP1 mRNA in the Exosomes. *Front. Physiol.* 9, 1357. doi:10.3389/fphys.2018.01357

Hsu, H. S., Liu, C. C., Lin, J. H., Hsu, T. W., Hsu, J. W., Su, K., et al. (2017). Involvement of ER Stress, PI3K/AKT Activation, and Lung Fibroblast Proliferation in Bleomycin-Induced Pulmonary Fibrosis. *Sci. Rep.* 7 (1), 14272. doi:10.1038/s41598-017-14612-5

Kakazu, E., Mauer, A. S., Yin, M., and Malhi, H. (2016a). Hepatocytes Release Ceramide-Enriched Pro-inflammatory Extracellular Vesicles in an IRE1α-dependent Manner. *J. Lipid Res.* 57 (2), 233–245. doi:10.1194/jlr.M063412

Kakazu, E., Mauer, A. S., Yin, M., and Malhi, H. (2016b). Hepatocytes Release Ceramide-Enriched Pro-inflammatory Extracellular Vesicles in an IRE1α-dependent Manner. *J. Lipid Res.* 57 (2), 233–245. doi:10.1194/jlr.M063412

Kwon, O. C., Lee, E. J., Chang, E. J., Youn, J., Ghang, B., Hong, S., et al. (2018). IL-17A+GM-CSF+ Neutrophils Are the Major Infiltrating Cells in Interstitial Lung Disease in an Autoimmune Arthritis Model. *Front. Immunol.* 9, 1544. doi:10.3389/fimmu.2018.01544

Lee, K. I., Su, C. C., Fang, K. M., Wu, C. C., Wu, C. T., and Chen, Y. W. (2020). Ultrafine Silicon Dioxide Nanoparticles Cause Lung Epithelial Cells Apoptosis via Oxidative Stress-Activated PI3K/Akt-Mediated Mitochondria- and Endoplasmic Reticulum Stress-dependent Signaling Pathways. *Sci. Rep.* 10 (1), 9928. doi:10.1038/s41598-020-66644-z

Lee, T. H., Yeh, C. F., Lee, Y. T., Shih, Y. C., Chen, Y. T., Hung, C. T., et al. (2020a). Fibroblast-enriched Endoplasmic Reticulum Protein TXNDC5 Promotes Pulmonary Fibrosis by Augmenting TGFβ Signaling through TGFBR1 Stabilization. *Nat. Commun.* 11 (1), 4254. doi:10.1038/s41467-020-18047-x

Lee, T. H., Yeh, C. F., Lee, Y. T., Shih, Y. C., Chen, Y. T., Hung, C. T., et al. (2020b). Fibroblast-enriched Endoplasmic Reticulum Protein TXNDC5 Promotes Pulmonary Fibrosis by Augmenting TGFβ Signaling through TGFBR1 Stabilization. *Nat. Commun.* 11 (1), 4254. doi:10.1038/s41467-020-18047-x

Li, G., Jin, F., Du, J., He, Q., Yang, B., and Luo, P. (2019). Macrophage-secreted TSLP and MMP9 Promote Bleomycin-Induced Pulmonary Fibrosis. *Toxicol. Appl. Pharmacol.* 366, 10–16. doi:10.1016/j.taap.2019.01.011

Li, W., Li, Y., Guan, S., Fan, J., Cheng, C. F., Bright, A. M., et al. (2007). Extracellular Heat Shock Protein-90alpha: Linking Hypoxia to Skin Cell Motility and Wound Healing. *EMBO J.* 26 (5), 1221–1233. doi:10.1038/sj.emboj.7601579

Li, W., Sahu, D., and Tsen, F. (2012). Secreted Heat Shock Protein-90 (Hsp90) in Wound Healing and Cancer. *Biochim. Biophys. Acta* 1823 (3), 730–741. doi:10.1016/j.bbamcr.2011.09.009

Liu, J., Fan, L., Yu, H., Zhang, J., He, Y., Feng, D., et al. (2019). Endoplasmic Reticulum Stress Causes Liver Cancer Cells to Release Exosomal miR-23a-3p and Up-Regulate Programmed Death Ligand 1 Expression in Macrophages. *Hepatology* 70 (1), 241–258. doi:10.1002/hep.30607

Martinez, F. J., Collard, H. R., Pardo, A., Raghu, G., Richeldi, L., Selman, M., et al. (2017). Idiopathic Pulmonary Fibrosis. *Nat. Rev. Dis. Primers* 3, 17074. doi:10.1038/nrdp.2017.74

Matsuzaki, S., Hiratsuka, T., Taniguchi, M., Shingaki, K., Kubo, T., Kiya, K., et al. (2015). Physiological ER Stress Mediates the Differentiation of Fibroblasts. *PLoS One* 10 (4), e0123578. doi:10.1371/journal.pone.0123578

Merkel, A., Chen, Y., and George, A. (2019). Endocytic Trafficking of DMP1 and GRP78 Complex Facilitates Osteogenic Differentiation of Human Periodontal Ligament Stem Cells. *Front. Physiol.* 10, 1175. doi:10.3389/fphys.2019.01175

Peñaranda-Fajardo, N. M., Meijer, C., Liang, Y., Dijkstra, B. M., Aguirre-Gamboa, R., den Dunnen, W. F. A., et al. (2019). ER Stress and UPR Activation in Glioblastoma: Identification of a Noncanonical PERK Mechanism Regulating GBM Stem Cells through SOX2 Modulation. *Cell Death Dis.* 10 (10), 690. doi:10.1038/s41419-019-1934-1

Penke, L. R., Speth, J. M., Dommeti, V. L., White, E. S., Bergin, I. L., and Peters-Golden, M. (2018). FOXM1 Is a Critical Driver of Lung Fibroblast Activation and Fibrogenesis. *J. Clin. Invest.* 128 (6), 2389–2405. doi:10.1172/JCI87631

Richeldi, L., Collard, H. R., and Jones, M. G. (2017). Idiopathic Pulmonary Fibrosis. *Lancet* 389 (10082), 1941–1952. doi:10.1016/S0140-6736(17)30866-8

Sanchez, J., Carter, T. R., Cohen, M. S., and Blagg, B. S. J. (2020). Old and New Approaches to Target the Hsp90 Chaperone. *Curr. Cancer Drug Targets* 20 (4), 253–270. doi:10.2174/1568009619666191202101330

Shi, J., Yu, J., Zhang, Y., Wu, L., Dong, S., Wu, L., et al. (2019). PI3K/Akt Pathway-Mediated HO-1 Induction Regulates Mitochondrial Quality Control and Attenuates Endotoxin-Induced Acute Lung Injury. *Lab. Invest.* 99 (12), 1795–1809. doi:10.1038/s41374-019-0286-x

Shuda, M., Kondoh, N., Imazeki, N., Tanaka, K., Okada, T., Mori, K., et al. (2003). Activation of the ATF6, XBP1 and Grp78 Genes in Human Hepatocellular Carcinoma: a Possible Involvement of the ER Stress Pathway in Hepatocarcinogenesis. *J. Hepatol.* 38 (5), 605–614. doi:10.1016/s0168-8278(03)00029-1

Song, M., Bode, A. M., Dong, Z., and Lee, M. H. (2019a). AKT as a Therapeutic Target for Cancer. *Cancer Res.* 79 (6), 1019–1031. doi:10.1158/0008-5472.CAN-18-2738

Song, M., Peng, H., Guo, W., Luo, M., Duan, W., Chen, P., et al. (2019b). Cigarette

Smoke Extract Promotes Human Lung Myofibroblast Differentiation by the Induction of Endoplasmic Reticulum Stress. *Respiration* 98 (4), 347–356. doi:10.1159/000502099

Tanimura, A., Miyoshi, K., Horiguchi, T., Hagita, H., Fujisawa, K., and Noma, T. (2018). Mitochondrial Activity and Unfolded Protein Response Are Required for Neutrophil Differentiation. *Cell. Physiol. Biochem.* 47 (5), 1936–1950. doi:10.1159/000491464

Trepel, J., Mollapour, M., Giaccone, G., and Neckers, L. (2010). Targeting the Dynamic HSP90 Complex in Cancer. *Nat. Rev. Cancer* 10 (8), 537–549. doi:10.1038/nrc2887

van Lidth de Jeude, J. F., Spaan, C. N., Meijer, B. J., Smit, W. L., Soeratram, T. T. D., Wielenga, M. C. B., et al. (2018). Heterozygosity of Chaperone Grp78 Reduces Intestinal Stem Cell Regeneration Potential and Protects against Adenoma Formation. *Cancer Res.* 78 (21), 6098–6106. doi:10.1158/0008-5472.CAN-17-3600

Wan, H., Xie, T., Xu, Q., Hu, X., Xing, S., Yang, H., et al. (2019). Thy-1 Depletion and Integrin β3 Upregulation-Mediated PI3K-Akt-mTOR Pathway Activation Inhibits Lung Fibroblast Autophagy in Lipopolysaccharide-Induced Pulmonary Fibrosis. *Lab. Invest.* 99 (11), 1636–1649. doi:10.1038/s41374-019-0281-2

Wang, H., Yu, Z., Huo, S., Chen, Z., Ou, Z., Mai, J., et al. (2018). Overexpression of ELF3 Facilitates Cell Growth and Metastasis through PI3K/Akt and ERK Signaling Pathways in Non-small Cell Lung Cancer. *Int. J. Biochem. Cel. Biol.* 94, 98–106. doi:10.1016/j.biocel.2017.12.002

Wang, Y., Lin, Y., Wang, L., Zhan, H., Luo, X., Zeng, Y., et al. (2020). TREM2 Ameliorates Neuroinflammatory Response and Cognitive Impairment via PI3K/AKT/FoxO3a Signaling Pathway in Alzheimer's Disease Mice. *Aging (Albany NY)* 12, 20862–20879. doi:10.18632/aging.104104

Wolters, P. J., Collard, H. R., and Jones, K. D. (2014). Pathogenesis of Idiopathic Pulmonary Fibrosis. *Annu. Rev. Pathol.* 9, 157–179. doi:10.1146/annurev-pathol-012513-104706

Xu, W., Wu, Y., Hu, Z., Sun, L., Dou, G., Zhang, Z., et al. (2019). Exosomes from Microglia Attenuate Photoreceptor Injury and Neovascularization in an Animal Model of Retinopathy of Prematurity. *Mol. Ther. Nucleic Acids* 16, 778–790. doi:10.1016/j.omtn.2019.04.029

Yao, L., Zhao, H., Tang, H., Liang, J., Liu, L., Dong, H., et al. (2016). The Receptor for Advanced Glycation End Products Is Required for β-catenin Stabilization in a Chemical-Induced Asthma Model. *Br. J. Pharmacol.* 173 (17), 2600–2613. doi:10.1111/bph.13539

Yao, X., Tu, Y., Xu, Y., Guo, Y., Yao, F., and Zhang, X. (2020). Endoplasmic Reticulum Stress-Induced Exosomal miR-27a-3p Promotes Immune Escape in Breast Cancer via Regulating PD-L1 Expression in Macrophages. *J. Cel. Mol. Med.* 24 (17), 9560–9573. doi:10.1111/jcmm.15367

Yoshida, H. (2007). ER Stress and Diseases. *FEBS J.* 274 (3), 630–658. doi:10.1111/j.1742-4658.2007.05639.x

Zhang, G., Liu, Z., Ding, H., Zhou, Y., Doan, H. A., Sin, K. W. T., et al. (2017). Tumor Induces Muscle Wasting in Mice through Releasing Extracellular Hsp70 and Hsp90. *Nat. Commun.* 8 (1), 589. doi:10.1038/s41467-017-00726-x

Zhou, X., Wen, Y., Tian, Y., He, M., Ke, X., Huang, Z., et al. (2019). Heat Shock Protein 90α-dependent B-Cell-2-Associated Transcription Factor 1 Promotes Hepatocellular Carcinoma Proliferation by Regulating MYC Proto-Oncogene C-MYC mRNA Stability. *Hepatology* 69 (4), 1564–1581. doi:10.1002/hep.30172

6

Gypenosides Attenuate Pulmonary Fibrosis by Inhibiting the AKT/mTOR/c-Myc Pathway

Suqing Liu[1†], *Qingqing Yang*[1,2†], *Binbin Dong*[3], *Chunhui Qi*[4], *Tao Yang*[5], *Ming Li*[1], *Shan He*[1], *Baojun Liu*[6*] and *Jinfeng Wu*[1*]

[1]Department of Dermatology, Huashan Hospital, Fudan University, Shanghai, China, [2]Shanghai Public Health Clinical Center, Fudan University, Shanghai, China, [3]Department of Pediatrics, Huashan Hospital North, Fudan University, Shanghai, China, [4]Department of Respiratory Medicine, Qingpu District Traditional Chinese Medicine Hospital, Institute of Integrative Medicine, Fudan University, Shanghai, China, [5]Department of Cardiovascular Disease, Institute of Cardiovascular Disease of Integrated Traditional Chinese and Western Medicine, Shuguang Hospital Affiliated to Shanghai University of Traditional Chinese Medicine, Shanghai, China, [6]Department of Integrative Medicine, Huashan Hospital, Fudan University, Shanghai, China

***Correspondence:**
Baojun Liu
lbj825@163.com
Jinfeng Wu
wujinfeng21@163.com

†These authors have contributed equally to this work

Gypenosides (Gyps), the major active constituents isolated from *Gynostemma pentaphyllum*, possess anti-inflammatory and antioxidant activities. Previous studies have demonstrated that Gyps displayed potent ameliorative effects on liver fibrosis and renal fibrosis. In this study, we found that Gyps significantly reduced the mortality of bleomycin-induced pulmonary fibrosis mice (40% mortality rate of mice in the model group versus 0% in the treatment group). Masson staining showed that Gyps could reduce the content of collagen in the lung tissue of pulmonary fibrosis mice Masson staining and immunohistochemistry demonstrated that the expression of the collagen gene α-SMA and fibrosis gene Col1 markedly decreased after Gyps treatment. The active mitosis of fibroblasts is one of the key processes in the pathogenesis of fibrotic diseases. RNA-seq showed that Gyps significantly inhibited mitosis and induced the G2/M phase cell cycle arrest. The mTOR/c-Myc axis plays an important role in the pathological process of pulmonary fibrosis. RNA-seq also demonstrated that Gyps inhibited the mTOR and c-Myc signaling in pulmonary fibrosis mice, which was further validated by Western blot and immunohistochemistry. AKT functions as an upstream molecule that regulates mTOR. Our western blot data showed that Gyps could suppress the activation of AKT. In conclusion, Gyps exerted anti-pulmonary fibrosis activity by inhibiting the AKT/mTOR/c-Myc pathway.

Keywords: gypenosides, pulmonary fibrosis, AKT, mTOR, c-Myc

INTRODUCTION

Pulmonary fibrosis (PF) is a chronic, progressive, and lethal interstitial lung disease, with a poor prognosis and median survival of 3–5 years after diagnosis (Masefield et al., 2019). PF is characterized by inflammation, fibroblast/myofibroblast proliferation, and the activation of alveolar epithelial cells with excessive extracellular matrix (ECM) deposition in the lung parenchyma (Wolters et al., 2014). Current pharmacological therapies include glucocorticoids, immunosuppressive drugs, and anti-fibrotic agents; however, none of them can improve the survival of patients with PF (Richeldi et al., 2017). To date, there are only two drugs approved by the U.S. Food and Drug Administration (FDA) for the treatment of PF: nintedanib and pirfenidone (Yamazaki et al., 2021). These two small molecule drugs target receptor tyrosine kinase (RTK) and the transforming growth factor (TGF-β), respectively. Although they can slow down the progression of PF, the high cost and strong toxic effects on the liver and kidneys limit their clinical application (Yang et al., 2019). In recent years, traditional Chinese medicine (TCM) has shown unique efficacies in the treatment of PF (Chen DQ. et al., 2018). Owing to the characteristics of multi-components, multi-targets, and multi-level interactions, TCM can improve the survival and life quality of the patients with PF disease to a certain extent (Wang et al., 2020).

The pathogenesis of PF is not well elucidated (Spagnolo et al., 2021). Increasing evidences showed that the progressive pulmonary scarring and lung function declining induced by the lung epithelial injury and aberrant fibroblast proliferation were involved in the pathogenesis of PF (Martinez et al., 2017). Currently, it is believed that PF originates from the repeated injury and aberrant repair of the alveolar epithelial cells (Sgalla et al., 2018). Repeatedly injured alveolar epithelial cells secrete PF-related growth factors, such as the connective tissue growth factor (CTGF), transforming growth factor β1 (TGF-β1), and insulin-like growth factors (IGF-1), which activate the phosphatidylinositol 3-kinase (PI3K)/AKT signaling pathway through binding to the corresponding receptors on the lung fibroblast membrane, to promote lung fibroblast proliferation and collagen synthesis and induce the epithelial-to-mesenchymal transition (EMT) (Phan et al., 2021). As a downstream target of the PI3K/AKT signaling pathway, excessive activation of mTOR in the alveolar epithelium exacerbates bleomycin (BLM)-induced PF in mice (Cong et al., 2020). Moreover, c-Myc, a star transcription factor in the downstream of mTOR, can stimulate fibroblast proliferation in the presence of growth factors (Lawrence and Nho, 2018).

Gypenosides (Gyps), the saponin extracts of *Gynostemma pentaphyllum*, have been extensively studied in fibrosis diseases, such as liver fibrosis and renal fibrosis, for their anti-inflammatory, anti-fibrotic, antioxidant, and anti-apoptotic effects (Nguyen et al., 2021). In this study, we evaluated that Gyps attenuated BLM-induced PF in mice through mediating the AKT/mTOR/c-Myc pathway.

MATERIALS AND METHODS

Instrument and Chromatographic Conditions

Chromatography was performed using a Dionex Ultimate 3000 ultra-high-performance liquid chromatography (HPLC) system from Thermo Fisher Scientific (Waltham, MA, United States) and an ACQUITY UPLC HSS T3 column (2.1 mm × 100 mm, 1.8 μm, Waters Corp., Milford, MA, United States). The components were eluted with a gradient elution system consisting of 0.1% formic acid aqueous solution (A) and acetonitrile (B). The mobile phase gradient elution was programmed as follows: 0–12 min, 5% B–95% B; 12–14 min, 95% B; 14.01 min, 5% B; and 14.01–16 min, 5% B. The mobile phase flow rate was 0.3 ml/min, and the column temperature was maintained at 45°C.

Mass spectrometric detection was performed using a quadrupole mass spectrometer equipped with electrospray ionization (HESI) in the positive and negative mode under the following operating parameters: the ion source was operated with a capillary voltage set to 3.5 kV (ESI+) and 2.8 kV (ESI-), the capillary temperature at 320 °C, the auxiliary gas heating temperature at 35°C, sheath gas (nitrogen) flow at 80 AU, and auxiliary gas (nitrogen) flow at 13 AU, respectively. Data acquisition was performed full-scan, selective ion monitoring (SIM) mode in the range of m/z 80–1,200.

Preparation of Standard Solutions and Sample Solutions

The mixture of a standard stock solution containing above eight compounds (ginsenoside Rb1, ginsenoside Rd, rutin, quercetin, kaempferol, gypenoside XLIX, ombuoside, and ombuin) was prepared in methanol at 1 μg/ml. Furthermore, the chemical constituents of the total saponin extract of *Gynostemma pentaphyllum* (Gypenosides, Gyps) was extracted by ultrasonicating in methanol for 30 min at 250 W and 40 kHz. Then, 100 μL aliquot of the sample solution which was filtered by a 0.22 μm millipore filter was injected into the chromatographic systems for analysis.

Reagents

Primary antibodies against mice α-SMA, Col1, c-Myc, INSC, AKT, p-AKT, mTOR, p-mTOR, and β-actin were purchased from Abcam (Cambridge, United Kingdom), and secondary antibodies were obtained from Yeasen Biotech Co., Ltd. (Shanghai, China). Gyps were bought from Ronghe Co., Ltd. (Shanghai, China). BLM was supplied by MCE (Shanghai, China).

Animal Experimental Procedure

Six-week-old female C57BL/6 J mice were purchased from Vital River Laboratory Animal Technology Co. (Beijing, China). All mice were housed in a pathogen-free facility at the animal room of the Shanghai Public Health Clinical Center. The mice were raised at proper humidity (60 ± 2%) and temperature (25 ± 2°C) and allowed free access to food and water. All animal experimental procedures were reviewed and approved by the animal ethics committee of the Shanghai Public Health Clinical Center (permit number: 2020-A037-01). Twenty-five mice were assigned to three groups at random: the control group (5 mice), BLM group (10 mice), and Gyps-treated group (10 mice). For BLM and Gyps-treated group, mice were anesthetized and then intratracheally injected with BLM at a dose of 3 mg/kg to induce the fibrotic response at day 0. The control group received intratracheal injection of the same amount of saline. The Gyps were administered daily from day 1 to day 20 by gavage at a dose of 200 mg/kg in the Gyps-treated group. The BLM group was given the same amount of saline by gavage. Mice were sacrificed on day 21. Briefly, the heart was perfused with PBS through the right ventricle until the lung was clear of blood after anesthetized. The right lung tissue was isolated for Western blot assay and

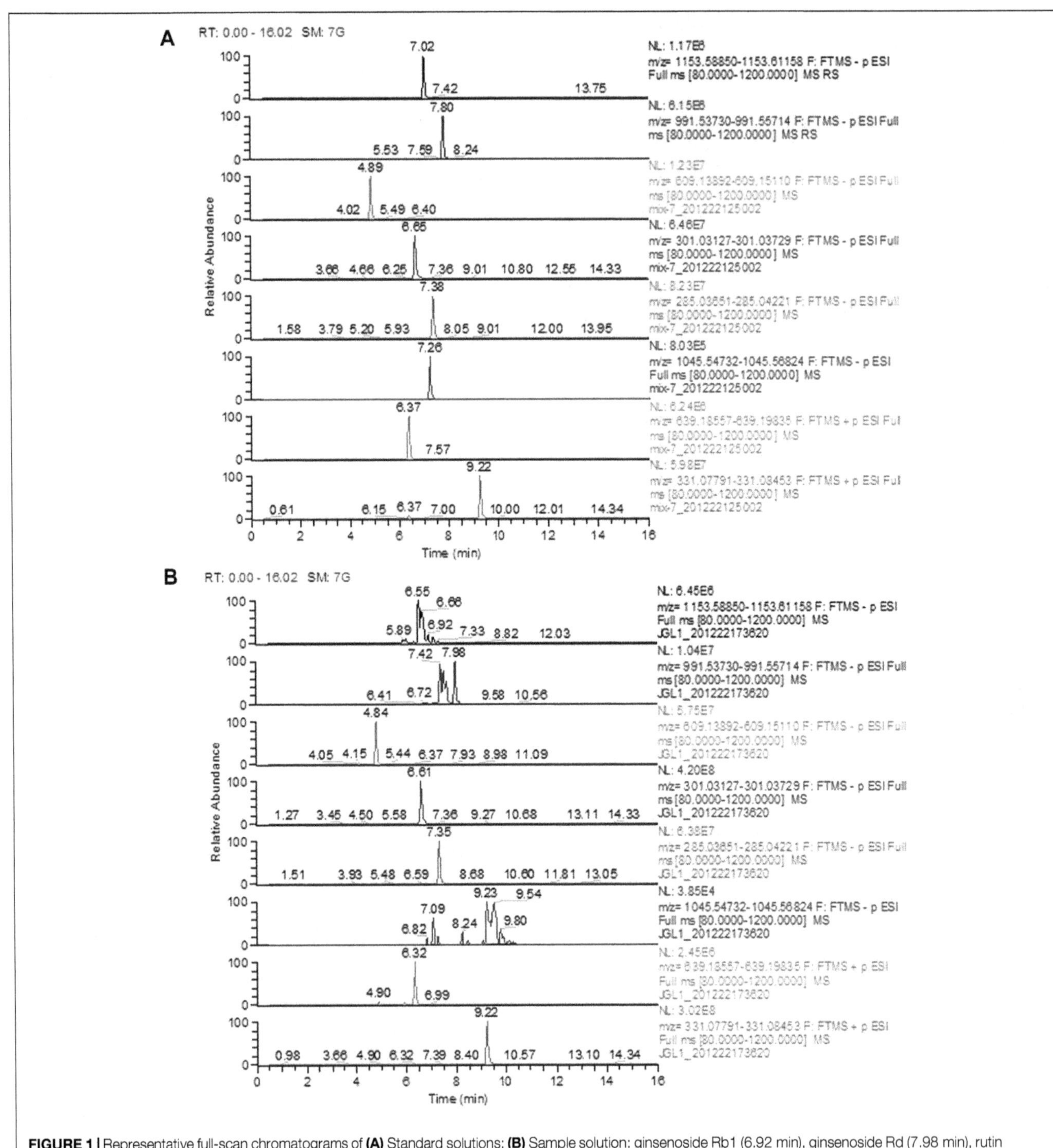

FIGURE 1 | Representative full-scan chromatograms of **(A)** Standard solutions; **(B)** Sample solution: ginsenoside Rb1 (6.92 min), ginsenoside Rd (7.98 min), rutin (4.84 min), quercetin (6.61 min), kaempferol (7.35 min), gypenoside XLIX (7.26 min), ombuoside (6.32 min), and ombuin (9.22 min).

RNA-sequencing, and the left lung tissue was harvested for histology assay.

Histology and Immunohistochemistry

Histology and immunohistochemistry assays were performed and analyzed, as described in our previous article (Li Q. et al., 2020). Briefly, after being fixed with 4% formaldehyde, the left lung was paraffin-embedded and sliced into 4–6 um thick sections. Deparaffinized sections were stained with hematoxylin and eosin (HE) and followed by staining with Masson's trichrome and periodic acid–Schiff (PAS). Immunohistochemical analysis was performed on 4-μm formalin-fixed sections using the primary antibody against α-SMA, Col1, and c-Myc.

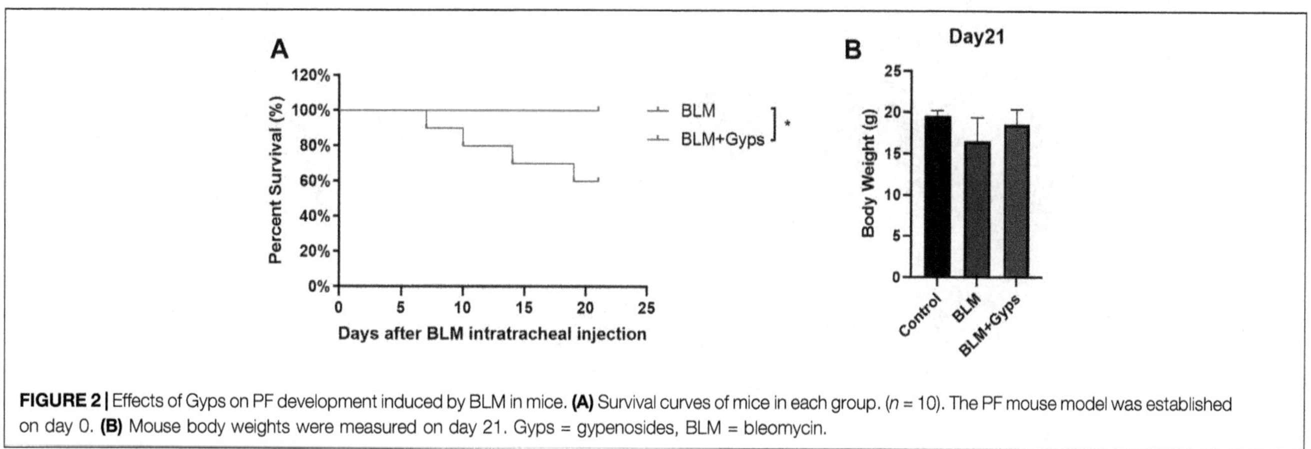

FIGURE 2 | Effects of Gyps on PF development induced by BLM in mice. **(A)** Survival curves of mice in each group. (n = 10). The PF mouse model was established on day 0. **(B)** Mouse body weights were measured on day 21. Gyps = gypenosides, BLM = bleomycin.

Western Blot

Total protein was extracted from lung tissue homogenates using the RIPA reagent (Beyotime Biotechnology, lnc, JiangSu, China) supplemented with 1% PMSF (Beyotime) and separated through electrophoresing on 10% SDS-PAGE gels (30μg/lane). The separated protein was transferred to the polyvinylidene difluoride (PVDF) membranes (Merck Millipore, lnc., Darmstadt, Germany) and subsequently blocked with 5% skimmed milk. The targeted protein was probed with antibodies against INSC, AKT, p-AKT, mTOR, p-mTOR, and β-actin (all from Abcam, Cambridge, United Kingdom). After an incubation step with horseradish peroxidase (HRP)-conjugated secondary antibodies, the bands were visualized using an enhanced chemiluminescence kit (Merck Millipore).

RNA Sequencing Analysis

Total RNA of the lung tissue was isolated using the miRNeasy Micro Kit (Qiagen, Hilden, Germany), and the concentration and purity of RNA were detected by using a Bioanalyzer 4200 (Agilent, Santa Clara, CA, United States). RNA-seq analysis was performed, as described in our previous article (Li H. et al., 2020).

Statistical Analysis

Statistical analysis was performed by GraphPad Prism 8 software (GraphPad Software, Inc., San Diego, CA). Data were analyzed by student's t-test or one-way *ANOVA* which were followed by Turkey's *post hoc* analysis for the comparison of two or more independent groups, respectively. Survival data were analyzed using Kaplan–Meier survival analysis. A p value less than 0.05 was regarded as a statistically significant difference.

RESULTS

UPLC Chromatograms of Gyps

The chromatograms of mixed standards and Gyps were illustrated in **Figure 1**. The contents of ginsenoside Rb1, ginsenoside Rd, rutin, quercetin, kaempferol, gypenoside XLIX, ombuoside, and ombuin in Gyps were approximately detected to be 0.01713, 0.02351, 0.07513, 0.09762, 0.01106, 0.00017, 0.05242, and 0.08317%, respectively.

Gyps Enhanced the Survival Rate of BLM-Induced PF Mice

As shown in **Figure 2A**, the death of BLM-induced PF mice occurred from day 7 after BLM intratracheal injection, and Kaplan–Meier survival curves demonstrated that BLM-induced PF mice treated with Gyps had a significantly higher survival rate than those treated with saline (100 vs. 60% 21-days survival, log-rank test, $p < 0.05$, **Figure 2A**). However, there was no significant difference in the body weight among the three groups on day 21 (**Figure 2B**).

Gyps Ameliorated Pulmonary Inflammation and Fibrosis

The normal alveolar structure was maintained in the control group (**Figure 3A**). Twenty-one days after BLM injection, HE and Masson's trichrome staining showed a remarkably thick alveolar wall and collapse of alveolar septa, inflammatory cell infiltration, loss of lung architecture, and excess deposition of collagen in the BLM-treated group compared with the control group, whereas treatment with Gyps markedly attenuated the injury of lung architecture and the deposition of collagen caused by BLM (**Figures 3A,B,E,F**). The effects of Gyps on the BLM-induced collagen deposition and alveolar fibrosis in the lungs were further investigated by immunohistochemistry assay. The data showed that BLM upregulated the expressions of the collagen gene α-SMA and fibrosis gene Col1 in the lung tissue compared with the control group, while the expressions of α-SMA and Col1 in the lung tissue of Gyps-treated mice were significantly lower than those in the model mice (**Figures 3C,D,G,H**).

Gyps Alleviated PF by Inhibiting Mitosis

We then performed RNA-seq of the RNA isolated from the lung tissues to further explore the possible mechanisms. As demonstrated in **Figure 4A**, 11,852 downregulated transcripts and 1927 upregulated transcripts were found in the Gyps-treated

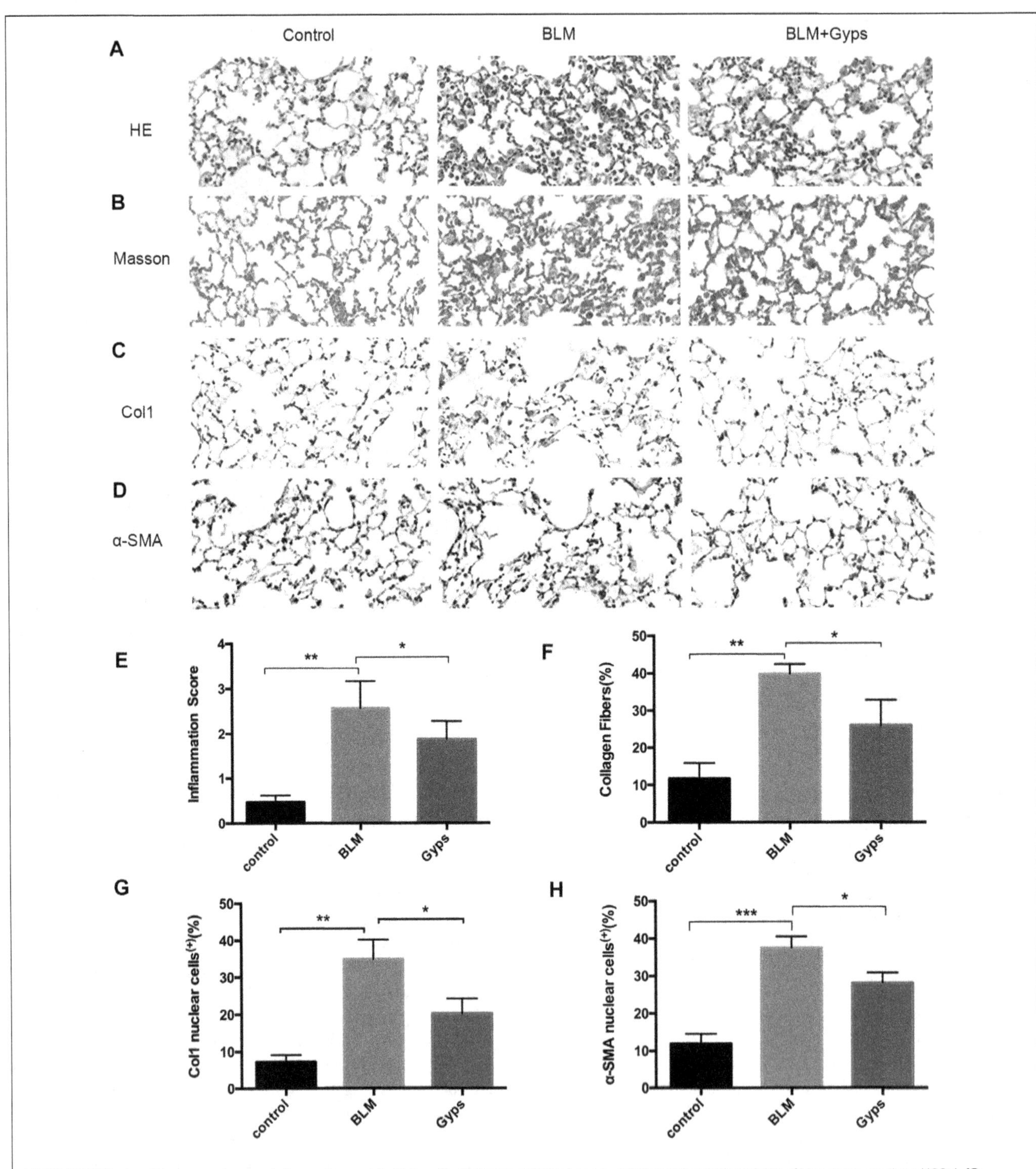

FIGURE 3 | Effects of Gyps on pulmonary inflammation and fibrillation. **(A, B)** Representative images of HE and Masson's staining of lung tissue sections (400×). **(C, D)** Immunohistochemistry was used to analyze the expression levels of Col1 and α-SMA (400×). **(E–H)** Quantitation of the data presented in panel **(A–D)**. Gyps = gypenosides, BLM = bleomycin. ***p < 0.001, **p < 0.01, compared with control; *p < 0.05 compared with BLM.

group compared with the BLM group (n = 5 mice/group). Gene set enrichment analysis of the downregulated transcripts enriched in the Hallmark gene sets (**Figure 4B**) illustrated that mitotic spindle-related transcripts (top 1 ranked) were significantly downregulated in the Gyps-treated group in comparison with the BLM group. It has been reported that the active mitosis of fibroblasts was one of the key processes in the pathogenesis of fibrotic diseases (Adamson, 1984; Tomcik et al., 2016). INSC functions as an adapter protein that was involved in spindle orientation during mitosis (Culurgioni and Mapelli, 2013). As

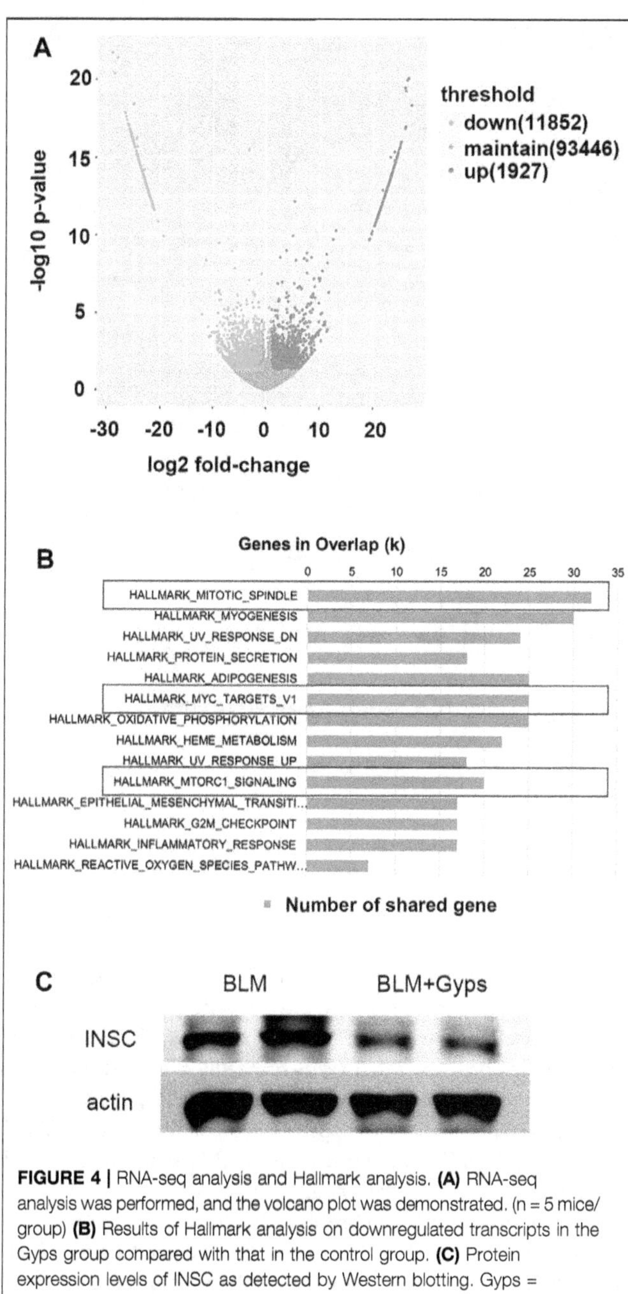

FIGURE 4 | RNA-seq analysis and Hallmark analysis. **(A)** RNA-seq analysis was performed, and the volcano plot was demonstrated. (n = 5 mice/group) **(B)** Results of Hallmark analysis on downregulated transcripts in the Gyps group compared with that in the control group. **(C)** Protein expression levels of INSC as detected by Western blotting. Gyps = gypenosides, BLM = bleomycin.

shown in **Figure 4C**, Gyps treatment significantly decreases the expressions of INSC, which was highly expressed in the BLM group. We also found that Gyps induced the G2/M cell cycle arrest (ranked 12) (**Figure 4C**).

Gyps Inhibited Mitosis by Repressing the mTOR/c-Myc Axis in PF Mice

As demonstrated in **Figure 4B**, the Hallmark analysis also indicated that Myc (ranked 6) and mTORC1 (ranked 10) signaling-related genes were notably inhibited after Gyps treatment. Myc family has a central role in orchestrating cell proliferation (Chen H. et al., 2018). The mTORC1 controls cell growth and metabolism in response to nutrients, energy levels, and growth factors (Yang et al., 2017). c-Myc is one of the key target genes of mTOR, and mTOR and c-Myc form an axis. They are highly related to the mitotic process (Cianfanelli et al., 2015). Our IHC analysis showed that Gyps inhibited the expression of c-Myc in BLM-injected mice (**Figures 5A,B**). Meanwhile, we found that Gyps administration obviously inhibited the BLM-induced increase of p-mTOR by Western blot assay (**Figure 5C**).

Gyps Inhibited the mTOR/c-Myc Axis by Regulating PI3K/AKT Signaling

PI3K/AKT signaling is one of the key cellular signaling pathways which regulate cell proliferation, growth, metabolism, and motility. mTOR and c-Myc are the downstream proteins of PI3K/AKT signaling (Alzahrani, 2019). Thus, we detected the expressions of p-PI3K, PI3K, p-AKT, and AKT in the lung tissues and found (**Figure 5D**) that the expression of p-PI3K and p-AKT in BLM-induced PF mice showed a significant increase compared with that of the control group. Interestingly, the expressions of p-PI3K and p-AKT were markedly reduced after treating with Gyps, which demonstrated that Gyps could suppress the mTOR/c-Myc axis by inactivating PI3K/AKT signaling.

DISCUSSION

Gyps, the total saponins extracted from *Gynostemma pentaphyllum*, were widely used for anti-inflammation, antioxidant, antitumor, and immune enhancement. The anti-fibrotic effects of Gyps have been reported in multiple fibrotic diseases including liver fibrosis, renal fibrosis, and Graves' ophthalmopathy (Chen et al., 2017; Li H. et al., 2020; Liu Q. et al., 2021). In this study, we first reported that Gyps could alleviate BLM-induced pulmonary fibrosis in mice. We found eight major components in Gyps, among which ginsenoside Rb1, rutin, quercetin, kaempferol, and gypenoside XLIX have been reported to have anti-fibrotic effects (Hou et al., 2014; Verma et al., 2017; Wu et al., 2017; Avila-Carrasco et al., 2019; Liu et al., 2019; Bai et al., 2020; Liu et al., 2020; Liu H. et al., 2021). Based on our *in vivo* data, 40% of PF mice died, while none of the Gyps treated PF mice died. This indicated that Gyps could significantly improve the survival rate of PF mice and had a good promise for the treatment of pulmonary fibrosis. However, administration of Gyps could not attenuate the effects of BLM on body weight loss in PF mice. It might be because most of the low-weight PF mice died.

PF is characterized by increased fibroblast proliferation and ECM protein deposition by myofibroblasts under the control of pro-fibrogenic stimuli such as TGF-β1 (Davies et al., 2012). Based on the analysis of RNA-seq, the Gyps-treated group showed the most significant improvement in mitosis and promoted G2/M cell cycle arrest. In the future, the *in vitro* experiment should be carried out to verify if Gyps could directly inhibit mitosis in pulmonary fibroblasts. It has been reported that some non–SMAD-mediated pathways including PI3K/AKT, RhoA,

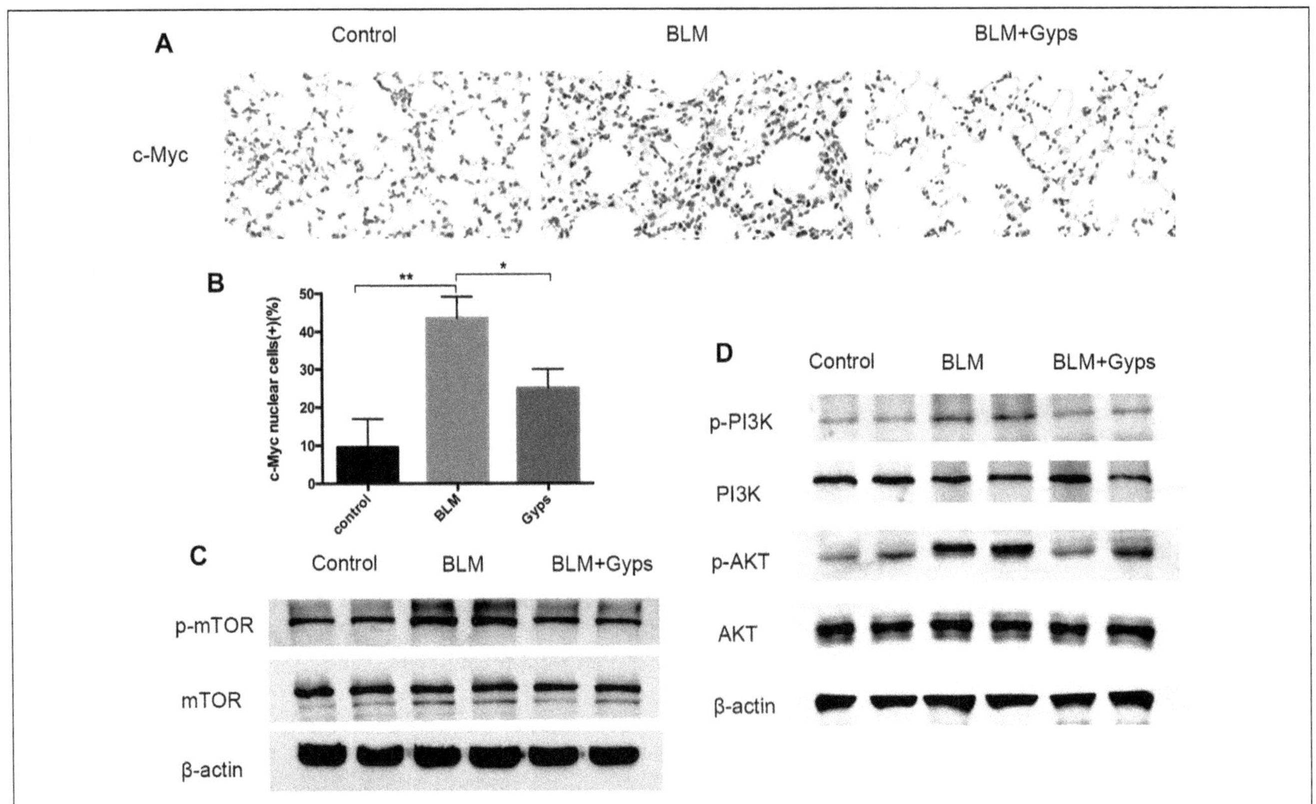

FIGURE 5 | Expressions of c-Myc, p-mTOR, mTOR, p-PI3K, PI3K, p-AKT, and AKT in the mouse model. **(A)** c-Myc Immunohistochemical staining (400×). **(B)** Quantitation of the data presented in panel **(A)**. **(C, D)** Protein expression levels of p-mTOR, mTOR, p-PI3K, PI3K, p-AKT, and AKT as detected by Western blotting. Gyps = gypenosides, BLM = bleomycin. ***$p < 0.001$, **$p < 0.01$, compared with control; *$p < 0.05$ compared with BLM.

PAR6, and MAPK pathways could lead to EMT in the fibrotic process (Cho et al., 2007; Willis and Borok, 2007). PI3K is an intracellular phosphatidylinositol kinase, which has serine/threonine kinase and phosphatidylinositol kinase activities (Yang et al., 2020). AKT is a serine/threonine kinase and is directly activated in response to PI3K which functions as an important regulator of cell growth, survival, and glucose metabolism (Barrett et al., 2012). Yuan et al. reported that miR-410 induces EMT through activating the PI3K/mTOR pathway in non–small cell lung cancer (Yuan et al., 2020). Recent studies have shown that the phosphorylation of AKT was increased in human pulmonary fibroblasts induced by BLM and was also increased in radiation-induced PF (Ma et al., 2020a; Ma et al., 2020b). The atypical serine/threonine kinase mTOR is the key downstream target molecule of AKT and functions as an important regulator of cell growth, metabolism, and immunity (Hua et al., 2019). c-Myc, a star transcription factor in the downstream of mTOR, can stimulate fibroblast proliferation in the presence of growth factors (Lawrence and Nho, 2018). Decreased c-Myc expression mediated fibronectin and collagen deposition into the extracellular matrix and attenuated cell proliferation in the fibrosis process (Valiente-Alandi et al., 2018). Shin et al. revealed that the AKT inhibitor LY294002 blocked the expressions of p-AKT and c-Myc in HepG2 cells and found that the compound K induced apoptosis in hepatocellular carcinoma cells *via* inhibition of AKT/mTOR/c-Myc signaling (Shin et al., 2021). Liu et al. reported Gyps-induced apoptosis of renal cell carcinoma cells through regulating the PI3K/AKT/mTOR signaling pathway. (Liu H. et al., 2021). In the present study, we demonstrated that Gyps markedly inhibited the AKT/mTOR/c-Myc pathway in pulmonary fibrosis (**Figure 6**).

Many growth factors are upstream regulators of PI3K/AKT signaling, such as CTGF, TGF-β1, and IGF-1, which are reported to be involved in the pathological process of PF. Gyps were reported to protect orbital fibroblasts in Graves' ophthalmopathy *via* downregulating TGF-β–induced fibrotic mediators (Li H. et al., 2020). In another study, researchers reported that Gyps ameliorated CCl_4-induced liver fibrosis *via* inhibiting TGF-β1 signaling and consequently inhibiting the differentiation of hepatic progenitor cells into myofibroblasts (Chen et al., 2017). In a unilateral ureteral obstruction-induced tubulointerstitial damage and fibrosis model, the expressions of TGF-β1 and CTGF were significantly reduced by Gyps treatment, and the Smad7 expression was elevated by Gyps treatment (Li Q. et al., 2020). In the future, we will determine if Gyps could affect the upstream regulators of PI3K/AKT signaling in PF.

EMT, inflammatory response, and reactive oxygen species (ROS) pathways are involved in the pathological process of PF (Wolters et al., 2014). EMT is a process in which epithelial cells gradually acquire a mesenchymal (fibroblast-like) cell phenotype (Bartis et al., 2014). A previous study reported that in a repetitive

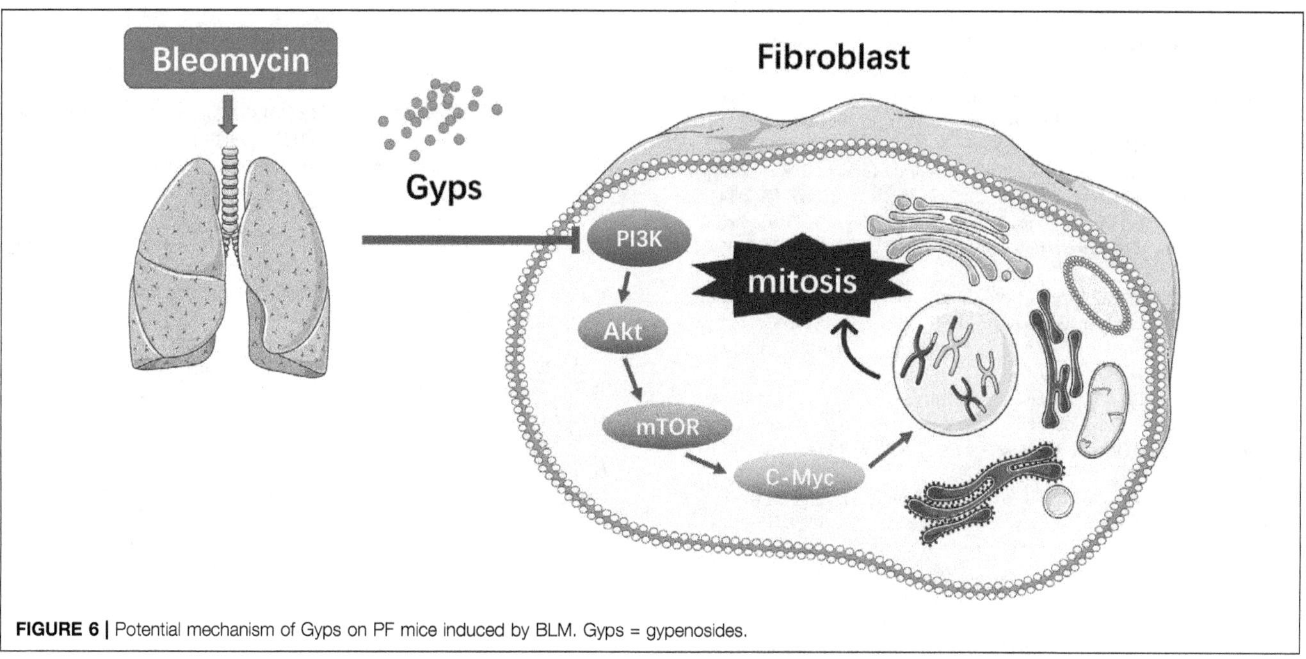

FIGURE 6 | Potential mechanism of Gyps on PF mice induced by BLM. Gyps = gypenosides.

bleomycin injury PF model, about 50% of S100A4+ fibroblasts were epithelial-derived using genetic fate tracking (Johnson et al., 2011). It was reported that polyhexamethylene guanidine-phosphate infiltrated into the lungs in the form of aerosol particles would induce an airway barrier injury by generating ROS, releasing fibrotic inflammatory cytokines, and triggering a wound-healing response, thus leading to pulmonary fibrosis (Kim et al., 2016). Our RNA-seq data suggested that Gyps had anti-inflammatory, antioxidative, and anti-EMT effects (ranked 11, 13, and 14, respectively) in PF mice. Further studies are needed to confirm the above effects of Gyps in PF.

In conclusion, we revealed that Gyps attenuated PF development in mice, and the potential mechanism was due to inhibiting the AKT/mTOR/c-Myc axis. Gyps might be a promising candidate drug for the treatment of pulmonary fibrosis.

AUTHOR CONTRIBUTIONS

SL performed a part of experiments, analyzed data, and wrote the manuscript. QY, BD, and TY assisted in experiments and data acquisition. SH, ML, and CQ assisted in manuscript preparation. JW planned experiments, supervised experiments, and assisted in data analysis. BL initiated experiments and provided funding and intellectual input to data interpretation. All authors read and approved all versions of the manuscript.

REFERENCES

Adamson, I. Y., and Bowden, D. H. (1984). Role of Polymorphonuclear Leukocytes in Silica-Induced Pulmonary Fibrosis. *Am. J. Pathol.* 117, 37–43. doi:10.1289/ehp.845525

Alzahrani, A. S. (2019). PI3K/Akt/mTOR Inhibitors in Cancer: At the Bench and Bedside. *Semin. Cancer Biol.* 59, 125–132. doi:10.1016/j.semcancer.2019.07.009

Avila-Carrasco, L., Majano, P., Sánchez-Tomẻro, J. A., Selgas, R., López-Cabrera, M., Aguilera, A., et al. (2019). Natural Plants Compounds as Modulators of Epithelial-to-Mesenchymal Transition. *Front. Pharmacol.* 10, 715. doi:10.3389/fphar.2019.00715

Bai, L., Li, A., Gong, C., Ning, X., and Wang, Z. (2020). Protective Effect of Rutin Against Bleomycin Induced Lung Fibrosis: Involvement of TGF-β1/α-SMA/Col I and III Pathway. *Biofactors* 46, 637–644. doi:10.1002/biof.1629

Barrett, D., Brown, V. I., Grupp, S. A., and Teachey, D. T. (2012). Targeting the PI3K/AKT/mTOR Signaling axis in Children with Hematologic Malignancies. *Paediatr. Drugs* 14, 299–316. doi:10.2165/11594740-000000000-00000

Bartis, D., Mise, N., Mahida, R. Y., Eickelberg, O., and Thickett, D. R. (2014). Epithelial-mesenchymal Transition in Lung Development and Disease: Does it Exist and Is it Important?. *Thorax* 69, 760–765. doi:10.1136/thoraxjnl-2013-204608

Chen, D. Q., Feng, Y. L., Cao, G., and Zhao, Y. Y. (2018a). Natural Products as a Source for Antifibrosis Therapy. *Trends Pharmacol. Sci.* 39, 937–952. doi:10.1016/j.tips.2018.09.002

Chen, H., Liu, H., and Qing, G. (2018b). Targeting Oncogenic Myc as a Strategy for Cancer Treatment. *Signal. Transduct Target. Ther.* 3, 5. doi:10.1038/s41392-018-0008-7

Chen, J., Li, X., Hu, Y., Liu, W., Zhou, Q., Zhang, H., et al. (2017). Gypenosides Ameliorate Carbon Tetrachloride-Induced Liver Fibrosis by Inhibiting the Differentiation of Hepatic Progenitor Cells into Myofibroblasts. *Am. J. Chin. Med.* 45, 1061–1074. doi:10.1142/S0192415X17500574

Cho, H. J., Baek, K. E., Saika, S., Jeong, M.-J., and Yoo, J. (2007). Snail is Required for Transforming Growth Factor-Beta-Induced Epithelial-Mesenchymal Transition by Activating PI3 Kinase/Akt Signal Pathway. *Biochem. Biophys. Res. Commun.* 353, 337–343. doi:10.1016/j.bbrc.2006.12.035

Cianfanelli, V., Fuoco, C., Lorente, M., Salazar, M., Quondamatteo, F., Gherardini, P. F., et al. (2015). AMBRA1 Links Autophagy to Cell Proliferation and Tumorigenesis by Promoting C-Myc Dephosphorylation and Degradation. *Nat. Cel Biol* 17, 20–30. doi:10.1038/ncb3072

Cong, L. H., Li, T., Wang, H., Wu, Y. N., Wang, S. P., Zhao, Y. Y., et al. (2020). IL-17A-producing T Cells Exacerbate fine Particulate Matter-Induced Lung Inflammation and Fibrosis by Inhibiting PI3K/Akt/mTOR-Mediated Autophagy. *J. Cel Mol Med* 24, 8532–8544. doi:10.1111/jcmm.15475

Culurgioni, S., and Mapelli, M. (2013). Going Vertical: Functional Role and Working Principles of the Protein Inscuteable in Asymmetric Cell Divisions.

Cell Mol Life Sci 70, 4039–4046. doi:10.1007/s00018-013-1319-z

Davies, E. R., Haitchi, H. M., Thatcher, T. H., Sime, P. J., Kottmann, R. M., Ganesan, A., et al. (2012). Spiruchostatin A Inhibits Proliferation and Differentiation of Fibroblasts from Patients with Pulmonary Fibrosis. *Am. J. Respir. Cel Mol Biol* 46, 687–694. doi:10.1165/rcmb.2011-0040OC

Hou, Y.-L., Tsai, Y.-H., Lin, Y.-H., and Chao, J. C.-J. (2014). Ginseng Extract and Ginsenoside Rb1 Attenuate Carbon Tetrachloride-Induced Liver Fibrosis in Rats. *BMC Complement Altern Med.* 14, 415. doi:10.1186/1472-6882-14-415

Hua, H., Kong, Q., Zhang, H., Wang, J., Luo, T., and Jiang, Y. (2019). Targeting mTOR for Cancer Therapy. *J. Hematol. Oncol.* 12, 71. doi:10.1186/s13045-019-0754-1

Johnson, J. R., Roos, A., Berg, T., Nord, M., and Fuxe, J. (2011). Chronic Respiratory Aeroallergen Exposure in Mice Induces Epithelial-Mesenchymal Transition in the Large Airways. *PLoS One* 6, e16175. doi:10.1371/journal.pone.0016175

Kim, H. R., Lee, K., Park, C. W., Song, J. A., Shin, D. Y., Park, Y. J., et al. (2016). Polyhexamethylene Guanidine Phosphate Aerosol Particles Induce Pulmonary Inflammatory and Fibrotic Responses. *Arch. Toxicol.* 90, 617–632. doi:10.1007/s00204-015-1486-9

Lawrence, J., and Nho, R. (2018). The Role of the Mammalian Target of Rapamycin (mTOR) in Pulmonary Fibrosis. *Int. J. Mol. Sci.* 19, E778. doi:10.3390/ijms19030778

Li, H., Ma, C., Liu, W., He, J., and Li, K. (2020a). Gypenosides Protect Orbital Fibroblasts in Graves Ophthalmopathy via Anti-inflammation and Anti-fibrosis Effects. *Invest. Ophthalmol. Vis. Sci.* 61, 64. doi:10.1167/iovs.61.5.64

Li, Q., Sun, J., Cao, Y., Liu, B., Li, L., Mohammadtursun, N., et al. (2020b). Bu-Shen-Fang-Chuan Formula Attenuates T-Lymphocytes Recruitment in the Lung of Rats with COPD through Suppressing CXCL9/CXCL10/CXCL11-CXCR3 axis. *Biomed. Pharmacother.* 123, 109735. doi:10.1016/j.biopha.2019.109735

Liu, H., Li, X., Duan, Y., Xie, J. B., and Piao, X. L. (2021a). Mechanism of Gypenosides of Gynostemma Pentaphyllum Inducing Apoptosis of Renal Cell Carcinoma by PI3K/AKT/mTOR Pathway. *J. Ethnopharmacol* 271, 113907. doi:10.1016/j.jep.2021.113907

Liu, H., Yu, H., Cao, Z., Gu, J., Pei, L., and Jia, M. (2019). Kaempferol Modulates Autophagy and Alleviates Silica-Induced Pulmonary Fibrosis. *DNA Cell Biol.* 38, 1418–1426. doi:10.1089/dna.2019.4941

Liu, Q., Chen, X., Kan, M., Yang, J., Gong, Q., Jin, R., et al. (2021b). Gypenoside XLIX Loaded Nanoparticles Targeting Therapy for Renal Fibrosis and its Mechanism. *Eur. J. Pharmacol.* 910, 174501. doi:10.1016/j.ejphar.2021.174501

Liu, X., Chen, J., Sun, N., Li, N., Zhang, Z., Zheng, T., et al. (2020). Ginsenoside Rb1 Ameliorates Autophagy Via the AMPK/mTOR Pathway in Renal Tubular Epithelial Cells *In Vitro* and *In Vivo*. *Int. J. Biol. Macromol.* 163, 996–1009. doi:10.1016/j.ijbiomac.2020.07.060

Martinez, F. J., Collard, H. R., Pardo, A., Raghu, G., Richeldi, L., Selman, M., et al. (2017). Idiopathic Pulmonary Fibrosis. *Nat. Rev. Dis. Primers* 3, 17074. doi:10.1038/nrdp.2017.74

Masefield, S., Cassidy, N., Ross, D., Powell, P., and Wells, A. (2019). Communication Difficulties Reported by Patients Diagnosed with Idiopathic Pulmonary Fibrosis and Their Carers: a European Focus Group Study. *ERJ Open Res.* 5, 00055–02019. doi:10.1183/23120541.00055-2019

Ma, W., Li, M., Ma, H., Li, W., Liu, L., Yin, Y., et al. (2020a). Protective Effects of GHK-Cu in Bleomycin-Induced Pulmonary Fibrosis *Via* Anti-Oxidative Stress and Anti-Inflammation Pathways. *Life Sciences* 241, 117139. doi:10.1016/j.lfs.2019.117139

Ma, Z., Yu, R., Zhu, Q., Sun, L., Jian, L., Wang, X., et al. (2020b). CXCL16/CXCR6 Axis Promotes Bleomycin-Induced Fibrotic Process in MRC-5 Cells *via* the PI3K/AKT/FOXO3a Pathway. *International Immunopharmacology* 81, 106035. doi:10.1016/j.intimp.2019.106035

Nguyen-Ngoc, H., Quy Ha, T. K., Yang, J. L., Tung Pham, H. T., and Oh, W. K. (2021). Triterpenoids from the Genus Gynostemma: Chemistry and Pharmacological Activities. *J. Ethnopharmacol* 268, 113574. doi:10.1016/j.jep.2020.113574

Phan, T. H. G., Paliogiannis, P., Nasrallah, G. K., Giordo, R., Eid, A. H., Fois, A. G., et al. (2021). Emerging Cellular and Molecular Determinants of Idiopathic Pulmonary Fibrosis. *Cel Mol Life Sci* 78, 2031–2057. doi:10.1007/s00018-020-03693-7

Richeldi, L., Collard, H. R., and Jones, M. G. (2017). Idiopathic Pulmonary Fibrosis. *Lancet* 389, 1941–1952. doi:10.1016/S0140-6736(17)30866-8

Sgalla, G., Iovene, B., Calvello, M., Ori, M., Varone, F., and Richeldi, L. (2018). Idiopathic Pulmonary Fibrosis: Pathogenesis and Management. *Respir. Res.* 19, 32. doi:10.1186/s12931-018-0730-2

Shin, N., Lee, H. J., Sim, D. Y., Im, E., Park, J. E., Park, W. Y., et al. (2021). Apoptotic Effect of Compound K in Hepatocellular Carcinoma Cells via Inhibition of Glycolysis and Akt/mTOR/c-Myc Signaling. *Phytother Res.* 35, 3812–3820. doi:10.1002/ptr.7087

Spagnolo, P., Kropski, J. A., Jones, M. G., Lee, J. S., Rossi, G., Karampitsakos, T., et al. (2021). Idiopathic Pulmonary Fibrosis: Disease Mechanisms and Drug Development. *Pharmacol. Ther.* 222, 107798. doi:10.1016/j.pharmthera.2020.107798

Tomcik, M., Palumbo-Zerr, K., Zerr, P., Sumova, B., Avouac, J., Dees, C., et al. (2016). Tribbles Homologue 3 Stimulates Canonical TGF-β Signalling to Regulate Fibroblast Activation and Tissue Fibrosis. *Ann. Rheum. Dis.* 75, 609–616. doi:10.1136/annrheumdis-2014-206234

Valiente-Alandi, I., Potter, S. J., Salvador, A. M., Schafer, A. E., Schips, T., Carrillo-Salinas, F., et al. (2018). Inhibiting Fibronectin Attenuates Fibrosis and Improves Cardiac Function in a Model of Heart Failure. *Circulation* 138, 1236–1252. doi:10.1161/CIRCULATIONAHA.118.034609

Verma, S., Kalita, B., Bajaj, S., Prakash, H., Singh, A. K., and Gupta, M. L. (2017). A Combination of Podophyllotoxin and Rutin Alleviates Radiation-Induced Pneumonitis and Fibrosis through Modulation of Lung Inflammation in Mice. *Front Immunol.* 8, 658. doi:10.3389/fimmu.2017.00658

Wang, W., Liu, Z., Niu, J., Yang, H., Long, Q., Liu, H., et al. (2020). Feibi Recipe Reduced Pulmonary Fibrosis Induced by Bleomycin in Mice by Regulating BRP39/IL-17 and TGFβ1/Smad3 Signal Pathways. *Evid. Based Complement. Alternat Med.* 2020, 5814658. doi:10.1155/2020/5814658

Willis, B. C., and Borok, Z. (2007). TGF-Beta-Induced EMT: Mechanisms and Implications for Fibrotic Lung Disease. *Am. J. Physiol. Lung Cell Mol. Physiol.* 293, L525–534. doi:10.1152/ajplung.00163.2007

Wolters, P. J., Collard, H. R., and Jones, K. D. (2014). Pathogenesis of Idiopathic Pulmonary Fibrosis. *Annu. Rev. Pathol.* 9, 157–179. doi:10.1146/annurev-pathol-012513-104706

Wu, L., Zhang, Q., Mo, W., Feng, J., Li, S., Li, J., et al. (2017). Quercetin Prevents Hepatic Fibrosis by Inhibiting Hepatic Stellate Cell Activation and Reducing Autophagy *via* the TGF-β1/Smads and PI3K/Akt Pathways. *Sci. Rep.* 7, 9289. doi:10.1038/s41598-017-09673-5

Yamazaki, R., Nishiyama, O., Saeki, S., Sano, H., Iwanaga, T., and Tohda, Y. (2021). Initial Therapeutic Dose of Corticosteroid for an Acute Exacerbation of IPF Is Associated with Subsequent Early Recurrence of Another Exacerbation. *Sci. Rep.* 11, 5782. doi:10.1038/s41598-021-85234-1

Yang, D. C., Li, J. M., Xu, J., Oldham, J., Phan, S. H., Last, J. A., et al. (2019). Tackling MARCKS-PIP3 Circuit Attenuates Fibroblast Activation and Fibrosis Progression. *FASEB J.* 33, 14354–14369. doi:10.1096/fj.201901705R

Yang, H., Jiang, X., Li, B., Yang, H. J., Miller, M., Yang, A., et al. (2017). Mechanisms of mTORC1 Activation by RHEB and Inhibition by PRAS40. *Nature* 552, 368–373. doi:10.1038/nature25023

Yang, L., Shi, P., Zhao, G., Xu, J., Peng, W., Zhang, J., et al. (2020). Targeting Cancer Stem Cell Pathways for Cancer Therapy. *Signal. Transduct Target. Ther.* 5, 8. doi:10.1038/s41392-020-0110-5

Yuan, Y., Liao, H., Pu, Q., Ke, X., Hu, X., Ma, Y., et al. (2020). miR-410 Induces Both Epithelial-Mesenchymal Transition and Radioresistance through Activation of the PI3K/mTOR Pathway in Non-small Cell Lung Cancer. *Signal. Transduct Target. Ther.* 5, 85. doi:10.1038/s41392-020-0182-2

7

Targeting Chitinase 1 and Chitinase 3-Like 1 as Novel Therapeutic Strategy of Pulmonary Fibrosis

Suh-Young Lee[1,2], Chang-Min Lee[1], Bing Ma[1], Suchitra Kamle[1], Jack A. Elias[1], Yang Zhou[1] and Chun Geun Lee[1]**

[1]Molecular Microbiology and Immunology, Brown University, 185 Meeting St., Providence, RI, United States, [2]Devision of Allergy and Clinical Immunology, Department of Internal Medicine, Seoul National University Hospital, Seoul, South Korea

***Correspondence:**
Yang Zhou
yang_zhou@brown.edu
Chun Geun Lee
chun_lee@brown.edu

Chitinase 1 (CHIT1) and chitinase 3-like-1 (CHI3L1), two representative members of 18-Glycosyl hydrolases family, are significantly implicated in the pathogenesis of various human diseases characterized by inflammation and remodeling. Notably, dysregulated expression of CHIT1 and CHI3L1 was noted in the patients with pulmonary fibrosis and their levels were inversely correlated with clinical outcome of the patients. CHIT1 and CHI3L1, mainly expressed in alveolar macrophages, regulate profibrotic macrophage activation, fibroblast proliferation and myofibroblast transformation, and TGF-β signaling and effector function. Although the mechanism or the pathways that CHIT1 and CHI3L1 use to regulate pulmonary fibrosis have not been fully understood yet, these studies identify CHIT1 and CHI3L1 as significant modulators of fibroproliferative responses leading to persistent and progressive pulmonary fibrosis. These studies suggest a possibility that CHIT1 and CHI3L1 could be reasonable therapeutic targets to intervene or reverse established pulmonary fibrosis. In this review, we will discuss specific roles and regulatory mechanisms of CHIT1 and CHI3L1 in profibrotic cell and tissue responses as novel therapeutic targets of pulmonary fibrosis.

Keywords: chitinase 1, chitinase-like proteins, chitinase 3-like 1, pulmonary fibrosis, foxo3, tgfbrap1

INTRODUCTION

Pulmonary fibrosis is a devastating lung disease that affects up to 200,000 people in the US alone. Idiopathic Pulmonary Fibrosis (IPF) is the most common form of pulmonary fibrosis and has a poor life expectancy (2 to 3 years of median survival) after diagnosis (Michaelson et al., 2000; Ley et al., 2011). Currently, there are two FDA approved therapeutic drugs for PF: pirfenidone (Esbriet®) and nintedanib (Ofev or Vargatef®). These drugs provide substantial benefits by slowing disease progression, but they do not relive symptom or improve quality of life and are associated with severe side effects and prohibitively high cost. Additionally, available treatments do not reverse lung damage incurred during fibrotic progression, necessitating early treatments prior to the destruction of normal lung architecture. The only curative treatment for PF is a high-risk lung transplant and life-long anti-rejection treatments. However, lung transplants are associated with extreme morbidity and recipients often succumb to fibrotic rejection within 5–10 years of the transplant. Therefore, new drug or methods of prevention and treatment of PF are critically needed.

IPF is a progressive lung disease characterized by epithelial damage, fibroproliferative matrix deposition and parenchymal remodeling (Raghu, 1998; Selman et al., 2001; Krein and Winston, 2002). Although extensive epidemiological studies suggested that environmental and occupational exposure to noxious materials or particulate matters such as silica, air pollution, cigarette smoke or certain drugs cause fibrosis, the exact etiology of PF has largely remained "idiopathic". TGF-β1 is believed to play an important role in this dysregulation because it is expressed in an exaggerated fashion in IPF where, in contrast to controls, a sizable percentage is biologically active (Khalil et al., 1996; Khalil et al., 2001; Xu et al., 2003). The important role that TGF-β1 may play in this disorder can be seen in studies that demonstrate that TGF-β1 is a critical mediator of pulmonary fibrosis after bleomycin injury (Nakao et al., 1999; Yehualaeshet et al., 2000) and that high dose adenoviral TGF-β1 transfer or lung-specific transgenic expression causes progressive pulmonary fibrosis *in vivo* (Sime et al., 1997; Kelly et al., 2003; Lee et al., 2004) and IPF-like fibroblastic foci *in vitro* explants (Xu et al., 2003). However, the factors that control these TGF-β1 responses that allow TGF-β1 to contribute to the pathogenesis of pulmonary fibrosis are still poorly understood.

Recent studies identified that chitinase 1 (CHIT1) and chitinase 3-like-1 (CHI3L1), two representative members of 18-Glycosyl hydrolase (18-GH) family, are significantly implicated in the pathogenesis of various human diseases characterized by inflammation and remodeling (Kanneganti et al., 2012; Hong et al., 2018; Zhao et al., 2020). Dysregulated expression of CHIT1 and CHI3L1 was noted in the patients with pulmonary fibrosis and their levels were inversely correlated with clinical outcome of the patients (Lee et al., 2012; Zhou et al., 2014). The macrophages are the major cells expressing CHIT1 and CHI3L1, and *in vitro* and *in vivo* studies demonstrated their regulatory roles in profibrotic macrophage activation, fibroblast proliferation, myofibroblast transformation, and TGF-β signaling and effector function (Lee et al., 2012; Zhou et al., 2014; Zhou et al., 2015; Lee et al., 2019). Preclinical studies using animal model of pulmonary fibrosis further demonstrated that both CHIT1 and CHI3L1 are sufficient and required for fibroproliferative responses. These studies suggest a possibility of re-programing of these profibrotic cells to reverse established pulmonary fibrosis by intervention of CHIT1 and or CHI3L1. Here we will overview the recent progress that revealed a new paradigm on the pathogenesis of pulmonary fibrosis and will discuss a new therapeutic strategy by targeting both CHIT1 and CHI3L1.

Current Therapeutics Being Used in the Patients With Pulmonary Fibrosis

Most clinical trials have been conducted on the patients with IPF based international multidisciplinary consensus classification of idiopathic interstitial pneumonias (Demedts and Costabel, 2002). Since the role of specific inflammatory cells in the pathogenesis of fibrosis is controversial (Gauldie, 2002; Strieter, 2002), anti-inflammatory agents represented by corticosteroids did not show a significant effect in the treatment of IPF (Richeldi et al., 2003). In addition, considering the risk of potential side effects, long-term, systemic use of high-dose anti-inflammatory drugs are not recommended. Even with combinatorial approaches using multiple drugs, prednisone, azathioprine, and N-acetylcysteine (NAC), rather increased the risk of death and hospitalization in IPF patients compared to the patients with placebo (Idiopathic Pulmonary Fibrosis Clinical Research et al., 2012). Anticoagulant warfarin did not show a benefit in the treatment of patients with progressive IPF (Noth et al., 2012). Ambrisentan, a selective endothelin receptor antagonist, was not effective in treating IPF and may be associated with an increased risk for disease progression and respiratory hospitalizations (Raghu et al., 2013). Imatinib, a serine/threonine kinase inhibitor, also did not affect survival or lung function (Daniels et al., 2010). Thus, these drugs either in single or combinational uses are not strongly recommended for the patients with IPF in the current guidelines (Raghu et al., 2015). The use of phosphodiesterase-5 inhibitor (Sildenafil) and dual endothelin receptor antagonists (Macitenta and Bosentan) were considered to use in certain cases of IPF patients with pulmonary arterial hypertension, but recent clinical studies did not show significant benefits of these drugs to these patients (Lee and Song, 2020; Kang and Song, 2021).

The currently recommended FDA-approved drugs for IPF are pirfenidone and nintedanib. Both pirfenidone and nintedanib have been shown to slow the lung function deterioration. Pirfenidone is a small synthetic molecule with antifibrotic properties. It reduce the expression of TGF-β in the lung and inhibits the recruitment of fibrocytes to the lung in bleomycin-induced lung fibrosis model (Myllärniemi and Kaarteenaho, 2015). In a phase II study, significantly reduced loss of VC was demonstrated in patients with pirfenidone (Taniguchi et al., 2010). Following phase III studies showed a beneficial effect on reduction in decline of FVC for pirfenidone compared to placebo (Noble et al., 2011; King et al., 2014). Nintedanib is an inhibitor of the *Src* family of tyrosine kinases, that inhibits VEGF and PDGF receptors (Myllärniemi and Kaarteenaho, 2015). Nintedanib inhibited proliferation, migration, and transformation of fibroblasts to myofibroblasts (Wollin et al., 2015). In two replicate phase 3 trials, nintedanib reduced the decline in FVC, which is consistent with a slowing of disease progression (Richeldi et al., 2014). There is no head-to-head comparison study performed between pirfenidone and nintedanib. Since currently available antifibrotic drugs cannot control or reverse the disease status, but only slow the loss of lung function, there is a strong need for effective, and less-toxic therapeutic methods available for the patients with pulmonary fibrosis.

Major Cellular and Tissue Factors Implicated in Pathogenesis of Pulmonary Fibrosis

Tissue fibrosis is a major cause of morbidity in pulmonary fibrosis. As a normal repair response, fibrosis is a series of process of cellular damage caused by various conditions that initiate inflammation, recruitments of inflammatory cells, followed by final tissue repair and termination of inflammation. Loss of regulatory signals and imbalance in the process of wound healing leads to aberrant activation of repair response, causing pathologic fibrosis in various organs including lung, resulting in a disease state (Wilson and Wynn, 2009). Since excellent review articles detailing the molecules and signaling pathways involved in the pathogenesis of pulmonary fibrosis are already available (Micallef et al., 2012; Wolters et al., 2014; Sgalla et al., 2018; Strykowski and Adegunsoye, 2021), in this section, we only focus on the discussion of major factors leading to pathologic fibrosis, that can be also regulated by CHIT1 or CHI3L1 in the development and progression of pulmonary fibrosis. Pulmonary fibrosis comprises a number of different etiologies and pathologies with completely different clinical features and therapeutic responses. Accordingly, there are significant limitations in identifying common pathogenetic mechanisms of pulmonary fibrosis. This is particularly true for *in vitro* cell or *in vivo* preclinical animal models of pulmonary fibrosis, since currently no preclinical models are exactly representing the characteristic cellular and tissue responses of IPF and other interstitial lung disease (ILD). In addition, so far relatively small number of human studies with dysregulated expression of CHIT1 and/or CHI3L1 in the patients with IPF and ILD add certain limitations in direct clinical translation of preclinical data. With these limitations in mind, here the molecular and mechanistic implications of CHIT1 and CHI3L1 as potential therapeutic targets are discussed based on up-to-dated and common lung pathologies of pulmonary fibrosis.

Myofibroblasts

Compared to normal wound healing, excessive accumulation of myofibroblasts plays a key role in fibrotic tissue responses. Activated myofibroblasts expressing α-smooth muscle actin (SMA), collagens and other extracellular matrix noted at sites of fibrotic foci are one of the pathologic hallmarks of pulmonary fibrosis. Although multiple types of cells which include resident interstitial fibroblasts, circulating fibrocytes or progenitor cells, epithelial cells and endothelial pericytes have been thought as sources of myofibroblasts (Zent and Guo, 2018; Hung, 2020), the exact origin of myofibroblasts in fibrotic foci is still largely elusive. Recent single cell RNAseq analysis identified different subsets of fibroblasts which have distinct expression profile and nature in the development of fibrotic cellular and tissue responses (Tsukui et al., 2020). The fibroblasts isolated from the lungs of progressive IPF with expression of PD-L1 or specific integrin receptors, such as αvβ6, demonstrated higher invasiveness compared to normal lung fibroblasts (Chen et al., 2016; Geng et al., 2019). Thus, understanding the exact origin, differentiation, and activation mechanism(s) of invasive fibroblasts/myofibroblasts would be essential for the development of effective therapeutics against pulmonary fibrosis with invasive and progressive nature. While the myofibroblasts noted in the normal repair process are known to be removed from the sites of normal wound healing through apoptotic cell death response, the invasive myofibroblasts at site of pathologic fibrosis are resistant to dying out (Hinz and Lagares, 2020). Thus, either de-differentiate of the invasive myofibroblasts to normal fibroblasts through reprogramming or the induction of apoptosis of myofibroblasts could be a reasonable therapeutic strategy to reverse established fibrosis in the patients with IPF.

Profibrotic Macrophages

In addition to myofibroblasts, recent studies also revealed a new regulatory role of inflammatory and immune cells in the development and resolution of pathologic fibrosis. Notably, specific subset of macrophages called as "profibrotic macrophages" were identified in the lungs of IPF patients as well as in the animal models of pulmonary fibrosis (Misharin et al., 2017; Aran et al., 2019; Ayaub et al., 2021). These macrophages, originated from circulating monocytes but not form tissue resident macrophages, contribute to fibrotic tissue response through expression of profibrotic growth factors and cytokines as well as extracellular matrix proteins. Recent *in vivo* single cell and bulk RNA sequencing analysis revealed impressive phenotype changes in the development of profibrotic macrophages from the circulating monocytes to interstitial and resident alveolar macrophages according to the progress of fibrosis (Misharin et al., 2017; Aran et al., 2019; Ayaub et al., 2021). These studies strongly suggest that profibrotic macrophages play a critical role not only in the initiation but also progression and resolution of pathologic fibrosis. The impressive plasticity of the macrophages also supports a possibility of re-programming of the macrophages to reverse profibrotic to non-profibrotic macrophages as a therapeutic strategy of pulmonary fibrosis. Recent studies identified that Bcl2 coupled with Carnitine palmitoyltransferase 1a (Cpt1a), the mitochondrial rate-limiting enzyme for fatty acid β-oxidation, confers apoptosis resistance of macrophages at site of pathologic fibrosis and dysregulated fibrotic remodeling (Gu et al., 2021). Thus, further identification of the factors or the pathways regulating the recruitment, activation and clearance of profibrotic macrophages will be essential to understand the process of pathologic fibrosis as well as for the development of therapeutics to reverse established progressive pulmonary fibrosis.

Collagens and Extracellular Matrix

The pathologic hallmark of pulmonary fibrosis is excessive accumulation of various types of collagens and other extracellular matrix proteins. Traditionally, collagen accumulation at sites of pathologic fibrosis is considered as a result of imbalance between newly generated collagens vs. collagen degradation. On this regard, the prevailing hypothesis was that either deficiencies of collagen degrading enzyme matrix metalloproteinases (MMPs) or the excess of tissue inhibitors of metalloproteinases (TIMPs), that result into the dysregulated collagen accumulation (Pardo et al., 2016). However, in contrast to our expectation, recent preclinical studies using targeted null mutant mice demonstrated that MMP-9 or MMP-12 did not show significant impact on the bleomycin induced pulmonary fibrosis (Craig et al., 2015). In addition, TIMP1 null mutant mice also did not reduce collagen accumulation in the lungs of animal models of pulmonary fibrosis (Kim et al., 2005). These studies suggest that other intrinsic and extrinsic factors are implicated in the regulation of collagen accumulation in the lung. Recent studies brought attention to the increased collagen stability at sites of pathologic fibrosis compared to normal wound healing. The deficiency of Lysyl oxidase (LOX) or Lysyl Oxidase-like Proteins (LOX/Ls) significantly reduced collagen accumulation in lungs of murine model of pulmonary fibrosis, since processed collagen (cross-linked collagen) could not be efficiently degraded by collagen degrading enzymes (Tjin et al., 2017; Bellaye et al., 2018). Collagens with certain epigenetic changes were noted only in the lungs of IPF patients, further support this notion that aberrant collagens are generated and accumulated in the lungs of pulmonary fibrosis (Merl-Pham et al., 2019). The expression and the stability of the collagens can be also regulated by transcriptional factors or microRNA, such as mir29, that directly binds to collagen RNAs or other mechanism of posttranscriptional modifications (Yano et al., 2018). These studies further suggest a possibility that collagen modifying enzymes or interacting proteins contribute to the excessive accumulation of collagens in the lungs of patients with pulmonary fibrosis.

TGF-β Expression and Signaling

Many signaling pathways that regulate cell differentiation, migration, and transition are implicated in the pathology of pulmonary fibrosis (Chanda et al., 2019). Among these, TGF-β signaling pathway has long been considered as a key player in initiation and progression of pulmonary fibrosis (Yue et al., 2010). TGF-β induces epithelial or endothelial mesenchymal transition (EMT and EndoMT), fibroblast proliferation and myofibroblast transformation through canonical and noncanonical signaling molecules such as Smads, PI3K-AKT, and MAPK (Kasai et al., 2005; Kim et al., 2006; Hashimoto et al., 2010). TGF-β also known to play a significant role in resolution of fibrosis in the process of normal healing by inducing apoptosis of cells responsible for pathologic fibrosis (Müller et al., 1997; Tschopp et al., 1998). However, factors or pathways regulating effector function of TGF-β between normal repair vs. pathologic fibrosis are not still clearly understood.

Role of CHIT1 in the Pathogenesis of Pulmonary Fibrosis

Although mammals do not have chitin or chitin synthase, substantial levels of chitinases and chitinase-like proteins (CLP) are noted in the circulation as well as in local tissues (Lee et al., 2009; Lee et al., 2011; Cho et al., 2015). CHIT1, a major enzymatically active true chitinase, is produced, stored, and secreted by macrophages and neutrophils (van Eijk et al., 2005) and plays important roles in innate immune homeostasis (Elias et al., 2005). This can be appreciated in the pivotal roles it plays in host defenses against chitin-containing pathogens such as fungi, protozoa and insects (Boot et al., 2001). As a sensitive biomarker of macrophage activation, dysregulated expression of CHIT1 in the circulation or local tissue has been reported in a variety of human diseases including Gaucher's disease, diabetes, sarcoidosis, inflammatory bowel disease, atherosclerosis, Alzheimer's disease, NASH and prostate cancer (Kanneganti et al., 2012; Elmonem et al., 2016). Recent studies also demonstrated that CHIT1 is dysregulated in lung diseases characterized by inflammation and remodeling such as bacterial infection, asthma, COPD and pulmonary fibrosis (Lee et al., 2012; Cho et al., 2015; James et al., 2016; Hong et al., 2018; Sharma et al., 2018; Lee et al., 2019). Recent human and preclinical studies demonstrated that CHIT1 plays an important role in the pathogenesis of both IPF and scleroderma-associated interstitial lung disease (SSc-ILD) (Lee et al., 2012; Lee et al., 2019). These studies further identified specific signaling pathways and interacting partners that CHIT1 uses to contribute to the pathogenesis of pulmonary fibrosis.

CHIT1 Expression in Human Lung Fibrosis

Significant increases in the expression of CHIT1 were noted in lungs of the patients with SSc-ILD as well as in the IPF patients (Lee et al., 2012; Lee et al., 2019). The increased levels of CHIT1 activities in the serum of the patients with SSc-ILD and they are inversely correlated with lung function and overall survival (Lee et al., 2012; Lee et al., 2019). Immunohistochemistry (IHC) analysis localized macrophages as the major cells expressing CHIT1. Modestly increased expression of CHIT1 was also noted in epithelial cells and other interstitial parenchymal cells in the lungs of IPF patients. Interestingly, single cell RNASeq transcriptome analysis on multiple cohorts of IPF patients identified subset of macrophages that highly express CHIT1 and that distinctly overlaps with macrophage populations from the patients with IPF but not with normal controls or COPD patients (**Figure 1**). These studies suggest a significant implication of CHIT1 in the pathogenesis of pulmonary fibrosis as a factor of macrophage differentiation.

CHIT1 in Profibrotic Macrophage Differentiation

As discussed above, profibrotic macrophage activation significantly contribute to the development of pulmonary fibrosis (Wynn and Vannella, 2016; Lee et al., 2018). Since the macrophages are the major cells expressing CHIT1 in IPF lungs, it is reasonable to assume that CHIT1 could plays an important role in profibrotic macrophage differentiation. In support of this notion, *in vitro* macrophages differentiation studies using alveolar macrophages isolated from wild type and CHIT1 null mutant mice, demonstrated that CHIT1 plays a critical role in recombinant (r) IL-4 or rTGF-β stimulated fibrotic macrophage activation (profibrotic macrophages activation) with characteristic expression of cell surface markers of CD206, CD204 CD163, Col1a1, Col3a1. On the other hand, rIFN-γ stimulated iNOS expression was not altered with null mutation of CHIT1. These studies strongly support a notion that CHIT1 contributes to the development of profibrotic, alternative macrophage activation, but not with classical activation. However, the specific mechanism(s) or pathways that CHIT1 uses to regulate macrophage activation remains to be determined.

CHIT1 in Fibroblasts Proliferation and Myofibroblast Transformation

Fibroblasts are the major effector cells responsible for fibrotic tissue responses in that TGF-β1 plays an essential role. In *in vitro* studies using normal human lung fibroblasts (NHLF), CHIT1 enhanced TGF-β1-stimulated fibroblast proliferation and myofibroblasts transformation while CHIT1 itself did not significantly alter at fibroblasts proliferation (Lee et al., 2012; Lee et al., 2019). Similarly, CHIT1 itself did not alter fibroblast differentiation into myofibroblasts as assessed by α-smooth

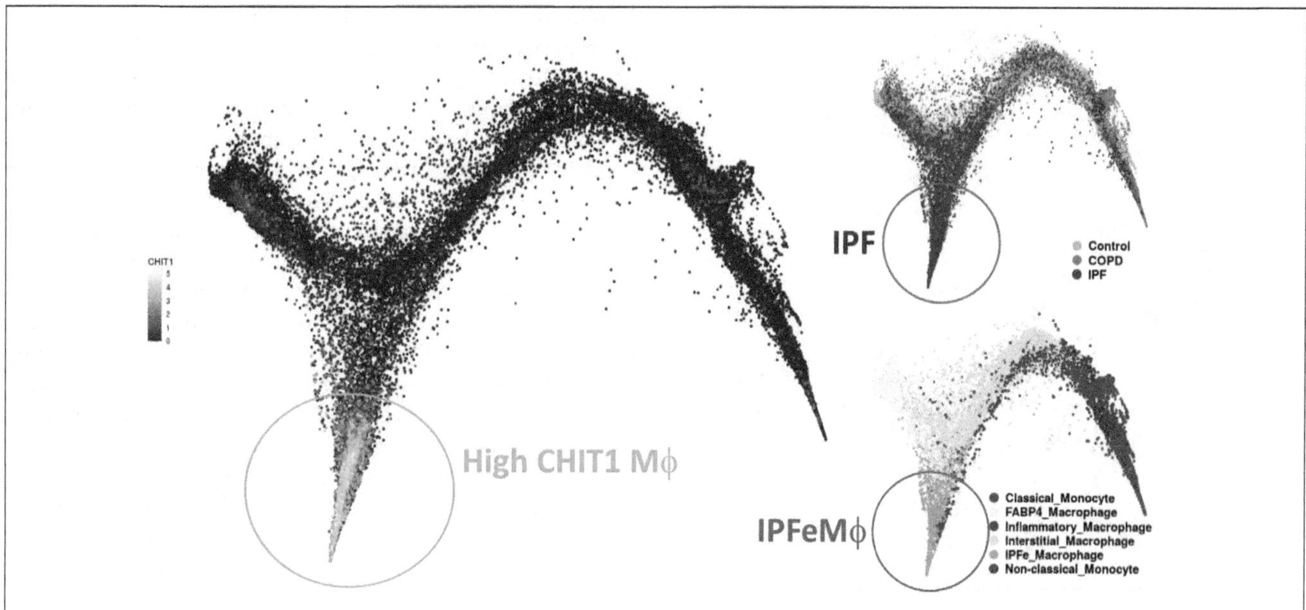

FIGURE 1 | UMAP (uniform manifold approximation and projection) clustering of lung macrophages in patients with IPF evaluated by single cell RNAseq analysis. Highly CHIT1 expressing macrophages (green, left) are overlapping with macrophage subset of patients with IPF (dark brown, upper right) but not with control or COPD patients (blue or bright brown, right upper). It is also notable that most of these CHIT1 expressing macrophages are significantly overlapping with IPF expanded macrophages (IPFeMϕ) (Blue, right lower), the distinct subset of profibrotic macrophages noted in IPF patients. Publicly available RNAseq data (http://www.ipfcellatlas.com/; Single cell RNA-seq, 2021, Ivan Rosas group) was re-plotted for CHIT1 expressing macrophages.

muscle actin (α-SMA) expression but did augment the ability of TGF-β1 to enhance α-SMA accumulation (Lee et al., 2019). This result suggests that CHIT1 enhances TGF-β1-stimulated fibroblast proliferation and myofibroblast transformation.

CHIT1 in TGF-β-Stimulated Pulmonary Fibrosis and its Signaling

Studies employing WT and CHIT1 null mutant mice demonstrated that the ability of TGF-β1 to stimulate ECM proteins including fibronectin, type 1 collagen, and other ECM molecules in a CHIT1 dependent manner (Lee et al., 2012). On the other hand, the exaggerated fibrotic responses were noted in lungs from the mice in which CHIT1 and TGF-β1 were simultaneously expressed compared to the mice in which each was expressed individually (Lee et al., 2019). They demonstrated that transgenic TGF-β1 increased canonical Smad2/3 and noncanonical MAPK/Erk, and Akt activation compared to wild type control mice, and these TGF-β stimulated signaling was further enhanced in lungs of CHIT1 and TGF-β1 double transgenic mice (Lee et al., 2019). These studies suggest that CHIT1 is required and sufficient for the development of pulmonary fibrosis in that TGF-β1 plays a critical role.

CHIT1 Interacts With Tgfbrap1 and FoxO3 as a Mechanism to Enhance TGF-β Signaling

Since CHIT1 can be found in both extracellular and intracellular compartments, it is reasonable to assume specific receptors or interacting partners are mediating CHIT1 effects in the lung. On this regard, potential CHIT1 binding partners were first defined using a yeast 2 hybrid (Y2H) screening assay with a lung cDNA library (Lee et al., 2019). This approach identified transforming growth factor receptor beta associate protein 1 (Tgfbrap1) and forkhead box O3 (FoxO3) as CHIT1-interacting proteins. Tgfbrap1 has been reported to be a chaperone for Smad signaling (Wurthner et al., 2001) and FoxO3 is a transcription factor for multiple genes that play critical roles in metabolism, cellular stress response, tissue remodeling, and disease progression (Nho and Hergert, 2014; Webb et al., 2016). Recently, FoxO3 was reported as a key regulator of pulmonary fibrosis (Al-Tamari et al., 2018). The co-immunoprecipitation (Co-IP) and immunoblot (IB) assay and double immunohistochemistry (IHC) evaluations of cells transfected with CHIT1, Tgfbrap1 and FoxO3 demonstrated significant molecular interactions between CHIT1 and Tgfbrap1 or FoxO3 (Lee et al., 2019). In these evaluations, it is interesting to note that the CHIT1 negatively regulates the expression of Smad7, one of the inhibitor smads, through interaction with FoxO3, that potentially provide positive feedback loop to further enhance TGF-β signaling and effector fucntion through CHIT-Tgfbrap1 interactions.

In summary, recent studies strongly support an important role of CHIT1 in the pathogenesis of pulmonary fibrosis *via* modulation of TGF-β1 signaling and effector function. They also highlight that CHIT1 uses Tgfbrap1 and FoxO3 as interacting partners to regulate canonical and non-canonical TGF-β1 signaling and Smad7 expression as schematically illustrated in **Figure 2**. These studies provide strong supportive evidence for introducing CHIT1 inhibitor(s) as a novel therapeutic drug for pulmonary fibrosis. However, details of protein-protein interactions between CHIT1 and its interacting partners and their specific role in profibrotic macrophage and fibroblasts activation remain to be determined.

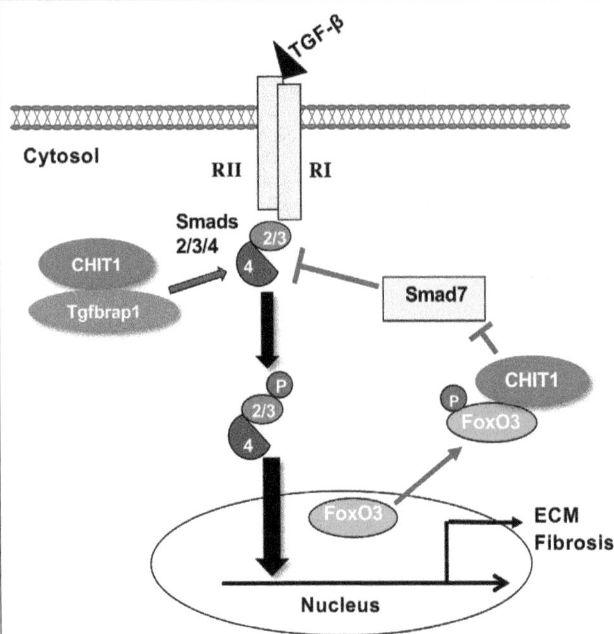

FIGURE 2 | Suggested pathway that chitinase 1 uses to regulate TGF-β signaling. Chitinase 1 (CHIT1) binds with transforming growth factor beta receptor associated protein 1 (Tgfbrap1), enhances the canonical receptor mediated Smads2/3 signaling potentially through recruiting of Co-Smad4. CHIT1 also interacts with transcription factor forkhead box O3 (FoxO3) that reduces the nuclear FoxO3 and that results into decreased the Smad7 expression. RI, TGF-β receptor 1; RII, TGF-β receptor 2; p, phosphorylation; ECM, extracellular matrix proteins.

Role and Mechanism of CHI3L1 in the Regulation of Pulmonary Fibrosis

CHI3L1 (also referred to as YKL-40 in human and Chil1/BRP-39 in mice (Lee and Elias, 2010)), a prototype of chitinase-like proteins, binds to chitin but does not cleave it (Lee et al., 2009). The importance of CHI3L1 can be readily appreciated in the diseases characterized by inflammation and remodeling in which CHI3L1 excess has been documented (Recklies et al., 2002; Sohn et al., 2010; Areshkov et al., 2012; Dela Cruz et al., 2012). In many of these disorders, CHI3L1 is likely produced as a protective response based on its ability to simultaneously decrease epithelial cell apoptosis while stimulating fibroproliferative repair. In patients with IPF, high serum and lung levels of CHI3L1 can be detected and are associated with poor survival (Korthagen et al., 2011; Lee et al., 2011). These findings support the major role of CHI3L1 in fibroproliferative responses including pulmonary fibrosis. However, the roles of CHI3L1 in these diseases have not been fully elucidated because the biologic functions of CHI3L1 and the mechanisms by which they are mediated have only recently begun to be studied.

CHI3L1 Expression in Human Lung Fibrosis

CHI3L1 is implicated as a serum biomarker in diseases with fibrosis, inflammation, and tissue remodeling. In IPF, serum and BALF CHI3L1 levels are significantly higher in IPF patients than in controls, and increased CHI3L1 expression was observed in alveolar macrophages and bronchiolar epithelial cells adjacent to fibrotic lesions (Furuhashi et al., 2010). Importantly, the circulatory levels of CHI3L1 are inversely correlated with prognosis of the patients. Recent epidemiologic studies including 85 patients with IPF, and 126 controls demonstrated that high serum and BALF CHI3L1 levels are associated with poor survival: IPF patients with high serum or high BALF CHI3L1 levels had significantly shorter survival than those with low CHI3L1 levels in serum or BALF (Korthagen et al., 2011). Notably, in patients with both low serum and low BALF CHI3L1 levels, no IPF related mortality was observed, suggesting that serum CHI3L1 could be a useful prognostic marker (Korthagen et al., 2011). Consistent with these reports, a significant increase in both quantities and percentages of CHI3L1-expresssing macrophages and epithelial cells in IPF lungs. In addition, in a cohort of 64 IPF patients and 42 age-matched controls, CHI3L1 levels were elevated in patients with IPF, and high levels of CHI3L1 are associated with severe disease progression as defined by lung transplantation or death (Zhou et al., 2014). Since then, numerus studies have showed that the serum CHI3L1 levels are increased in patients with other types of ILD, including connective tissue-related ILD (Hozumi et al., 2017; Furukawa et al., 2019; Jiang et al., 2019), sarcoidosis (Johansen et al., 2005; Kruit et al., 2007), cryptogenic tissue pneumonia (Korthagen et al., 2014; Long et al., 2017), asbestosis-ILD (Väänänen et al., 2017), and idiopathic nonspecific interstitial (Korthagen et al., 2014; Long et al., 2017).

CHI3L1 and its Receptors

Because CHI3L1 lacks enzymatic activity, recent studies were undertaken to identify if CHI3L1 mediates its effector functions through novel cell surface receptors. Yeast Two Hybrid (Y2H) screening and other binding and cellular approaches demonstrate that CHI3L1 binds to, signals and confers tissue responses *via* at least two receptor complexes: IL-13Rα2 (and its beta subunit transmembrane protein 219 (TMEM 219)) and CRTH2 (Chemoattractant Receptor-homologous molecule expressed on Th2 cells) (He et al., 2013; Zhou et al., 2015). These studies further revealed that IL-13Rα2/TMEM219 is expressed on lung epithelial cells and mediates CHI3L1's protective effects against cell death. On the other hand, CHI3L1 interacts with CRTH2 and promotes fibrosis *via* a mechanism that involves fibroblast proliferation and matrix deposition.

CRTH2 is a G-protein coupled receptor that binds with Prostaglandin D2 (PGD2). The interactions between CHI3L1 and CRTH2 have been further verified with co-Immunoprecipitation and immunoblot assay and co-localization immunohistochemistry (IHC) (Zhou et al., 2015). CRTH2 played an important role in augmenting CHI3L1-medaited fibroproliferative responses because collagen accumulation and extracellular gene expression were significantly reduced in the mice lacking CRTH2 or in mice treated with a CRTH2 inhibitor (Cay10471) (Zhou et al., 2015). Consistent with these findings, a recent study indicated that CRTH2 contributed to the development of fibrosis in kidney (Ito et al., 2012).

Gal-3 is a β-galactoside–binding lectin with pro-fibrotic effects (Young et al., 2006; Cullinane et al., 2014; Li et al., 2014). Further studies demonstrate that Gal-3 interferes with CHI3L1 signaling by competing for IL-13Rα2 binding. As a result, Gal-3 diminishes the anti-apoptotic effects of CHI3L1 in epithelial cells while increasing macrophage Wnt/ß-catenin signaling (Zhou et al., 2018). Therefore, Gal-3 contributes to the exaggerated injury and fibroproliferative repair response by altering the anti-apoptotic and fibroproliferative effects of CHI3L1 and its receptors.

Geng et al. demonstrated that CHI3L1 physically interacts with CD44, a cell-surface transmembrane glycoprotein involved in cell growth, survival, and differentiation. They elegantly showed that the interaction between CHI3L1 and CD44 activated the Erk and Akt pathways, along with phosphorylation of β-catenin (Geng et al., 2018). Other potential CHI3L1 receptors/binding partners include heparin and heparin-like molecules (Ngernyuang et al., 2018), and hyaluronic acid (Nishikawa and Millis, 2003; Zheng et al., 2005). However, the specific roles of CD44, heparin-like molecules, and hyaluronic acid and their interactions with CHI3L1 in the pathogenesis of pulmonary fibrosis remain to be determined.

CHI3L1 and cells Implicated in the Pathogenesis of Pulmonary Fibrosis

Abundant data indicate that profibrotic macrophages (traditionally called as M2 alternatively activated macrophages) play an important role in the development of lung fibrosis. Macrophages remain as a major cellular source of CHI3L1 production in IPF lungs (Furuhashi et al., 2010; Zhou et al., 2014). Murine bleomycin lung fibrosis model showed a predominant shift toward alternative macrophage activation in CHI3L1 overexpressing Tg mice, and eradication of these profibrotic macrophages is sufficient to reduce tissue fibrosis (Zhou et al., 2014). Consistently, $CD206^+$ alternatively activated, profibrotic macrophages are increased in the IPF lung, and circulating monocytes of IPF patients exhibit increased expression of alternative activation marker CD206 (Zhou et al., 2014).

The role of CHI3L1 on fibroblast proliferation/differentiation was explored using a three-dimensional cell culture model (Zhou et al., 2014). These studies demonstrated that, in contrast to unstimulated cells, fibroblasts grown in the presence of recombinant CHI3L1 showed increased cell density, and increased proliferation. Additionally, the addition of CHI3L1 was sufficient to modestly induce α-SMA detection in MRC5 cells cultured in this model, and a contractile fibroblast phenotype was observed as shown by the shrinking and rupture of the matrix slices (Zhou et al., 2014). It was reported that the CD44, a putative receptor for CHI3L1 (Cohen et al., 2017), mediates invasive fibroblasts phenotypes leading to severe lung fibrosis (Li et al., 2011). Recent studies reported that CHI3L1 induces the expression of PD-L1 in various lung cells (Ma et al., 2021) and the increased expression of PD-L1 is a major characteristic of transformed and invasive fibroblasts (Geng et al., 2019). These findings show that CHI3L1 directly regulates fibroblast proliferation, and to a smaller extent, myofibroblast transformation with invasive nature, thereby demonstrating a role for CHI3L1 in the regulation of all three phases of the fibroblast-mediated fibrotic responses.

The role of Gal-3 and its interactions with CHI3L1 and/or its receptor components in fibroproliferative repair response was explored in macrophages and fibroblasts. These studies demonstrate that Gal-3 is up-regulated in murine models of pulmonary fibrosis. Interestingly, these studies demonstrated spatial differences in its cellular and tissue effects: Extracellular Gal-3 drives epithelial apoptosis when in the extracellular space while intracellular accumulation of Gal3 in fibroblasts and macrophages stimulates fibroblast proliferation, myofibroblast differentiation and profibrotic macrophage differentiation (Zhou et al., 2018).

CHI3L1 and its Receptors in Hermansky-Pudlak Syndrome-Associated Lung Fibrosis

Hermansky-Pudlack Syndrome (HPS) is a rare, genetic, multisystem disorder characterized by oculocutaneous albinism (OCA), bleeding diathesis, immunodeficiency, granulomatous colitis, and pulmonary fibrosis (Gahl and Huizing, 2012). Ten genetic subtypes (HPS1-10) have been described with each mutation affecting the function of lysosome-related organelles (LROs) (Schinella et al., 1980; Anderson et al., 2003). The dysfunction of melanosomes accounts for the oculocutaneous albinism and visual impairment found in all HPS patients ((Gahl et al., 1998)). The dysfunction of platelet dense granules accounts for the bleeding disorder that is often the presenting complaint of the disease ((Hermansky and Pudlak, 1959; Gahl et al., 1998)). Ceroid deposition also occurs in multiple organs, and inflammatory bowel disease has been reported in various subtypes of HPS (Schinella et al., 1980; Mahadeo et al., 1991; Parker et al., 1997; Tsilou et al., 2004). Pulmonary Fibrosis has been appreciated in HPS-1 and HPS-4 patients, whose genetic defects are in biogenesis of lysosome-related organelle complex 3 (BLOC-3), which includes HPS1 and HPS4 proteins, and, less commonly, HPS-2 patients (Brantly et al., 2000; Anderson et al., 2003; Chiang et al., 2003; Li et al., 2004; Carmona-Rivera et al., 2013). Due to the untreatable and progressive nature of the pulmonary fibrosis of HPS, this complication is the leading cause of death (Pierson et al., 2006). However, there is no way to predict in which HPS-1 or HPS-4 patients are at risk for lung disease, or which patients will progress most rapidly. In addition, although it is known that murine genetic models of HPS-1 manifest exaggerated injury and fibroproliferative repair responses to fibrogenic agents like bleomycin (Young et al., 2007), the mechanism(s) by which LRO-related defects in trafficking lead to injury and fibrosis have not been adequately defined.

Zhou et al. found that in HPS, levels of CHI3L1 are higher in patients with HPS-PF in comparison with patients without pulmonary fibrosis, where higher levels are associated with greater disease severity (Zhou et al., 2015). In murine models, the animals with BLOC-3 mutation have a defect in the ability of CHI3L1 to restrain epithelial cell death, yet CHI3L1 exhibits exaggerated fibroproliferative effects, promoting fibrosis by

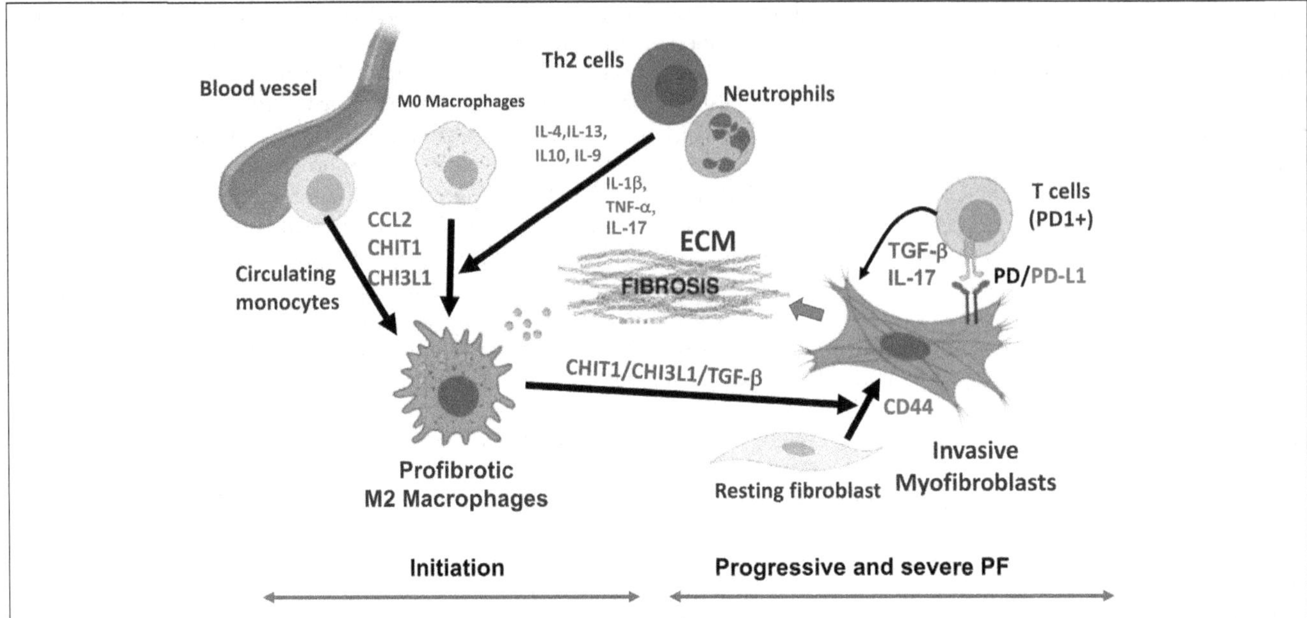

FIGURE 3 | Schematic illustration of hypothetical pathway leading to the development of profibrotic macrophages and invasive fibroblasts in the pathogenesis of pulmonary fibrosis (PF). Although multiple cells and mediators are involved in this process, implication of CHIT1/CHI3L1 and PD-1/PD-L1 axis are highlighted as major players in the development of profibrotic macrophages and invasive fibroblasts/myofibroblasts leading to progressive and severe pulmonary fibrosis through suggested heterocellular interactions. As indicated, fibrotic macrophages are recruited from the circulatory monocytes potentially through CCL2, CHIT1 or CHI3L1 then develops to alternatively activated profibrotic macrophages that highly expressing CHIT1, CHI3L1 and TGF-β. These mediators synergistically interact to transform resting fibroblasts to myofibroblasts with invasive nature through CD44. PD-L1 expressing invasive fibroblasts interact with PD-1 (+) T cells that further induce the profibrotic mediators including TGF-β and IL-17, that resulted into fibrotic tissue response with excessive extracellular matrix (ECM) accumulation. Th2 cytokines (IL-4, IL-13, IL-10, and IL-9) and proinflammatory cytokines (IL-1β, TNF-α, and IL-17) from TH2 cells and neutrophils can also contribute to profibrotic macrophage activation and subsequent fibroblasts proliferation and activation leading to pulmonary fibrosis (*The image is created with BioRender.com*).

inducing alternative macrophage activation and fibroblast proliferation (Zhou et al., 2015). The two distinctive features of CHI3L1 are mediated by trafficking of two CHI3LI receptors, IL-13Rα2 and CRTH2. The increase of apoptosis results from the abnormal localization of IL-13Rα2, which is caused by the dysfunction of BLOC-3. Fibrotic effects were caused by interactions between CHI3L1 and CRTH2 receptors which traffic normally (Zhou et al., 2015). These studies suggest that CHI3L1 and its receptors are dysregulated and play critical roles in the generation and progression of lung fibrosis associated with HPS. In addition, these responses are largely mediated by CRTH2, which may serve as a therapeutic target. Multiple clinical trials were designed to assess the effects of CRTH2 antagonism on asthma control. Future studies will be required to explore the possibility of repurposing these small molecular CRTH2 antagonists for HPS-PF treatment.

Strong evidence has indicated a critical role of Gal-3 in the development of HPS-PF. In samples from HPS-1 patients, AT2 cells, alveolar macrophages, and fibroblasts have high levels of Gal-3 expression and intracellular accumulation. It is speculated that the accumulation of Gal-3 in the cells of HPS individuals can be explained by the abnormal trafficking in the endosomal recycling compartment, which can contribute to fibrogenesis in HPS-PF (Cullinane et al., 2014). Consistently, murine studies have found that Gal-3 has increased levels in the extracellular space, traffics abnormally, and accumulates in lung fibroblasts and macrophages. Extracellular Gal-3 stimulates epithelial apoptosis and intracellular Gal-3 enhances fibroblast survival and proliferation as well as myofibroblast and macrophage differentiation. It can be speculated that Gal-3-based therapies may very well act in an additive or synergistic manner with interventions that augment membrane expression of IL-13Rα2 or block CRTH2. Additional investigations will be required to assess the utility of each of these approaches.

CHIT1/CHI3L1 in Collagen Stability and Bioactivity

As discussed above, ChIT1 and CHI3L1 distinctly contribute to pulmonary fibrosis using unique receptors or interacting molecules and signaling pathways. However, CHIT1 and CHI3L1 also have similar regulatory functions in the development of profibrotic macrophage activation, fibroblasts proliferation and myofibroblasts differentiation, the major hallmarks of pulmonary fibrosis. These studies suggest a possibility that CHIT1 and CHI3L1 can share specific biologic function that are independent of their receptors or interacting partners. Both CHIT1 and CHI3L1, as members of 18 Glycosyl hydrolase family, contain carbohydrate binding domain or motif (CBD or CBM) that has a binding ability with various forms of carbohydrates including chitin, hyaluronan and collagens (Crasson et al., 2017). Studies also suggest that the CBD is a critical region determining the biologic activity of CHIT1 and CHI3L1 (Chen et al., 2011; Crasson et al., 2017). However, the details of physical binding between CHIT1 or CHI3L1 with collagens through CBD and its effect on the profibrotic macrophage activation or myofibroblast transformation remain to be determined.

CHIT1/CHI3L1 as Modifiers of TGF-β Expression and its Signaling

As discussed earlier, TGF-β is a potent profibrotic cytokine that mediates pulmonary fibrosis especially associated with profibrotic activity of CHIT1. It is interesting to note that CHI3L1 was also reported to increase the expression of TGF-β and its signaling in the lung (He et al., 2013). This means that both CHIT1 and CHI3L1 could modulate the effector function of TGF-β possibly through synergistic fashion where these moieties are co-expressed. However, the interactions between these two in the pathogenesis of pulmonary fibrosis has not been determined. Since other genes, such as Wilms' tumor 1 (WT-1) or transforming growth factor alpha (TGF-α), also significantly regulate the expression and or signaling of TGF-β directly or indirectly, indued fibrotic tissue responses especailly in distal areas of lung (Madala et al., 2014; Sontake et al., 2018). If this is the case, whether and how the CHIT1/CHI3L1 axis is implicated in the development both parenchymal and subpleural fibrosis by activating TGF-β signaling would be an interesting question to be determined.

CHIT1/CHI3L1 in Heterocellular Crosstalk in Progressive Pulmonary Fibrosis

As discussed before, IPF is a disease characterized by the excessive accumulation of extracellular matrix (ECM) in the lung parenchyma with an unchecked, vicious cycle of repeated injury and abnormal repair responses. Thus, it is reasonable to speculate that there could be a temporal association between the emergence of profibrotic macrophages and invasive fibroblasts during the progression of pulmonary fibrosis and a potential positive feedback loop to generate a pathologic progressive fibrosis. If this is the case, the heterocellular crosstalk between "profibrotic macrophages" and "invasive fibroblasts" could be the major component of the profibrotic microenvironment responsible for progressive pulmonary fibrosis. In addition, the PD-1/PD-L1 axis is another fibrosis regulatory mechanism that consists of a positive feedback loop between PD-L1$^+$ invasive fibroblasts and PD-1$^+$CD4$^+$ T cells and contributes to progressive fibrosis through enhanced expression of TGF-β and IL-17 (Celada et al., 2018). Since CHIT1 and CHI3L1 play an essential role in these processes, targeting CHIT1 or CHI3L1 or both would be an effective therapeutic strategy that potentially blocks or reverses ongoing fibrosis as schematically illustrated in **Figure 3**.

SUMMARY

Recently, increasing number of studies are demonstrating that chitinase and chitinase like proteins (C/CLPs) represented by CHIT1 and CHI3L1 are significantly implicated in the pathogenesis of various human diseases including pulmonary fibrosis. However, the C/CLPs biology underlying specific pathologic process of the diseases has not been fully understood. A substantial body of literatures are strongly support that both CHIT1 and CHI3L1 contribute to the development and progression of pulmonary fibrosis through regulation of profibrotic macrophage activation and/or invasive myofibroblast differentiation. However, no data are currently available to support whether CHIT1 and CHI3L1 regulation of fibroproliferative cellular and tissue responses occurs in an independent manner or dependently each other. Since CHI3L1 does not have enzyme activity while retaining binding capacity with same substrates that CHIT1 uses, we speculate that CBD, not catalytic domain, is likely to function as a major domain responsible for profibrotic activities. Thus, development of antifibrotic therapeutics against CBD would be a reasonable strategy to block bioactivities of CHIT1 and CHI3L1. In addition, further mechanistic understanding on the putative receptors and interacting partners of CHIT1 and CHI3L1 in profibrotic macrophage activation and invasive fibroblast differentiation and their heterocellular interactions will be crucial for the development of effective therapeutics targeting CHIT1 and CHI3L1 for the patients with progressive pulmonary fibrosis.

AUTHOR CONTRIBUTIONS

Conception and design: YZ, CL; Data collection: S-YL, C-ML, BM, and SK; Analysis and interpretation: JAE, YZ, and CL; Drafting the manuscript for important intellectual content: S-YL, YZ, CL.

REFERENCES

Al-Tamari, H. M., Dabral, S., Schmall, A., Sarvari, P., Ruppert, C., Paik, J., et al. (2018). FoxO3 an Important Player in Fibrogenesis and Therapeutic Target for Idiopathic Pulmonary Fibrosis. *EMBO Mol. Med.* 10 (2), 276–293. doi:10.15252/emmm.201606261

Anderson, P. D., Huizing, M., Claassen, D. A., White, J., and Gahl, W. A. (2003). Hermansky-Pudlak Syndrome Type 4 (HPS-4): Clinical and Molecular Characteristics. *Hum. Genet.* 113 (1), 10–17. doi:10.1007/s00439-003-0933-5

Aran, D., Looney, A. P., Liu, L., Wu, E., Fong, V., Hsu, A., et al. (2019). Reference-based Analysis of Lung Single-Cell Sequencing Reveals a Transitional Profibrotic Macrophage. *Nat. Immunol.* 20 (2), 163–172. doi:10.1038/s41590-018-0276-y

Areshkov, P. O., Avdieiev, S. S., Balynska, O. V., Leroith, D., and Kavsan, V. M. (2012). Two Closely Related Human Members of Chitinase-like Family, CHI3L1 and CHI3L2, Activate ERK1/2 in 293 and U373 Cells but Have the

Different Influence on Cell Proliferation. *Int. J. Biol. Sci.* 8 (1), 39–48. doi:10.7150/ijbs.8.39

Ayaub, E., Poli, S., Ng, J. J., Adams, T. S., Schupp, J. C., Quesada-Arias, L. D., et al. (2021). Single Cell RNA-Seq and Mass Cytometry Reveals a Novel and a Targetable Population of Macrophages in Idiopathic Pulmonary Fibrosis. *bioRxiv.* doi:10.1101/2021.01.04.425268

Bellaye, P. S., Shimbori, C., Upagupta, C., Sato, S., Shi, W., Gauldie, J., et al. (2018). Lysyl Oxidase-like 1 Protein Deficiency Protects Mice from Adenoviral Transforming Growth Factor-B1-Induced Pulmonary Fibrosis. *Am. J. Respir. Cel Mol Biol* 58 (4), 461–470. doi:10.1165/rcmb.2017-0252OC

Boot, R. G., Blommaart, E. F., Swart, E., Ghauharali-van der Vlugt, K., Bijl, N., Moe, C., et al. (2001). Identification of a Novel Acidic Mammalian Chitinase Distinct from Chitotriosidase. *J. Biol. Chem.* 276 (9), 6770–6778. doi:10.1074/jbc.M009886200

Brantly, M., Avila, N. A., Shotelersuk, V., Lucero, C., Huizing, M., and Gahl, W. A. (2000). Pulmonary Function and High-Resolution CT Findings in Patients with an Inherited Form of Pulmonary Fibrosis, Hermansky-Pudlak Syndrome, Due to Mutations in HPS-1. *Chest* 117 (1), 129–136. doi:10.1378/chest.117.1.129

Carmona-Rivera, C., Simeonov, D. R., Cardillo, N. D., Gahl, W. A., and Cadilla, C. L. (2013). A Divalent Interaction between HPS1 and HPS4 Is Required for the Formation of the Biogenesis of Lysosome-Related Organelle Complex-3 (BLOC-3). *Biochim. Biophys. Acta* 1833 (3), 468–478. doi:10.1016/j.bbamcr.2012.10.019

Celada, L. J., Kropski, J. A., Herazo-Maya, J. D., Luo, W., Creecy, A., Abad, A. T., et al. (2018). PD-1 Up-Regulation on CD4+ T Cells Promotes Pulmonary Fibrosis through STAT3-Mediated IL-17A and TGF-B1 Production. *Sci. Transl Med.* 10 (460), eaar8356. doi:10.1126/scitranslmed.aar8356

Chanda, D., Otoupalova, E., Smith, S. R., Volckaert, T., De Langhe, S. P., and Thannickal, V. J. (2019). Developmental Pathways in the Pathogenesis of Lung Fibrosis. *Mol. Aspects Med.* 65, 56–69. doi:10.1016/j.mam.2018.08.004

Chen, C. C., Llado, V., Eurich, K., Tran, H. T., and Mizoguchi, E. (2011). Carbohydrate-binding Motif in Chitinase 3-like 1 (CHI3L1/YKL-40) Specifically Activates Akt Signaling Pathway in Colonic Epithelial Cells. *Clin. Immunol.* 140 (3), 268–275. doi:10.1016/j.clim.2011.04.007

Chen, H., Qu, J., Huang, X., Kurundkar, A., Zhu, L., Yang, N., et al. (2016). Mechanosensing by the α6-integrin Confers an Invasive Fibroblast Phenotype and Mediates Lung Fibrosis. *Nat. Commun.* 7, 12564. doi:10.1038/ncomms12564

Chiang, P. W., Oiso, N., Gautam, R., Suzuki, T., Swank, R. T., and Spritz, R. A. (2003). The Hermansky-Pudlak Syndrome 1 (HPS1) and HPS4 Proteins Are Components of Two Complexes, BLOC-3 and BLOC-4, Involved in the Biogenesis of Lysosome-Related Organelles. *J. Biol. Chem.* 278 (22), 20332–20337. doi:10.1074/jbc.M300090200

Cho, S. J., Weiden, M. D., and Lee, C. G. (2015). Chitotriosidase in the Pathogenesis of Inflammation, Interstitial Lung Diseases and COPD. *Allergy Asthma Immunol. Res.* 7 (1), 14–21. doi:10.4168/aair.2015.7.1.14

Cohen, N., Shani, O., Raz, Y., Sharon, Y., Hoffman, D., Abramovitz, L., et al. (2017). Fibroblasts Drive an Immunosuppressive and Growth-Promoting Microenvironment in Breast Cancer via Secretion of Chitinase 3-like 1. *Oncogene* 36 (31), 4457–4468. doi:10.1038/onc.2017.65

Craig, V. J., Zhang, L., Hagood, J. S., and Owen, C. A. (2015). Matrix Metalloproteinases as Therapeutic Targets for Idiopathic Pulmonary Fibrosis. *Am. J. Respir. Cel Mol Biol* 53 (5), 585–600. doi:10.1165/rcmb.2015-0020TR

Crasson, O., Courtade, G., Léonard, R. R., Aachmann, F. L., Legrand, F., Parente, R., et al. (2017). Human Chitotriosidase: Catalytic Domain or Carbohydrate Binding Module, Who's Leading HCHT's Biological Function. *Sci. Rep.* 7 (1), 2768. doi:10.1038/s41598-017-02382-z

Cullinane, A. R., Yeager, C., Dorward, H., Carmona-Rivera, C., Wu, H. P., Moss, J., et al. (2014). Dysregulation of Galectin-3. Implications for Hermansky-Pudlak Syndrome Pulmonary Fibrosis. *Am. J. Respir. Cel Mol Biol* 50 (3), 605–613. doi:10.1165/rcmb.2013-0025OC

Daniels, C. E., Lasky, J. A., Limper, A. H., Mieras, K., Gabor, E., Schroeder, D. R., et al. (2010). Imatinib Treatment for Idiopathic Pulmonary Fibrosis: Randomized Placebo-Controlled Trial Results. *Am. J. Respir. Crit. Care Med.* 181 (6), 604–610. doi:10.1164/rccm.200906-0964OC

Dela Cruz, C. S., Liu, W., He, C. H., Jacoby, A., Gornitzky, A., Ma, B., et al. (2012). Chitinase 3-like-1 Promotes Streptococcus Pneumoniae Killing and Augments Host Tolerance to Lung Antibacterial Responses. *Cell Host Microbe* 12 (1), 34–46. doi:10.1016/j.chom.2012.05.017

Demedts, M., and Costabel, U. (2002). ATS/ERS International Multidisciplinary Consensus Classification of the Idiopathic Interstitial Pneumonias. *Eur. Respir. J.* 19 (5), 794–796. doi:10.1183/09031936.02.00492002

Elias, J. A., Homer, R. J., Hamid, Q., and Lee, C. G. (2005). Chitinases and Chitinase-like Proteins in T(H)2 Inflammation and Asthma. *J. Allergy Clin. Immunol.* 116 (3), 497–500. doi:10.1016/j.jaci.2005.06.028

Elmonem, M. A., van den Heuvel, L. P., and Levtchenko, E. N. (2016). Immunomodulatory Effects of Chitotriosidase Enzyme. *Enzyme Res.* 2016, 2682680. doi:10.1155/2016/2682680

Furuhashi, K., Suda, T., Nakamura, Y., Inui, N., Hashimoto, D., Miwa, S., et al. (2010). Increased Expression of YKL-40, a Chitinase-like Protein, in Serum and Lung of Patients with Idiopathic Pulmonary Fibrosis. *Respir. Med.* 104 (8), 1204–1210. doi:10.1016/j.rmed.2010.02.026

Furukawa, T., Matsui, K., Kitano, M., Yokoyama, Y., Sekiguchi, M., Azuma, N., et al. (2019). Relationship between YKL-40 and Pulmonary Arterial Hypertension in Systemic Sclerosis. *Mod. Rheumatol.* 29 (3), 476–483. doi:10.1080/14397595.2018.1480256

Gahl, W., and Huizing, M. (2012). "Hermansky-Pudlak Syndrome," in *GeneReviews at GeneTests: Medical Genetics Information Resource* (Seattle, WA: University of Washington), 1997–2010. Available at: http://www.genetests.org.

Gahl, W. A., Brantly, M., Kaiser-Kupfer, M. I., Iwata, F., Hazelwood, S., Shotelersuk, V., et al. (1998). Genetic Defects and Clinical Characteristics of Patients with a Form of Oculocutaneous Albinism (Hermansky-Pudlak Syndrome). *N. Engl. J. Med.* 338 (18), 1258–1264. doi:10.1056/NEJM199804303381803

Gauldie, J. (2002). Pro: Inflammatory Mechanisms Are a Minor Component of the Pathogenesis of Idiopathic Pulmonary Fibrosis. *Am. J. Respir. Crit. Care Med.* 165 (9), 1205–1206. doi:10.1164/rccm.2202054

Geng, B., Pan, J., Zhao, T., Ji, J., Zhang, C., Che, Y., et al. (2018). Chitinase 3-like 1-CD44 Interaction Promotes Metastasis and Epithelial-To-Mesenchymal Transition through β-catenin/Erk/Akt Signaling in Gastric Cancer. *J. Exp. Clin. Cancer Res.* 37 (1), 208. doi:10.1186/s13046-018-0876-2

Geng, Y., Liu, X., Liang, J., Habiel, D. M., Kulur, V., Coelho, A. L., et al. (2019). PD-L1 on Invasive Fibroblasts Drives Fibrosis in a Humanized Model of Idiopathic Pulmonary Fibrosis. *JCI Insight* 4 (6). doi:10.1172/jci.insight.125326

Gu, L., Surolia, R., Larson-Casey, J. L., He, C., Davis, D., Kang, J., et al. (2021). Targeting Cpt1a-Bcl-2 Interaction Modulates Apoptosis Resistance and Fibrotic Remodeling. *Cell Death Differ.* doi:10.1038/s41418-021-00840-w

Hashimoto, N., Phan, S. H., Imaizumi, K., Matsuo, M., Nakashima, H., Kawabe, T., et al. (2010). Endothelial-mesenchymal Transition in Bleomycin-Induced Pulmonary Fibrosis. *Am. J. Respir. Cel Mol Biol* 43 (2), 161–172. doi:10.1165/rcmb.2009-0031OC

He, C. H., Lee, C. G., Dela Cruz, C. S., Lee, C. M., Zhou, Y., Ahangari, F., et al. (2013). Chitinase 3-like 1 Regulates Cellular and Tissue Responses via IL-13 Receptor α2. *Cell Rep* 4 (4), 830–841. doi:10.1016/j.celrep.2013.07.032

Hermansky, F., and Pudlak, P. (1959). Albinism Associated with Hemorrhagic Diathesis and Unusual Pigmented Reticular Cells in the Bone Marrow: Report of Two Cases with Histochemical Studies. *Blood* 14 (2), 162–169. doi:10.1182/blood.v14.2.162.162

Hinz, B., and Lagares, D. (2020). Evasion of Apoptosis by Myofibroblasts: a Hallmark of Fibrotic Diseases. *Nat. Rev. Rheumatol.* 16 (1), 11–31. doi:10.1038/s41584-019-0324-5

Hong, J. Y., Kim, M., Sol, I. S., Kim, K. W., Lee, C. M., Elias, J. A., et al. (2018). Chitotriosidase Inhibits Allergic Asthmatic Airways via Regulation of TGF-β Expression and Foxp3+ Treg Cells. *Allergy* 73 (8), 1686–1699. doi:10.1111/all.13426

Hozumi, H., Fujisawa, T., Enomoto, N., Nakashima, R., Enomoto, Y., Suzuki, Y., et al. (2017). Clinical Utility of YKL-40 in Polymyositis/dermatomyositis-Associated Interstitial Lung Disease. *J. Rheumatol.* 44 (9), 1394–1401. doi:10.3899/jrheum.170373

Hung, C. (2020). Origin of Myofibroblasts in Lung Fibrosis. *Curr. Tissue Microenviron. Rep.* 1 (4), 155–162. doi:10.1007/s43152-020-00022-9

Idiopathic Pulmonary Fibrosis Clinical Research, N., Raghu, G., Anstrom, K. J., King, T. E., Jr., Lasky, J. A., and Martinez, F. J. (2012). Prednisone, Azathioprine, and N-Acetylcysteine for Pulmonary Fibrosis. *N. Engl. J. Med.* 366 (21), 1968–1977. doi:10.1056/NEJMoa1113354

Ito, H., Yan, X., Nagata, N., Aritake, K., Katsumata, Y., Matsuhashi, T., et al. (2012). PGD2-CRTH2 Pathway Promotes Tubulointerstitial Fibrosis. *J. Am. Soc. Nephrol.* 23 (11), 1797–1809. doi:10.1681/ASN.2012020126

James, A. J., Reinius, L. E., Verhoek, M., Gomes, A., Kupczyk, M., Hammar, U., et al. (2016). Increased YKL-40 and Chitotriosidase in Asthma and Chronic Obstructive Pulmonary Disease. *Am. J. Respir. Crit. Care Med.* 193 (2), 131–142. doi:10.1164/rccm.201504-0760OC

Jiang, L., Wang, Y., Peng, Q., Shu, X., Wang, G., and Wu, X. (2019). Serum YKL-40 Level Is Associated with Severity of Interstitial Lung Disease and Poor Prognosis in Dermatomyositis with Anti-MDA5 Antibody. *Clin. Rheumatol.* 38 (6), 1655–1663. doi:10.1007/s10067-019-04457-w

Johansen, J. S., Milman, N., Hansen, M., Garbarsch, C., Price, P. A., and Graudal, N. (2005). Increased Serum YKL-40 in Patients with Pulmonary Sarcoidosis-Aa Potential Marker of Disease Activity? *Respir. Med.* 99 (4), 396–402. doi:10.1016/j.rmed.2004.09.016

Kang, J., and Song, J. W. (2021). Effect of Sildenafil Added to Antifibrotic Treatment in Idiopathic Pulmonary Fibrosis. *Sci. Rep.* 11 (1), 17824. doi:10.1038/s41598-021-97396-z

Kanneganti, M., Kamba, A., and Mizoguchi, E. (2012). Role of Chitotriosidase (Chitinase 1) under normal and Disease Conditions. *J. Epithel Biol. Pharmacol.* 5, 1–9. doi:10.2174/1875044301205010001

Kasai, H., Allen, J. T., Mason, R. M., Kamimura, T., and Zhang, Z. (2005). TGF-beta1 Induces Human Alveolar Epithelial to Mesenchymal Cell Transition (EMT). *Respir. Res.* 6, 56. doi:10.1186/1465-9921-6-56

Kelly, M., Kolb, M., Bonniaud, P., and Gauldie, J. (2003). Re-evaluation of Fibrogenic Cytokines in Lung Fibrosis. *Curr. Pharm. Des.* 9 (1), 39–49. doi:10.2174/1381612033392341

Khalil, N., O'Connor, R. N., Flanders, K. C., and Unruh, H. (1996). TGF-beta 1, but Not TGF-Beta 2 or TGF-Beta 3, Is Differentially Present in Epithelial Cells of Advanced Pulmonary Fibrosis: an Immunohistochemical Study. *Am. J. Respir. Cel Mol Biol* 14 (2), 131–138. doi:10.1165/ajrcmb.14.2.8630262

Khalil, N., Parekh, T. V., O'Connor, R., Antman, N., Kepron, W., Yehaulaeshet, T., et al. (2001). Regulation of the Effects of TGF-Beta 1 by Activation of Latent TGF-Beta 1 and Differential Expression of TGF-Beta Receptors (T Beta R-I and T Beta R-II) in Idiopathic Pulmonary Fibrosis. *Thorax* 56 (12), 907–915. doi:10.1136/thorax.56.12.907

Kim, K. H., Burkhart, K., Chen, P., Frevert, C. W., Randolph-Habecker, J., Hackman, R. C., et al. (2005). Tissue Inhibitor of Metalloproteinase-1 Deficiency Amplifies Acute Lung Injury in Bleomycin-Exposed Mice. *Am. J. Respir. Cel Mol Biol* 33 (3), 271–279. doi:10.1165/rcmb.2005-0111OC

Kim, K. K., Kugler, M. C., Wolters, P. J., Robillard, L., Galvez, M. G., Brumwell, A. N., et al. (2006). Alveolar Epithelial Cell Mesenchymal Transition Develops *In Vivo* during Pulmonary Fibrosis and Is Regulated by the Extracellular Matrix. *Proc. Natl. Acad. Sci. U S A.* 103 (35), 13180–13185. doi:10.1073/pnas.0605669103

King, T. E., Jr., Bradford, W. Z., Castro-Bernardini, S., Fagan, E. A., Glaspole, I., Glassberg, M. K., et al. (2014). A Phase 3 Trial of Pirfenidone in Patients with Idiopathic Pulmonary Fibrosis. *N. Engl. J. Med.* 370 (22), 2083–2092. doi:10.1056/NEJMoa1402582

Korthagen, N. M., van Moorsel, C. H., Barlo, N. P., Ruven, H. J., Kruit, A., Heron, M., et al. (2011). Serum and BALF YKL-40 Levels Are Predictors of Survival in Idiopathic Pulmonary Fibrosis. *Respir. Med.* 105 (1), 106–113. doi:10.1016/j.rmed.2010.09.012

Korthagen, N. M., van Moorsel, C. H., Zanen, P., Ruven, H. J., and Grutters, J. C. (2014). Evaluation of Circulating YKL-40 Levels in Idiopathic Interstitial Pneumonias. *Lung* 192 (6), 975–980. doi:10.1007/s00408-014-9647-9

Krein, P. M., and Winston, B. W. (2002). Roles for Insulin-like Growth Factor I and Transforming Growth Factor-Beta in Fibrotic Lung Disease. *Chest* 122 (6 Suppl. l), 289S–293S. doi:10.1378/chest.122.6_suppl.289s

Kruit, A., Grutters, J. C., Ruven, H. J., van Moorsel, C. C., and van den Bosch, J. M. (2007). A CHI3L1 Gene Polymorphism Is Associated with Serum Levels of YKL-40, a Novel Sarcoidosis Marker. *Respir. Med.* 101 (7), 1563–1571. doi:10.1016/j.rmed.2006.12.006

Lee, C. G., Cho, S. J., Kang, M. J., Chapoval, S. P., Lee, P. J., Noble, P. W., et al. (2004). Early Growth Response Gene 1-mediated Apoptosis Is Essential for Transforming Growth Factor Beta1-Induced Pulmonary Fibrosis. *J. Exp. Med.* 200 (3), 377–389. doi:10.1084/jem.20040104

Lee, C. G., Da Silva, C. A., Dela Cruz, C. S., Ahangari, F., Ma, B., Kang, M. J., et al. (2011). Role of Chitin and Chitinase/chitinase-like Proteins in Inflammation, Tissue Remodeling, and Injury. *Annu. Rev. Physiol.* 73, 479–501. doi:10.1146/annurev-physiol-012110-142250

Lee, C. G., and Elias, J. A. (2010). Role of Breast Regression protein-39/YKL-40 in Asthma and Allergic Responses. *Allergy Asthma Immunol. Res.* 2 (1), 20–27. doi:10.4168/aair.2010.2.1.20

Lee, C. G., Hartl, D., Lee, G. R., Koller, B., Matsuura, H., Da Silva, C. A., et al. (2009). Role of Breast Regression Protein 39 (BRP-39)/chitinase 3-like-1 in Th2 and IL-13-induced Tissue Responses and Apoptosis. *J. Exp. Med.* 206 (5), 1149–1166. doi:10.1084/jem.20081271

Lee, C. G., Herzog, E. L., Ahangari, F., Zhou, Y., Gulati, M., Lee, C. M., et al. (2012). Chitinase 1 Is a Biomarker for and Therapeutic Target in Scleroderma-Associated Interstitial Lung Disease that Augments TGF-B1 Signaling. *J. Immunol.* 189 (5), 2635–2644. doi:10.4049/jimmunol.1201115

Lee, C. M., Cho, S. J., Cho, W. K., Park, J. W., Lee, J. H., Choi, A. M., et al. (2018). Laminin α1 Is a Genetic Modifier of TGF-B1-Stimulated Pulmonary Fibrosis. *JCI insight* 3 (18), e99574. doi:10.1172/jci.insight.99574

Lee, C. M., He, C. H., Park, J. W., Lee, J. H., Kamle, S., Ma, B., et al. (2019). Chitinase 1 Regulates Pulmonary Fibrosis by Modulating TGF-B/smad7 Pathway via TGFBRAP1 and FOXO3. *Life Sci. Alliance* 2 (3). doi:10.26508/lsa.201900350

Lee, J., and Song, J. U. (2020). The Clinical Efficacy of Pulmonary Hypertension-specific Agents in Idiopathic Pulmonary Fibrosis: Systematic Review and Meta-Analysis of Randomized Controlled Clinical Trials. *J. Korean Med. Sci.* 35 (8), e48–e. doi:10.3346/jkms.2020.35.e48

Ley, B., Collard, H. R., and King, T. E., Jr (2011). Clinical Course and Prediction of Survival in Idiopathic Pulmonary Fibrosis. *Am. J. Respir. Crit. Care Med.* 183 (4), 431–440. doi:10.1164/rccm.201006-0894CI

Li, L. C., Li, J., and Gao, J. (2014). Functions of Galectin-3 and its Role in Fibrotic Diseases. *J. Pharmacol. Exp. Ther.* 351 (2), 336–343. doi:10.1124/jpet.114.218370

Li, W., Rusiniak, M. E., Chintala, S., Gautam, R., Novak, E. K., and Swank, R. T. (2004). Murine Hermansky-Pudlak Syndrome Genes: Regulators of Lysosome-Related Organelles. *Bioessays* 26 (6), 616–628. doi:10.1002/bies.20042

Li, Y., Jiang, D., Liang, J., Meltzer, E. B., Gray, A., Miura, R., et al. (2011). Severe Lung Fibrosis Requires an Invasive Fibroblast Phenotype Regulated by Hyaluronan and CD44. *J. Exp. Med.* 208 (7), 1459–1471. doi:10.1084/jem.20102510

Long, X., He, X., Ohshimo, S., Griese, M., Sarria, R., Guzman, J., et al. (2017). Serum YKL-40 as Predictor of Outcome in Hypersensitivity Pneumonitis. *Eur. Respir. J.* 49 (2). doi:10.1183/13993003.01924-2015

Ma, B., Akosman, B., Kamle, S., Lee, C-M., Koo, J. S., Lee, C. G., et al. (2021). Chitinase 3-like-1 Stimulates PD-L1 and Other Immune Checkpoint Inhibitors. *bioRxiv.* doi:10.1101/2021.01.15.426788

Madala, S. K., Korfhagen, T. R., Schmidt, S., Davidson, C., Edukulla, R., Ikegami, M., et al. (2014). Inhibition of the αvβ6 Integrin Leads to Limited Alteration of TGF-α-Induced Pulmonary Fibrosis. *Am. J. Physiol. Lung Cel Mol Physiol* 306 (8), L726–L735. doi:10.1152/ajplung.00357.2013

Mahadeo, R., Markowitz, J., Fisher, S., and Daum, F. (1991). Hermansky-Pudlak Syndrome with Granulomatous Colitis in Children. *J. Pediatr.* 118 (6), 904–906. doi:10.1016/s0022-3476(05)82204-8

Merl-Pham, J., Basak, T., Knüppel, L., Ramanujam, D., Athanason, M., Behr, J., et al. (2019). Quantitative Proteomic Profiling of Extracellular Matrix and Site-specific Collagen post-translational Modifications in an *In Vitro* Model of Lung Fibrosis. *Matrix Biol. Plus* 1, 100005. doi:10.1016/j.mbplus.2019.04.002

Micallef, L., Vedrenne, N., Billet, F., Coulomb, B., Darby, I. A., and Desmoulière, A. (2012). The Myofibroblast, Multiple Origins for Major Roles in normal and Pathological Tissue Repair. *Fibrogenesis Tissue Repair* 5 (Suppl. 1), S5–S. doi:10.1186/1755-1536-5-S1-S5

Michaelson, J. E., Aguayo, S. M., and Roman, J. (2000). Idiopathic Pulmonary Fibrosis: a Practical Approach for Diagnosis and Management. *Chest* 118 (3), 788–794. doi:10.1378/chest.118.3.788

Misharin, A. V., Morales-Nebreda, L., Reyfman, P. A., Cuda, C. M., Walter, J. M., McQuattie-Pimentel, A. C., et al. (2017). Monocyte-derived Alveolar Macrophages Drive Lung Fibrosis and Persist in the Lung over the Life Span. *J. Exp. Med.* 214 (8), 2387–2404. doi:10.1084/jem.20162152

Müller, M., Strand, S., Hug, H., Heinemann, E. M., Walczak, H., Hofmann, W. J., et al. (1997). Drug-induced Apoptosis in Hepatoma Cells Is Mediated by the CD95 (APO-1/Fas) Receptor/ligand System and Involves Activation of Wild-type P53. *J. Clin. Invest.* 99 (3), 403–413. doi:10.1172/JCI119174

Myllärniemi, M., and Kaarteenaho, R. (2015). Pharmacological Treatment of Idiopathic Pulmonary Fibrosis - Preclinical and Clinical Studies of Pirfenidone, Nintedanib, and N-Acetylcysteine. *Eur. Clin. Respir. J.* 2. doi:10.3402/ecrj.v2.26385

Nakao, A., Fujii, M., Matsumura, R., Kumano, K., Saito, Y., Miyazono, K., et al. (1999). Transient Gene Transfer and Expression of Smad7 Prevents Bleomycin-Induced Lung Fibrosis in Mice. *J. Clin. Invest.* 104 (1), 5–11. doi:10.1172/JCI6094

Ngernyuang, N., Yan, W., Schwartz, L. M., Oh, D., Liu, Y. B., Chen, H., et al. (2018). A Heparin Binding Motif Rich in Arginine and Lysine Is the Functional Domain of YKL-40. *Neoplasia* 20 (2), 182–192. doi:10.1016/j.neo.2017.11.011

Nho, R. S., and Hergert, P. (2014). FoxO3a and Disease Progression. *World J. Biol. Chem.* 5 (3), 346–354. doi:10.4331/wjbc.v5.i3.346

Nishikawa, K. C., and Millis, A. J. (2003). gp38k (CHI3L1) Is a Novel Adhesion and Migration Factor for Vascular Cells. *Exp. Cel Res* 287 (1), 79–87. doi:10.1016/s0014-4827(03)00069-7

Noble, P. W., Albera, C., Bradford, W. Z., Costabel, U., Glassberg, M. K., Kardatzke, D., et al. (2011). Pirfenidone in Patients with Idiopathic Pulmonary Fibrosis (CAPACITY): Two Randomised Trials. *Lancet* 377 (9779), 1760–1769. doi:10.1016/S0140-6736(11)60405-4

Noth, I., Anstrom, K. J., Calvert, S. B., de Andrade, J., Flaherty, K. R., Glazer, C., et al. (2012). A Placebo-Controlled Randomized Trial of Warfarin in Idiopathic Pulmonary Fibrosis. *Am. J. Respir. Crit. Care Med.* 186 (1), 88–95. doi:10.1164/rccm.201202-0314OC

Pardo, A., Cabrera, S., Maldonado, M., and Selman, M. (2016). Role of Matrix Metalloproteinases in the Pathogenesis of Idiopathic Pulmonary Fibrosis. *Respir. Res.* 17, 23. doi:10.1186/s12931-016-0343-6

Parker, M. S., Rosado Shipley, W., de Christenson, M. L., Slutzker, A. D., Carroll, F. E., Worrell, J. A., et al. (1997). The Hermansky-Pudlak Syndrome. *Ann. Diagn. Pathol.* 1 (2), 99–103. doi:10.1016/s1092-9134(97)80014-7

Pierson, D. M., Ionescu, D., Qing, G., Yonan, A. M., Parkinson, K., Colby, T. C., et al. (2006). Pulmonary Fibrosis in Hermansky-Pudlak Syndrome. A Case Report and Review. *Respiration* 73 (3), 382–395. doi:10.1159/000091609

Raghu, G. (1998). in *Fishman's Pulmonary Diseases and Disorders*. Editors A. P. Fishman, J. A. Elias, J. A. Fishman, M. A. Grippi, R. KL, and R. M. Senior (N.Y., N.Y.: McGraw-Hill), 1037–1053.

Raghu, G., Behr, J., Brown, K. K., Egan, J. J., Kawut, S. M., Flaherty, K. R., et al. (2013). Treatment of Idiopathic Pulmonary Fibrosis with Ambrisentan: a Parallel, Randomized Trial. *Ann. Intern. Med.* 158 (9), 641–649. doi:10.7326/0003-4819-158-9-201305070-00003

Raghu, G., Rochwerg, B., Zhang, Y., Garcia, C. A., Azuma, A., Behr, J., et al. (2015). An Official ATS/ERS/JRS/ALAT Clinical Practice Guideline: Treatment of Idiopathic Pulmonary Fibrosis. An Update of the 2011 Clinical Practice Guideline. *Am. J. Respir. Crit. Care Med.* 192 (2), e3–19. doi:10.1164/rccm.201506-1063ST

Recklies, A. D., White, C., and Ling, H. (2002). The Chitinase 3-like Protein Human Cartilage Glycoprotein 39 (HC-Gp39) Stimulates Proliferation of Human Connective-Tissue Cells and Activates Both Extracellular Signal-Regulated Kinase- and Protein Kinase B-Mediated Signalling Pathways. *Biochem. J.* 365 (Pt 1), 119–126. doi:10.1042/BJ20020075

Richeldi, L., Davies, H. R., Ferrara, G., and Franco, F. (2003). Corticosteroids for Idiopathic Pulmonary Fibrosis. *Cochrane Database Syst. Rev.* 3, CD002880. doi:10.1002/14651858.CD002880

Richeldi, L., du Bois, R. M., Raghu, G., Azuma, A., Brown, K. K., Costabel, U., et al. (2014). Efficacy and Safety of Nintedanib in Idiopathic Pulmonary Fibrosis. *N. Engl. J. Med.* 370 (22), 2071–2082. doi:10.1056/NEJMoa1402584

Schinella, R. A., Greco, M. A., Cobert, B. L., Denmark, L. W., and Cox, R. P. (1980). Hermansky-Pudlak Syndrome with Granulomatous Colitis. *Ann. Intern. Med.* 92 (1), 20–23. doi:10.7326/0003-4819-92-1-20

Selman, M., King, T. E., and Pardo, A. (2001). Idiopathic Pulmonary Fibrosis: Prevailing and Evolving Hypotheses about its Pathogenesis and Implications for Therapy. *Ann. Intern. Med.* 134 (2), 136–151. doi:10.7326/0003-4819-134-2-200101160-00015

Sgalla, G., Iovene, B., Calvello, M., Ori, M., Varone, F., and Richeldi, L. (2018). Idiopathic Pulmonary Fibrosis: Pathogenesis and Management. *Respir. Res.* 19 (1), 32. doi:10.1186/s12931-018-0730-2

Sharma, L., Amick, A. K., Vasudevan, S., Lee, S. W., Marion, C. R., Liu, W., et al. (2018). Regulation and Role of Chitotriosidase during Lung Infection with *Klebsiella pneumoniae*. *J. Immunol.* 201 (2), 615–626. doi:10.4049/jimmunol.1701782

Sime, P. J., Xing, Z., Graham, F. L., Csaky, K. G., and Gauldie, J. (1997). Adenovector-mediated Gene Transfer of Active Transforming Growth Factor-Beta1 Induces Prolonged Severe Fibrosis in Rat Lung. *J. Clin. Invest.* 100 (4), 768–776. doi:10.1172/JCI119590

Sohn, M. H., Kang, M. J., Matsuura, H., Bhandari, V., Chen, N. Y., Lee, C. G., et al. (2010). The Chitinase-like Proteins Breast Regression Protein-39 and YKL-40 Regulate Hyperoxia-Induced Acute Lung Injury. *Am. J. Respir. Crit. Care Med.* 182 (7), 918–928. doi:10.1164/rccm.200912-1793OC

Sontake, V., Kasam, R. K., Sinner, D., Korfhagen, T. R., Reddy, G. B., White, E. S., et al. (2018). Wilms' Tumor 1 Drives Fibroproliferation and Myofibroblast Transformation in Severe Fibrotic Lung Disease. *JCI Insight* 3 (16). doi:10.1172/jci.insight.121252

Strieter, R. M. (2002). Con: Inflammatory Mechanisms Are Not a Minor Component of the Pathogenesis of Idiopathic Pulmonary Fibrosis. *Am. J. Respir. Crit. Care Med.* 165 (9), 1206–1208. doi:10.1164/rccm.2202055

Strykowski, R., and Adegunsoye, A. (2021). Molecular Pathways in Idiopathic Pulmonary Fibrosis Pathogenesis: Transcending Barriers to Optimally Targeted Pharmacotherapies. *EBioMedicine* 67, 103373. doi:10.1016/j.ebiom.2021.103373

Taniguchi, H., Ebina, M., Kondoh, Y., Ogura, T., Azuma, A., Suga, M., et al. (2010). Pirfenidone in Idiopathic Pulmonary Fibrosis. *Eur. Respir. J.* 35 (4), 821–829. doi:10.1183/09031936.00005209

Tjin, G., White, E. S., Faiz, A., Sicard, D., Tschumperlin, D. J., Mahar, A., et al. (2017). Lysyl Oxidases Regulate Fibrillar Collagen Remodelling in Idiopathic Pulmonary Fibrosis. *Dis. Model. Mech.* 10 (11), 1301–1312. doi:10.1242/dmm.030114

Tschopp, J., Irmler, M., and Thome, M. (1998). Inhibition of Fas Death Signals by FLIPs. *Curr. Opin. Immunol.* 10 (5), 552–558. doi:10.1016/s0952-7915(98)80223-9

Tsilou, E. T., Rubin, B. I., Reed, G. F., McCain, L., Huizing, M., White, J., et al. (2004). Milder Ocular Findings in Hermansky-Pudlak Syndrome Type 3 Compared with Hermansky-Pudlak Syndrome Type 1. *Ophthalmology* 111 (8), 1599–1603. doi:10.1016/j.ophtha.2003.12.058

Tsukui, T., Sun, K. H., Wetter, J. B., Wilson-Kanamori, J. R., Hazelwood, L. A., Henderson, N. C., et al. (2020). Collagen-producing Lung Cell Atlas Identifies Multiple Subsets with Distinct Localization and Relevance to Fibrosis. *Nat. Commun.* 11 (1), 1920. doi:10.1038/s41467-020-15647-5

Väänänen, T., Lehtimäki, L., Vuolteenaho, K., Hämäläinen, M., Oksa, P., Vierikko, T., et al. (2017). Glycoprotein YKL-40 Levels in Plasma Are Associated with Fibrotic Changes on HRCT in Asbestos-Exposed Subjects. *Mediators Inflamm.* 2017, 1797512. doi:10.1155/2017/1797512

van Eijk, M., van Roomen, C. P., Renkema, G. H., Bussink, A. P., Andrews, L., Blommaart, E. F., et al. (2005). Characterization of Human Phagocyte-Derived Chitotriosidase, a Component of Innate Immunity. *Int. Immunol.* 17 (11), 1505–1512. doi:10.1093/intimm/dxh328

Webb, A. E., Kundaje, A., and Brunet, A. (2016). Characterization of the Direct Targets of FOXO Transcription Factors throughout Evolution. *Aging Cell* 15 (4), 673–685. doi:10.1111/acel.12479

Wilson, M. S., and Wynn, T. A. (2009). Pulmonary Fibrosis: Pathogenesis, Etiology and Regulation. *Mucosal Immunol.* 2 (2), 103–121. doi:10.1038/mi.2008.85

Wollin, L., Wex, E., Pautsch, A., Schnapp, G., Hostettler, K. E., Stowasser, S., et al. (2015). Mode of Action of Nintedanib in the Treatment of Idiopathic Pulmonary Fibrosis. *Eur. Respir. J.* 45 (5), 1434–1445. doi:10.1183/09031936.00174914

Wolters, P. J., Collard, H. R., and Jones, K. D. (2014). Pathogenesis of Idiopathic Pulmonary Fibrosis. *Annu. Rev. Pathol. Mech. Dis.* 9 (1), 157–179. doi:10.1146/annurev-pathol-012513-104706

Wurthner, J. U., Frank, D. B., Felici, A., Green, H. M., Cao, Z., Schneider, M. D., et al. (2001). Transforming Growth Factor-Beta Receptor-Associated Protein 1 Is a Smad4 Chaperone. *J. Biol. Chem.* 276 (22), 19495–19502. doi:10.1074/jbc.M006473200

Wynn, T. A., and Vannella, K. M. (2016). Macrophages in Tissue Repair, Regeneration, and Fibrosis. *Immunity* 44 (3), 450–462. doi:10.1016/j.immuni.2016.02.015

Xu, Y. D., Hua, J., Mui, A., O'Connor, R., Grotendorst, G., and Khalil, N. (2003). Release of Biologically Active TGF-(beta)1 by Alveolar Epithelial Cells Results in Pulmonary Fibrosis. *Am. J. Physiol. (Lung Cel Mol Physiol).* 285, L527–L539. doi:10.1152/ajplung.00298.2002

Yano, H., Hamanaka, R., Nakamura-Ota, M., Zhang, J. J., Matsuo, N., and

Yoshioka, H. (2018). Regulation of Type I Collagen Expression by microRNA-29 Following Ionizing Radiation. *Radiat. Environ. Biophys.* 57 (1), 41 54. doi:10.1007/s00411-017-0723-4

Yehualaeshet, T., O Connor, R., Begleiter, A., Murphy-Ullrich, J. E., Silverstein, R., and Khalil, N. (2000). A CD36 Synthetic Peptide Inhibits Bleomycin-Induced Pulmonary Inflammation and Connective Tissue Synthesis in the Rat. *Am. J. Respir. Cel Mol Biol* 23 (2), 204–212. doi:10.1165/ajrcmb.23.2.4089

Young, L. R., Borchers, M. T., Allen, H. L., Gibbons, R. S., and McCormack, F. X. (2006). Lung-restricted Macrophage Activation in the Pearl Mouse Model of Hermansky-Pudlak Syndrome. *J. Immunol.* 176 (7), 4361–4368. doi:10.4049/jimmunol.176.7.4361

Young, L. R., Pasula, R., Gulleman, P. M., Deutsch, G. H., and McCormack, F. X. (2007). Susceptibility of Hermansky-Pudlak Mice to Bleomycin-Induced Type II Cell Apoptosis and Fibrosis. *Am. J. Respir. Cel Mol Biol* 37 (1), 67–74. doi:10.1165/rcmb.2006-0469OC

Yue, X., Shan, B., and Lasky, J. A. (2010). TGF-β: Titan of Lung Fibrogenesis. *Curr. Enzym Inhib.* 6 (2). doi:10.2174/10067

Zent, J., and Guo, L.' W. (2018). Signaling Mechanisms of Myofibroblastic Activation: Outside-In and Inside-Out. *Cell Physiol Biochem* 49 (3), 848–868. doi:10.1159/000493217

Zhao, T., Su, Z., Li, Y., Zhang, X., and You, Q. (2020). Chitinase-3 Like-Protein-1 Function and its Role in Diseases. *Signal. Transduct Target. Ther.* 5 (1), 201. doi:10.1038/s41392-020-00303-7

Zheng, M., Cai, W. M., Zhao, J. K., Zhu, S. M., and Liu, R. H. (2005). Determination of Serum Levels of YKL-40 and Hyaluronic Acid in Patients with Hepatic Fibrosis Due to Schistosomiasis Japonica and Appraisal of Their Clinical Value. *Acta Trop.* 96 (2-3), 148–152. doi:10.1016/j.actatropica.2005.07.009

Zhou, Y., He, C. H., Herzog, E. L., Peng, X., Lee, C. M., Nguyen, T. H., et al. (2015). Chitinase 3-like-1 and its Receptors in Hermansky-Pudlak Syndrome-Associated Lung Disease. *J. Clin. Invest.* 125 (8), 3178–3192. doi:10.1172/JCI79792

Zhou, Y., He, C. H., Yang, D. S., Nguyen, T., Cao, Y., Kamle, S., et al. (2018). Galectin-3 Interacts with the CHI3L1 Axis and Contributes to Hermansky-Pudlak Syndrome Lung Disease. *J. Immunol.* 200 (6), 2140–2153. doi:10.4049/jimmunol.1701442

Zhou, Y., Peng, H., Sun, H., Peng, X., Tang, C., Gan, Y., et al. (2014). Chitinase 3-like 1 Suppresses Injury and Promotes Fibroproliferative Responses in Mammalian Lung Fibrosis. *Sci. Transl Med.* 6 (240), 240ra76. doi:10.1126/scitranslmed.3007096

8

Tetrandrine Modulates Rheb-mTOR Signaling-Mediated Selective Autophagy and Protects Pulmonary Fibrosis

Yuanyuan Liu†, Wenshan Zhong†, Jinming Zhang†, Weimou Chen, Ye lu, Yujie Qiao, Zhaojin Zeng, Haohua Huang, Shaoxi Cai and Hangming Dong**

Department of Respiratory and Critical Care Medicine, Chronic Airways Diseases Laboratory, Nanfang Hospital, Southern Medical University, Guangzhou, China

***Correspondence:**
Hangming Dong
dhm@smu.edu.cn
Shaoxi Cai
caishaox@fimmu.com

†These authors have contributed equally to this work

Idiopathic pulmonary fibrosis is a progressive fatal disease characterized by interstitial remodeling, with high lethality and a lack of effective medical therapies. Tetrandrine has been proposed to present anti-fibrotic effects, but the efficacy and mechanisms have not been systematically evaluated. We sought to study the potential therapeutic effects and mechanisms of tetrandrine against lung fibrosis. The anti-fibrotic effects of tetrandrine were evaluated in bleomycin-induced mouse models and TGF-β1-stimulated murine lung fibroblasts. We performed Chromatin Immunoprecipitation (ChIP), Immunoprecipitation (IP), and mRFP-GFP-MAP1LC3B adenovirus construct to investigate the novel mechanisms of tetrandrine-induced autophagy. Tetrandrine decreased TGF-β1-induced expression of α-smooth muscle actin, fibronectin, vimentin, and type 1 collagen and proliferation in fibroblasts. Tetrandrine restored TGF-β1-induced impaired autophagy flux, accompanied by enhanced interaction of SQSTM1 and MAP1LC3-II. ChIP studies revealed that tetrandrine induced autophagy via increasing binding of NRF2 and SQSTM1 promoter. Furthermore, tetrandrine inhibited TGF-β1-induced phosphorylation of mTOR by reducing activation of Rheb. *In vivo* tetrandrine suppressed the bleomycin-induced expression of fibrotic markers and improved pulmonary function. Our data suggest that protective effect of tetrandrine against lung fibrosis might be through promoting Rheb-mTOR and NRF2-SQSTM1 mediated autophagy. Tetrandrine may thus be potentially employed as a novel therapeutic medicine against IPF.

Keywords: lung fibrosis, tetrandrine, autophagy, mTOR, COL-I

INTRODUCTION

Idiopathic pulmonary fibrosis is a prototype of chronic, progressive, and fibrotic lung disease, characterized by repetitive injury of the lung epithelium, activation and proliferation of (myo) fibroblasts, and accumulation of extracellular matrix (King et al., 2011; Hutchinson et al., 2015). Despite this high unmet clinical need, only two anti-fibrotics drugs, Pirfenidone and nintedanib, have been approved to be effective in slowing down the decline of lung function in IPF patients. However, neither agent stops the progression of IPF (King et al., 2014; Richeldi et al., 2014). Thus, there is a tremendous interest in investigating the pathological mechanisms underlying IPF in order to identify novel therapies.

Tetrandrine (TET) is a low-toxicity drug extracted from the plant Stephania tetrandra S. Moore (Fenfangji) of the menispermaceae (Bhagya and Chandrashekar 2016). Previous studies have reported that TET could exert anti-fibrotic effects on multiple organs, primarily by interfering with autophagy (Wang et al., 2015). In addition, TET had also been identified as an effective inducer of autophagy (Liu et al., 2017). However, the mechanism underlying the protective effects of TET on lung fibrosis remains unclear.

Autophagy is the process in which cells degrade internal constituents for the maintenance of cellular homeostasis (Barth et al., 2010) and is known to participate in removing ubiquitinated proteins (Ciani et al., 2003). SQSTM1/p62 is a signaling hub and a critical selective autophagy receptor (Lippai and Low 2014). Intriguingly, autophagy deficit, a common feature of many diseases, plays an important role in various fibrotic diseases, including liver, kidney, and pulmonary fibrosis (Patel et al., 2012; Araya et al., 2013). Transforming growth factor β1 (TGF-β1) is one of the major profibrotic cytokines in fibrosis diseases that could inhibit autophagy during myofibroblast differentiation in lung fibroblasts (Sosulski et al., 2015). Furthermore, autophagy may contribute to the degradation of COL1/collagen I to alleviate fibrosis (Moscat and Diaz-Meco 2009; Sosulski et al., 2015).

The purpose of the current study was to analyze the anti-fibrotic effect of TET on TGF-β1-induced fibroblast transdifferentiation and bleomycin-induced murine lung fibrosis. We demonstrate that TET therapy decreases fibrotic markers *in vitro* and *in vivo*. These protective effects of TET on pulmonary fibrosis are associated with activation of autophagy through promoting NRF2-SQSTM1 axis and Rheb-mTOR signaling. Taken together, our findings provide important proof-of-concept evidence that activation autophagy induced by TET could be used as a novel pharmacological approach for treatment of human IPF.

MATERIALS AND METHODS

Culture of Lung Fibroblasts

Primary mouse lung fibroblasts (pMLFs) were isolated from the lungs obtained from C57BL/6J mice and maintained in DMEM supplemented with 10% FBS and penicillin–streptomycin. pMLFs were isolated using a method described previously (Bueno et al., 2015). Briefly, mouse lungs were minced into 1–2 mm^3 pieces and incubated in calcium- and magnesium-free Hanks' balanced salt solution (HBSS) containing 1,000 U/ml collagenase A for 30 min, and after washing with HBSS, then add 0.25% trypsin-EDTA for 20 min at 37°C with shaking. The dissociated cells were centrifuged and cultured in DMEM supplemented with 10% FBS for 1 h, and then adherent fibroblasts were rinsed with HBSS and cultured in DMEM supplemented with 10% FBS and penicillin–streptomycin. More than 95% of the cells were morphologically fibroblasts and stained with vimentin, and no cells were stained with CD45. The fibroblasts were used between culture passages 3 and 6.

Human lung fibroblast line IMR90 was purchased from American Type Culture Collection (Manassas, VA). IMR90 were maintained in DMEM supplemented with 10% FBS, 100 units/mL penicillin, and 100 g/ml streptomycin in 5% CO_2 and 95% humidity at 37°C.

Cell Viability Assay

Cell viability was measured by a cell counting Kit-8 (CCK8) assay (Dojindo, Japan). Cells were seeded in 200 µl of growth medium at a density of 8×10^3 cells per well in 96-well plates. Cells were treated with or without TET for 24 h. Following the manufacturer's recommendations, 10 µl CCK-8 solution was added per well for 2 h before the end of incubation at 37°C. Cell viability was measured at an absorbance of 450 nm.

Transfection of siRNA and Plasmids

Different siRNA oligos were obtained from Gene Pharma (Shanghai, China), and the sequences were listed in **Supplementary Table S1**. Plasmids for Rheb overexpression were purchased from Hanbio (Shanghai, China) and the sequence is shown in **Supplementary Table S1**. Cells were transfected with the appropriate siRNA oligos or plasmid with Lipofectamine 3,000 (Invitrogen, CA, United States), according to the manufacturer's protocol. After 48 h, cells were further stimulated with different reagents. The successfully transfected clones were confirmed by western blotting.

Tandem Fluorescent-mRFP-GFP-MAP1LC3B-Adenovirus Transduction of pMLFs

pMLFs were transfected with a tandem fluorescent-mRFP-GFP-MAP1LC3B-adenovirus (HanBio, HB-AP2100001) that expresses a specific marker of autophagosome formation to detect autophagy, according to the manufacturer's instructions (Hariharan et al., 2011). With this tandem construct, autophagosomes and autolysosomes are labelled with yellow (mRFP and GFP) and red (mRFP only) signals, respectively. Five fields were chosen from 3 different cell preparations. GFP- and mRFP-expressing spots, which were indicated by fluorescent puncta and DAPI-stained nuclei, were counted manually. The number of spots per cell was determined by dividing the total number of spots by the number of nuclei in each field.

Immunofluorescence Assay

The immunofluorescence assay was performed as described previously (Ohashi et al., 2015). Cells were seeded on a confocal dish for 24 h. After treatment, cells were fixed with 4% paraformaldehyde for 15 min in phosphate-buffered saline (PBS), followed by permeabilization for 10 min with Triton X-100–containing buffer. Antibodies was used for immunofluorescence assays. Then, cells were incubated for 12 h at 4°C with corresponding antibodies. Next, cells were washed with PBS and incubated with Alexa Fluor 594 anti-Rat (1:200) and Alexa Fluor 488 anti-mouse (1:200) (Life Technologies, CA, United States) at room temperature

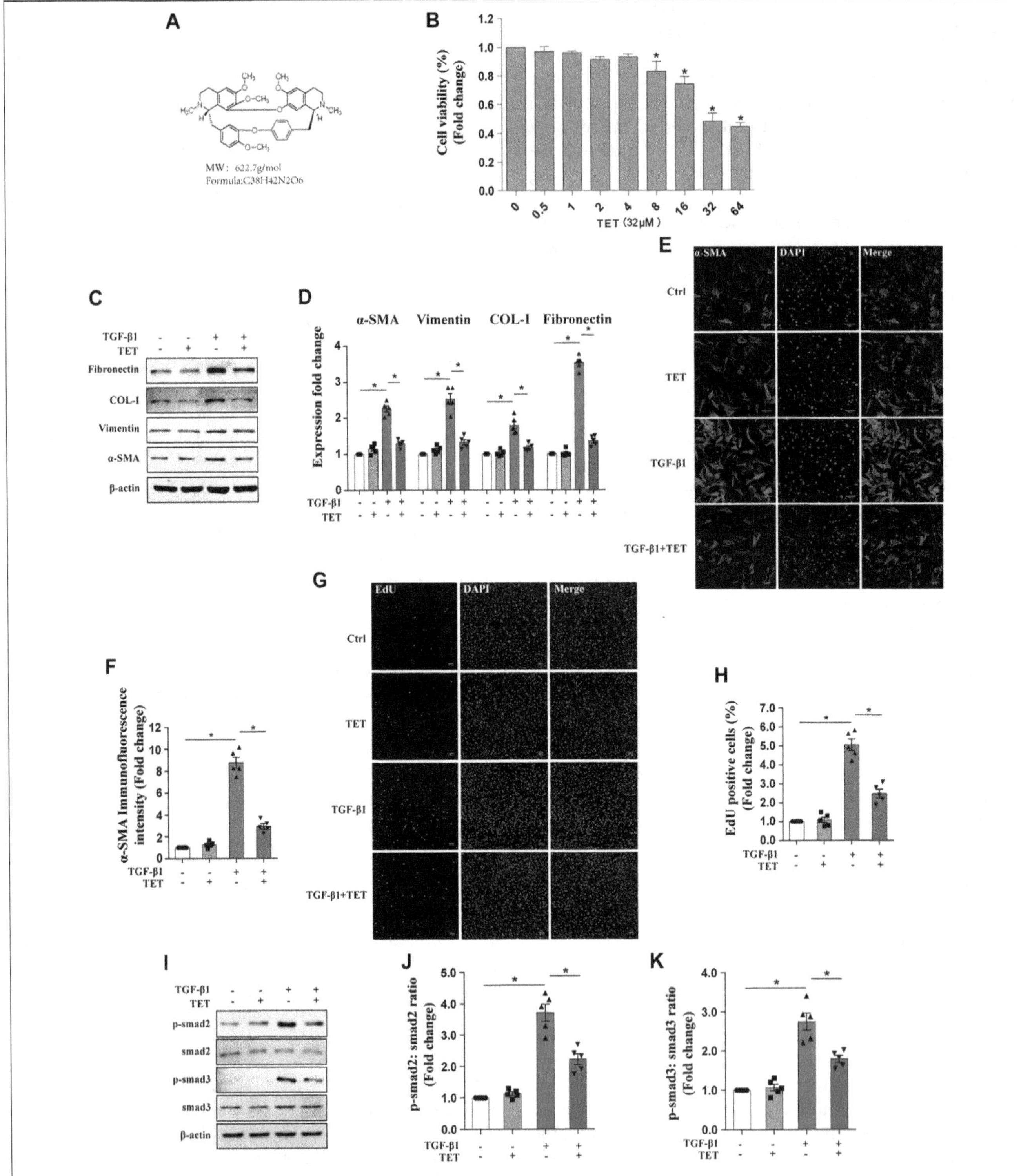

FIGURE 1 | Tetrandrine suppresses TGF-β1-induced myofibroblasts differentiation, proliferation, and ECM deposition in primary MLFs. **(A)** Chemical structure of TET. Its Molecular formation is $C_{38}H_{42}N_2O_6$. **(B)** Primary MLFs were incubated with various indicated concentrations of TET for 24 h and subjected to CCK8 assay to assess cell viability. One-way ANOVA with Dunnett's multiple comparison test: *$p < 0.05$ comparison to TET = 0 μM group value: *$p < 0.05$. **(C,D)** Primary MLFs were pretreated with DMSO or TET (4 μM) for 1 h and stimulated with or without TGF-β1 (10 ng/ml) for 24 h. Representative immunoblot analysis **(C)** and quantitative analysis **(D)** show the expression of ECM deposition (fibronectin, COL-I), myofibroblasts transdifferentiation (vimentin, α-SMA). **(E,F)** Representative Immunofluorescence monitored by confocal microscopy **(E)** and quantitative analysis **(F)** show the expression of α-SMA (red) in Primary MLFs. Blue staining indicates nuclei Scale bars: 100 μM. **(G,H)** Representative Immunofluorescence **(G)** and quantitative analysis **(H)** of *EdU* -positive cell proportion show the proliferation marker (*EdU:* 5-ehtynal-2′-deoxyuridine) in myofibroblast. Scale bars: 100 μM. **(I-K)** Representative immunoblot analysis **(I)** and quantitative analysis **(J,K)** show the expression of TGF-β/smad pathway markers (p-smad2, smad2, p-smad3, smad3) in primary MLFs. *p* values were determined by two-way ANOVA with Tukey's multiple comparison test (n = 5): *$p < 0.05$.

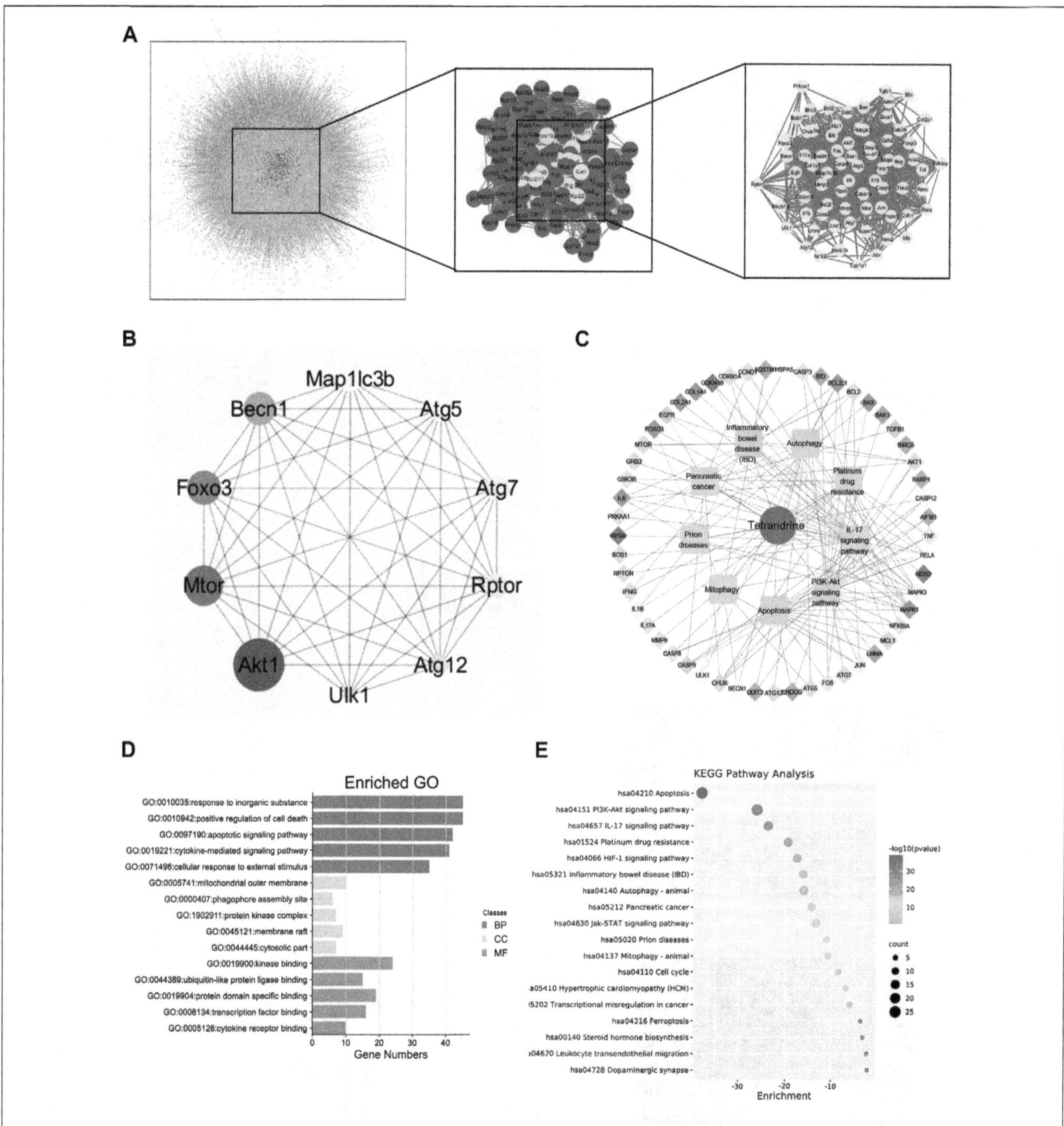

FIGURE 2 | Analysis of TET's targets on pulmonary fibrosis based on network pharmacology. **(A)** protein—protein interaction (PPI) networks of active ingredients of TET for the treatment of pulmonary fibrosis. Each node represents the relevant genes, the edge means line thickness indicates the strength of data support. **(B)** Hub top 10 genes in PPI network, the lighter the color, the higher the score; the larger the diameter, the higher the score. **(C)** Representative networks assembled by predicted TET targets. Diamonds in various colors nodes represent the targets for TET identified through target mapping. Green nodes represent signaling pathways or processes. Targets are connected with pathways or processes with inner circle in the corresponding color. **(D)** The GO analysis was discovered with the top five enriched conditions in the biological process (BP), cell component (CC), and molecular function (MF) categories. **(E)** KEGG pathways of target genes.

for 2 h afterwards. The nuclei of the cells were stained with DAPI (Invitrogen). Images were taken on an Olympus FV1000 Confocal Laser Scanning Microscope (Tokyo, Japan). The following antibodies were used: MAP1LC3B (CST, 2775s, 83506S), SQSTM1 (proteintech, 18420-1-AP, 66184-1-AP), Anti-alpha smooth muscle Actin (Abcam, ab7817), Cleaved caspase-3 (CST, 9664s), ubiquitin (Proteintech, 10201-2-AP), Phospho-4E-BP1 (Thr37/46) (236B4) (CST, 2855T), LAMP2 (Abcam, Ab13524), Collagen1 (Affinitiy, AF7001).

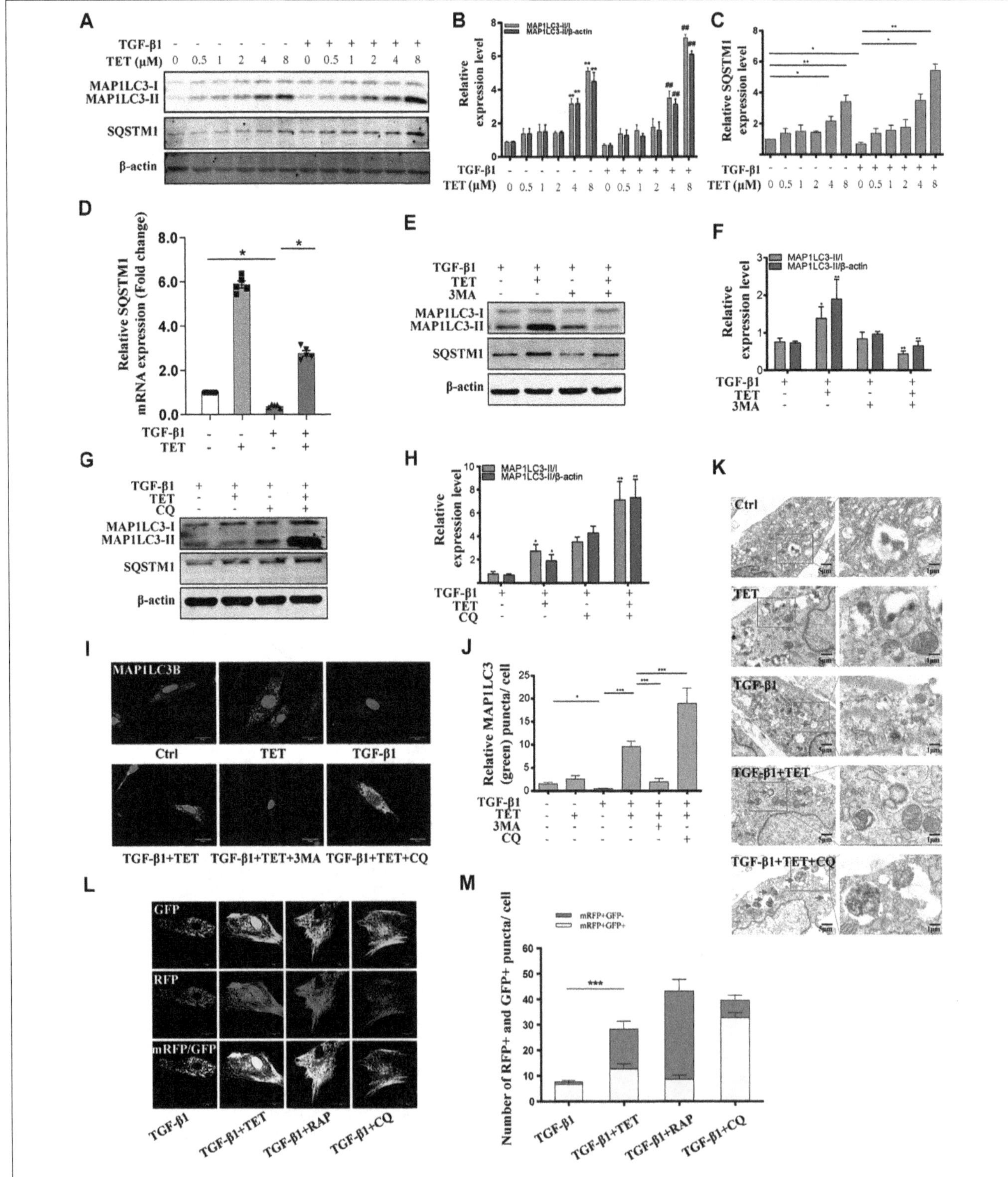

FIGURE 3 | TET restores TGF-β1-induced impaired autophagy in primary MLFs. **(A-C)** Primary MLFs were pretreated with TET for indicated concentrations for 1 h and then subsequently stimulated with or without TGF-β1 (10 ng/ml) for 24 h. Representative immunoblot analysis **(A)** and quantitative analysis **(B–C)** showed the expression of autophagy (MAP1LC3-I/II, SQSTM1) markers and β-actin (loading control). Values in bar graph are presented as means ± SEM (n = 5). Two-way ANOVA: $^{*}p < 0.05$, $^{**}p < 0.01$, versus the control group; $\#p < 0.05$, $\#\#p < 0.01$, versus the TGF-β1 group. **(D)** Primary MLFs were pretreated with DMSO or TET (4 μM) for 1 h and stimulated with or without TGF-β1 (10 ng/ml) for 24 h. Representative of qPCR analysis showed the mRNA expression of SQSTM1. **(E,F)** Primary MLFs were exposed to TGF-β1 (10 ng/ml) for 24 h. In some experimental groups, cells were treated with TET (4 μM), 3-methyladenine (3 MA: 500 nM). Immunoblot assays **(E)** and densitometric analysis **(F)** showed the expression of autophagic markers. **(G,H)** Primary MLFs were treated with TGF-β1 (10 ng/ml) in the presence/absence of TET

(Continued)

FIGURE 3 | (4 μM) or chloroquine (CQ: 20 μM). The protein sample were collected 24 h after the treatment. The levels of autophagic markers were examined with immunoblotting **(G)**. Relative levels of autophagic markers were determined by densitometry and normalized to β-actin levels (H). **(I,J)** Primary MLFs were treated with TGF-β1 (0 or 10 ng/ml) for 24 h in the presence/absence of TET (4 μM), 3 MA (500 nM), or CQ (20 μM). Representative images of immunofluorescence monitored by confocal microscopy **(I)** and quantification **(J)** showed the expression of autophagic marker (MAP1LC3B). Green staining is MAP1LC3B, blue staining indicates nuclei. Scale bars: 20 μm. **(K)** The transmission electron microscopy images showed numerous double-membraned cytoplasmic vacuolation (arrows). Scale bars: left panels, 5 μm; right panels, 1 m. **(L,M)** Primary MLFs were transfected with mRFP-GFP-LC3B plasmids for 48 h and treated with TGF-β1 (10 ng/ml) for 24 h in the presence/absence of TET (4 μM), rapamycin (RAP: 50 nM) or CQ (20 μM). Representative immunofluorescent images showed mRFP (green), GFP (red) and merged mRFP and GFP (yellow) puncta **(L)**. Scale bars: 10 μm. Quantification of red (mRFP + GFP−) and yellow (mRFP + GFP+) puncta per cell (M). Values in bar graph are presented as means ± SEM (n = 5). Two-way ANOVA with Tukey's multiple comparison test (n = 5): *$p < 0.05$, **$p < 0.01$, **$p < 0.01$, ***$p < 0.001$.

Network Pharmacology and Bioinformatics Analysis

Pulmonary fibrosis-related genes were obtained from Comparative Toxicogenomics database (CTD, http://ctdbase.org/) and DisGeNET (a database of gene-disease associations, https://www.disgenet.org/) using the term "pulmonary fibrosis," followed by filtering with the term "*Homo sapiens.*" Potential targets of TET were obtained from the Swiss target prediction (http://www.swisstargetprediction.ch/) and pubchem (https://pubchem.ncbi.nlm.nih.gov/). A total of 74 potential human targets were obtained and the official gene names were obtained from Uniprot (http://www.uniprot.org/) by confining the species to "*Homo sapiens.*" Subsequently, various ID forms of the targets were transformed into UniProt IDs. The Search Tool for the Retrieval of Interacting Genes (STRING) database (https://string-db.org/) supplies each predicted PPI information as well as the data which have actually been experimentally confirmed. Then, we seek out the intersection through Cytoscape-Bisogenet (3.7.2) and screen out the top 10 key genes. The functional pathways of TET related to pulmonary fibrosis were analyzed using the Kyoto Encyclopedia of Genes and Genomes (KEGG) pathway and gene ontology (GO) enrichment evaluation based upon the database for annotation, Visualization and Integrated Discovery (DAVID) version 6.8 (https://david.ncifcrf.gov/). *p*-value was calculated in these two enrichment analyses, and $p < 0.05$ suggests the enrichment degree was statistically significant and the pathway results would certainly be necessary functional mechanisms of pulmonary fibrosis.

Western blotting and Co-Immunoprecipitation

Total cell lysates were obtained using the Total Protein Extraction Kit (KeyGen Biotech, China) according to the manufacturer's instructions. Proteins were subjected to SDS-PAGE, transferred to PVDF membranes, and probed with various primary antibodies and LICOR: fluorescence-labeled secondary antibodies (#926-68071, 926-32,210). Blots were visualized using a LICOR Odyssey fluorescent imaging system (LICOR Biotechnology) finally. For co-immunoprecipitation, protein extracts from MLFs were incubated with indicated primary antibody overnight at 4°C. The immune-complexes were cleared with Protein A/G Magnetic Beads (Thermo Scientific). Input lysates were run simultaneously with the IP samples on 10% polyacrylamide gels and visualized with LICOR Odyssey Scanner. Antibodies used were: anti-β-actin (Proteintech, 66009-1-Ig), anti-phospho-mTOR (Ser2448; Cell Signaling Technology, 5536S), anti-Phospho-P70 (Thr389; Cell Signaling Technology, 9236S), anti-Phospho-4E-BP1 (Thr37/46; Cell Signaling Technology, 2855T), anti-phospho-smad3 (Ser423/425; Cell Signaling Technology, 9520T), anti-phospho-smad2 (Ser465/Ser467; Cell Signaling Technology, 18338T), anti-MAP1LC3-I/II (Cell Signaling Technology, 2775S), anti-cleaved caspase3 (Cell Signaling Technology, 9664S), anti-α-SMA (Abcam, ab32575), anti-fibronectin (Abcam, ab2413), Anti-Rheb (Santa Cruz, sc-271509), anti-SQSTM1 (Proteintech, 18420-1-AP), anti-4E-BP1 (Proteintech, 60246-Ig), anti-p70(S6K) (Proteintech, 14485AP), anti-mTOR (Proteintech, 20657-1-AP), anti-ATG7 (Proteintech, 10088-2-AP), anti-vimentin (Proteintech, 10366-1-AP), anti-IgG (Proteintech, B900610), anti-smad3 (Proteintech, 25494-1-AP), anti-smad 2 (Proteintech, 12570-1-AP), anti-Col-I (Affinity, AF7001) Ubiquitin (Proteintech, 10201-2-AP).

Chromatin Immunoprecipitation Assay

The immunoprecipitation (ChIP) assay in MLFs was performed using the SimpleChIP Enzymatic Chromatin IP Kit (CST, 9003) according to the manufacturer's protocol. Approximately 4×10^6 cells were used for each immunoprecipitation. Chromatin was immunoprecipitated with the immunoglobulin G (CST, #2729; as a negative control) or NRF2 (Genetex, #GTX103322). In all, 10% total DNA was used for input evaluation. DNA enrichment in the ChIP samples was determined by reverse transcription and semi-quantitative PCR (RT-PCR) with PrimeScript™ RT reagent Kit with gDNA Eraser (Takara, China) and a LightCycler 96 Instrument (Roche) following the manufacturer's protocol. PCR products of immunoprecipitated and input samples were analyzed on a 2% agarose gel. Specific primer sets for the SQSTM1 locus are shown as follow: SQSTM1_P1 forward: ATTCTGCCCTGCATGTCTT, reverse: GCCTTCTAGGTATGGTCCTTTC; SQSTM1_P2 forward: TGGCCGAGCCTTGAATTAG, reverse: GCACCTGCCTAGTATGTGTT.

RNA Extraction and Quantitative Real-Time PCR

Total RNA was extracted from cells with the TRIzol reagent (Takara, Dalian, China). The quantity and quality of RNA

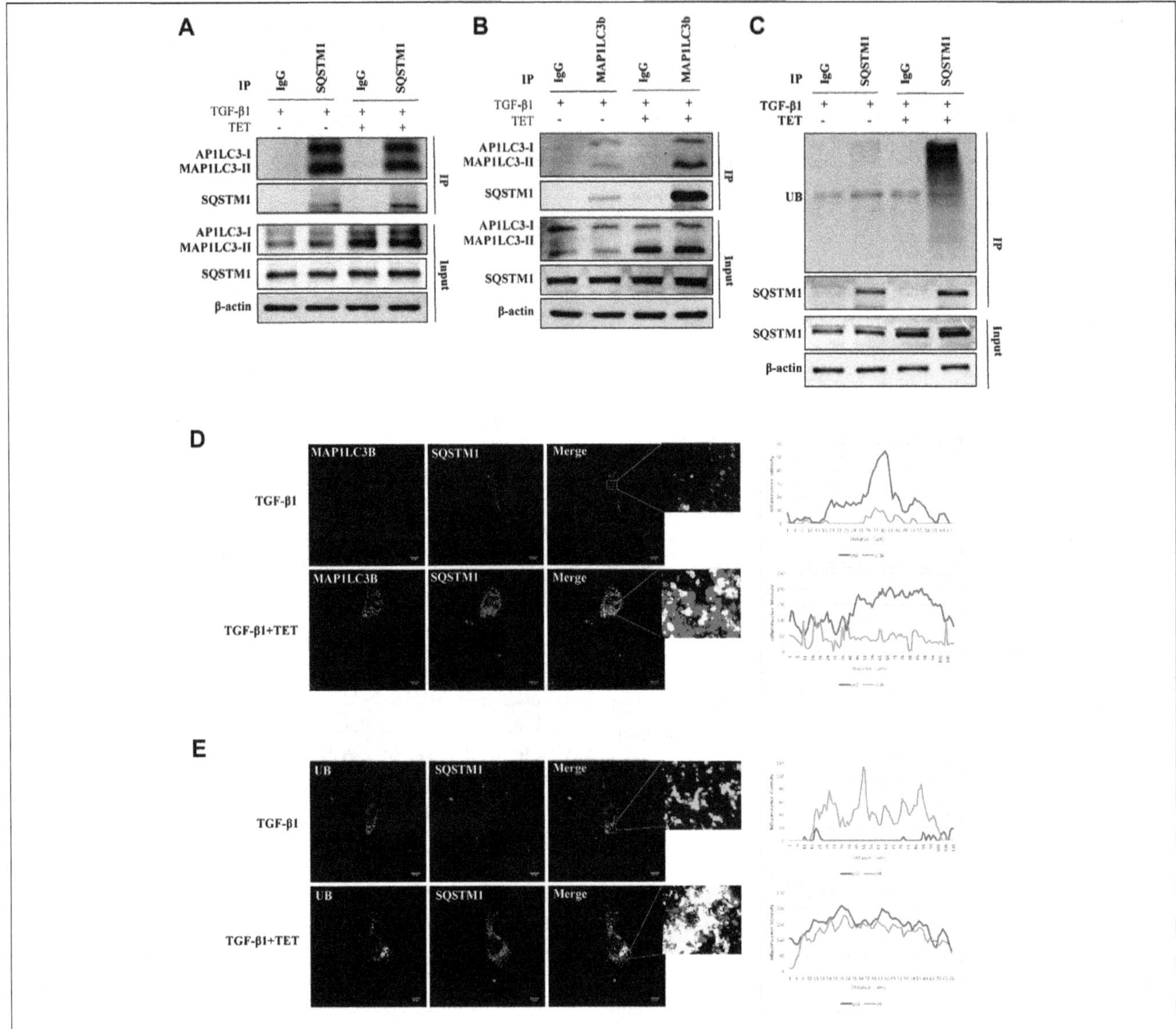

FIGURE 4 | TET promotes the interaction of SQSTM1 with MAP1LC3B and with ubiquitinated protein. Primary MLFs were pretreated with TET or DMSO for 1 h and then subsequently stimulated with TGF-β1 for 24 h. **(A,B)** Co-immunoprecipitation (Co-IP) assays with SQSTM1 and MAP1LC3-I/II. Samples before (Input) and after (IP) immunopurification were analyzed by immunoblotting using SQSTM1 and MAP1LC3-I/II antibodies. **(C)** Co-IP assays with SQSTM1 and ubiquitinated protein. Samples were analyzed by immunoblotting using SQSTM1 and ubiquitin (UB) antibodies. **(D)** Confocal microscopy analysis of co-localization of MAP1LC3B and SQSTM1 in primary MLFs. The representative single optical sections and merge images are shown in the right panel. In these representative images, MAP1LC3B is visualized in green, SQSTM1 in red. Scale bars: 10 μm. **(E)** Confocal microscopy analysis of co-localization of UB and SQSTM1. Scale bars: 10 μm. UB is visualized in green, SQSTM1 in red.

were determined using a Nanodrop 2000 spectrophotometer (Thermo Fisher Scientific), and then RNA was reverse transcribed using iScript™ cDNA synthesis kit (Biorad; 1708890) according to the manufacturer's instructions. The qPCR was performed using TaqMan® universal PCR Master Mix (Fisher Scientific; 4304437) on a StepOnePlus™ Real-Time PCR System (Thermo Fisher Scientific) in 20 μl reaction. Relative mRNA levels were calculated using the $2^{-\Delta\Delta CT}$ method normalized against β-actin in each reaction. The following primers were used, Actb, forward: GTGACGTTG ACATCCGTAAAGA, reverse: GCCGGACTCATCGTACTC C; SQSTM1, forward: ATGTGGAACATGGAGGGAAGA, reverse: GGAGTTCACCTGTAGATGGGT; Rheb, forward: GGTCTGTGGGAAAGTCCTCAT, reverse: GGTGAACGT GTTCTCTATGGTT.

Bleomycin-Induced Lung Fibrosis Model and Treatment With Tetrandrine

All animal experiments were conducted according to Southern Medical University Animal Welfare, and research protocols were approved by the Institutional Animal Care and

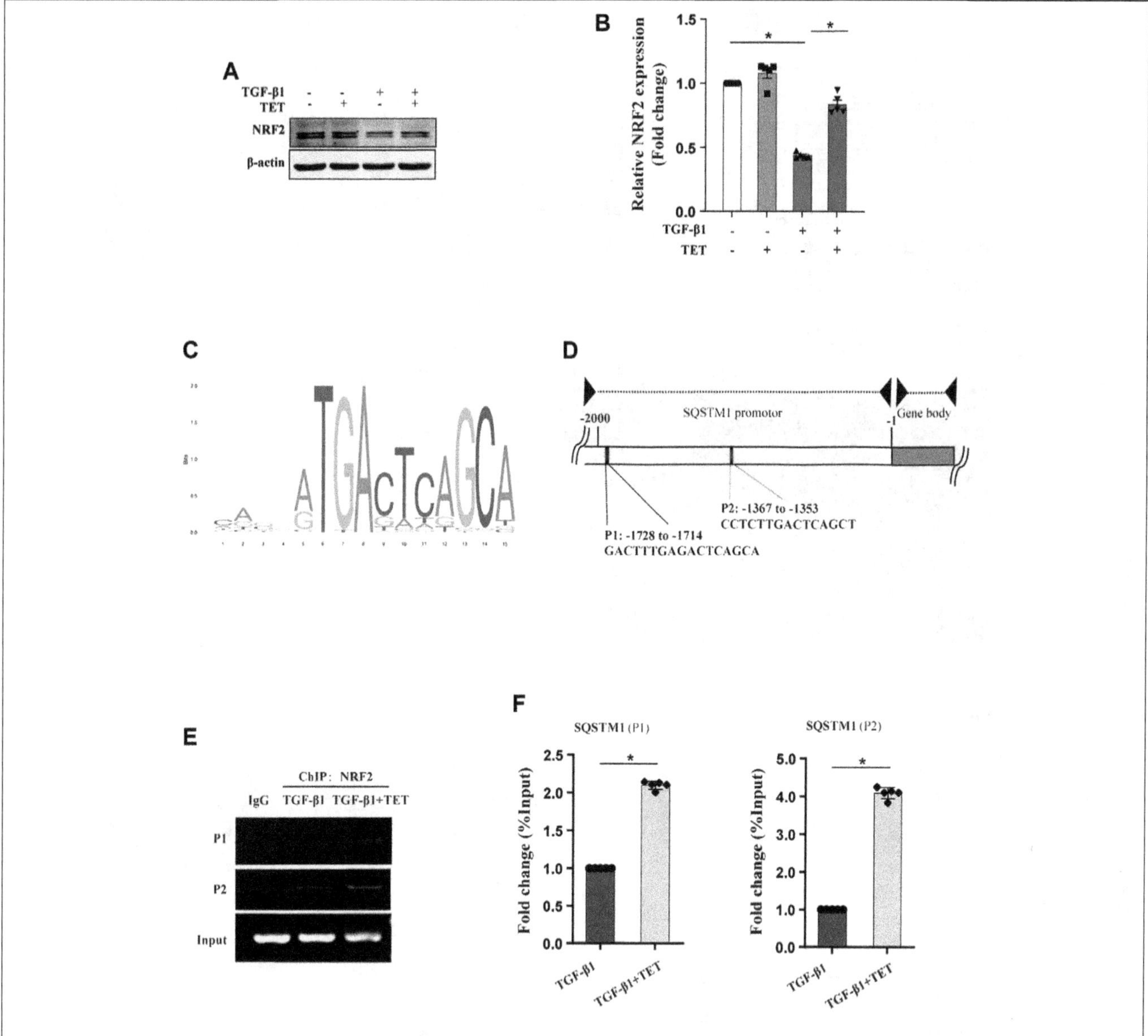

FIGURE 5 | TET regulates the transcription of SQSTM1 through NRF2. Primary MLFs were treated with TGF-β1 (0 or 10 ng/ml) for 24 h in the presence/absence of TET (4 μM). **(A,B)** Immunoblot assays **(A)** and densitometric analysis **(B)** showed the expression of NRF2. **(C)** Identification of SQSTM1 promoter-containing genes in the mouse genome by the FIMO software tool. **(D)** Schematic representation of the SQSTM1 promotor region. PCR primers used for amplification (P1 and P2) are shown in the underneath schematic representation. **(E)** ChIP-PCR analysis to showing the association of NRF2 with the SQSTM1 promotor in MLFs. *RT-PCR* products were resolved by agarose gel electrophoresis. **(F)** *Statistical analysis* was obtained. Values in bar graph are presented as means ± SEM (n = 5). Two-way ANOVA followed by Tukey's multiple comparisons test was used for statistical analysis of **(B)** and Student's t-test was used for **(F)**. $^{*}p < 0.05$.

Use Committee of Southern Medical University. Mice were housed four mice per cage in a specific pathogen-free room with a 12 h light/dark schedule at 25°C ± 1°C and were fed an autoclaved chow diet and water ad libitum. An established mammalian model of idiopathic pulmonary fibrosis (IPF) was utilized as described in previous publications. Six- to eight-week-old C57BL/6 female mice (16–20 g) were anesthetized (2,2,2-tribromoethanol, Sigma-Aldrich) and then injected intratracheally with prepared bleomycin sulfate (5 U kg^{-1}) (Hanhui pharmaceuticals co., LTD.) in sterile PBS (volume was varied between 80 and 100 μl depending on the body weight). Control mice were injected with 100 μl of sterile PBS. Body weights were monitored throughout each study. Each experimental group consisted of at least five animals.

To quantitate fibrosis during longitudinal studies, lungs were harvested at 21 days after bleomycin instillation and assayed as described below. To test the prevention efficacy of TET in our modeling of IPF, TET (20 mg kg^{-1}, Sigma-Aldrich) or vehicle (equal volume of 0.1% sodium carboxymethyl cellulose) were administered by intraperitoneal injection at every other day after bleomycin administration, and the mice were sacrificed at day 21. For

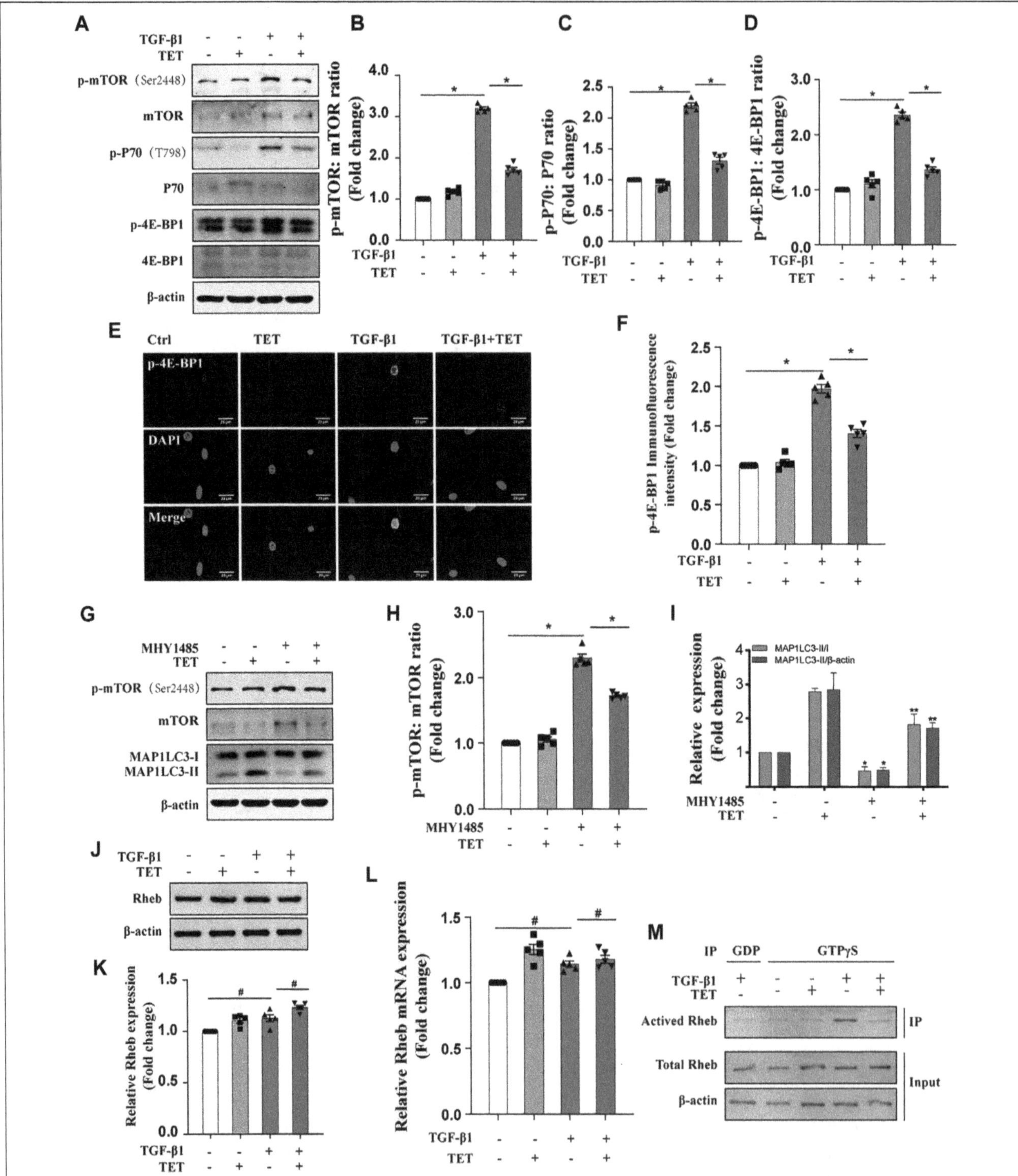

FIGURE 6 | TET activates autophagy by inhibiting Rheb/mTORC1 signaling. **(A–D)** Effect of TET on mTOR activation. Immunoblot **(A)** and quantitative analysis **(B–D)** showed the expression level of mTOR phosphorylation (p-mTOR), *mTOR* downstream substrates (p-P70, p-4E-BP1). **(E,F)** Representative images of immunofluorescence monitored by confocal microscopy **(J)** and quantitative analysis **(K)** showed the expression of p-4E-BP1. Green staining is p-4E-BP1, blue staining indicates nuclei. Scale bars: 20 μm. **(G–I)** Effect of mTOR activation on autophagy regulation. Primary MLFs were cotreated with TET (4 μM) and MHY1485 (5 μM) for 24 h. Immunoblot (G) and quantitative analysis **(H–I)** showed the expression of autophagy markers (MAP1LC3-I/II, SQSTM1), mTOR activation (mTOR, p-mTOR). **(J,K)** Effect of TET on the expression of Rheb protein. Representative immunoblot analysis **(J)** and quantitative analysis **(K)** show the expression of Rheb protein. **(L)** Representative of qPCR analysis showed the mRNA expression of Rheb. **(M)** Effect of TET on Rheb activation. Co-immunoprecipitation was performed using agarose beads conjugated to an antibody directed against the GTPγS and GDP. Immunoblot analysis was performed to check for protein expression of activated Rheb (Rheb/GTP), total Rheb. Total Rheb includes the inactive GDP-Bound form (GDP) and activated Rheb (Rheb/GTP). Values in bar graph are presented as means ± SEM (n = 5). Two-way ANOVA with Tukey's multiple comparison test (n = 5). $^{*}p < 0.05$.

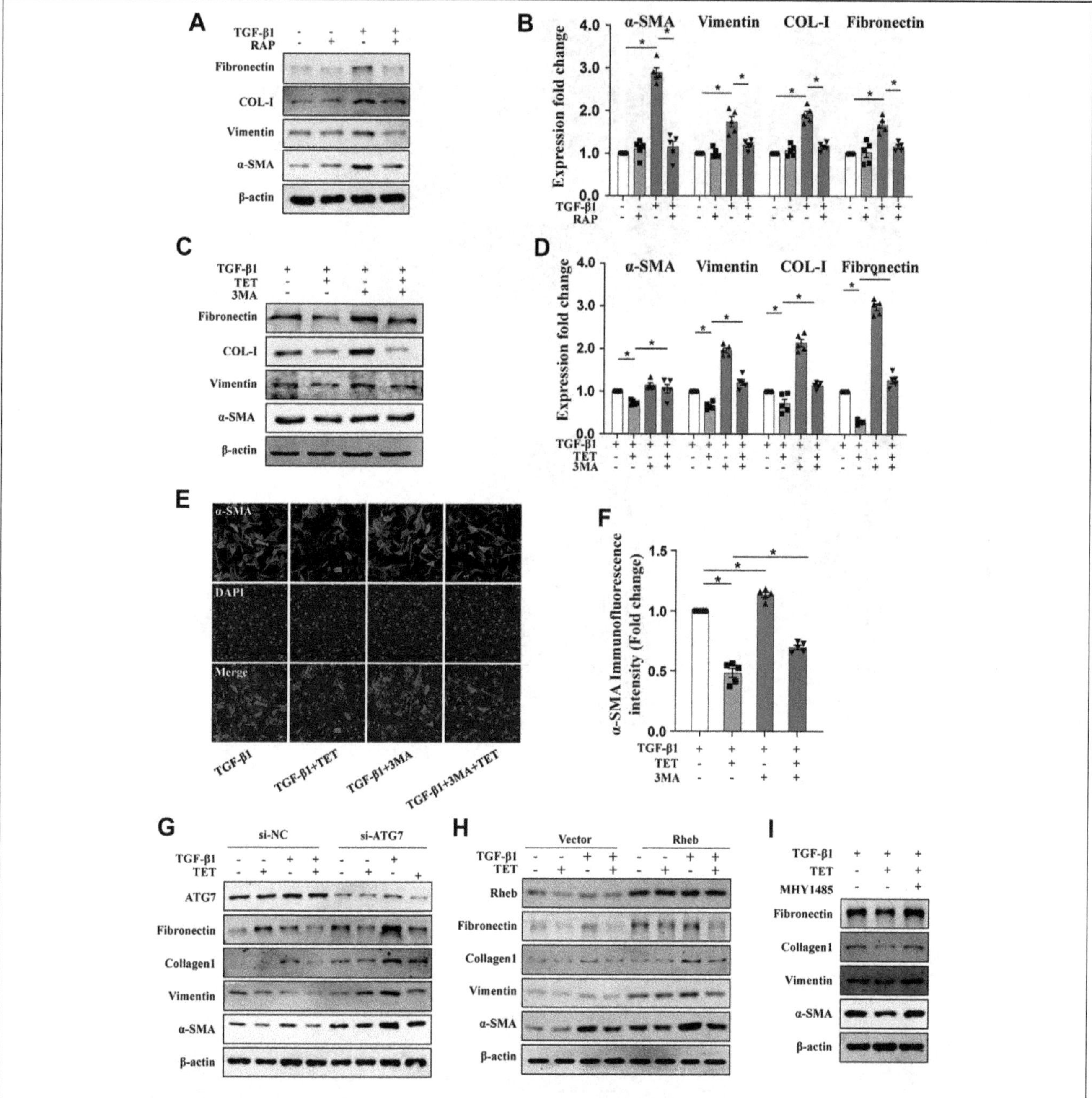

FIGURE 7 | TET improves pulmonary fibrosis by activating autophagy through Rheb/mTOR in MLFs. Primary MLFs were treated with TGF-β1 (0 or 10 ng/ml) for 24 h in the presence/absence of TET (4 μM), 3 MA (500 nM), RAP (50 nM), or MHY1485 (a small molecule mTOR activator, 5 μM). **(A,B)** Representative immunoblot analysis **(A)** and quantitative analysis **(B)** showed the expression of fibrosis-associated proteins. **(C,D)** The effect of autophagy on TGF-β1-induced primary MLFs. Immunoblot **(C)** and quantitative analysis **(D)** showed the expression of ECM deposition, myofibroblasts transdifferentiation markers. **(E,F)** Confocal microscopy images **(E)** and relative fluorescence intensity of α-SMA **(F)**. α-SMA was visualized in green, DAPI-stained nuclei in blue. Scale bars: 50 μm. **(G)** MLFs transfected with nonspecific nonsilencing negative siRNA control (*si-NC*) or ATG7 small interfering *RNA* (*si*-ATG7) for 48 h were treated with TET and TGF-β1. Representative immunoblot analysis showed the expression of fibrosis-associated proteins. **(H)** Cells transfected with the empty vector plasmid (vector) or Rheb overexpression plasmid (Rheb) for 48 h and then incubated with TET and TGF-β1. Immunoblot of fibrosis-associated proteins. **(I)** TET-attenuated fibrosis was associated with mTOR activation. Immunoblot showed the expression of fibrosis-associated proteins. Values in bar graph are presented as means ± SEM (n = 5). Two-way ANOVA with Tukey's multiple comparison test (n = 5). *$p < 0.05$.

delayed therapy studies, induction of IPF was initiated as described above, and TET (20 mg kg^{-1} or 40 mg kg^{-1}) was intraperitoneally injected every other day beginning on day 8. Lungs were harvested on day 21 and assayed as described below (day 0 was taken as the day of bleomycin administration).

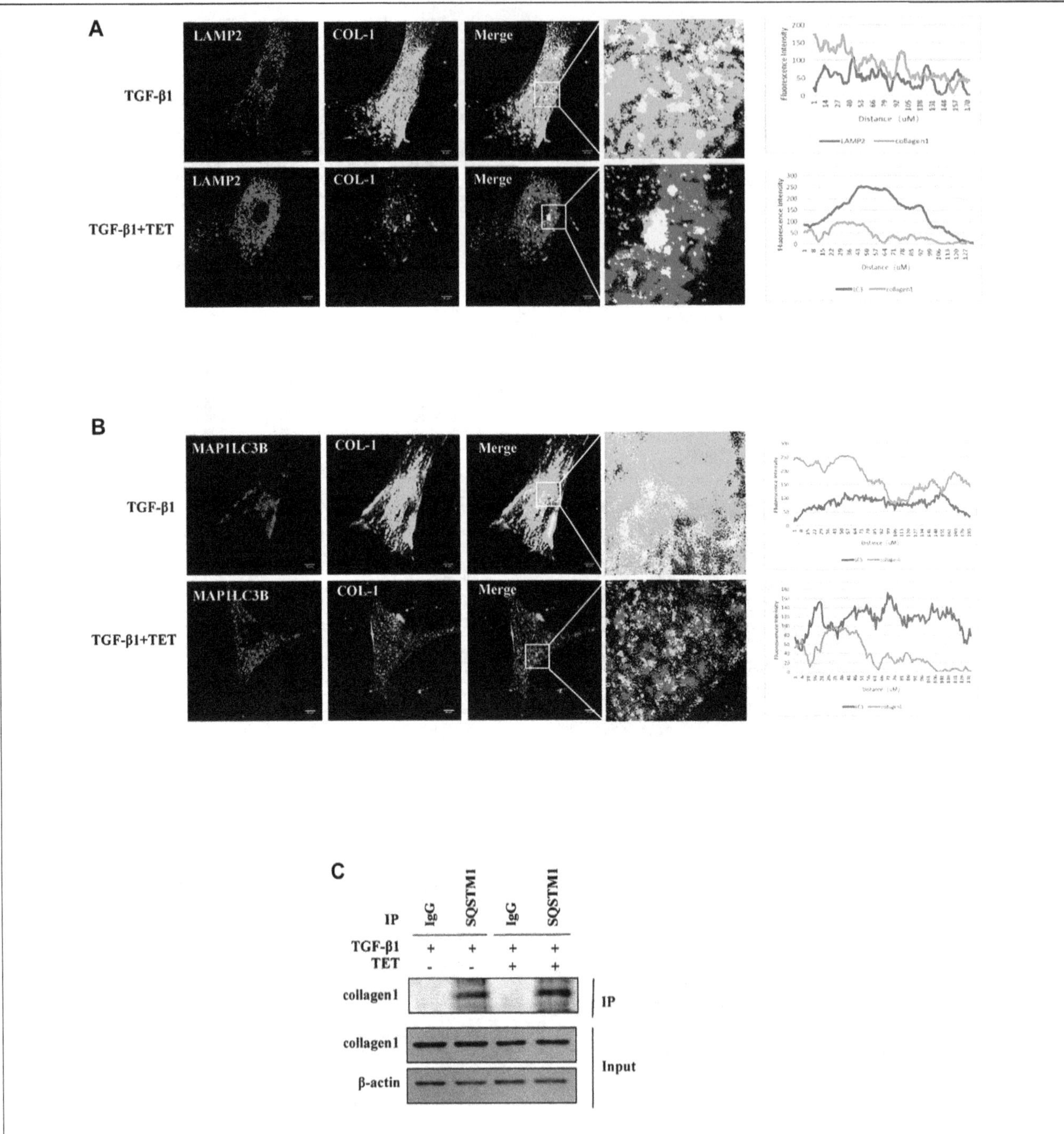

FIGURE 8 | Col-I is degraded by autophagy. Primary MLFs treated with DMSO or TET for 1 h and then subsequently simulated with TGF-β1 for an additional 24 h. **(A)** Confocal microscopy analysis of colocalization of LAMP2 (lysosomal markers, red) and COL-I (green). The representative single optical sections and merge images are shown. Scale bar: 10 μm. **(B)** Confocal microscopy analysis of colocalization of MAP1LC3B (red) and COL-I (green). The representative single optical sections and merge images are shown. Scale bar: 10 μM. **(C)** Co-immunoprecipitation (Co-IP) assays with SQSTM1 and COL-I. Samples before (Input) and after (IP) immunopurification were analyzed by immunoblotting.

Pulmonary Function Assay

At endpoint, at least five mice from each group were anesthetized with 2,2,2-tribromoethanol in saline, tracheotomized below the larynx, and intubated with a tracheal cannula. After the surgery, the mice were placed inside the plethysmographic chamber and the cannula was connected to the machine. Pulmonary function was measured by pulmonary function test system (BUXCO, United States). The system's software automatically records and displays the pulmonary function parameters.

Immunoanalysis and Histopathology

Formalin-fixed, paraffin-embedded (FFPE) tissue blocks obtained from mouse models were sectioned at 5 mm. For immunohistochemistry, the FFPE unstained slides were deparaffinized through standard methods. Paraffin embedded sections of mouse lung tissue were pretreated in citrate buffer pH6 for 20 min for antigen retrieval. Sections were then incubated with corresponding antibodies. For murine fibrosis assessment, FFPE lung tissue blocks were sectioned at 5 mm and subjected to haematoxylin and eosin and Masson's trichrome staining. Sections were reviewed by a blinded pathologist and approximately half of the specimens were scored by a second blinded pathologist to confirm agreement. Specimens were scored according to an eight-tier, modified Ashcroft scale (Hübner et al., 2008).

Hydroxyproline Assay

Lung hydroxyproline content was analyzed using a hydroxyproline assay kit (#A030-2, Nanjing Jianchen Bioengineering Institute, China) according to the manufacturer's instructions.

MATERIALS

Dimethyl sulfoxide (DMSO) and chloroquine (CQ) were obtained from Sigma-Aldrich (St. Louis, MO, United States). TGF-β1 were purchased from R&D Systems, Inc. (Minneapolis, MN, United States). 3-Methyladenine (3 MA) and MHY1485 were purchased from MedChemExpress (United States).

Data and Statistical Analysis

All data were analyzed blinded and presented as scatter plots showing each single data point representing the number of independent values and means ± SEM using bars and whiskers. Group sizes in the animal experiment were $n \geq 5$. The number of included data per group was mentioned in the figure legends. After testing values for normal distribution using Kolmogorov-Smirnov test, data were analyzed by: (1) Two-tailed t tests for comparison of two group means, using nonparametric analysis (Wilcoxon or Mann-Whitney) for $n = 5$; (2) One-way analysis of variance (ANOVA) followed by Dunnett's multiple comparisons test was used for multiple comparisons to control for concentration of TET dose effects; (3) Two-way ANOVA followed by Tukey post hoc tests for three or more group means with two factors. Non-parametric data were analyzed by Dunnett's multiple comparison test. Post hoc tests were run only if F achieved $p < 0.05$ and there was no significant variance in homogeneity. Differences between group means were considered statistically significant at the level of $p < 0.05$. Statistical analysis was performed using GraphPad Prism eight for Windows software (version 8.4.2, GraphPad software Inc, San Diego, CA, United States). The data and statistical analysis comply with the recommendations on experimental design and analysis in pharmacology (Curtis, Alexander et al., 2018).

RESULTS

Tetrandrine Inhibited TGF-β1-Induced Myofibroblasts Differentiation, ECM Deposition, and Proliferation

Fibroblast differentiation is critical pathogenesis processes in IPF (Baek et al., 2012). Previous studies have reported anti-fibrotic effects of TET (chemical structure shown in **Figure 1A**) in multiple organs (Yin et al., 2007; Teng et al., 2015). However, whether TET is capable of deactivating differentiated myofibroblasts and resolving fibrosis is not well known. We confirmed that 50% inhibition of cell growth was not achieved until TET concentration at 32 μM in primary mouse lung fibroblasts (pMLFs) or 32 μM in IMR90 cells (**Figure 1B, Supplementary Figure S1A**). Western blots and Immunofluorescence (IF) revealed that the expressions of fibronectin, type 1 collagen, vimentin, and α-SMA were all increased in pMLFs and IMR90 cells by stimulation with TGF-β1, indicating fibroblast differentiation and excessive matrix protein production. The effects of TGF-β1 were blocked by administration of TET (**Figures 1C–F, Supplementary Figures S1B–E**). Moreover, Numbers of *EdU* (+) cells after TGF-β1 exposure were significantly reduced by TET treatment for pMLFs (**Figures 1G,H**). TGF-β1-induced Smad2/3 activation indicated by Smad2/3 phosphorylation was blocked by TET in pMLFs (**Figures 1I–K**). Taken together, these results suggest that TET suppresses fibroblast differentiation and proliferation.

Potential Target Genes and Network Analysis of TET Treatment for Pulmonary Fibrosis

To elucidate the potential anti-fibrotic mechanisms of TET, we conducted an integrated systems pharmacology approach as previously described (Klionsky et al., 2007). We compared the respective gene-expression profiles of TET (from LINCS) to that of IPF and identified 74 target genes in IPF lungs visualized using Cytoscape (**Figure 2A**). Ten hub genes (AKT1, mTOR, Foxo3, Beclin1, MAP1LC3B, ATG5, ATG7, Rptor, ATG12, and ULK1) were identified in protein-protein interaction (PPI) networks (**Figure 2B**). We performed GO and KEGG pathway enrichment analysis of above gene sets using Cytoscape. The top enriched biological process is cell metabolism and the top cell component is membrane composition (**Figure 2D**). Interestingly, PI3K/AKT signaling, apoptosis, and autophagy are the top enriched gene ontology terms in KEGG pathway enrichment analysis (**Figures 2C–E**). Thus, the above data suggest that TET may relieve pulmonary fibrosis by regulating apoptosis and/or autophagy pathway.

TET Restored TGF-β1-Induced Impaired Autophagy in MLFs

To test whether TET regulates autophagy pathway in lung fibrosis, we administered TET to TGF-β1-induced MLFs and

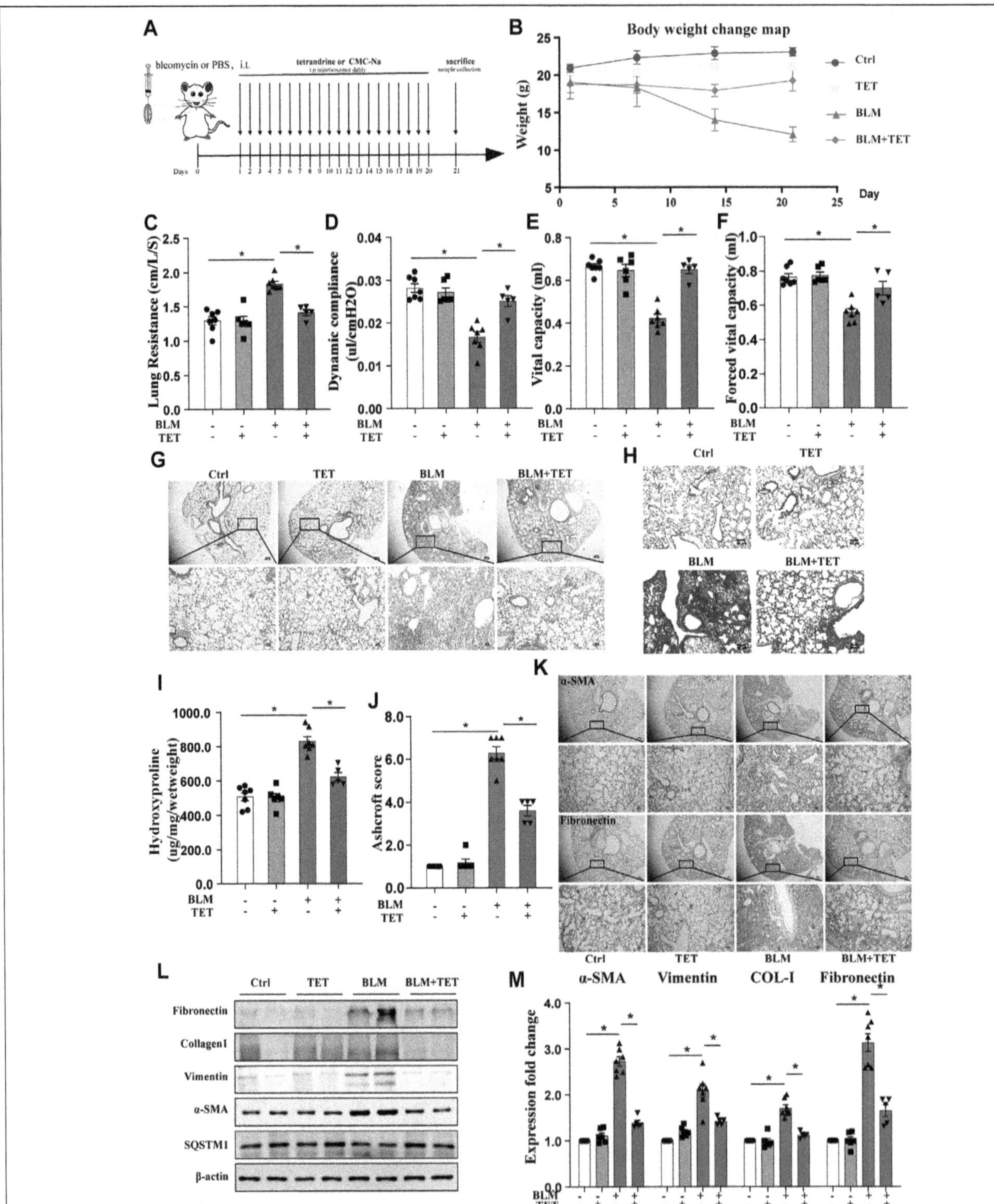

FIGURE 9 | TET treatment protects against pulmonary fibrosis induced by bleomycin. Mice, were treated prophylactically with either vehicle (sodium carboxymethyl cellulose, i. p, daily) or TET (20 mg $kg^{-1} \cdot d^{-1}$, i.p.) starting on Day 1 after receiving a single intratracheal administration of BLM. The control group received intratracheal PBS. **(A)** Schematic diagram of the time course of TET treatment in a mouse model of BLM-induced pulmonary fibrosis. **(B)** Changes in body weight were presented relative to the initial weight. **(C-F)** The pulmonary function parameters were measured by pulmonary function test. **(G)** Lung tissue was sectioned at day 21 and performed HE staining. Scale bar of top images: 100 μm, below images: 40 μm. **(H)** Lung tissues were stain with Masson trichrome staining. Scale bars: 40 μm. **(I)** Ashcroft scores were analyzed. **(J)** Hydroxyproline (HYP) expression of each group by hydroxyproline assay. **(K)** The protein expression of α-SMA (left images) and fibronectin (right images) in lung sample were examined by immunohistochemical staining. Scale bar of top images: 100 μm. Scale bar of below images: 40 μm. **(L-M)** Lung tissues were treated as described in (A) and subjected to immunoblots of fibrosis and autophagy-associated proteins(L) and densitometric analysis was obtained **(M)**. The data were presented as the means ± SEM (n ≥ 5). Two-way ANOVA followed by Dunnett's multiple comparisons test was used for statistical analysis. $^{*}p < 0.05$.

evaluated the extent of autophagic flux. Conversion of MAP1LC3-I to MAP1LC3-II was decreased in fibroblasts by stimulation with TGF-β1, indicating impaired autophagy. The effects of TGF-β1 were reversed by co-administration of TET in a dose-dependent manner (**Figures 3A,B**). SQSTM1, a cargo receptor protein, is degraded upon the delivery of ubiquitinated proteins to autophagosomes (Mauvezin and Neufeld 2015). We found that inhibition of the autophagy flux with chloroquine (CQ, which blocks fusion of autophagosomes and lysosomes) "TET regulated SQSTM1 in both autophagy dependent and independent manner" following treatment with TET induced the cytosolic accumulation of the SQSTM1 protein (**Figure 3G**). This observation indicates that the SQSTM1 protein is regulated by TET partially in an autophagy dependent manner. However, the inhibition of autophagy initiation by 3 MA treatment also induced the accumulation of the SQSTM1 protein (**Figure 3E**). Based on the above results, we believe that the increase in SQSTM1 by TET is likely to occur at the transcription regulation, rather than just a consequence of autophagic inhibition. Further, we observed that mRNA level of SQSTM1 is significantly upregulated by TET through PCR experiment (**Figure 3D**), which could positively contribute to the TET-induced autophagic flux. It is indicated that TET regulated SQSTM1 in both autophagy dependent and independent manner. Similarly, Immunofluorescence results indicated that the TET-induced punctate staining of MAP1LC3B was significantly increased after treatment with CQ, and the effect of TET was suppressed by 3-MA in TGF-β1-treated fibroblasts. (**Figures 3I,J**). Transmission electron microscopy (TEM) further supported the induction of autophagy by TET in TGF-β1-stimulated fibroblasts (**Figure 3K**). To further demonstrate whether TET restores TGF-β1-induced impaired autophagy, a double tagged MAP1LC3 (mRFP-GFP) plasmid was used to examine autophagic flux. Notably, consistent with rapamycin (RAP, a representative autophagy promotor), TET treatment increased red fluorescence (red, autolysosomes), whereas CQ treatment accumulated yellow fluorescence (yellow, autophagosomes) in TGF-β1-induced MLFs (**Figures 3L,M**).

In order to validate the relevance of TET with apoptosis in lung fibrosis, we examined the expression of cleaved-caspase3. The results show that TET did not affect the expression of cleaved-caspase3 (**Supplementary Figures S2A–E**). Additionally, TET did not induce apoptosis as shown on flow cytometry and TUNEL assay (**Supplementary Figures S2F–H**). These findings indicated that TET did activate autophagic flux characterized by SQSTM1 accumulation.

TET Activated SQSTM1-Mediated Selective Autophagy

The prevailing view is that ubiquitin-tagged misfolded proteins are assembled into aggregates by SQSTM1 (selective autophagy receptor), and the aggregates are then engulfed and degraded by autolysosomes (Svenning and Johansen, 2013). Interaction between selective autophagy receptors and MAP1LC3B is the molecular basis for selective autophagy. We next test whether TET induce autophagy in a SQSTM1 dependent manner. Our IP results show that TET treatment enhanced interaction of SQSTM1 and MAP1LC3B in TGF-β1-induced fibroblast (**Figures 4A,B**). Furthermore, the binding of SQSTM1 to ubiquitylated protein was significantly increased by TET (**Figure 4C**). Similarly, TET treatment efficiently enhanced the colocalization of SQSTM1 and MAP1LC3B and induced the SQSTM1-recruited cargos to autophagosomes (**Figures 4D,E**). Together, TET positively regulated selective autophagy via targeting SQSTM1.

NRF2 Regulated SQSTM1 Transcription Involved in TET-Induced Selective Autophagy

It has been demonstrated that both protein and mRNA expression of SQSTM1 were increased by TET, partially independent of autophagy pathway. We aim to investigate how TET regulates SQSTM1. Previous research suggested that transcription factor NRF2 can bind to promoter of SQSTM1, leading to promoted SQSTM1 transcription. We found that expression of NRF2 was decreased by TGF-β1, but increased by treatment with TET in fibroblasts (**Figures 5A,B**). To further confirm that SQSTM1 is regulated by NRF2, we performed ChIP for endogenous NRF2 in primary MLFs and analyzed the enrichment of NRF2 at the transcription start site (TSS). Firstly, using NCBI website and JASPAR programs, we analyzed the SQSTM1 promoter sequence to predict transcription factor binding sites (**Figures 5C,D**). Our data showed that TET increased enrichment of NRF2 at binding sites of SQSTM1 in TGF-β1-stimulated fibroblasts (**Figures 5E,F**).

TET Activated SQSTM1-Mediated Selective Autophagy via Rheb-mTOR Signaling

The mTOR kinase is a key regulator of autophagy induction (Hu et al., 2015). As our results show, TET significantly suppressed TGF-β1-induced mTOR activation and phosphorylation of P70 and 4E-BP1 (**Figures 6A–D**). Similarly, 4E-BP1 inhibition by TET was confirmed by immunofluorescent staining (**Figures 6E,F**). To investigate the role of mTOR during TET-induced autophagy, fibroblasts were treated with MHY1485, an activator of mTOR, after TET stimulation. Importantly, TET enhanced conversion of MAP1LC3-I to MAP1LC3-II, and this effect was reduced by MHY1485 (**Figures 6G–I**). These results suggest that TET-induced autophagy is related to the inhibition of mTOR signaling pathway.

Previous studies suggest mTOR activation is regulated by Rheb, a Ras-like small guanosine triphosphatase (GTPase) (Goordan et al., 2011; Narita et al., 2011). However, both the total Rheb protein and mRNA expression was not reduced by TET (**Figures 6J–L**). We next determined the Rheb activity by Co-IP. Our results showed that TET reduces Rheb activity in TGF-β1-stimulated fibroblasts (**Figure 6M**), suggesting TET negatively regulates Rheb activity but not protein or mRNA

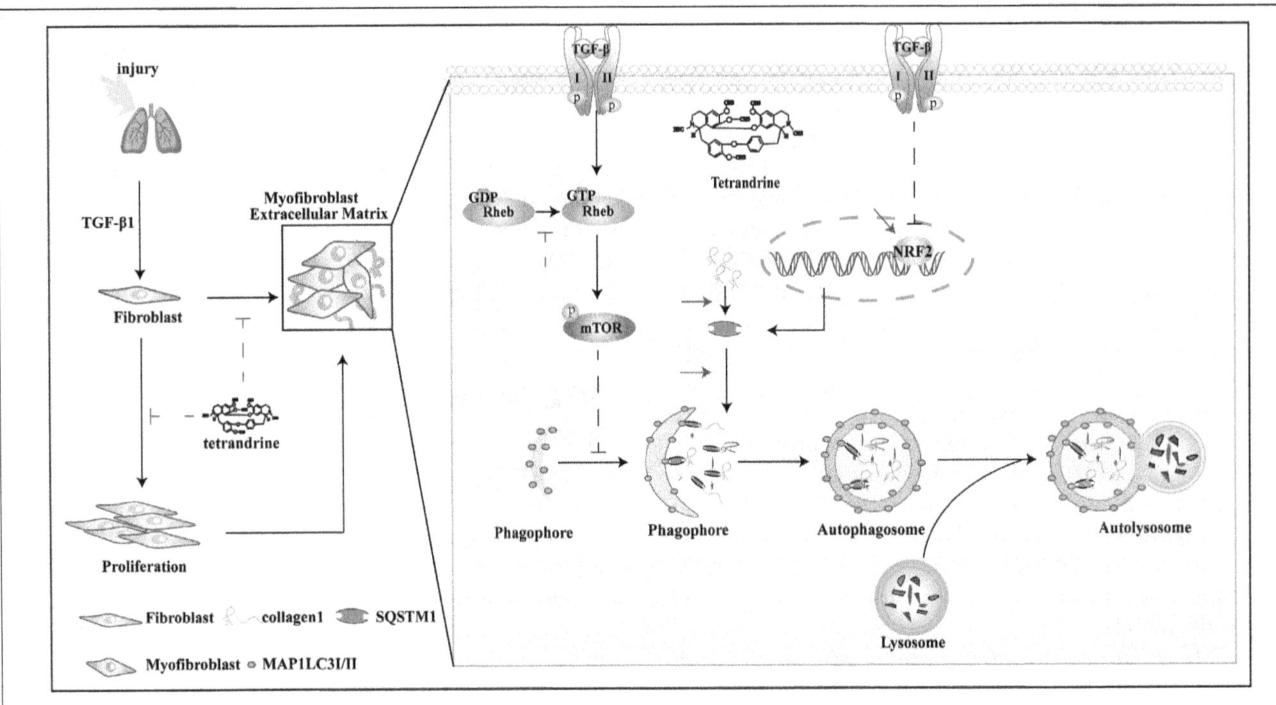

FIGURE 10 | Underlying mechanism of TET against pulmonary fibrosis through SQSTM1-mediated activation of autophagy. See the text for details.

expression. Taken together, TET activated autophagy through Rheb-mTOR signaling.

TET Attenuated TGF-β1-Induced Myofibroblasts Differentiation and Proliferation by Inducing Autophagy *In Vitro*

To further examine whether autophagy induction contributes to TET-mediated protective effects in lung fibrosis, we performed pharmacological and transgenic approaches to inhibit autophagy and detected fibrotic markers. The addition of Rapamycin (autophagy inducer as a positive control) downregulated expression of fibrotic markers in fibroblasts stimulated by TGF-β1 (**Figures 7A,B**). These results supported that autophagy inducers can attenuate lung fibrosis. We observed that fibronectin, collagen type I, vimentin, and α-SMA were all decreased by TET in TGF-β1-induced fibroblasts, and this effect was blocked by 3 MA (**Figures 7C–F**). Furthermore, silencing of ATG7 caused efficient downregulation of ATG7 protein expression compared with a non-silencing control and markedly inhibited TET-decreased expression of fibrotic markers in fibroblasts (**Figure 7G**). To test whether Rheb/mTOR signaling controls fibroblasts transdifferentiation, Rheb was overexpressed in fibroblasts. The effects of TET on suppressing fibrotic markers induced by TGF-β 1 was lost when Rheb is overexpressed (**Figure 7H**). Additionally, TET reduced TGF-β1-stimulated fibrotic expression, which was blocked by MHY1485, a small molecule activator of mTOR (**Figure 7I**). Taken together, TET attenuates lung fibrosis through inducing autophagy.

Type I Collagen Is Degraded by TET-Induced Autophagy

As shown before, TET presented a significant decrease in the steady-state levels of collagen inducing by TGF-β 1. However, the mechanism is unknown. Since previous data indicated that intracellular Col-I could degrade by lysosome (Sosulski et al., 2015) we hypothesized that Col-I is degraded by autophagy. The addition of TET increased the appearance of lysosomes and the colocalization of Col-I and lysosomes in TGF-β1-stimulated fibroblasts, indicating lysosomal degradation of Col-I (**Figure 8A**). Similarly, there are more endogenous Col-I colocalized with autophagosomes in cells treated with TET after TGF-β 1 stimulation (**Figure 8B**), further confirming that Col-I is degraded by autophagy. Interestingly, TET improved interaction of Col-I and SQSTM1 in TGF-β 1-induced fibroblasts (**Figure 8C**). These results suggest that Col-I is delivered to the lysosome *via* SQSTM1 for degradation during TET-induced autophagy.

TET Attenuated Lung Fibrosis in bleomycin-Induced Mouse Models Through Activating Autophagy

TET is a safe and widely used agent for silicosis and has therapeutic potential to restore cell metabolic homeostasis (Zhang et al., 2018). We explored whether TET can accelerate the resolution of fibrosis in the bleomycin (BLM)-induced lung fibrosis model. We treated mice with BLM at day 0 and started daily TET treatment from day 1–21 after BLM administration to examined the preventative effects of TET on pulmonary fibrosis (**Figure 9A**). Notably, TET attenuated BLM-induced mice body weight loss and impaired pulmonary function (**Figures 9B–F**). TET therapy significantly alleviated pulmonary fibrosis including improvement of the disordered lung structure and reduction of collagen deposition (**Figures 9G–J**). Histology and immunohistochemistry showed diminished amounts of collagen and α -SMA were seen in TET treatment group compared with BLM group (**Figure 9K**). Consistent with the histological analysis, immunoblotting showed that TET blocked the increase of extracellular matrix (ECM) deposition and α-SMA protein in BLM-challenged mice (**Figures 9L–M**). Importantly, these effects of TET are accompanied with autophagy activation (**Figure 9L**).

We also examined the therapeutic effects of TET on pulmonary fibrosis (**Supplementary Figure S4A**). These results demonstrated significant reduction in several fibrosis-related changes, including total lung hydroxyproline, histologic change, ECM deposition, and weight loss (**Supplementary Figure S4B–F**). These data indicated that TET activated autophagy to blunt bleomycin-induced lung fibrosis, suggesting a further potential therapeutic effect of TET on pulmonary fibrosis.

DISCUSSION

TET, originally isolated from Chinese herbs but now produced synthetically, has been tested for clinical trials and found to be effective against silicosis and lung cancer (Bhagya and Chandrashekar 2016). However, whether TET has anti-fibrotic activity and its potential mechanisms have not been systematically evaluated. In this study, we provide evidences that TET can resolve pulmonary fibrosis through inhibiting myofibroblast differentiation, proliferation, and ECM deposition. We found that TET can enhance the interaction of SQSTM1 with MAP1LC3-II and ubiquitinated proteins due to NRF2-mediated SQSTM1 transcription and Rheb-mTOR signaling activation, thus dramatically inducing SQSTM1-selective autophagy and directly leading to Col-I degradation in lysosome (**Figure 10**). This is the first report that showed the potential new mechanisms involved in TET-induced selective autophagy in the context of lung fibrosis.

TET therapy significantly attenuated experimental lung injury and produced similar therapeutic results in animal models of cardiac and liver injury. In a previous study, inhalation of TET could alleviate pulmonary fibrosis in a mouse model (Su et al., 2020). However, its precise role and its therapeutic utility in IPF remains unclear. Our results further explore the therapeutic role of TET on lung fibrosis. TET therapy effectively improved pulmonary function and decreased fibrotic markers in two mouse models. Specially, our data suggest that TET may play a role in reversing established pulmonary fibrosis. This is indicated by our observation that delayed administration of TET at day 8 after BLM-induced pulmonary fibrosis inhibits the procession of pulmonary fibrosis. Similarly, TET inhibits TGF-β1-induced fibroblast differentiation, proliferation, and ECM deposition *in vitro*. Impressively, TET therapy did not induce apoptosis, in contrast with previous studies (Liu et al., 2011), because the TET dose we used is not high to 30 μM. We suggest a more safe and effective concentration in lung fibrosis.

Network pharmacology studies emphasize the paradigm shift from "one target, one drug" to "network target, multicomponent therapeutics," highlighting a holistic thinking also shared by traditional Chinese medicine (TCM) (Li et al., 2014). Through network pharmacology analysis we found that the anti-fibrotic effect of TET may be related to autophagy. Previous studies using lung biopsies from IPF patients reported a diminution of autophagy (Patel et al., 2012; Araya et al., 2013) and some from animal model illustrated that TGF-β1 could mediate dysfunction of the autophagy response during lung fibrosis (Sosulski et al., 2015). Herein, we impart an appreciation for TET-mediated regulation of the autophagic response in TGF-β1-induced MLFs. Our findings demonstrated that TET may restrain differentiation of lung fibroblasts and ECM deposition through increasing autophagy flux. Furthermore, TET increased autophagy flux, MAP1LC3-II/SQSTM1 dependent ubiquitinated protein recycling, and lysosome degradation of Col-I. This study connects autophagy and protein homeostasis to lung fibrosis. Nevertheless, the redundancy of mechanism of TET that regulate lysosome homeostasis needs to be investigated, as protein metabolism is a complex process that involves multiple interacting signaling pathways (Araya and Nishimura 2010).

SQSTM1 serves as multifunctional regulator of cell signaling involved in selective autophagy (Svenning and Johansen, 2013; Lamark et al., 2017). Both MAP1LC3-II and SQSTM1 are required to maintain autophagy flux that promoted recruitment of SQSTM1-associated ubiquitinated proteins towards autophagosome-lysosome degradation. Interestingly, TET treatment significantly increases protein levels of SQSTM1 and MAP1LC3-II in TGF-β1-induced MLFs. It is important to confirm that the SQSTM1 mRNA level has not changed if the SQSTM1 protein level is used an indicator of autophagy flux. We provide evidence that TET dramatically increases mRNA expression of SQSTM1 in TGF-β1-induced MLFs. In addition, CQ, a lysosome inhibitor, can further increase protein levels of SQSTM1 at present of TET. This observation indicates that the SQSTM1 regulation is likely to occur at the level of transcription rather than due to the SQSTM1 protein accumulation as a consequence of autophagic inhibition. The increase in SQSTM1 expression by TET seemed to be autophagy-independent manner, but could positively contribute to the TET-induced autophagic flux. Previous studies suggest that TGF-β1-induced impaired autophagy is a critical pathogenesis of IPF, major in SQSTM1 gene repression. Emerging studies have found that NRF2 binds to the antioxidant response element (ARE) of the SQSTM1 promoter, leading to increase SQSTM1 transcription (Liu et al., 2007).

NRF2, a critical transcription factor, has a major anti-oxidant and anti-inflammatory effect. During stress conditions, NRF2 dissociates from Keap1 and translocates into the nucleus to regulate target genes through binding to ARE in their promoters (Hayes and McMahon 2009; Iso et al., 2016). However, the interaction of NRF2 and SQSTM1 is not confirmed in lung fibrosis. We show TET enhances the association between NRF2 and SQSTM1 and executes its anti-fibrosis effect via NRF2-SQSTM1pathway. Besides, defects in SQSTM1 may contribute to the deregulation in NRF2 activity seen in myofibroblasts and pulmonary fibrosis (Ichimura et al., 2013; Bian et al., 2018). Thus, up-regulation of SQSTM1 by TET may provide dual protection to TGF-β1-induced MLFs through facilitating both selective autophagy and the NRF2-mediated antioxidant response. Moreover, further investigations are required to clarify the involvement of NRF2 in the SQSTM1 transcription.

The Ras homolog enriched in the brain gene (Rheb) is ubiquitously expressed in mammalian cells and encodes proteins that play an important role in regulating cell growth and survival (Bai et al., 2007). Rheb exists either in an active GTP-bound state or an inactive GDP-bound state and only Rheb-GTP activates the rapamycin complex 1 (TORC1) (Goordan et al., 2011). Rheb/mTORC1 signaling plays a critical role for fibroblast activation in kidney fibrosis (Jiang et al., 2013). Our results show that TET inhibits the activity of Rheb by stimulating the conversion of Rheb-GTP to Rheb-GDP to repress mTOR signaling. Rheb activates mTOR signaling, including increased p-p70S6K and p-4E-BP1 (Huang and Manning 2008). Some studies provide strong support that mTORC1 signaling induces canonical Smad activation via 4E-BP1 phosphorylation which strongly promotes the profibrotic effect of TGF-β1 (Jiang et al., 2013). Indeed, TET inhibits mTORC1- 4E-BP1 signaling in TGF-β1-induced MLFs. Based on above data, we demonstrate that TET decreased collagen deposition induced by TGF-β1, partially through mTORC1/4E-BP1 signaling.

On the other hand, mTORC1 has been well established as the key negative regulator of autophagy, *via* suppression of the ULK1 complex at the initiation of autophagy (Yu et al., 2010). In this section, our data indicate TET can induce autophagy by inhibiting mTORC1 signaling pathway. Although mTORC1 is inactivated during autophagy initiation, it can be reactivated when energy supplies through the degradation of autolysosomal products at the end of autophagy flux. Interestingly, we found that TET can significantly increase the number of lysosomes which might be because of reactivated mTORC1. Its reaction is required for the reformation of functional lysosomes (Yu et al., 2010). Previous studies have been suggested that mTORC1 directly phosphorylates TFEB, a master transcriptional regulator of lysosomal and autophagy genes (Settembre et al., 2011). Taken together, TET induces autophagy by inactivating mTORC1 to supply more energy, then might reactivate mTORC1 in time-dependent manner to improve lysosome cycle. Nevertheless, further experiments will need to be performed to support this assumption.

Additionally, intracellular degradation of Col-I via autophagy indicates a critical role of autophagy in collagen homeostasis (Kim et al., 2012). We provide evidence TET improves co-localization Col-I with LAMP2 and MAP1LC3-II. Among these, we suggest TET reduced Col-I accumulation by dragging Col-1-LC3 complex into the lysosome for degradation. Therefore, our study provides initial evidence that TET -mediated degradation of Col-I through autophagy was partially resistance to pulmonary fibrosis.

In summary, TET, a monomeric component of traditional Chinese medicine, ameliorates BLM-induced experimental lung fibrosis. In addition, our results showed that TET exerts antifibrotic effects via NRF2/SQSTM1 signaling and Rheb/ mTORC1 pathway mediated autophagy. Furthermore, TET can promote SQSTM1 transcription by NRF2. This study shows a novel mechanism that NRF2 and SQSTM1 play fundamental roles through regulating autophagy in lung fibrosis. Based on these findings, TET should be considered as a therapeutic option for IPF patients.

AUTHOR CONTRIBUTIONS

YL and WZ designed and performed experiments, analyzed data, interpreted the results and wrote the manuscript. JZ, WC, and YeL performed experiments and analyzed data. YQ, ZZ, and HH performed experiments. HD and SC designed and supervised the study, interpreted the results, wrote, and edited the manuscript.

REFERENCES

Araya, J., and Nishimura, S. L. (2010). Fibrogenic Reactions in Lung Disease. *Annu. Rev. Pathol.* 5, 77–98. doi:10.1146/annurev.pathol.4.110807.092217

Araya, J., Kojima, J., Takasaka, N., Ito, S., Fujii, S., Hara, H., et al. (2013). Insufficient Autophagy in Idiopathic Pulmonary Fibrosis. *Am. J. Physiol. Lung Cel Mol Physiol.* 304 (1), L56–L69. doi:10.1152/ajplung.00213.2012

Baek, H. A., Kim, D. S., Park, H. S., Jang, K. Y., Kang, M. J., Lee, D. G., et al. (2012). Involvement of Endoplasmic Reticulum Stress in Myofibroblastic Differentiation of Lung Fibroblasts. *Am. J. Respir. Cel Mol Biol* 46 (6), 731–739. doi:10.1165/rcmb.2011-0121OC

Bai, X., Ma, D., Liu, A., Shen, X., Wang, Q. J., Liu, Y., et al. (2007). Rheb Activates mTOR by Antagonizing its Endogenous Inhibitor, FKBP38. *Science* 318 (5852), 977–980. doi:10.1126/science.1147379

Barth, S., Glick, D., and Macleod, K. F. (2010). Autophagy: Assays and Artifacts. *J. Pathol.* 221 (2), 117–124. doi:10.1002/path.2694

Bhagya, N., and Chandrashekar, K. R. (2016). Tetrandrine--A Molecule of Wide Bioactivity. *Phytochemistry* 125, 5–13. doi:10.1016/j.phytochem.2016.02.005

Bian, C., Qin, W. J., Zhang, C. Y., Zou, G. L., Zhu, Y. Z., Chen, J., et al. (2018). Thalidomide (THD) Alleviates Radiation Induced Lung Fibrosis (RILF) via Down-Regulation of TGF-β/Smad3 Signaling Pathway in an Nrf2-dependent Manner. *Free Radic. Biol. Med.* 129, 446–453. doi:10.1016/j.freeradbiomed.2018.10.423

Bueno, M., Lai, Y. C., Romero, Y., Brands, J., St Croix, C. M., Kamga, C., et al. (2015). PINK1 Deficiency Impairs Mitochondrial Homeostasis and Promotes Lung Fibrosis. *J. Clin. Invest.* 125 (2), 521–538. doi:10.1172/JCI74942

Ciani, B., Layfield, R., Cavey, J. R., Sheppard, P. W., and Searle, M. S. (2003). Structure of the Ubiquitin-Associated Domain of P62 (SQSTM1) and Implications for Mutations that Cause Paget's Disease of Bone. *J. Biol. Chem.* 278 (39), 37409–37412. doi:10.1074/jbc.M307416200

Curtis, M. J., Alexander, S., Cirino, G., Docherty, J. R., George, C. H., Giembycz, M. A., et al. (2018). Experimental Design and Analysis and Their Reporting II: Updated and Simplified Guidance for Authors and Peer Reviewers. *Br. J. Pharmacol.* 175 (7), 987–993. doi:10.1111/bph.14153

Goordan., S. M., Hoogeveen-Westerveld, M., Cheng, C., van Woerden, G. M., Mozaffari, M., Post, L., et al. (2011). Rheb Is Essential for Murine Development. *Mol. Cel Biol* 31 (8), 1672–1678. doi:10.1128/MCB.00985-10

Hariharan, N., Zhai, P., Sadoshima, J., and signaling, r. (2011). Oxidative Stress

Stimulates Autophagic Flux during Ischemia/reperfusion. *Antioxid. Redox Signal.* 14 (11), 2179–2190. doi:10.1089/ars.2010.3488

Hayes, J. D., and McMahon, M. (2009). NRF2 and KEAP1 Mutations: Permanent Activation of an Adaptive Response in Cancer. *Trends Biochem. Sci.* 34 (4), 176–188. doi:10.1016/j.tibs.2008.12.008

Hübner, R. H., Gitter, W., El Mokhtari, N. E., Mathiak, M., Both, M., Bolte, H., et al. (2008). Standardized Quantification of Pulmonary Fibrosis in Histological Samples. *Biotechniques* 44 (4), 507–11. doi:10.2144/000112729

Hu, B., Zhang, Y., Jia, L., Wu, H., Fan, C., Sun, Y., et al. (2015). Binding of the Pathogen Receptor HSP90AA1 to Avibirnavirus VP2 Induces Autophagy by Inactivating the AKT-MTOR Pathway. *Autophagy* 11 (3), 503–515. doi:10.1080/15548627.2015.1017184

Huang, J., and Manning, B. D. (2008). The TSC1-TSC2 Complex: a Molecular Switchboard Controlling Cell Growth. *Biochem. J.* 412 (2), 179–190. doi:10.1042/BJ20080281

Hutchinson, J., Fogarty, A., Hubbard, R., and McKeever, T. (2015). Global Incidence and Mortality of Idiopathic Pulmonary Fibrosis: a Systematic Review. *Eur. Respir. J.* 46 (3), 795–806. doi:10.1183/09031936.00185114

Ichimura, Y., Waguri, S., Sou, Y. S., Kageyama, S., Hasegawa, J., Ishimura, R., et al. (2013). Phosphorylation of P62 Activates the Keap1-Nrf2 Pathway during Selective Autophagy. *Mol. Cel* 51 (5), 618–631. doi:10.1016/j.molcel.2013.08.003

Iso, T., Suzuki, T., Baird, L., Yamamoto, M., and Biology, C. (2016). Absolute Amounts and Status of the Nrf2-Keap1-Cul3 Complex within Cells. *Mol. Cel Biol* 36 (24), 3100–3112. doi:10.1128/MCB.00389-16

Jiang, L., Xu, L., Mao, J., Li, J., Fang, L., Zhou, Y., et al. (2013). Rheb/mTORC1 Signaling Promotes Kidney Fibroblast Activation and Fibrosis. *J. Am. Soc. Nephrol.* 24 (7), 1114–1126. doi:10.1681/ASN.2012050476

Kim, S. I., Na, H. J., Ding, Y., Wang, Z., Lee, S. J., and Choi, M. E. (2012). Autophagy Promotes Intracellular Degradation of Type I Collagen Induced by Transforming Growth Factor (TGF)-β1. *J. Biol. Chem.* 287 (15), 11677–11688. doi:10.1074/jbc.M111.308460

King, T. E., Bradford, W. Z., Castro-Bernardini, S., Fagan, E. A., Glaspole, I., Glassberg, M. K., et al. (2014). A Phase 3 Trial of Pirfenidone in Patients with Idiopathic Pulmonary Fibrosis. *N. Engl. J. Med.* 370 (22), 2083–2092. doi:10.1056/NEJMoa1402582

King, T. J., Noble, P. W., and Bradford, W. Z. (2011). Idiopathic Pulmonary Fibrosis. *Lancet (London, England)* 378 (9807), 1949–1961. doi:10.1055/b-0034-74199

Klionsky, D. J., Cuervo, A. M., and Seglen, P. O. (2007). Methods for Monitoring Autophagy from Yeast to Human. *Autophagy* 3 (3), 181–206. doi:10.4161/auto.3678

Lamark, T., Svenning, S., and Johansen, T. (2017). Regulation of Selective Autophagy: the p62/SQSTM1 Paradigm. *Essays Biochem.* 61 (6), 609–624. doi:10.1042/EBC20170035

Li, S., Fan, T. P., Jia, W., Lu, A., and Zhang, W. (2014). Network Pharmacology in Traditional Chinese Medicine. *Evid. Based Complement. Alternat Med.* 2014, 138460. doi:10.1155/2014/138460

Lippai, M., and Lőw, P. (2014). The Role of the Selective Adaptor P62 and Ubiquitin-like Proteins in Autophagy. *Biomed. Res. Int.* 2014, 832704. doi:10.1155/2014/832704

Liu, Y., Kern, J. T., Walker, J. R., Johnson, J. A., Schultz, P. G., and Luesch, H. (2007). A Genomic Screen for Activators of the Antioxidant Response Element. *Proc. Natl. Acad. Sci. U S A.* 104 (12), 5205–5210. doi:10.1073/pnas.0700898104

Liu, C., Gong, K., Mao, X., and Li, W. (2011). Tetrandrine Induces Apoptosis by Activating Reactive Oxygen Species and Repressing Akt Activity in Human Hepatocellular Carcinoma. *Int. J. Cancer* 129 (6), 1519–1531. doi:10.1002/ijc.25817

Liu, T., Zhang, Z., Yu, C., Zeng, C., Xu, X., Wu, G., et al. (2017). Tetrandrine Antagonizes Acute Megakaryoblastic Leukaemia Growth by Forcing Autophagy-Mediated Differentiation. *Br. J. Pharmacol.* 174 (23), 4308–4328. doi:10.1111/bph.14031

Mauvezin, C., and Neufeld, T. P. (2015). Bafilomycin A1 Disrupts Autophagic Flux by Inhibiting Both V-ATPase-Dependent Acidification and Ca-P60A/SERCA-dependent Autophagosome-Lysosome Fusion. *Autophagy* 11 (8), 1437–1438. doi:10.1080/15548627.2015.1066957

Moscat, J., and Diaz-Meco, M. T. (2009). p62 at the Crossroads of Autophagy, Apoptosis, and Cancer. *Cell* 137 (6), 1001–1004. doi:10.1016/j.cell.2009.05.023

Narita, M., Young, A. R., Arakawa, S., Samarajiwa, S. A., Nakashima, T., Yoshida, S., et al. (2011). Spatial Coupling of mTOR and Autophagy Augments Secretory Phenotypes. *Science* 332 (6032), 966–970. doi:10.1126/science.1205407

Ohashi, A., Ohori, M., Iwai, K., Nakayama, Y., Nambu, T., Morishita, D., et al. (2015). Aneuploidy Generates Proteotoxic Stress and DNA Damage Concurrently with P53-Mediated post-mitotic Apoptosis in SAC-Impaired Cells. *Nat. Commun.* 6, 7668. doi:10.1038/ncomms8668

Patel, A. S., Lin, L., Geyer, A., Haspel, J. A., An, C. H., Cao, J., et al. (2012). Autophagy in Idiopathic Pulmonary Fibrosis. *PLoS One* 7 (7), e41394. doi:10.1371/journal.pone.0041394

Richeldi, L., du Bois, R. M., Raghu, G., Azuma, A., Brown, K. K., Costabel, U., et al. (2014). Efficacy and Safety of Nintedanib in Idiopathic Pulmonary Fibrosis. *N. Engl. J. Med.* 370 (22), 2071–2082. doi:10.1056/NEJMoa1402584

Settembre, C., Di Malta, C., Polito, V. A., Garcia Arencibia, M., Vetrini, F., Erdin, S., et al.(2011). TFEB Links Autophagy to Lysosomal Biogenesis. *Science* 332 (6036), 1429–1433. doi:10.1126/science.1204592

Sosulski, M. L., Gongora, R., Danchuk, S., Dong, C., Luo, F., and Sanchez, C. G. (2015). Deregulation of Selective Autophagy during Aging and Pulmonary Fibrosis: the Role of TGFβ1. *Aging cell* 14 (5), 774–783. doi:10.1111/acel.12357

Su, W., Liang, Y., Meng, Z., Chen, X., Lu, M., Han, X., et al. (2020). Inhalation of Tetrandrine-Hydroxypropyl-β-Cyclodextrin Inclusion Complexes for Pulmonary Fibrosis Treatment. *Mol. Pharm.* 17 (5), 1596–1607. doi:10.1021/acs.molpharmaceut.0c00026

Svenning, S., and Johansen, T. (2013). Selective Autophagy. *Essays Biochem.* 55, 79–92. doi:10.1042/bse0550079

Teng, G., Svystonyuk, D., Mewhort, H. E., Turnbull, J. D., Belke, D. D., Duff, H. J., et al. (2015). Tetrandrine Reverses Human Cardiac Myofibroblast Activation and Myocardial Fibrosis. *Am. J. Physiol. Heart Circ. Physiol.* 308 (12), H1564–H1574. doi:10.1152/ajpheart.00126.2015

Wang, H., Liu, T., Li, L., Wang, Q., Yu, C., Liu, X., et al. (2015). Tetrandrine is a Potent Cell Autophagy Agonist via Activated Intracellular Reactive Oxygen Species. *Cell Biosci* 5, 4. doi:10.1186/2045-3701-5-4

Yin, M. F., Lian, L. H., Piao, D. M., and Nan, J. X. (2007). Tetrandrine Stimulates the Apoptosis of Hepatic Stellate Cells and Ameliorates Development of Fibrosis in a Thioacetamide Rat Model. *World J. Gastroenterol.* 13 (8), 1214–1220. doi:10.3748/wjg.v13.i8.1214

Yu, L., McPhee, C. K., Zheng, L., Mardones, G. A., Rong, Y., Peng, J., et al. (2010). Termination of Autophagy and Reformation of Lysosomes Regulated by mTOR. *Nature* 465 (7300), 942–946. doi:10.1038/nature09076

Zhang, Z., Liu, T., Yu, M., Li, K., and Li, W. (2018). The Plant Alkaloid Tetrandrine Inhibits Metastasis via Autophagy-dependent Wnt/β-Catenin and Metastatic Tumor Antigen 1 Signaling in Human Liver Cancer Cells. *J. Exp. Clin. Cancer Res.* 37 (1), 7. doi:10.1186/s13046-018-0678-6

9

Dec1 Deficiency Ameliorates Pulmonary Fibrosis through the PI3K/AKT/GSK-3β/β-Catenin Integrated Signaling Pathway

Xingxing Hu[1†], Menglin Zou[1†], Lan Ni[1†], Mingyang Zhang[1], Weishuai Zheng[1], Bing Liu[1] and Zhenshun Cheng[1,2*]*

[1]Department of Respiratory and Critical Care Medicine, Zhongnan Hospital of Wuhan University, Wuhan, China, [2]Wuhan Research Center for Infectious Diseases and Cancer, Chinese Academy of Medical Sciences, Wuhan, China

***Correspondence:**
Bing Liu
bingliu@whu.edu.cn
Zhenshun Cheng
zhenshun_cheng@126.com

[†]These authors have contributed equally to this work and share first authorship

Tissue remodeling/fibrosis is a main feature of idiopathic pulmonary fibrosis (IPF), which results in the replacement of normal lung parenchyma with a collagen-rich extracellular matrix produced by fibroblasts and myofibroblasts. Epithelial-mesenchymal transition (EMT) in type 2 lung epithelial cells is a key process in IPF, which leads to fibroblasts and myofibroblasts accumulation and excessive collagen deposition. DEC1, a structurally distinct class of basic helix-loop-helix proteins, is associated with EMT in cancer. However, the functional role of DEC1 in pulmonary fibrosis (PF) remains elusive. Herein, we aimed to explore DEC1 expression in IPF and bleomycin (BLM)-induced PF in mice and the mechanisms underlying the fibrogenic effect of DEC1 in PF *in vivo* and *in vitro* by *Dec1*-knockout (*Dec1*$^{-/-}$) mice, knockdown and overexpression of *DEC1* in alveolar epithelial cells (A549 cells). We found that the expression of DEC1 was increased in IPF and BLM-injured mice. More importantly, *Dec1*$^{-/-}$ mice had reduced PF after BLM challenge. Additionally, DEC1 deficiency relieved EMT development and repressed the PI3K/AKT/GSK-3β/β-catenin integrated signaling pathway in mice and in A549 cells, whereas *DEC1* overexpression *in vitro* had converse effects. Moreover, the PI3K/AKT and Wnt/β-catenin signaling inhibitors, LY294002 and XAV-939, ameliorated BLM-meditated PF *in vivo* and relieved EMT *in vivo* and *in vitro*. These pathways are interconnected by the GSK-3β phosphorylation status. Our findings indicated that during PF progression, DEC1 played a key role in EMT via the PI3K/AKT/GSK-3β/β-catenin integrated signaling pathway. Consequently, targeting DEC1 may be a potential novel therapeutic approach for IPF.

Keywords: pulmonary fibrosis, differentiated embryonic chondrocyte expressed gene 1, epithelial-mesenchymal transition, PI3K/AKT/GSK-3β/β-catenin integrated signaling pathway, bleomycin, TGF-β1

INTRODUCTION

Idiopathic pulmonary fibrosis (IPF), the most common type of idiopathic interstitial pneumonia (IIP), is a chronic, irreversible and typically fatal fibrotic lung disease, which is characterized by overproduction and disorganized deposition of extracellular matrix (ECM) proteins, together with abnormal proliferation of mesenchymal cells, ultimately leading to distortion of pulmonary architecture and impairment of pulmonary functions (Okamoto et al., 2011; Wolters et al.,

2018). The incidence and prevalence of IPF reportedly range from 2 to 30 cases per 100,000 person-years and 10–60 cases per 100,000 people, respectively. The disease has a grave prognosis with an estimated median survival time of 3–5 years following diagnosis if untreated (Martinez et al., 2017). Currently, only two drugs, nintedanib and pirfenidone, are FDA-approved for the treatment of IPF, but they only reduce the rate of lung function decline, and they may have several serious side effects (Kasam et al., 2020). At present, the pathogenesis of IPF is poorly understood. Therefore, it is necessary to investigate the precise mechanisms underlying IPF and identify new antifibrotic therapeutic approaches.

In recent years, the proposed mechanisms involved in IPF have been reported to include epithelial cell dysfunction, fibroblast proliferation and excessive ECM production (Inoue et al., 2020). Dysregulation of type 2 alveolar epithelial cells (AEC2s) is thought to be central in fibrogenesis in IPF (Richeldi et al., 2017). Fibroblasts and myofibroblasts, which express the contractile protein, α-smooth muscle actin (α-SMA), and produce excessive ECM, are the key sources of ECM and are implicated in the pathogenesis of pulmonary fibrosis (PF). In the lung, myofibroblasts are mainly derived from activated lung fibroblasts. Additionally, it has been reported that epithelial microinjuries (of a yet unknown cause) trigger abnormal epithelial-mesenchymal interactions and pathogenesis of IPF(Fernandez and Eickelberg, 2012). More importantly, emerging evidence suggests that epithelial-mesenchymal transition (EMT) of alveolar epithelial cells contributes to the cellular origin of fibroblasts and myofibroblasts accumulation, ultimately resulting in the development of PF (Chen et al., 2013; Goldmann et al., 2018; Hill et al., 2019). EMT is a multifunctional process in which epithelial cells lose the epithelial phenotype and acquire the mesenchymal phenotype, accompanied by down-regulation of epithelial cell marker (e.g., E-cadherin) and upregulation of mesenchymal cell marker (e.g., N-cadherin and Vimentin), thereby promoting PF development (Thiery et al., 2009; Peng et al., 2020). A growing body of research has demonstrated that many signaling pathways are involved in the regulation of EMT induced during fibrosis (Gonzalez and Medici, 2014). Recently, several signaling pathways have been regarded as important regulators of EMT in IPF. These include phosphoinositide 3-kinase (PI3K)/AKT-, Wnt-, transforming growth factor-beta (TGF-β)- and vascular endothelial growth factor (VEGF)-dependent pathways (Yan et al., 2014). Hence, elucidation of the underlying molecular mechanism may ultimately be beneficial for obtaining innovative therapeutic strategies against IPF.

Human differentiated embryonic chondrocyte expressed gene 1 (DEC1), also known as BHLHE40/Stra13/Sharp2, belongs to a structurally distinct class of basic helix- loop-helix (bHLH) proteins (Sato et al., 2016). It has been considered as a signaling mediator of diverse physiological processes including circadian rhythmicity, immunity, proliferation, apoptosis, senescence, tumorigenesis, and fibrosis (Honma et al., 2002; Qian et al., 2008; Gallo et al., 2018; Jia et al., 2018; Jarjour et al., 2019; Le et al., 2019; Li et al., 2019). A previous study has reported that *Dec1* deficiency suppressed cardiac perivascular fibrosis in hypertrophic hearts induced by transverse aortic constriction (TAC), resulting in preserved cardiac function (Le et al., 2019). However, the significance of DEC1 in PF has never been investigated.

In this study, we aimed to elucidate the effects of DEC1 on bleomycin (BLM)-induced PF and EMT in mice, and on TGF-β1-induced EMT in A549 cells. Furthermore, we explored the underlying downstream signaling mechanisms regulated by DEC1 *in vivo* and *in vitro*.

MATERIALS AND METHODS

Reagents

Bleomycin was purchased from HANHUI PHARMACEUTICALS CO., LTD. (Zhejiang, China). Recombinant human TGF-β1 (Cat. No.: 100-21-2) was obtained from Peprotech (Rocky Hill, NJ, United States). The PI3K/AKT and Wnt/β-catenin pathway inhibitors, LY294002 (Cat. No.: HY-10108) and XAV-939 (Cat. No.: HY-15147), respectively, were obtained from MedChem Express (Monmouth Junction, NJ, United States). Dimethyl sulfoxide (DMSO) was purchased from Sigma–Aldrich (St. Louis, MO, United States). All other solvents used in this study were of an analytical grade or higher and acquired from commercial sources.

Human Samples

Lung tissues from IPF patients (n = 3) were collected in Zhongnan Hospital of Wuhan University. Three normal lung tissues from resection of cancer were used as control. Patients were diagnosed with IPF according to the American Thoracic Society (ATS)/European Respiratory Society (ERS) consensus diagnostic criteria (Raghu et al., 2018).

Gene Expression Omnibus (GEO) Database Analysis

Search for the keyword "IPF" in the GEO database, the website is https://www.ncbi.nlm.nih.gov/geo/. Identify the biochip data related to IPF, compare the IPF in the chip data with normal lung tissue, and analyze the differential expression of DEC1 between IPF and normal lung tissue. This study uses two gene chips (GSE53845 and GSE5774), of which the GSE53845 chip belongs to GPL6480 (Agilent-014850 Whole Human Genome Microarray 4 × 44K G4112F), including 40 cases of IPF and 8 cases of normal human lung tissue samples; GSE5774 chip belongs to GPL4225 (NIH- NIEHS/Agilent Human Familial IIP 43K array), including 26 cases of IIP and 9 cases of normal human lung tissue samples.

Animal Experiments

Experimental Animals

$Dec1^{+/-}$ (C57BL/6 background) male and female mice were acquired from Prof. Yang Jian (Nanjing Medical University, Nanjing, China), whose *Dec1*-knockout ($Dec1^{-/-}$) mice (RBRC04841) were originally obtained from RIKEN BioResource Center. $Dec1^{+/-}$ males and females were mated to obtain male WT ($Dec1^{+/+}$) and KO ($Dec1^{-/-}$) littermates for experiments. All healthy male mice, weighing 20–26 g (9–10 weeks old) were kept under pathogen-free conditions on a 12-h light/dark cycle, at a room temperature of 25 ± 2°C and a relative humidity of 55 ± 5%. Before the PF model was established, the mice underwent an acclimatization period of at least 1 week.

Murine Model of Pulmonary Fibrosis

To induce PF, mice were anesthetized with pentobarbital (6 ml/kg 1% pentobarbital) and treated once with 50 μL of 2.5 mg/kg BLM via intratracheal instillation on day 0. Mice in the control group received an equal volume of sterile saline.

Animal Experimental Groups

1) To investigate the effect of DEC1 on PF, EMT and the activity of the PI3K/AKT/GSK-3β/β-catenin integrated signaling pathway, mice were randomly divided into four groups: WT + control group, WT + BLM group, KO + control group and KO + BLM group. BLM was dissolved in saline.
2) To verify the participation of the PI3K/AKT/GSK-3β/β-catenin integrated signaling pathway in PF, mice were randomly assigned into four groups: WT + BLM group, WT + BLM + DMSO group, WT + BLM + LY294002 group and WT + BLM + XAV-939 group. Mice began to receive the inhibitors (LY294002 and XAV-939) or DMSO *via* intraperitoneal injection 1 day before the BLM administration and LY294002 was administrated every other day for 21 days (25 mg/kg per injection) and XAV-939 was injected once daily for 11 days (10 mg/kg per injection). DMSO (10%) diluted in saline was used as a control and to dissolve the inhibitors (LY294002 and XAV-939).

On day 21 after the BLM or 0.9% saline intervention, the mice were anesthetized with 1% pentobarbital sodium or sacrificed under CO2, and were then subjected to bronchoalveolar lavage, and finally the lung tissues were rapidly collected. The left lung tissues were fixed in 4% paraformaldehyde for histological analysis, and the right lung tissues were stored at −80°C until being used for the hydroxyproline assay, quantitative real-time PCR (qRT-PCR) and western blotting.

Cell Culture and Intervention

A549 cell line were purchased from the Type Culture Collection of the Chinese Academy of Sciences (Shanghai, China) and cultured in RPMI-1640 medium (Hyclone, UT, United States) supplemented with 10% fetal bovine serum (FBS) (Gibco, Waltham, MA, United States) and 1% antibiotics (100 μg/ml streptomycin and 100 μg/ml penicillin) at 37°C in a 5% CO_2 incubator.

To induce the EMT model *in vitro*, cells at 50–60% confluence were starved with serum-free medium for 12 h, and then subjected to recombinant human TGF-β1 (10 ng/ml) for 48 h. Cells were assigned into different groups as follows:

1) control group and TGF-β1 group.
2) shRNA-NC group, shRNA-*DEC1* group, TGF-β1 + shRNA-NC group and TGF-β1 + shRNA-*DEC1* group.
3) Vector group, *DEC1* cDNA group, *DEC1* cDNA + LY294002 group and *DEC1* cDNA + XAV-939 group. A549 cells were treated with LY294002 or XAV-939 for 1 h prior to the transfection with *DEC1* plasmids. LY294002 and XAV-939 were dissolved in 0.1% DMSO and diluted to 10 μM during cell treatment.

Cell Transfections

Lentiviruses containing short hairpin RNAs specially targeting *DEC1* (shRNA-*DEC1*) or the scramble control short hairpin RNA (shRNA-NC) were purchased from GeneChem (Shanghai, China). Cells were cultured for 24 h in a 6-well plate (8 × 10^4 cells/well), and then transfected with scrambled shRNA or DEC1 shRNA at a MOI of 40. After 8 h, the medium was replaced with 10% RPMI-1640 medium for 72 h when the cells reached 70–80% confluence. Then the cells were incubated with 3 μg/ml puromycin to select stable cell line. Knockdown efficiency was verified by western blotting. For *DEC1* overexpression plasmids construction and transfection, human *DEC1* cDNA was purchased from GeneChem (Shanghai, China). Transfection was carried out using the Lipo8000™ Transfection Reagent (Beyotime, Shanghai, China) according to the manufacturer's instructions. Overexpression efficiency was verified by western blotting.

Quantitative Real-Time PCR (qRT-PCR)

Total RNA was isolated using TRIzol (Invitrogen, Carlsbad, CA, United States) according to the manufacturer's instructions. RNA reverse transcription was conducted using ReverTra Ace qPCR RT Kit (TOYOBO, Osaka, Japan) and qPCR was performed using UltraSYBR Mixture (CWBIO, Beijing, China). The relative mRNA expression levels were measured on the basis of the Ct value and relative to the endogenous reference gene, *GAPDH*, in accordance with the $2^{-\Delta\Delta Ct}$ method.

The mouse primer sequences used in the study were listed as follows: DEC1: forward, 5′-CGTTGAAGCACGTGAAAG CA-3′, reverse, 5′-AAGTACCTC ACGGGCACAAG-3′; E-cadherin: forward, 5′-GACCG GAAGTGACTCGAAATG-3′, reverse, 5′-CCCTCGTAATCGAACAC CAAC-3′; Vimentin: forward, 5′-GCAGT ATGAAAGCGTGGCTG-3′, reverse, 5′-GCTCCAGGGACTCGTTAGTG-3′; α- SMA: forward, 5′-GGACGTACAACTGGTATTGTGC-3′, reverse, 5′-TCGGCAGTAGTC ACGAAGGA-3′; COL1A1: forward, 5′-GACGGGAGTTTCTCCTCGG G-3′, reverse, 5′-GGG ACCCTTAGGCCATTGTG-3′; COL1A2: forward, 5′-GGGCAAAA GAGAAGGATTGGTC-3′, reverse, 5′-AGCC ACAAGTGGTGCGAAT-3′; MMP2: forward, 5′-ACCTGAACACTTTC TATGGCTG-3′, reverse, 5′-CTTCCGCATGGTC TCGATG-3′; GAPDH: forward, 5′-TGAAGGGTGGAGCCAAAAG-3′, reverse, 5′-AGTCTTC TGGGTGGCAGTGAT-3′.

The human primer sequences used in the study were listed as follows: DEC1: forward, 5′-ATCCAGCGGACTTTCGCTC-3′, reverse, 5′-TAAT TGCGCCG ATCCTTTCTC-3′; E-cadherin: forward, 5′- GAGAACGCA TTGCCACATACAC-3′, reverse, 5′-GCACCTTCCATGACA GACCC-3′; Vimentin: forward, 5′- AGTCCACT

GAGTACCGGAGAC-3′, reverse, 5′- CATTTCACGCATCTG GCGTTC-3′; GAPDH: forward, 5′-GTCTCCTCTGACTTC AACAGCG-3′, reverse, 5′-ACCACCCTGTTG CTGTAGCCAA-3′.

Western Blotting

Proteins were extracted from lung tissues and A549 cells using RIPA lysis buffer (Sigma–Aldrich, St. Louis, MI, United States) supplemented with PMSF (Beyotime, Shanghai, China) and Phosphatase Inhibitor Cocktail (CWBIO). Tissue and cell lysates were centrifuged at 12,000 × *g* for 15 min at 4°C, and then the supernatants were immediately collected. Equal protein quantities were then subjected to 10% SDS-PAGE, transferred onto poly-vinylidene fluoride membranes (Millipore, Bedford, MA, United States), blocked with 5% skim milk for 1 h at room temperature, and then incubated with the indicated primary antibodies at 4°C overnight. The primary antibodies were as follows: DEC1 (NB100-1800SS, Novus, Centennial, CO, United States), E-cadherin (3,195, CST, Danvers, MA, United States), N-cadherin (13,116, CST), Vimentin (5,741, CST), AKT1/2/3 (ab179463, Abcam, Cambridge, MA, United States), p-AKT (Ser473) (4,060, CST), GSK-3β (ab32391, Abcam), p-GSK-3β (Ser9) (5,558, CST), β-catenin (ab32572, Abcam) and GAPDH (AS1039, Aspen, Wuhan, China). The membranes were then incubated with horseradish peroxidase-conjugated anti-rabbit secondary antibodies for 1 h at room temperature. Subsequently, the specific protein bands were visualized with an enhanced ECL kit (Thermo Fisher Scientific, Waltham, MA, United States), and then exposed to the electrochemiluminescence (ECL) system (Tanon, Shanghai, China).

Determination of Lung Hydroxyproline Level

To measure the total collagen content of the left lung, the hydroxyproline contents of lung tissues on day 21 after BLM administration were measured using the Hydroxyproline assay kit (Cat. No.: A030-2, Nanjing Jiancheng Bioengineering Institute, Nanjing, China) in accordance with the manufacturer's method.

Histopathology Analysis

The lung samples were fixed with 4% formaldehyde, followed by de-hydration and embedding in paraffin. The tissues were cut into 3-μm-thick transverse sections. Then, hematoxylin and eosin (H&E) and Masson's trichrome staining were performed using standard techniques. The degree of lung fibrosis was evaluated using the Ashcroft method (Ashcroft et al., 1988).

Immunofluorescence

For tissue Immunofluorescence (IF) staining, formalin-fixed and paraffin-embedded sections were deparaffinized in xylene, hydrated with an ethanol gradient and briefly washed with distilled water. Paraffin sections were placed in a repair box filled with EDTA antigen retrieval buffer (pH 8.0) and heated in a microwave oven for antigen retrieval. Next, the sections were incubated with goat serum for 30 min, followed by incubation with primary antibodies at 4°C overnight. The next day, the sections were incubated with different fluorescein-conjugated secondary antibodies for 50 min at room temperature in the dark, and nuclear staining with DAPI was performed for 10 min. Finally, images of IF staining were taken using a fluorescence microscope.

For cell IF staining, cells were plated and grown on sterilized glass coverslips. Cells were washed three times with cold PBS and fixed with 4% paraformaldehyde for 30 min, and then incubated with primary antibodies at 4°C overnight. Next, cells were incubated with fluorescein-labeled goat anti-rabbit secondary antibodies for 50 min at 37°C in the dark. Nuclear staining with DAPI was performed for 10 min. The cells were observed under a fluorescence microscope.

Statistical Analysis

All data in this study were analyzed with SPSS 21.0 or GraphPad Prism 8.0 and were presented as means ± SEM of at least three independent experiments. Student's *t*-test and one-way ANOVA were used for comparison between two or multiple groups. $p < 0.05$ was considered statistically significant.

RESULTS

DEC1 Is Increased in Idiopathic Pulmonary Fibrosis Patients and Bleomycin-Stimulated Pulmonary Fibrosis in Mice

Before we study the functional role of DEC1 in PF, we first measured the expression of DEC1 in lung tissues from IPF patients. Just as we expected, DEC1 expression was obviously increased in the lungs from IPF (**Figures 1A,B**). Additionally, we found that DEC1 was highly expressed in IPF and IIP patients by analyzing data from GEO database (GSE53845 and GSE5774) (**Figure 1C**). To further address our assumption, we examined DEC1 expression in the BLM-induced PF murine model. We noticed that BLM significantly upregulated the protein and mRNA expression of DEC1 in lung tissues (**Figures 1D–H**). Consequently, these results verify that the expression of DEC1 is obviously enhanced in IPF patients and BLM-induced mice.

Dec1 KO Ameliorates Bleomycin-Induced Pulmonary Fibrosis in Mice

The role of DEC1 in PF induced by BLM was investigated using *Dec1* KO (*Dec1*$^{-/-}$) mice. The genotypes of the mice were identified by the protocol provided by Nanjing Medical University (**Supplementary Figure S1A**). After WT and KO mice were administrated with BLM or saline for 21 days, lung tissues were collected for analysis. Firstly, WT mice exposed to BLM demonstrated obvious deposition of collagen in the lungs compared with saline-treated WT mice, whereas the collagen content was clearly reduced in BLM-induced KO mice (**Figures 2A,C**). To quantify lung fibrosis, we evaluated the Ashcroft score in the lung sections images. As shown in **Figure 2B**, BLM-induced WT mice attained a higher Ashcroft score compared with saline-treated WT mice, whereas BLM-

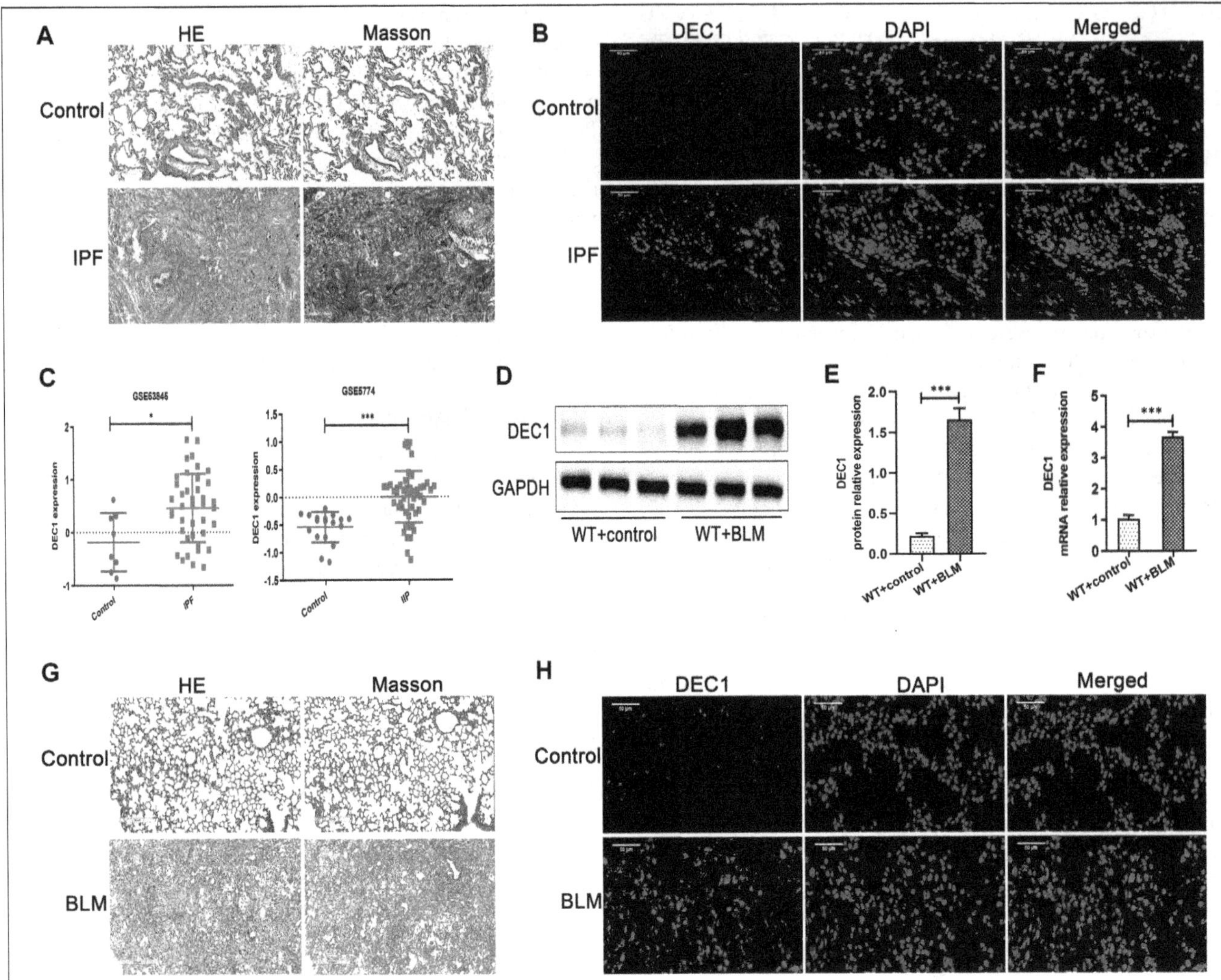

FIGURE 1 | DEC1 is increased in IPF patients and BLM-stimulated PF in mice. **(A)** Representative HE staining and Masson's trichrome staining of lung tissues from normal people and IPF patients. Scale bar = 200 μm $n = 3$. **(B)** Representative immunofluorescence staining of DEC1 (red) in the lung sections from normal people and IPF patients. Nuclei are stained with DAPI (blue). Scale bar = 50 μm $n = 3$. **(C)** The expression of DEC1 in the lung tissues from healthy people, IPF patients and IIP patients by analyzing GEO database. **(D)** The protein expression of DEC1 in the lung tissues were detected by western blotting. $n = 6$. **(E)** Statistical analysis of relative expression levels of proteins in **(D)**. **(F)** The mRNA expression of *DEC1* in the lung tissues were measured by qRT-PCR. $n = 6$. **(G)** Representative HE staining and Masson's trichrome staining of lung tissues in mice. Scale bar = 200 μm $n = 6$. **(H)** Representative immunofluorescence staining of DEC1 (red) in the lung tissues of mice. Nuclei are stained with DAPI (blue). Scale bar = 50 μm $n = 6$. All data are shown as the mean ± SEM. Statistical analysis was performed by student's t-test. $^{*}p < 0.05$, $^{**}p < 0.01$, $^{***}p < 0.001$, $^{ns}\ p > 0.05$.

induced KO mice acquired lower scores compared with BLM-induced WT mice. Furthermore, we evaluated the mRNA expression of several fibrosis-related markers in the different groups, such as *α-SMA*, *COL1A1*, *COL1A2*, and *MMP2*. BLM significantly induced the expression of these fibrosis-related markers in WT mice; however, this induced expression was attenuated in the KO mice (**Figure 2D**). The protein levels of α-SMA and collagen I were altered in accordance with the mRNA results above (**Figures 2E,F**). Namely, *Dec1* KO suppressed the expression of fibrosis-related markers in the BLM-induced PF model. To sum up, DEC1 expression is increased in the BLM-induced PF model in mice and *Dec1* KO ameliorates the BLM-induced PF, suggesting that DEC1 is involved in the development of BLM-induced PF.

Dec1 KO Inhibits EMT in the Bleomycin-Induced Pulmonary Fibrosis Murine Model

To investigate the mechanism involved in the development of PF *in vivo*, we examined the expression of the classic EMT-related markers, E-cadherin, N-cadherin and Vimentin, in the lung tissues of mice. EMT, the transition from an epithelial to a mesenchymal state, is one of the crucial processes in PF (Yang et al., 2019; Skibba et al., 2020). BLM induced the development of EMT in WT mice, which was associated with significant downregulation of the protein expression of the epithelial cell marker E-cadherin, and the upregulation of the protein level of the mesenchymal cell markers, N-cadherin and Vimentin. In

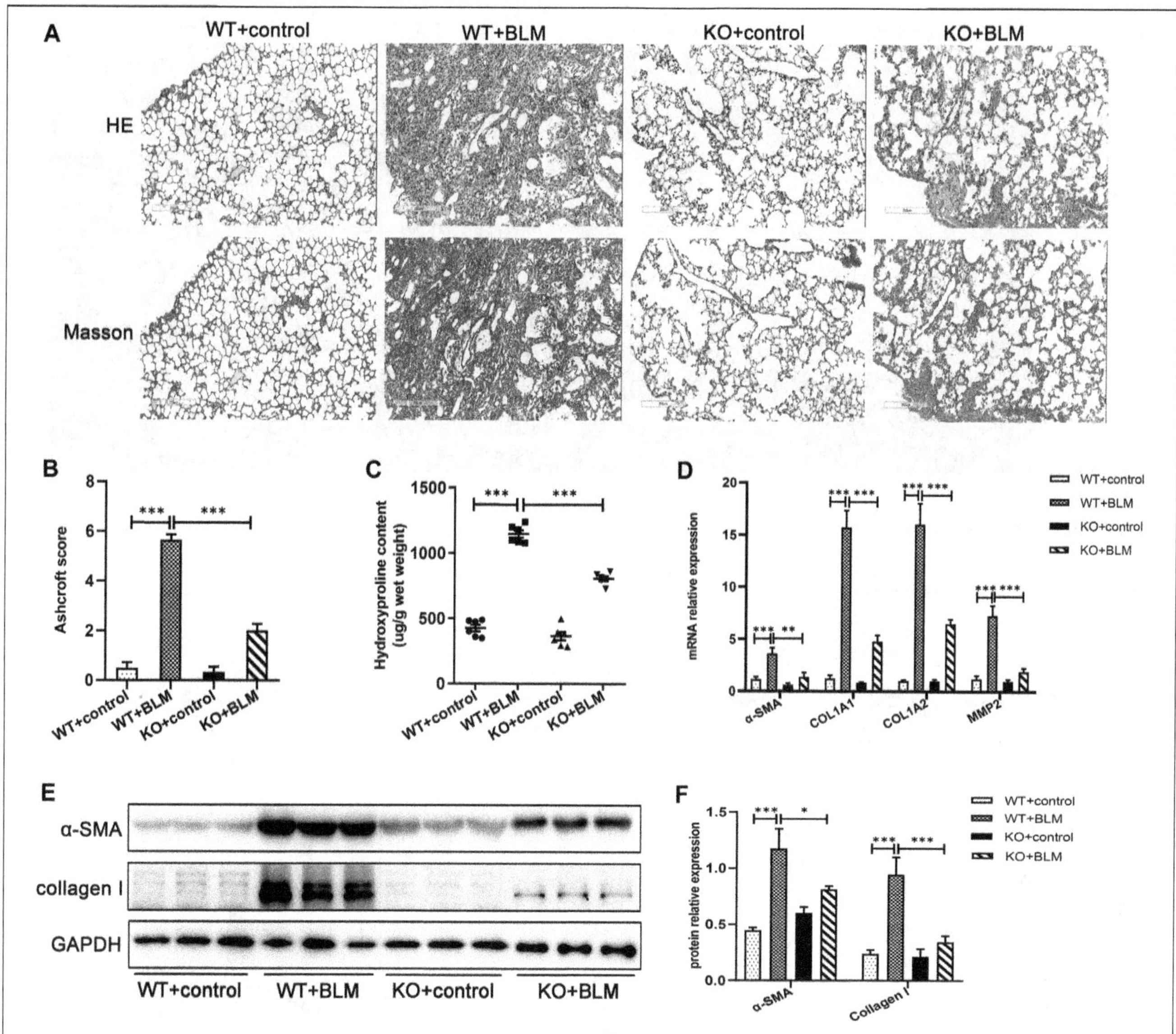

FIGURE 2 | *Dec1* KO ameliorates BLM-induced PF in mice. WT and KO mice were treated with a single intratracheal injection of BLM (2.5 mg/kg) or saline for 21 days. **(A)** Representative HE staining and Masson's trichrome staining of lung tissues in mice. Scale bar = 200 μm. **(B)** Ashcroft score was measured using the Ashcroft method. **(C)** Total collagen levels were assessed by measuring hydroxyproline content in the lung tissues of mice. **(D)** The mRNA expression of *α-SMA, COL1A1, COL1A* and *MMP2* in the lung tissues of mice were measured by qRT-PCR. **(E)** The protein expression of α-SMA and collagen I in the lung tissues of mice were detected by western blotting. **(F)** Statistical analysis of relative expression levels of proteins in E. $n = 6$. Data are shown as the mean ± SEM. Statistical analysis was performed by one-way ANOVA. $^{*}p < 0.05$, $^{**}p < 0.01$, $^{***}p < 0.001$, $^{ns}p > 0.05$.

contrast, the accumulation of E-cadherin was significantly increased and the expression of N-cadherin and Vimentin was obviously decreased in the BLM-induced *Dec1* KO mice compared with the BLM-induced WT mice (**Figures 3A–C**). Furthermore, the transcription levels of *E-cadherin* and *Vimentin* were regulated consistently with the corresponding protein results (**Figure 3D**). Additionally, as for TGF-β1 is a strong inducer of EMT, we made an examination of TGF-β1 in BALF, BLM significantly upregulated the concentration of TGF-β1 in mice BALF. However, TGF-β1 expression induced by BLM was attenuated in *Dec1*-knockout mice (**Figure 3E**). These results indicate that *Dec1* KO impedes the development of EMT in the BLM-induced PF model.

Dec1 KO Suppresses the Activation of the PI3K/AKT/GSK-3β/β-Catenin Signaling Pathway in the Bleomycin-Induced Pulmonary Fibrosis Murine Model

Next, we explored the specific signaling pathways involved in EMT during BLM-induced PF. To this end, we assessed the role of DEC1 in the PI3K/AKT/GSK-3β/β-catenin signaling pathway. We found that BLM upregulated AKT and GSK-3β phosphorylation and the level of β-catenin protein without obvious changes in the total AKT and GSK-3β expression levels in WT mice. In contrast, the levels of p-ser473-AKT,

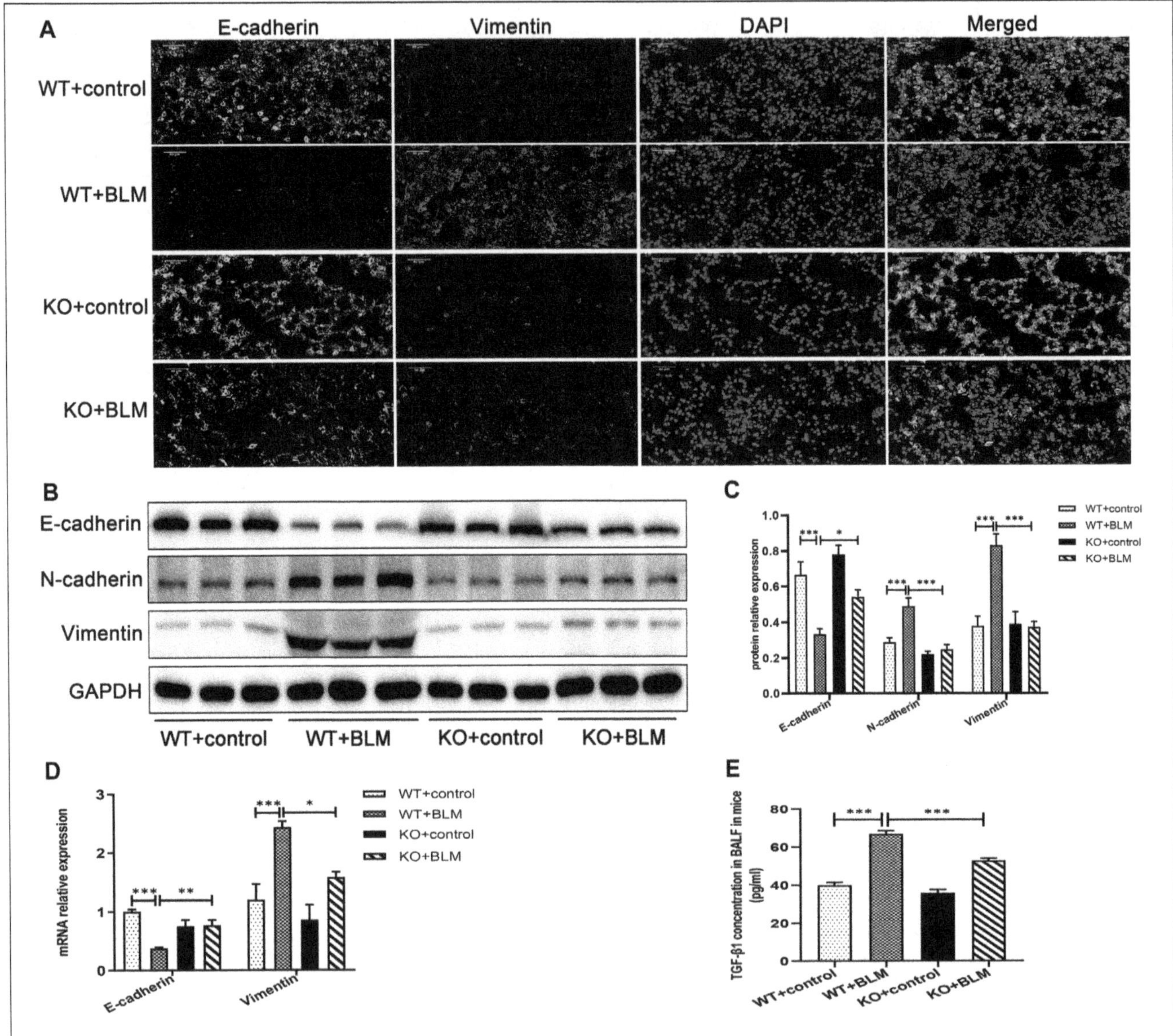

FIGURE 3 | *Dec1* KO inhibits EMT in the BLM-induced PF murine model. WT and KO mice were treated with a single intratracheal injection of BLM (2.5 mg/kg) or saline for 21 days. **(A)** Dual immunofluorescent analysis for E-cadherin and Vimentin expression in the lungs tissue of mice. Scale bar = 50 μm. **(B)** The protein expression of E-cadherin, N-cadherin and Vimentin in the lung tissues of mice were measured by western blotting. **(C)** Statistical analysis of relative expression levels of proteins in **(B)**. **(D)** The mRNA expression of *E-cadherin* and *Vimentin* in the lung tissues of mice were assessed by qRT-PCR. **(E)** TGF-β1 levels in BALF of mice. $n = 6$. Data are shown as the mean ± SEM. Statistical analysis was performed by one-way ANOVA. $^{*}p < 0.05$, $^{**}p < 0.01$, $^{***}p < 0.001$, $^{ns}p > 0.05$.

p-ser9-GSK3β and β-catenin were effectively decreased in BLM- induced KO mice, suggesting an involvement of the PI3K/AKT/GSK-3β/β-catenin signaling pathway in BLM-induced PF *in vivo* and that *Dec1* KO inhibits the activation of this BLM-induced pathway (**Figures 4A,B**).

Inhibition of the PI3K/AKT/GSK-3β/β-Catenin Signaling Pathway Relieved Bleomycin-Induced Pulmonary Fibrosis

To further clarify whether the PI3K/AKT/GSK-3β/β-catenin signaling pathway participates in EMT in the BLM-induced PF murine model, we examined the effect of LY294002 and XAV-939, potent inhibitors of the PI3K/AKT and Wnt/β-catenin signaling pathways, respectively, on lung fibrosis induced by BLM. Mice were administrated with LY294002, XAV-939 or DMSO. Interestingly, both LY294002 and XAV-939 ameliorated the degree of lung collagen deposition in the BLM-induced PF murine model (**Figures 5A–C**) and distinctly reversed the BLM-induced mRNA levels of the fibrosis-related markers, *α-SMA*, *COL1A1*, *COL1A2*, and *MMP2* (**Figure 5D**). Additionally, the changes in α-SMA and collagen I protein levels after intervening with LY294002 and XAV-939 were congruent with the mRNA results (**Figures 5E,F**). To further investigate the relationship between DEC1 and PI3K/AKT/GSK-3β/β-

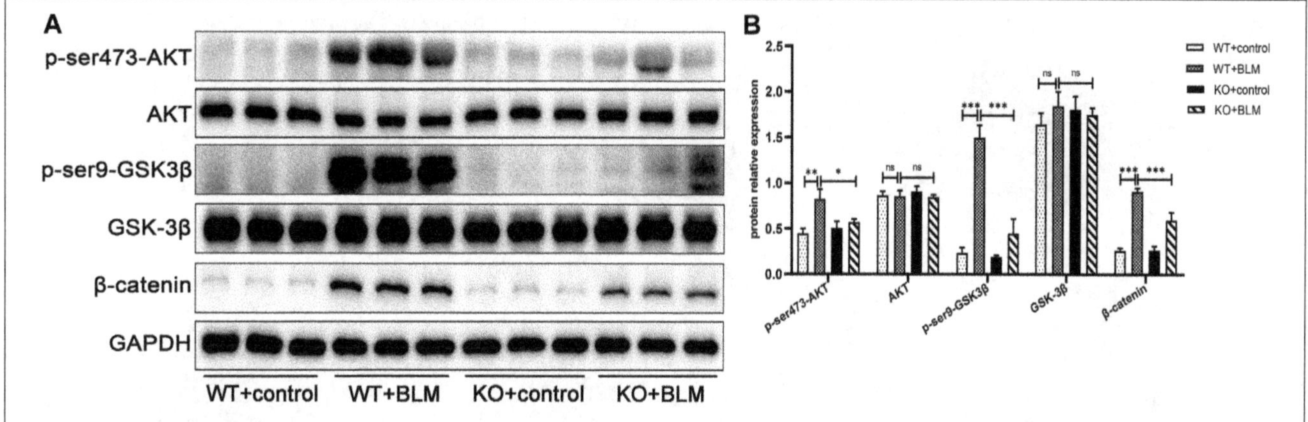

FIGURE 4 | *Dec1* KO suppresses the activation of the PI3K/AKT/GSK-3β/β-catenin signaling pathway in the BLM-induced PF murine model. WT and KO mice were treated with a single intratracheal injection of BLM (2.5 mg/kg) or saline for 21 days **(A)** The protein expression of p-ser473-AKT, AKT, p-ser9-GSK3β, GSK-3β and β-catenin in the lung tissues of mice were detected by western blotting. **(B)** Statistical analysis of relative expression levels of proteins in A. $n = 6$. Data are shown as the mean ± SEM. Statistical analysis was performed by one-way ANOVA. $^{*}p < 0.05$, $^{**}p < 0.01$, $^{***}p < 0.001$, $^{ns}p > 0.05$.

catenin signaling pathway, we detected the protein level of DEC1 under LY294002 and XAV-939 treatment. Importantly, both LY294002 and XAV-939 did not alter the BLM-induced protein level of DEC1 in lung tissues of mice (**Figures 5E,F**).

Inhibition of the PI3K/AKT/GSK-3β/β-Catenin Signaling Pathway Repressed Epithelial-Mesenchymal Transition in the Bleomycin-Induced Pulmonary Fibrosis Murine Model

Subsequently, we examined whether LY294002 and XAV-939 affect the EMT process induced by BLM. Consistent with our expectation, LY294002 and XAV-939 clearly suppressed BLM-induced EMT, showing elevated protein level of E-cadherin and reduced protein levels of N-cadherin and Vimentin (**Figures 6A,B**). The changes in *E-cadherin* and *Vimentin* mRNA levels were consistent with the changes in their protein level (**Figure 6C**). Furthermore, dual immunofluorescence for E-cadherin and Vimentin was performed to confirm the changed expression in lung tissues following the intervention with the two inhibitors (**Figure 6D**). Taken together, these data demonstrate that DEC1 plays an important role in BLM-induced PF and EMT *via* the PI3K/AKT/GSK-3β/β-catenin signaling pathway.

DEC1 Expression is Upregulated in TGF-β1-Induced EMT in A549 Cells

DEC1 has been reported to be involved in TGF-β1-induced EMT in PANC-1 cells (Wu et al., 2012). Additionally, our animal experiments demonstrated that *Dec1* KO ameliorated lung fibrosis by inhibiting EMT *in vivo*, hence, we examined the DEC1 expression in TGF-β1-induced A549 cells. Firstly, we observed that TGF-β1 successfully induced EMT. Compared with the control group, TGF-β1 downregulated the protein expression of E-cadherin, whereas it upregulated N-cadherin and Vimentin protein expression in A549 cells (**Figures 7A,B**). Furthermore, the mRNA levels of *E-cadherin* and *Vimentin* were altered similarly to the above protein results (**Figure 7C**). Secondly, TGF-β1 increased the protein expression levels of p-ser473-AKT and p-ser9-GSK3β and induced the accumulation of β-catenin without distinct changes in the total AKT and GSK-3β expression levels (**Figures 7D,E**), suggesting that TGF-β1 activated the PI3K/AKT/GSK-3β/β-catenin signaling pathway during the development of EMT. Thirdly, we assayed the DEC1 protein and mRNA expression levels in the two groups. An obviously higher level of DEC1 expression was found in the TGF-β1-induced group compared with the control group (**Figures 7F–H**). Additionally, dual immunofluorescence for E-cadherin and DEC1 confirmed that TGF-β1 downregulated the level of E-cadherin and upregulated DEC1 expression (**Figure 7I**).

DEC1 KD Suppresses TGF-β1-Induced Epithelial-Mesenchymal Transition in A549 Cells

Because DEC1 was significantly upregulated in TGF-β1-induced EMT in A549 cells, we further investigated whether DEC1 plays a significant role in the EMT process. We conducted experiments using the *DEC1* knockdown (KD) model, which was established by an shRNA lentiviral construct. The most effective shRNA, shRNA1-*DEC1*, was selected for the following experiments (**Supplementary Figures S1B,S1C**). We examined the changes in EMT-related markers in A549 cells after transfection with shRNA-*DEC1* lentiviruses. After TGF-β1 stimulation, shRNA-*DEC1* cells expressed higher protein level of E-cadherin and lower protein levels of N-cadherin and Vimentin compared with the shRNA-NC cells (**Figures 8A,B**). Additionally, the transcription levels of *E-cadherin* and *Vimentin* were changed in line with the protein results (**Figure 8C**). Moreover, the protein alterations in E-cadherin

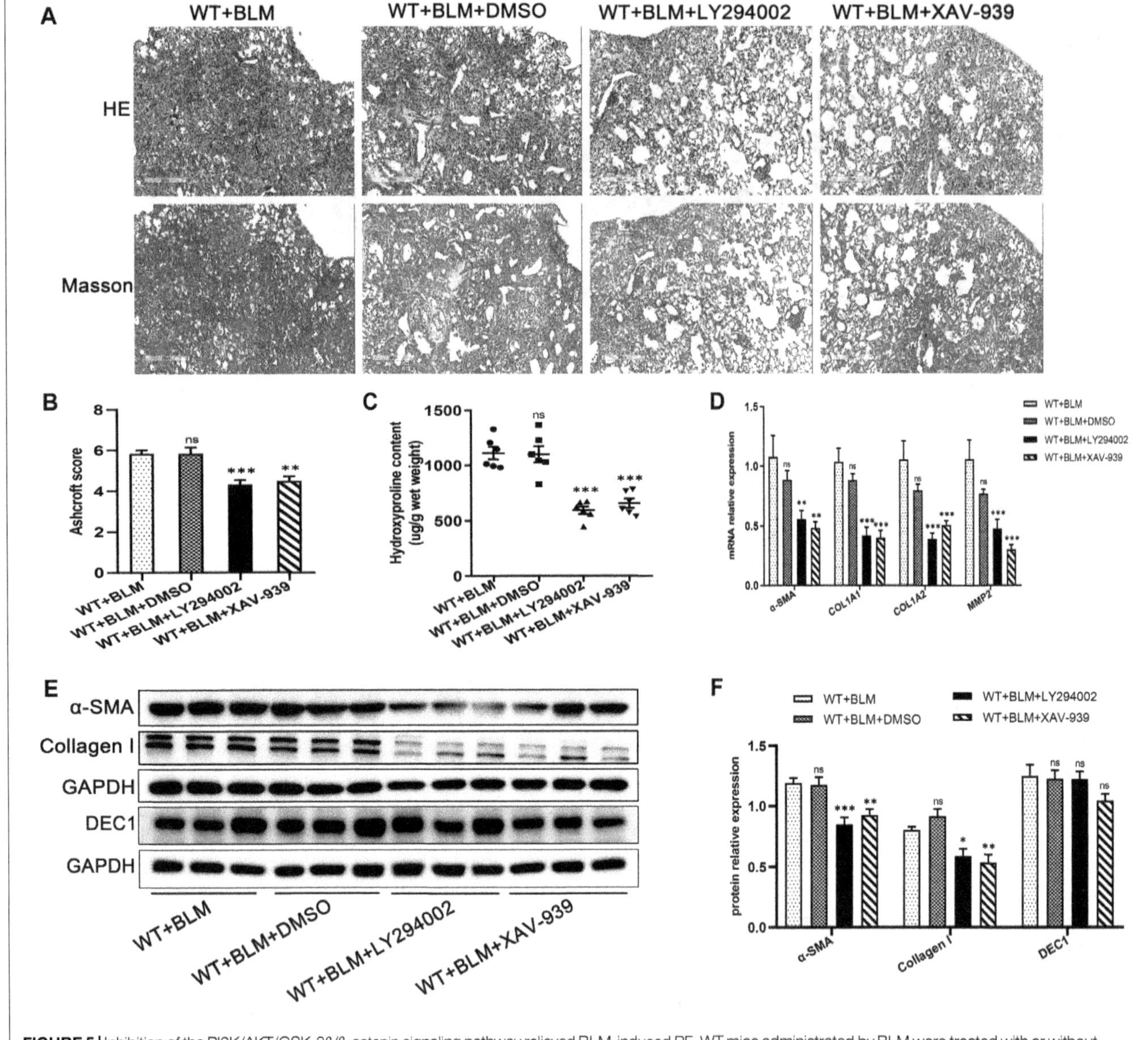

FIGURE 5 | Inhibition of the PI3K/AKT/GSK-3β/β-catenin signaling pathway relieved BLM-induced PF. WT mice administrated by BLM were treated with or without LY294002 or XAV-939 or DMSO for 21 days. **(A)** Representative HE staining and Masson's trichrome staining in the lung tissues in mice. Scale bar = 200 μm. **(B)** Ashcroft score was measured using the Ashcroft method. **(C)** Total collagen levels were assessed by measuring hydroxyproline content in the lung tissues of mice. **(D)** The mRNA expression of *α-SMA, COL1A1, COL1A*, and *MMP2* in the lung tissues of mice were measured by qRT-PCR. **(E)** The protein expression of α-SMA, collagen I and DEC1 in the lung tissues of mice were detected by western blotting. **(F)** Statistical analysis of relative expression levels of proteins in E. $n = 6$. Data are shown as the mean ± SEM. Statistical analysis was performed by one-way ANOVA. $^{*}p < 0.05$, $^{**}p < 0.01$, $^{***}p < 0.001$, $^{ns}p > 0.05$.

and Vimentin were once again confirmed by immunofluorescence (**Figure 8D**). Taken together, these results show that *DEC1* KD alleviates TGF-β1-induced EMT in A549 cells.

DEC1 KD Reduces the Activation of the PI3K/AKT/GSK-3β/β-Catenin Signaling Pathway in A549 Cells

In order to determine the mechanism of action of DEC1 in TGF-β1-stimulated EMT, we analyzed the expression of PI3K/AKT/GSK-3β/β-catenin signaling pathway-related molecules in TGF-β1-stimulated EMT model. Interestingly, we discovered that a combination treatment of shRNA-*DEC1* and TGF-β1 clearly decreased the levels of p-ser473-AKT, p-ser9-GSK3β and β-catenin compared with TGF-β1-induced shRNA-NC cells (**Figures 9A,B**). Moreover, the protein alterations in β-catenin were certified by immunofluorescence (**Figure 9C**). Above results indicate that *DEC1* KD represses the TGF-β1-induced activation of the PI3K/AKT/GSK-3β/β-catenin signaling pathway in A549 cells.

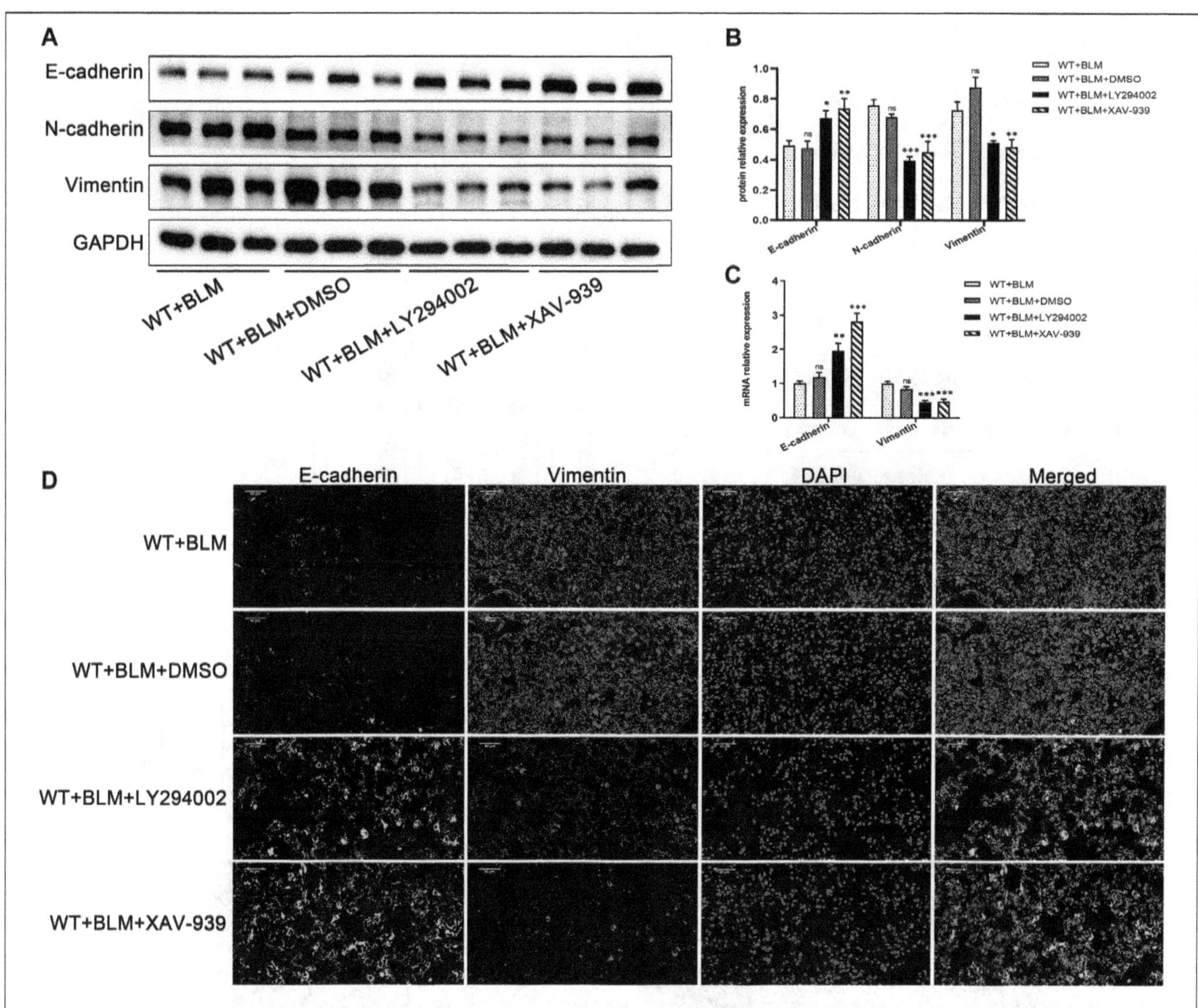

FIGURE 6 | Inhibition of the PI3K/AKT/GSK-3β/β-catenin signaling pathway repressed EMT in the BLM-induced pulmonary fibrosis murine model. WT mice administrated by BLM were treated with or without LY294002 or XAV-939 or DMSO for 21 days. **(A)** The protein expression of E-cadherin, N-cadherin and Vimentin in the lung tissues of mice were measured by western blotting. **(B)** Statistical analysis of relative expression levels of proteins in A. **(C)** The mRNA expression of *E-cadherin* and *Vimentin* in the lung tissues of mice were assessed by qRT-PCR. **(D)** Dual immunofluorescent analysis for E-cadherin and Vimentin expression in the lungs tissue of mice. Scale bar = 50 μm $n = 6$. Data are shown as the mean ± SEM. Statistical analysis was performed by one-way ANOVA. $^{*}p < 0.05$, $^{**}p < 0.01$, $^{***}p < 0.001$, $^{ns}p > 0.05$.

DEC1 Overexpression Induces Epithelial-Mesenchymal Transition and Activates the PI3K/AKT/GSK3β/β-Catenin Signaling Pathway in A549 Cells

To further verify the fibrogenic effect of DEC1 and the involvement of the PI3K/AKT/GSK-3β/β-catenin signaling pathway in EMT, we overexpressed DEC1 in A549 cells by *DEC1* plasmid and used the signaling pathway inhibitors, LY294002 and XAV-939. Overexpression plasmid successfully overexpressed DEC1 in A549 cells (**Supplementary Figures S1D,S1E**) and both inhibitors effectively reduced the phosphorylation levels of the corresponding proteins. More importantly, we observed that *DEC1* overexpression significantly reduced the protein expression of E-cadherin, whereas it enhanced the protein level of N-cadherin and Vimentin (**Figures 10A,B**). Moreover, *DEC1* overexpression distinctly increased the expression of p-ser473-AKT, p-ser9-GSK3β and β-catenin (**Figures 10C,D**). These results demonstrated that *DEC1* overexpression successfully induced EMT and activated the PI3K/AKT/GSK-3β/β-catenin signaling pathway. Meanwhile, cells were stimulated with inhibitors. Compared with the *DEC1* cDNA group, the expression of p-ser473-AKT, p-ser9-GSK3β and β-catenin was reduced by LY294002, and the expression of p-ser9-GSK3β and β-catenin was decreased by XAV-939. Furthermore, LY294002 and XAV-939 reversed the *DEC1* cDNA-induced EMT process, as evident from the increased protein levels of E-cadherin, whereas the distinctly decreased N-cadherin and Vimentin protein expression (**Figures 10A,B**). Additionally, the expression changes in E-cadherin,

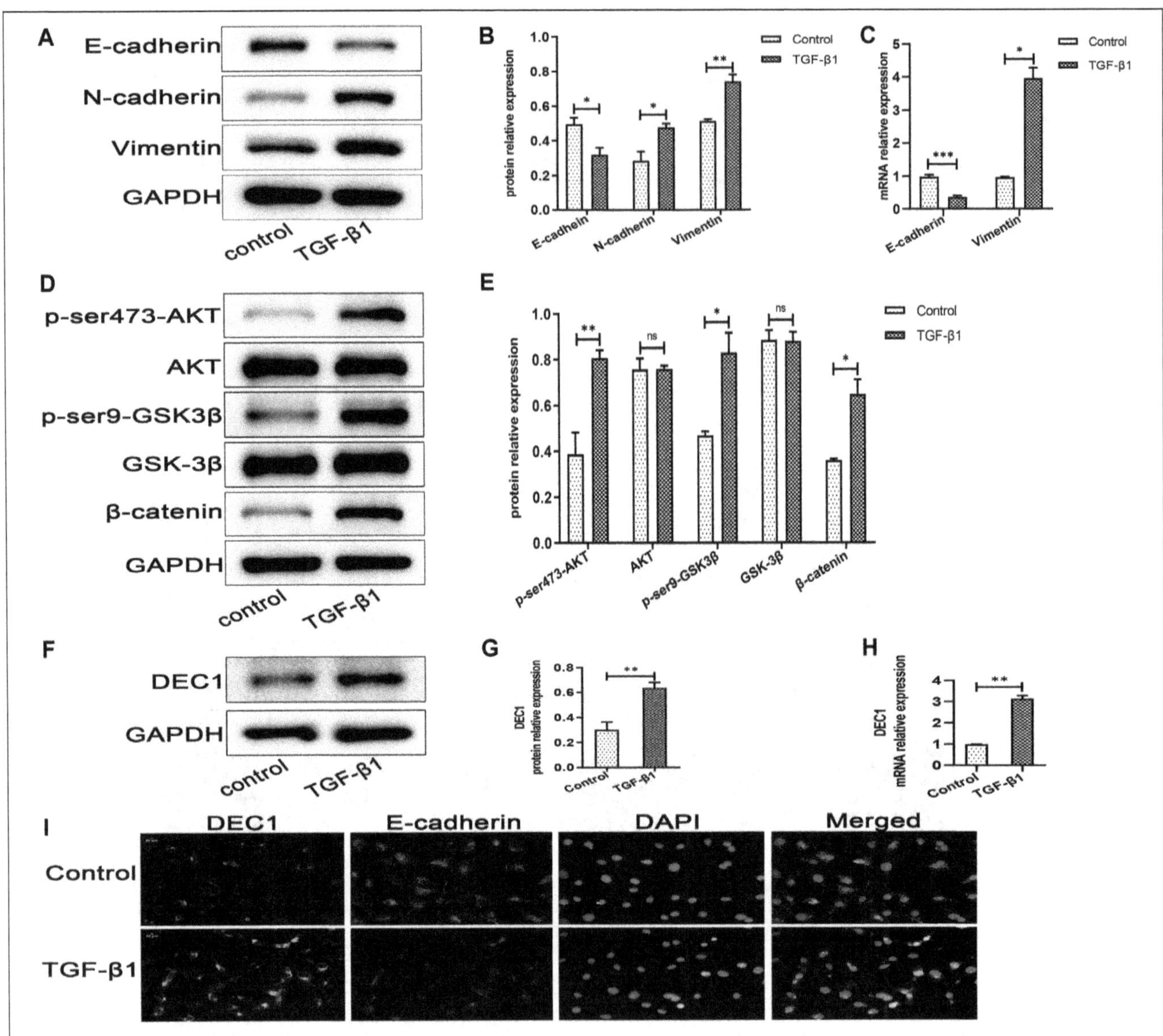

FIGURE 7 | DEC1 expression is upregulated in TGF-β1-induced EMT in A549 cells. A549 cells were treated with TGF-β1 for 48 h. **(A)** The protein expression of E-cadherin, N-cadherin and Vimentin in A549 cells were measured by western blotting. **(B)** Statistical analysis of relative expression levels of proteins in A. **(C)** The mRNA expression of *E-cadherin* and *Vimentin* in A549 cells were assessed by qRT-PCR. **(D)** The protein expression of p-ser473-AKT, AKT, p-ser9-GSK3β, GSK-3β and β-catenin in A549 cells were measured by western blotting. **(E)** Statistical analysis of relative expression levels of proteins in D. **(F)** The protein expression of DEC1 in A549 cells were detected by western blotting. **(G)** Statistical analysis of relative expression level of proteins in F. **(H)** The mRNA expression of *DEC1* in A549 cells were detected by qRT-PCR. **(I)** Dual immunofluorescent analysis for DEC1 and E-cadherin expression in A549 cells. Scale bar = 20 μm $n = 3$. Data are shown as the mean ± SEM. Statistical analysis was performed by student's t-test. $^{*}p < 0.05$, $^{**}p < 0.01$, $^{***}p < 0.001$, $^{ns}p > 0.05$.

Vimentin and β-catenin in these groups were further validated by immunofluorescence (**Figure 10E**). The findings in this study demonstrated that *DEC1* overexpression induced EMT, and this effect was dependent on the PI3K/AKT/GSK-3β/β-catenin signaling pathway activation.

DISCUSSION

IPF is a clinically common chronic fibrotic lung disease with unknown etiology, characterized by progressive PF, high disability rate and mortality (Richeldi et al., 2017). In this study, we demonstrated the role of DEC1 in the development of PF. The major findings of our study were that DEC1 was high expressed in IPF patients and BLM-challenged PF in mice. Moreover, *Dec1* KO markedly ameliorated PF in mice by inhibiting the EMT process in a BLM-induced PF model. Additionally, consistent with the *in vivo* results, *DEC1* KD suppressed TGF-β1-induced EMT, whereas *DEC1* overexpression induced EMT *in vitro*. Importantly, DEC1 regulated the activity of the PI3K/AKT/GSK-3β/β-catenin signaling pathway to regulate PF and the EMT process *in vivo*

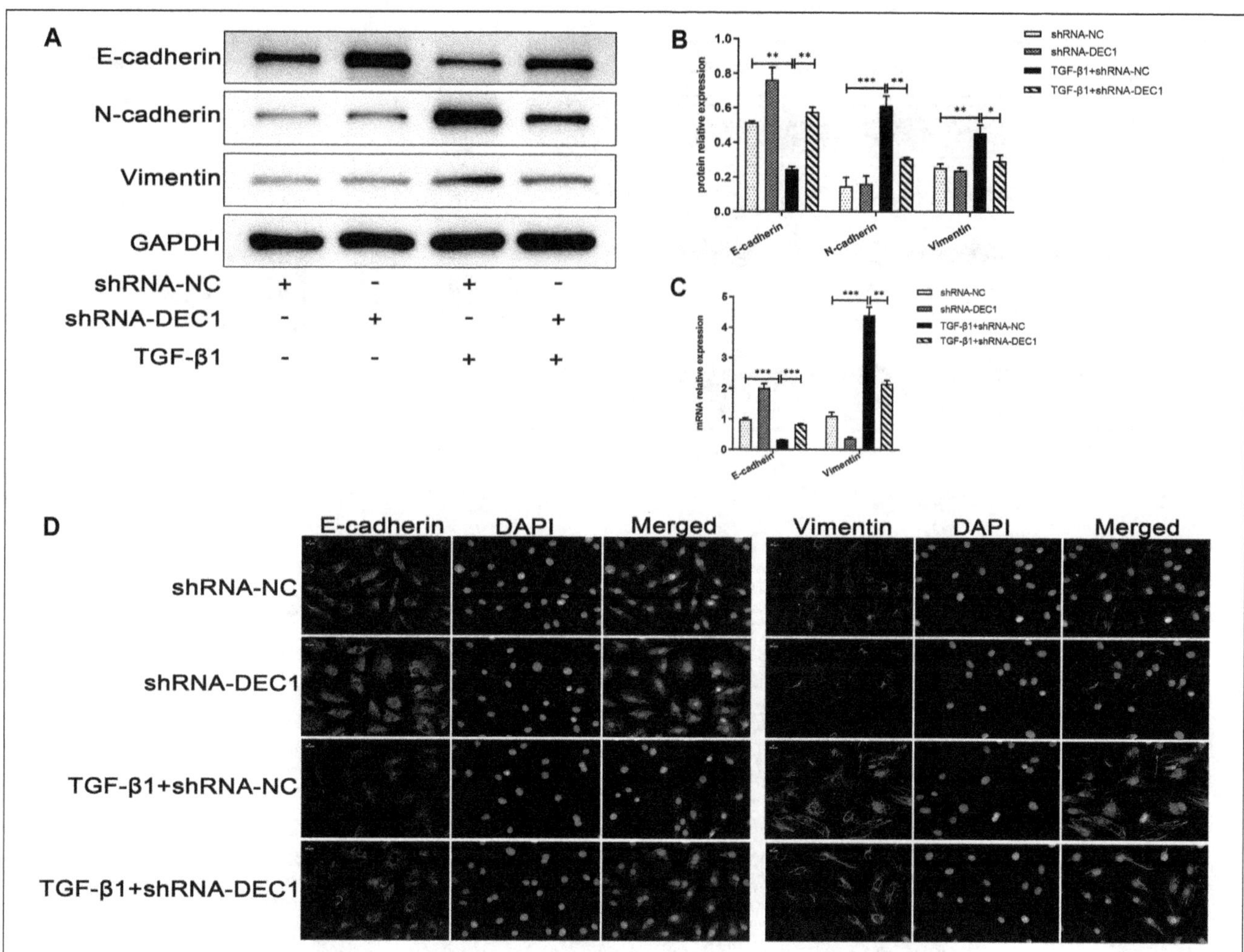

FIGURE 8 | *DEC1* KD suppresses TGF-β1-induced EMT in A549 cells. shRNA-NC and shRNA-*DEC1* A549 cells were treated with or without TGF-β1 for 48 h. **(A)** The protein expression of E-cadherin, N-cadherin and Vimentin in A549 cells were measured by western blotting. **(B)** Statistical analysis of relative expression levels of proteins in A. **(C)** The mRNA expression of *E-cadherin* and *Vimentin* in A549 cells were assessed by qRT-PCR. **(D)** Immunofluorescent analysis for E-cadherin and Vimentin expression in A549 cells. Scale bar = 20 μm $n = 3$. Data are shown as the mean ± SEM. Statistical analysis was performed by one-way ANOVA. $^{*}p < 0.05$, $^{**}p < 0.01$, $^{***}p < 0.001$, $^{ns}\ p > 0.05$.

and *in vitro*. These results support the notion that DEC1 plays an important role in PF.

Dec1 KO significantly attenuated BLM-induced PF. A single intratracheal dose of BLM in mice has been the most popular and best characterized animal model to investigate PF, which has provided valuable insight into the treatment of human IPF (Wollin et al., 2015; Glassberg et al., 2017). In previous studies, it has been shown that *Dec1* deficiency protects the heart from TAC-induced perivascular fibrosis through TGF-β1/pSmad3 and M1/M2 macrophage polarization (Le et al., 2019; Li et al., 2020). In this study, we evaluated whether DEC1 participates in the development of PF using *Dec1* KO mice. We found that *Dec1* KO distinctly alleviated BLM-induced PF. To the best of our knowledge, this is the first report showing that *Dec1* KO suppressed BLM-induced PF in mice. This observation implies that DEC1 plays a crucial role in development and progression of PF.

The precise molecular mechanisms by which DEC1 influences PF remain to be determined. We demonstrated that *Dec1* KO inhibited PF by impeding the EMT process *in vivo* and that *DEC1* KD repressed TGF-β1-induced EMT *in vitro*. In contrast, *DEC1* overexpression induced EMT *in vitro*. TGF-β1, a crucial mediator in tissue fibrosis, is a significant factor in promoting EMT and the development of PF (Akhurst and Hata, 2012; Aschner et al., 2020). We also found that *Dec1* KO alleviated BLM-induced upregulated expression of TGF-β1 in BALF in mice. The pathology of IPF has several characteristics including repetitive microscopic alveolar epithelial cell injury and dysregulated repair, unregulated proliferation and differentiation of fibroblasts into myofibroblasts, causing excessive ECM deposition, ultimately resulting in loss of parenchymal architecture and lung function (Borensztajn et al., 2013; Wollin et al., 2015). As reported previously, the origin of fibro-blasts and myofibroblasts in PF is still controversial; however, EMT in AEC2s is believed to be a significant source of the lung fibroblasts and myofibroblasts in PF (Willis et al.,

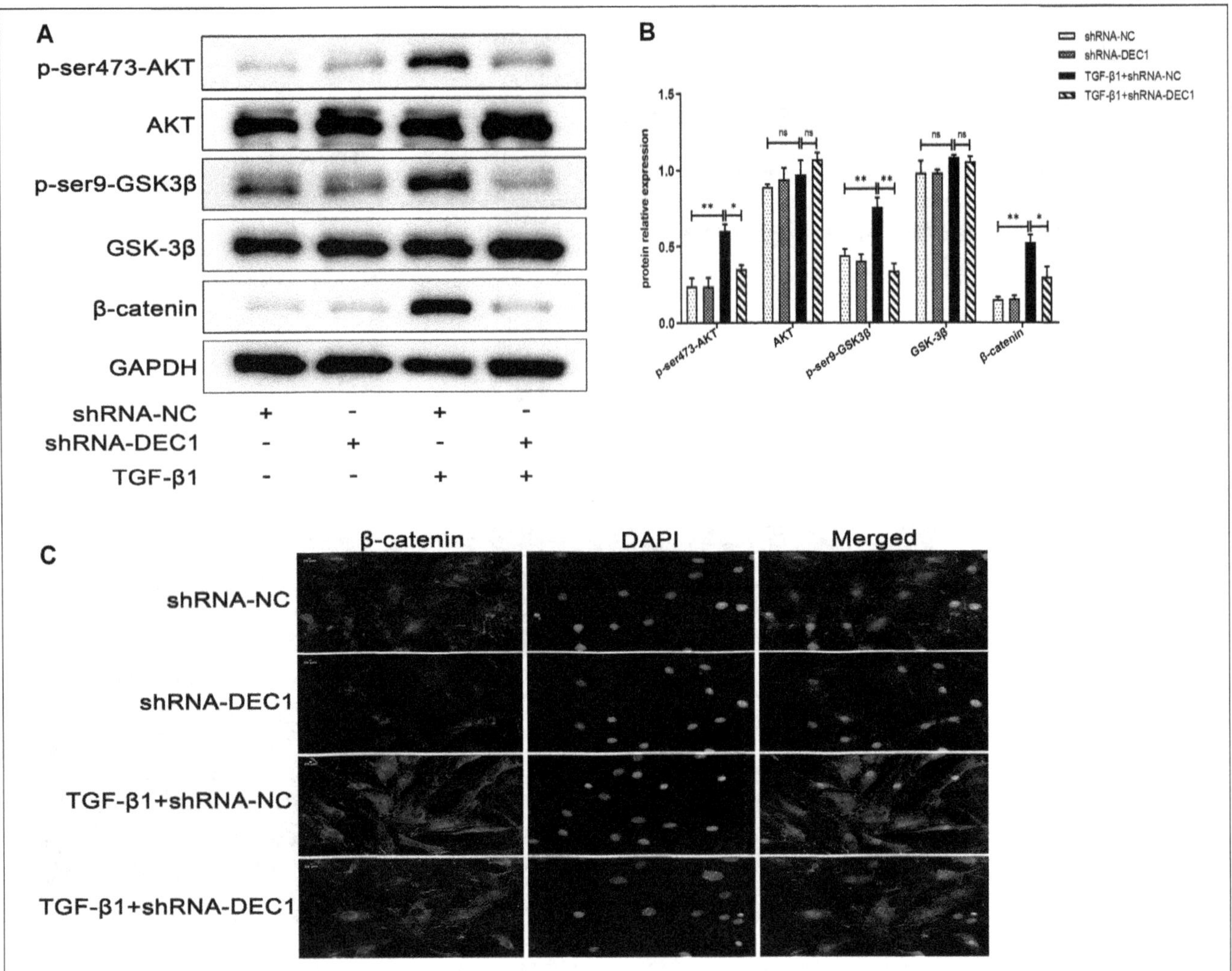

FIGURE 9 | *DEC1* KD reduces the activation of the PI3K/AKT/GSK-3β/β-catenin signaling pathway in A549 cells. shRNA-NC and shRNA-DEC1 A549 cells were treated with or without TGF-β1 for 48 h. **(A)** The protein expression of p-ser473-AKT, AKT, p-ser9- GSK3β, GSK-3β, and β-catenin in A549 cells were measured by western blotting. **(B)** Statistical analysis of relative expression levels of proteins in A. **(C)** Immuno-fluorescent analysis for β-catenin expression in A549 cells. Scale bar = 20 μm $n = 3$. Data are shown as the mean ± SEM. Statistical analysis was performed by one-way ANOVA. $^{*}p < 0.05$, $^{**}p < 0.01$, $^{***}p < 0.001$, $^{ns}\ p > 0.05$.

2006; Chapman, 2011). Several reports have suggested that EMT is an important mechanism in the development of PF (Zhang et al., 2019; Chen et al., 2020; Yang et al., 2020). TGF-β1, one of the major profibrotic cytokines in IPF, is widely used to induce EMT in epithelial cells to explore the mechanism of PF (Qian et al., 2019; Kim et al., 2020). Accumulating evidence indicated that DEC1 regulates diverse biological processes involving EMT in cancer (Wu et al., 2012; Asanoma et al., 2015; Xiong et al., 2016). Therefore, we established a lung fibrosis model in mice and an EMT model in A549 cells using BLM and TGF-β1, respectively. Consistent with previous studies, our results showed that EMT developed in the BLM-induced PF model; however, it was alleviated when *Dec1* was knocked out in mice. *In vitro*, we obtained a similar trend, whereby TGF-β1 induced EMT in A549 cells and *DEC1* KD reversed the TGF-β1-stimulated EMT. Moreover, *DEC1* overexpression alone successfully induced EMT. These findings support the notion that DEC1 plays a crucial part in PF by regulating the EMT process.

The mechanism by which DEC1 affects the EMT process in PF is unclear. Another important finding in our study is that hyperactivation of the PI3K/AKT/GSK-3β/β-catenin signaling pathway was responsible for development of PF and EMT *in vivo* and *in vitro*. EMT is a complex process with the potential involvement of multiple signaling pathways (Lamouille et al., 2014). The PI3K/AKT signaling pathway, one of the most important signal transduction pathways in cells, is involved in the regulation of the EMT process (Wei et al., 2019). Moreover, GSK-3β is a downstream effector of the PI3K/AKT pathway, and AKT inhibits its activity by phosphorylating it at Ser9. GSK-3β also plays a crucial role in β-catenin phosphorylation and degradation, and the transfer of β-catenin into the nucleus, in which it forms a

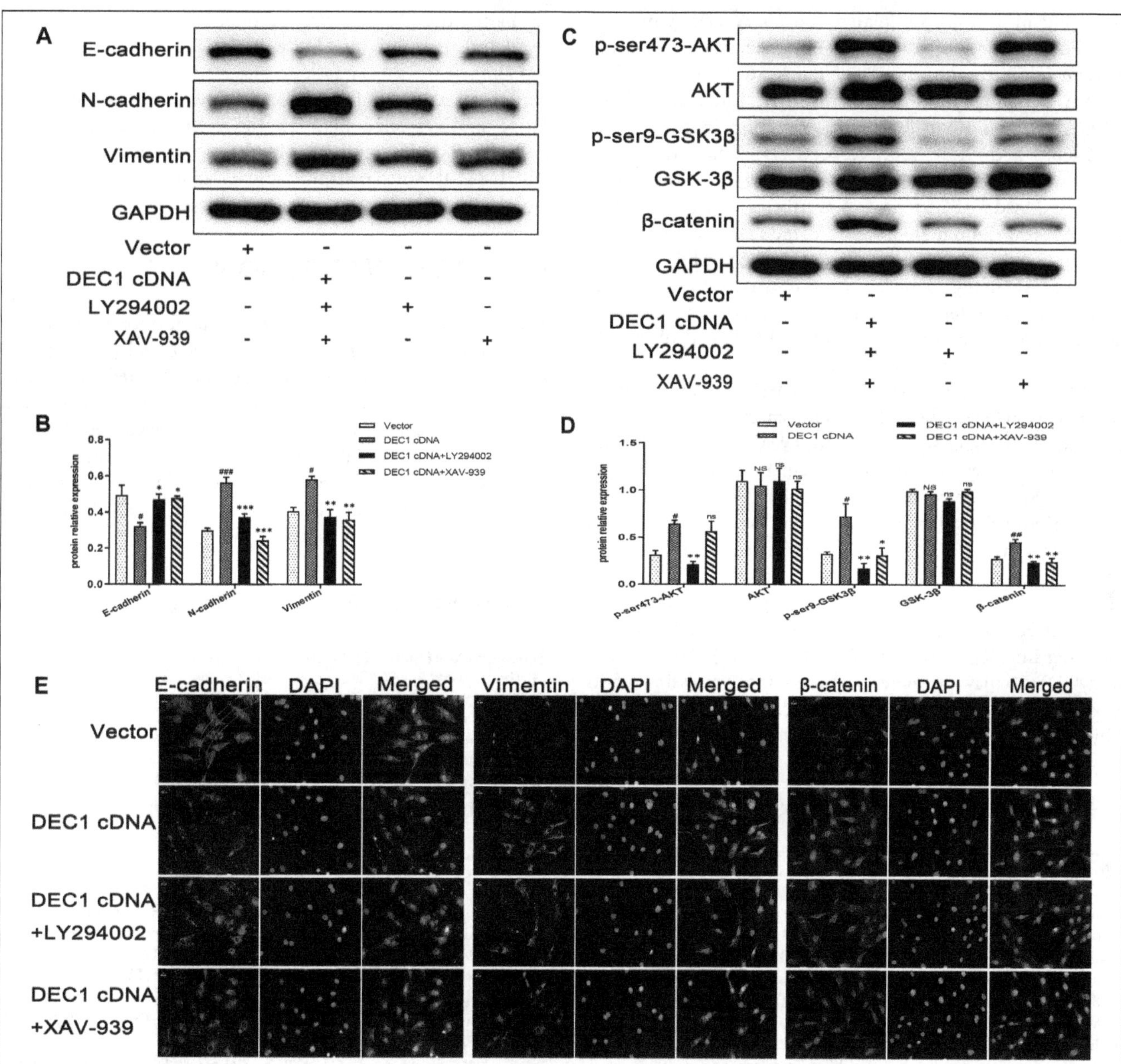

FIGURE 10 | *DEC1* overexpression induces EMT and activates the PI3K/AKT/GSK3β/β-catenin signaling pathway in A549 cells. A549 cells were treated with LY294002 or XAV-939 for 1 h prior to the transfection with *DEC1* overexpression plasmids. **(A)** The protein expression of E-cadherin, N-cadherin and Vimentin in A549 cells were measured by western blotting. **(B)** Statistical analysis of relative expression levels of proteins in A. **(C)** The protein expression of p-ser473-AKT, AKT, p-ser9-GSK3β, GSK-3β, and β-catenin in A549 cells were measured by western blotting. **(D)** Statistical analysis of relative expression levels of proteins in C. **(E)** Immunofluorescent analysis for E-cadherin, Vimentin and β-catenin expression in A549 cells. Scale bar = 20 μm $n = 3$. Data are shown as the mean ± SEM. Statistical analysis was performed by one-way ANOVA. $^{\#}p < 0.05$, $^{\#\#}p < 0.01$ and $^{NS}P > 0.05$ vs. Vector. $^{*}p < 0.05$, $^{**}p < 0.01$, $^{***}p < 0.001$ and $^{ns}p > 0.05$ vs. *DEC1* cDNA.

complex to activate target genes, such as E-cadherin, which is important in the development of EMT and fibrosis (Macdonald et al., 2009; Zheng et al., 2020). It has been documented that the PI3K/AKT signaling pathway and the Wnt/β-catenin signaling pathway are interconnected by the phosphorylation status of GSK-3β. The involvement of the PI3K/AKT/GSK-3β/β-catenin signaling pathway in EMT in gastric cancer cells has been reported and inhibition of this pathway suppresses EMT (Ge et al., 2018). However, the exact relationship between DEC1 and PI3K/AKT/GSK-3β/β-catenin signaling pathway has not been reported. A previous study has already showed that DEC1 deficiency led to a significant inhibition of PI3K/AKT/GSK3β signaling pathway. Additionally, LiCl, an agonist of Wnt/β-catenin signaling, could rescue the DA neuron loss of midbrain in the 6-month-old *Dec1* KO mice (Zhu et al., 2019). In this study, the PI3K/AKT/GSK-3β/β-catenin signaling pathway was clearly activated in BLM-treated mice, and in TGF-β1-stimulated and *DEC1* cDNA-induced cells. Furthermore, we found that DEC1 deficiency *in vivo* and *in vitro* inhibited the activity of the PI3K/AKT/GSK-3β/β-catenin signaling pathway. Interestingly, inhibition of the PI3K/AKT and Wnt/β-catenin signaling pathways by LY294002 and XAV-939, respectively, ameliorated the BLM-induced PF and EMT *in vivo*, and abated *DEC1* cDNA-induced EMT *in vitro*. Nevertheless, both LY294002 and XAV-939 did not alter the BLM-induced protein level of DEC1 in lung tissues of mice, suggesting PI3K/AKT/GSK-3β/β-catenin signaling pathway is a downstream of DEC1. Namely, DEC1 interacted with the PI3K/AKT and Wnt/β-catenin signaling pathways, leading to EMT, and ultimately giving rise to the development of PF.

DEC1 is a basic helix–loop–helix (BHLH) transcriptional factor. It is believed that DEC1 is a transcription factor that acts on a specific sequence. However, the transcription regulation mechanisms of DEC1 remain controversial (Jia et al., 2018), as one report suggested that DEC1 functions as a transcription activator through binding to the Sp1 element of its target genes (Li et al., 2006), whereas another report suggested it acts as a transcription repressor by directly binding to the E-box region of its target genes (Li et al., 2003). In addition, it has been documented that PI3K/AKT signaling interacts with Sp1 (Yan et al., 2015). Thus, in our study, DEC1 may promote or inhibit the expression of its target factors by acting on a specific sequence region, which is what we are going to investigate and confirm in the future.

In summary, the present study demonstrated two important findings. First, DEC1 exerted a considerable role in PF by regulating the EMT process. Second, DEC1 affected EMT by regulating the activity of the PI3K/AKT/GSK-3β/β-catenin signaling pathway. Thus, our findings give credence to the hypothesis that DEC1 is crucial in the pathogenesis of PF. These findings shed light on the better understanding of mechanisms regulating PF. Finally, our study indicates that DEC1 and the mechanism described above may be potential molecular therapeutic targets in IPF.

AUTHOR CONTRIBUTIONS

XH conceived and designed research, performed experiments, analyzed data and drafted manuscript. MeZ and LN conceived and designed research, prepared figures and edited and revised manuscript. MiZ and WZ performed experiments and interpreted results of experiments. BL conceived and designed research and edited and revised manuscript. ZC conceived and designed research, analyzed data, drafted manuscript and edited and revised manuscript. XH, MeZ, LN, MiZ, WZ, BL, and ZC approved final version of manuscript.

SUPPLEMENTARY MATERIAL

Supplementary Figure S1 | (A) The genotypes of the mice were detected by PCR. **(B)** The efficiency of DEC1 knockdown lentivirus containing short hairpin RNAs in A549 cells was assessed by western blotting. **(C)** Statistical analysis of relative expression level of DEC1 proteins in A549 cells in **(B)**. **(D)** The efficiency of DEC1 overexpression plasmids in A549 cells was assessed by western blotting. **(E)** Statistical analysis of relative expression level of DEC1 proteins in A549 cells in **(D)**. $n = 3$. Data are shown as the mean ± SEM. Statistical analysis was performed by one-way ANOVA. $^{*}p < 0.05$, $^{**}p < 0.01$, $^{***}p < 0.001$, ns $p > 0.05$.

REFERENCES

Akhurst, R. J., and Hata, A. (2012). Targeting the TGFβ Signalling Pathway in Disease. *Nat. Rev. Drug Discov.* 11 (10), 790–811. doi:10.1038/nrd3810

Asanoma, K., Liu, G., Yamane, T., Miyanari, Y., Takao, T., Yagi, H., et al. (2015). Regulation of the Mechanism of TWIST1 Transcription by BHLHE40 and BHLHE41 in Cancer Cells. *Mol. Cel. Biol.* 35 (24), 4096–4109. doi:10.1128/MCB.00678-15

Aschner, Y., Nelson, M., Brenner, M., Roybal, H., Beke, K., Meador, C., et al. (2020). Protein Tyrosine Phosphatase-α Amplifies Transforming Growth Factor-β-dependent Profibrotic Signaling in Lung Fibroblasts. *Am. J. Physiol. Lung Cel Mol Physiol* 319 (2), L294–L311. doi:10.1152/ajplung.00235.2019

Ashcroft, T., Simpson, J. M., and Timbrell, V. (1988). Simple Method of Estimating Severity of Pulmonary Fibrosis on a Numerical Scale. *J. Clin. Pathol.* 41 (4), 467–470. doi:10.1136/jcp.41.4.467

Borensztajn, K., Crestani, B., and Kolb, M. (2013). Idiopathic Pulmonary Fibrosis: from Epithelial Injury to Biomarkers-Iinsights from the Bench Side. *Respiration* 86 (6), 441–452. doi:10.1159/000357598

Chapman, H. A. (2011). Epithelial-mesenchymal Interactions in Pulmonary Fibrosis. *Annu. Rev. Physiol.* 73, 413–435. doi:10.1146/annurev-physiol-012110-142225

Chen, Y. C., Chuang, T. Y., Liu, C. W., Liu, C. W., Lee, T. L., Lai, T. C., et al. (2020). Particulate Matters Increase Epithelial-Mesenchymal Transition and Lung Fibrosis through the ETS-1/nf-κb-dependent Pathway in Lung Epithelial Cells. *Part. Fibre Toxicol.* 17 (1), 41. doi:10.1186/s12989-020-00373-z

Chen, Y. L., Zhang, X., Bai, J., Gai, L., Ye, X. L., Zhang, L., et al. (2013). Sorafenib Ameliorates Bleomycin-Induced Pulmonary Fibrosis: Potential Roles in the Inhibition of Epithelial-Mesenchymal Transition and Fibroblast Activation. *Cell Death Dis* 4, e665. doi:10.1038/cddis.2013.154

Fernandez, I. E., and Eickelberg, O. (2012). New Cellular and Molecular Mechanisms of Lung Injury and Fibrosis in Idiopathic Pulmonary Fibrosis. *Lancet* 380 (9842), 680–688. doi:10.1016/S0140-6736(12)61144-1

Gallo, C., Fragliasso, V., Donati, B., Torricelli, F., Tameni, A., Piana, S., et al. (2018). The bHLH Transcription Factor DEC1 Promotes Thyroid Cancer Aggressiveness by the Interplay with NOTCH1. *Cel Death Dis* 9 (9), 871. doi:10.1038/s41419-018-0933-y

Ge, H., Liang, C., Li, Z., An, D., Ren, S., Yue, C., et al. (2018). DcR3 Induces Proliferation, Migration, Invasion, and EMT in Gastric Cancer Cells via the PI3K/AKT/GSK-3β/β-catenin Signaling Pathway. *Onco Targets Ther.* 11, 4177–4187. doi:10.2147/OTT.S172713

Glassberg, M. K., Minkiewicz, J., Toonkel, R. L., Simonet, E. S., Rubio, G. A., Difede, D., et al. (2017). Allogeneic Human Mesenchymal Stem Cells in Patients with Idiopathic Pulmonary Fibrosis via Intravenous Delivery (AETHER): A Phase I Safety Clinical Trial. *Chest* 151 (5), 971–981. doi:10.1016/j.chest.2016.10.061

Goldmann, T., Zissel, G., Watz, H., Drömann, D., Reck, M., Kugler, C., et al. (2018). Human Alveolar Epithelial Cells Type II Are Capable of TGFβ-dependent Epithelial-Mesenchymal-Transition and Collagen-Synthesis. *Respir. Res.* 19 (1), 138. doi:10.1186/s12931-018-0841-9

Gonzalez, D. M., and Medici, D. (2014). Signaling Mechanisms of the Epithelial-Mesenchymal Transition. *Sci. Signal.* 7 (344), re8. doi:10.1126/scisignal.2005189

Hill, C., Li, J., Liu, D., Conforti, F., Brereton, C. J., Yao, L., et al. (2019). Autophagy Inhibition-Mediated Epithelial-Mesenchymal Transition Augments Local Myofibroblast Differentiation in Pulmonary Fibrosis. *Cel Death Dis* 10 (8), 591. doi:10.1038/s41419-019-1820-x

Honma, S., Kawamoto, T., Takagi, Y., Fujimoto, K., Sato, F., Noshiro, M., et al. (2002). Decl and Dec2 Are Regulators of the Mammalian Molecular Clock. *Nature* 419 (6909), 841–844. doi:10.1038/nature01123

Inoue, Y., Kaner, R. J., Guiot, J., Maher, T. M., Tomassetti, S., Moiseev, S., et al. (2020). Diagnostic and Prognostic Biomarkers for Chronic Fibrosing Interstitial Lung Diseases with a Progressive Phenotype. *Chest* 158 (2), 646–659. doi:10.1016/j.chest.2020.03.037

Jarjour, N. N., Schwarzkopf, E. A., Bradstreet, T. R., Shchukina, I., Lin, C. C., Huang, S. C., et al. (2019). Bhlhe40 Mediates Tissue-specific Control of Macrophage Proliferation in Homeostasis and Type 2 Immunity. *Nat. Immunol.* 20 (6), 687–700. doi:10.1038/s41590-019-0382-5

Jia, Y., Hu, R., Li, P., Zheng, Y., Wang, Y., and Ma, X. (2018). DEC1 Is Required for Anti-apoptotic Activity of Gastric Cancer Cells under Hypoxia by Promoting Survivin Expression. *Gastric Cancer* 21 (4), 632–642. doi:10.1007/s10120-017-0780-z

Kasam, R. K., Ghandikota, S., Soundararajan, D., Reddy, G. B., Huang, S. K., Jegga, A. G., et al. (2020). Inhibition of Aurora Kinase B Attenuates Fibroblast Activation and Pulmonary Fibrosis. *EMBO Mol. Med.* 12 (9), e12131. doi:10.15252/emmm.202012131

Kim, H. S., Yoo, H. J., Lee, K. M., Song, H. E., Kim, S. J., Lee, J. O., et al. (2020). Stearic Acid Attenuates Profibrotic Signalling in Idiopathic Pulmonary Fibrosis. *Respirology* 26, 255–263. doi:10.1111/resp.13949

Lamouille, S., Xu, J., and Derynck, R. (2014). Molecular Mechanisms of Epithelial-Mesenchymal Transition. *Nat. Rev. Mol. Cel Biol* 15 (3), 178–196. doi:10.1038/nrm3758

Le, H. T., Sato, F., Kohsaka, A., Bhawal, U. K., Nakao, T., Muragaki, Y., et al. (2019). Decl Deficiency Suppresses Cardiac Perivascular Fibrosis Induced by Transverse Aortic Constriction. *Int. J. Mol. Sci.* 20 (19), 4967. doi:10.3390/ijms20194967

Li, C., Zhu, B., Son, Y. M., Wang, Z., Jiang, L., Xiang, M., et al. (2019). The Transcription Factor Bhlhe40 Programs Mitochondrial Regulation of Resident CD8+ T Cell Fitness and Functionality. *Immunity* 51 (3), 491–e7. doi:10.1016/j.immuni.2019.08.013

Li, X., Le, H. T., Sato, F., Kang, T. H., Makishima, M., Zhong, L., et al. (2020). Decl Deficiency Protects the Heart from Fibrosis, Inflammation, and Myocardial Cell Apoptosis in a Mouse Model of Cardiac Hypertrophy. *Biochem. Biophys. Res. Commun.* 532 (4), 513–519. doi:10.1016/j.bbrc.2020.08.058

Li, Y., Xie, M., Song, X., Gragen, S., Sachdeva, K., Wan, Y., et al. (2003). DEC1 Negatively Regulates the Expression of DEC2 through Binding to the E-Box in the Proximal Promoter. *J. Biol. Chem.* 278 (19), 16899–16907. doi:10.1074/jbc.M300596200

Li, Y., Xie, M., Yang, J., Yang, D., Deng, R., Wan, Y., et al. (2006). The Expression of Antiapoptotic Protein Survivin Is Transcriptionally Upregulated by DEC1 Primarily through Multiple Sp1 Binding Sites in the Proximal Promoter. *Oncogene* 25 (23), 3296–3306. doi:10.1038/sj.onc.1209363

Macdonald, B. T., Tamai, K., and He, X. (2009). Wnt/beta-catenin Signaling: Components, Mechanisms, and Diseases. *Dev. Cel.* 17 (1), 9–26. doi:10.1016/j.devcel.2009.06.016

Martinez, F. J., Collard, H. R., Pardo, A., Raghu, G., Richeldi, L., Selman, M., et al. (2017). Idiopathic Pulmonary Fibrosis. *Nat. Rev. Dis. Primers* 3, 17074. doi:10.1038/nrdp.2017.74

Okamoto, M., Hoshino, T., Kitasato, Y., Sakazaki, Y., Kawayama, T., Fujimoto, K., et al. (2011). Periostin, a Matrix Protein, Is a Novel Biomarker for Idiopathic Interstitial Pneumonias. *Eur. Respir. J.* 37 (5), 1119–1127. doi:10.1183/09031936.00059810

Peng, L., Wen, L., Shi, Q. F., Gao, F., Huang, B., Meng, J., et al. (2020). Scutellarin Ameliorates Pulmonary Fibrosis through Inhibiting NF-Kb/nlrp3-Mediated Epithelial-Mesenchymal Transition and Inflammation. *Cel Death Dis* 11 (11), 978. doi:10.1038/s41419-020-03178-2

Qian, W., Cai, X., Qian, Q., Peng, W., Yu, J., Zhang, X., et al. (2019). lncRNA ZEB1-AS1 Promotes Pulmonary Fibrosis through ZEB1-Mediated Epithelial-Mesenchymal Transition by Competitively Binding miR-141-3p. *Cel Death Dis* 10 (2), 129. doi:10.1038/s41419-019-1339-1

Qian, Y., Zhang, J., Yan, B., and Chen, X. (2008). DEC1, a Basic helix-loop-helix Transcription Factor and a Novel Target Gene of the P53 Family, Mediates P53-dependent Premature Senescence. *J. Biol. Chem.* 283 (5), 2896–2905. doi:10.1074/jbc.M708624200

Raghu, G., Remy-Jardin, M., Myers, J. L., Richeldi, L., Ryerson, C. J., Lederer, D. J., et al. (2018). Diagnosis of Idiopathic Pulmonary Fibrosis. An Official ATS/ERS/JRS/ALAT Clinical Practice Guideline. *Am. J. Respir. Crit. Care Med.* 198 (5), e44–e68. doi:10.1164/rccm.201807-1255ST

Richeldi, L., Collard, H. R., and Jones, M. G. (2017). Idiopathic Pulmonary Fibrosis. *Lancet* 389 (10082), 1941–1952. doi:10.1016/S0140-6736(17)30866-8

Sato, F., Bhawal, U. K., Yoshimura, T., and Muragaki, Y. (2016). DEC1 and DEC2 Crosstalk between Circadian Rhythm and Tumor Progression. *J. Cancer* 7 (2), 153–159. doi:10.7150/jca.13748

Skibba, M., Drelich, A., Poellmann, M., Hong, S., and Brasier, A. R. (2020). Nanoapproaches to Modifying Epigenetics of Epithelial Mesenchymal Transition for Treatment of Pulmonary Fibrosis. *Front. Pharmacol.* 11, 607689. doi:10.3389/fphar.2020.607689

Thiery, J. P., Acloque, H., Huang, R. Y., and Nieto, M. A. (2009). Epithelial-mesenchymal Transitions in Development and Disease. *Cell* 139 (5), 871–890. doi:10.1016/j.cell.2009.11.007

Wei, R., Xiao, Y., Song, Y., Yuan, H., Luo, J., and Xu, W. (2019). FAT4 Regulates the EMT and Autophagy in Colorectal Cancer Cells in Part via the PI3K-AKT Signaling axis. *J. Exp. Clin. Cancer Res.* 38 (1), 112. doi:10.1186/s13046-019-1043-0

Willis, B. C., Dubois, R. M., and Borok, Z. (2006). Epithelial Origin of Myofibroblasts during Fibrosis in the Lung. *Proc. Am. Thorac. Soc.* 3 (4), 377–382. doi:10.1513/pats.200601-004TK

Wollin, L., Wex, E., Pautsch, A., Schnapp, G., Hostettler, K. E., Stowasser, S., et al. (2015). Mode of Action of Nintedanib in the Treatment of Idiopathic Pulmonary Fibrosis. *Eur. Respir. J.* 45 (5), 1434–1445. doi:10.1183/09031936.00174914

Wolters, P. J., Blackwell, T. S., Eickelberg, O., Loyd, J. E., Kaminski, N., Jenkins, G., et al. (2018). Time for a Change: Is Idiopathic Pulmonary Fibrosis Still Idiopathic and Only Fibrotic? *Lancet Respir. Med.* 6 (2), 154–160. doi:10.1016/S2213-2600(18)30007-9

Wu, Y., Sato, F., Yamada, T., Bhawal, U. K., Kawamoto, T., Fujimoto, K., et al. (2012). The BHLH Transcription Factor DEC1 Plays an Important Role in the Epithelial-Mesenchymal Transition of Pancreatic Cancer. *Int. J. Oncol.* 41 (4), 1337–1346. doi:10.3892/ijo.2012.1559

Xiong, J., Yang, H., Luo, W., Shan, E., Liu, J., Zhang, F., et al. (2016). The Anti-metastatic Effect of 8-MOP on Hepatocellular Carcinoma Is Potentiated by the Down-Regulation of bHLH Transcription Factor DEC1. *Pharmacol. Res.* 105, 121–133. doi:10.1016/j.phrs.2016.01.025

Yan, Y. X., Zhao, J. X., Han, S., Zhou, N. J., Jia, Z. Q., Yao, S. J., et al. (2015). Tetramethylpyrazine Induces SH-Sy5y Cell Differentiation toward the Neuronal Phenotype through Activation of the PI3K/Akt/Sp1/TopoIIβ Pathway. *Eur. J. Cel Biol.* 94 (12), 626–641. doi:10.1016/j.ejcb.2015.09.001

Yan, Z., Kui, Z., and Ping, Z. (2014). Reviews and Prospectives of Signaling Pathway Analysis in Idiopathic Pulmonary Fibrosis. *Autoimmun. Rev.* 13 (10), 1020–1025. doi:10.1016/j.autrev.2014.08.028

Yang, F., Hou, Z. F., Zhu, H. Y., Chen, X. X., Li, W. Y., Cao, R. S., et al. (2020). Catalpol Protects against Pulmonary Fibrosis through Inhibiting TGF-β1/Smad3 and Wnt/β-Catenin Signaling Pathways. *Front. Pharmacol.* 11, 594139. doi:10.3389/fphar.2020.594139

Yang, Y., Hu, L., Xia, H., Chen, L., Cui, S., Wang, Y., et al. (2019). Resolvin D1 Attenuates Mechanical Stretch-Induced Pulmonary Fibrosis via Epithelial-Mesenchymal Transition. *Am. J. Physiol. Lung Cel Mol Physiol* 316 (6), L1013–L1024. doi:10.1152/ajplung.00415.2018

Zhang, C., Zhu, X., Hua, Y., Zhao, Q., Wang, K., Zhen, L., et al. (2019). YY1 Mediates TGF-B1-Induced EMT and Pro-fibrogenesis in Alveolar Epithelial Cells. *Respir. Res.* 20 (1), 249. doi:10.1186/s12931-019-1223-7

Zheng, H., Yang, Z., Xin, Z., Yang, Y., Yu, Y., Cui, J., et al. (2020). Glycogen Synthase Kinase-3β: a Promising Candidate in the Fight against Fibrosis. *Theranostics* 10 (25), 11737–11753. doi:10.7150/thno.47717

Zhu, Z., Yichen, W., Ziheng, Z., Dinghao, G., Ming, L., Wei, L., et al. (2019). The Loss of Dopaminergic Neurons in DEC1 Deficient Mice Potentially Involves the Decrease of PI3K/Akt/GSK3β Signaling. *Aging (Albany NY)* 11 (24), 12733–12753. doi:10.18632/aging.102599

10

Anlotinib Inhibits PFKFB3-Driven Glycolysis in Myofibroblasts to Reverse Pulmonary Fibrosis

Weimou Chen[1†], Jinming Zhang[1†], Wenshan Zhong[1†], Yuanyuan Liu[1], Ye Lu[1], Zhaojin Zeng[1], Haohua Huang[1], Xuan Wan[1], Xiaojing Meng[2], Fei Zou[2], Shaoxi Cai[1] and Hangming Dong[1*]*

[1]*Chronic Airways Diseases Laboratory, Department of Respiratory and Critical Care Medicine, Nanfang Hospital, Southern Medical University, Guangzhou, China,* [2]*Guangdong Provincial Key Laboratory of Tropical Disease Research, Department of Occupational Health and Medicine, School of Public Health, Southern Medical University, Guangzhou, China*

***Correspondence:**
Hangming Dong
dhm@smu.edu.cn
Shaoxi Cai
hxkc@smu.edu.cn

[†]*These authors have contributed equally to this work*

Idiopathic pulmonary fibrosis (IPF) is a fatal disease in which the normal alveolar network is gradually replaced by fibrotic scars. Current evidence suggests that metabolic alterations correlate with myofibroblast activation in IPF. Anlotinib has been proposed to have antifibrotic effects, but the efficacy and mechanisms of anlotinib against lung fibrosis have not been systematically evaluated. The antifibrotic effects of anlotinib were evaluated in bleomycin-induced mouse models and transforming growth factor-beta 1 (TGF-β1)-stimulated lung fibroblasts. We measured lactate levels, 2-NBDG glucose uptake and the extracellular acidification rate (ECAR) to assess glycolysis in fibroblasts. RNA-protein coimmunoprecipitation (RIP) and polysome analyses were performed to investigate novel mechanisms of glycolytic reprogramming in pulmonary fibrosis. We found that anlotinib diminished myofibroblast activation and inhibited the augmentation of glycolysis. Moreover, we show that PCBP3 posttranscriptionally increases PFKFB3 expression by promoting its translation during myofibroblast activation, thus promoting glycolysis in myofibroblasts. Regarding mechanism, anlotinib exerts potent antifibrotic effects by downregulating PCBP3, reducing PFKFB3 translation and inhibiting glycolysis in myofibroblasts. Furthermore, we observed that anlotinib had preventative and therapeutic antifibrotic effects on bleomycin-induced pulmonary fibrosis. Therefore, we identify PCBP3 as a protein involved in the regulation of glycolysis reprogramming and lung fibrogenesis and propose it as a therapeutic target for pulmonary fibrosis. Our data suggest that anlotinib has antifibrotic effects on the lungs, and we provide a novel mechanism for this effect. Anlotinib may constitute a novel and potent candidate for the treatment of pulmonary fibrosis.

Keywords: pulmonary fibrosis, anlotinib, glycolysis, PFKFB3, PCBP3

Abbreviations: IPF, idiopathic pulmonary fibrosis; BLM, bleomycin; RBP, RNA binding protein; α-SMA, α-smooth muscle actin; ECM, extracellular matrix; PFKFB3, 6-phosphofructo-2-kinase/fructose-2, 6-bisphosphatase-3; F2, 6BP, fructose-2, 6-bisphosphate; PFK1, phosphofructokinase-1; TKI, tyrosine kinase inhibitor; VEGFR, vascular endothelial growth factor receptor; EGFR, epidermal growth factor receptor; FGFR, fibroblast growth factor receptor; PDGFR, platelet-derived growth factor receptor; TGF-β1, transforming growth factor-beta 1; TV, tidal volume; Cdyn, dynamic compliance; RI, resistance; HYP, hydroxyproline; IHC, immunohistochemical; H&E, Hematoxylin and eosin; MLF, mouse lung fibroblasts; PPI, protein-protein interaction; MAPK, mitogen-activated protein kinase; ECAR, extracellular acidification rate; siRNA, small interfering RNA; DMSO, dimethylsulfoxide; PBS, phosphate buffered saline; DMEM, Dulbecco's Modified Eagle Medium; FBS, fetal bovine serum; DAPI, 4′,6-diamidino-2-phenylindole.

INTRODUCTION

Fibrosis can develop in most organs and cause organ failure. The most common type of lung fibrosis is idiopathic pulmonary fibrosis (IPF), which is highly prevalent and associated with a dramatically increased disease burden worldwide (Wynn and Ramalingam, 2012; Hutchinson et al., 2015). Overall, the development of new therapeutics should be pursued. Currently, only pirfenidone and nintedanib have been approved as therapeutics for IPF (Taniguchi et al., 2010; Sato et al., 2017), and as both drugs have limited efficacy (Spagnolo and Maher, 2017), there is an urgent need to identify new potential therapeutic agents for IPF patients.

Upon chronic microinjury to the alveolar epithelium, fibroblast activation and transdifferentiation into myofibroblasts are among the first responses detectable at the site of damage (Plantier et al., 2018). Myofibroblasts are characterized by *de novo* expression of α-smooth muscle actin (α-SMA), the formation of stress fibers, and enhanced abilities to proliferate, migrate, and produce extracellular matrix (ECM) (Hinz, 2012; Hinz et al., 2012; Liu et al., 2021). These cells drive a wound-healing response that relies on the deposition of collagen-rich ECM and activates transforming growth factor-beta 1 (TGF-β1) signaling (Kenyon et al., 2003; Sapudom et al., 2015; Nigdelioglu et al., 2016). This transient response must be tightly controlled, otherwise it can become persistent and lead to excessive matrix accumulation and fibrosis. Understanding the molecular bases of fibroblast activation is therefore essential in identifying novel and efficient antifibrotic therapeutic targets to reduce the incidence, morbidity and mortality of people suffering from clinically refractory disorders, including IPF.

Metabolic perturbation is implicated in the pathogenesis of several kinds of tissue fibrosis (DeBerardinis and Thompson, 2012; Chen et al., 2018), including pulmonary fibrosis (Para et al., 2019; Bueno et al., 2020). To cope with the high energy demands of myofibroblasts, including increases in proliferation and matrix production, it is reasonable that activated myofibroblasts exhibit augmented aerobic glycolysis to meet additional bioenergetic and biosynthetic demands, even in oxygen-rich conditions, similar to observations in many cancer cells and other nonmalignant proliferating cells. A major driver of glycolysis is 6-phosphofructo-2-kinase/fructose-2,6-bisphosphatase-3 (PFKFB3), which produces fructose-2,6-bisphosphate (F2,6BP), the most potent allosteric activator of the glycolytic rate-limiting enzyme phosphofructokinase-1 (PFK1) (Van Schaftingen et al., 1982; Cao et al., 2019). Previous studies have shown that augmentation of aerobic glycolysis is an essential step during myofibroblast activation (Para et al., 2019). Ramping down glycolysis is effective in diminishing myofibroblast activation, thus limiting lung fibrosis. However, metabolism-based therapeutics for treating fibrotic disorders are still lacking.

Anlotinib (AL3818) hydrochloride is a novel multitargeted tyrosine kinase inhibitor (TKI) that targets the receptor tyrosine kinases vascular endothelial growth factor receptor (VEGFR) 1 thru 3, epidermal growth factor receptor (EGFR), fibroblast growth factor receptor (FGFR) 1 thru 4, platelet-derived growth factor receptor (PDGFR) α and β, and stem cell factor receptor (Sun et al., 2016; Xie et al., 2018). Many studies have reported the therapeutic effects of anlotinib in several diseases, such as nonsmall cell lung cancer (Liang et al., 2019), endometrial cancers (Taurin et al., 2018) and osteosarcoma (Liang et al., 2019). Interestingly, the targets of anlotinib are similar to those of nintedanib, a drug that has been approved for the treatment of IPF. A recent report suggested that intraperitoneal administration of anlotinib attenuates bleomycin-induced lung fibrosis in mice by suppressing the TGF-β signaling pathway (Ruan et al., 2020). Nevertheless, the mechanism by which anlotinib resolves lung fibrosis and whether anlotinib may be therapeutically used to improve lung function are not well understood.

In the current study, we analyzed the antifibrotic effect of anlotinib on TGF-β1-induced fibroblast transdifferentiation and bleomycin-induced pulmonary fibrosis. Our data suggest that anlotinib therapy decreases fibrotic markers *in vitro* and *in vivo*. The antifibrotic effect of anlotinib is associated with inhibition of PFKFB3-dependent glycolysis, which is posttranscriptionally regulated by the RNA binding protein PCBP3. These findings provide a theoretical basis for the clinical development and application of anlotinib for the treatment of pulmonary fibrosis.

MATERIALS AND METHODS

Isolation of Primary Mouse Fibroblast Cultures

Normal mouse primary fibroblasts were generated by culturing the lungs of C57BL/6 as previously described (Meng et al., 2014). The cells were cultured in Dulbecco's modified Eagle's medium (DMEM, Gibco, United States) supplemented with 15% fetal bovine serum (FBS, PAN, German). The cells were cultured at 37°C in 5% CO2 and 95% humidity. Unless specifically noted, all experiments were performed with cells at passage 3.

Cell Lines

Human lung fibroblast line IMR90 was purchased from American Type Culture Collection (Manassas, VA). IMR90 were maintained in DMEM supplemented with 10% FBS, 100 units/mL penicillin, and 100 g/ml streptomycin in 5% CO2 and 95% humidity at 37°C.

Western Blotting

Cells or dissected mouse lung tissue samples were lysed in ice-cold RIPA lysis buffer with protease inhibitors. Protein concentrations were determined using a BCA Protein Quantitative Analysis Kit (Fudebio-tech) after which protein samples were separated by 8–12% SDS-PAGE and transferred onto polyvinylidene difluoride membranes (Millipore). The membranes were then incubated at room temperature for 1 h in TBST containing 5% BSA. After blocking, the membranes were incubated with primary antibodies for 24 h at 4°C.The following primary antibodies were used: anti-Fibronectin (Abcam, ab268020); anti-Collagen I (affinity, AF7001); anti-alpha smooth muscle (Abcam, ab5694); anti-PFKFB3 (Abcam, ab181861); anti-Beta actin (proteintech, 66009-1-Ig); anti-Hexokinase 2 (proteintech, 22029-1-AP); anti-PKM2 (Proteintech, 15822-1-AP); anti-LDHA (Proteintech, 19987-1-AP); anti-LDHB (Proteintech, 14824-1-AP); and anti-PCBP3 (Abcam, ab154252). Then, the membranes were washed three times with TBST and incubated with donkey anti-rabbit IgG H&L (Abcam, ab175772) for

1 h at room temperature. The membranes were developed using the ECL method according to the manufacturer's instructions (Millipore) and detected on a GeneGnome XRQ chemiluminescence imaging system (Syngene). ImageJ was used to calculate the relative density of proteins.

Immunofluorescence Staining

The culture medium was washed away with PBS. The cultured cells were fixed with 4% paraformaldehyde for 30 min. Then, the samples were permeabilized with 0.5% Triton X-100 in PBS for 10 min, blocked with 1% BSA in PBS for 1 h at room temperature, and incubated with primary antibodies at 4°C overnight. The primary antibodies included anti- Fibronectin (Abcam, ab268020), anti-alpha smooth muscle (Abcam, ab5694) and anti-PCBP3 (Abcam, ab154252). Then, the cells were washed three times with PBS and incubated with goat anti-rabbit IgG/ Alexa Fluor 555-conjugated secondary antibodies (Biosynthesis, bs-0296GA488 and bs-0295G-AF555) for 1 h at room temperature followed by 10 min of DAPI (4',6-diamidino-2-phenylindole dihydrochloride) staining to visualize cell nuclei visualization as previously described (Chen et al., 2021).

Quantitative RT-PCR (qPCR)

Total RNA was isolated from primary mouse lung fibroblasts using RNA MiniPrep Kits (Zymo Research, R2050). Reverse transcription reactions were performed with a PrimeScriptTM II 1st strand cDNA synthesis Kit (Takara, 6210A/B) according to the manufacturer's recommendations. qPCR analysis was performed using a HiScript RT- SuperMix for qPCR kit (Vazyme, R223-01) with a CFX96 Touch Real-Time PCR Detection System. The mRNA levels of target genes were normalized to the β-actin mRNA level. Primers used for qPCR are listed in (**Table 1**).

Wound-Healing Migration Assay

Cells were seeded in six-well plates and grown until they reach 100% confluence. A "wound" was subsequently created with a sterile 100 μL pipette tip. The cells were pretreated with anlotinib (1 μM) for 3 h and then exposed to TGF-β1 (10 ng/ml) for an additional 24 h. After 24 h, the cells were fixed with 4% paraformaldehyde, and images were obtained using a fluorescence microscope. Wound area can be calculated by manually tracing the cell-free area in captured images using the ImageJ public domain software (NIH, Bethesda, MD).

Cell Proliferation Assay

Cell proliferation was determined by the CCK-8 Kit (Dojindo Laboratories) according to the manufacturer's instructions. Briefly, 10 μL of CCK-8 solution was added to cultured cells in each well, followed by incubation at 37°C for 1 h. The OD values were measured at 450 nm using a microplate reader. EdU staining was conducted using the BeyoClick™ EdU Cell Proliferation Kit with Alexa Fluor 594 (Beyotime, Cat. No: C00788L). Cells were washed with PBS. Fresh DMEM was added, and then, 10 μM EdU was added into the medium. The cells were incubated for 2 h at 37°C/5% CO2. After the incubation, the cells were washed with PBS to remove the DMEM and the free EdU probe. The cells were then fixed in 4% paraformaldehyde at room temperature for 30 min before being stained with DAPI for 3 min. After an additional wash in PBS, the cells were observed under Nikon ECLIPSE TS100 (Japan).

Glucose Uptake Assay

Primary mouse lung fibroblasts were pretreated with anlotinib (1 μM) for 3 h and then exposed to TGF-β1 (10 ng/ml) for an additional 24 h. Then, the four types of cells were detached and transferred to a 96-well plate in fresh growth medium at a density of 10,000 cells per well for the direct 2-NBDG glucose uptake assay. The cells were rinsed twice with PBS. Glucose uptake was initiated by the addition of 100 μM 2-NBDG to each well. After 30 min, the medium was removed. The plates were then rinsed with PBS, and the fluorescence was measured at an excitation wavelength of 485 nm and an emission wavelength of 535 nm.

Intracellular and Extracellular Lactate Analysis

To measure lactate production, cells were treated as described for the glucose uptake assay. One hundred thousand cells were then plated into a 12-well plate and incubated in DMEM containing 10% FBS for 10 h. To measure the secretion of lactate, the media were removed, and the cells were incubated in FBS-free DMEM. After incubation for 1 h, the supernatant was collected to measure lactate production (Biovision). The reaction mixture was incubated for 30 min at room temperature in the dark. The lactate levels were measured at 450 nm in a microplate reader and normalized to the protein concentrations. To measure the lactate levels in mouse lung tissue, 10 mg of lung tissues was isolated and homogenized in assay buffer (Biovision). The samples were centrifuged, and the soluble fractions were measured and normalized to the protein concentrations.

Extracellular Acidification Rate

The extracellular acidification rate (ECAR) was measured using the Agilent Seahorse XFp Extracellular Flux Analyzer (Seahorse Bioscience). Experiments were performed according to the manufacturer's instructions. ECAR were measured using Seahorse XF Glycolysis Stress Test Kit (Agilent Technologies). Briefly, cells were transfected or infected as in glucose uptake assay. The transfected cells were harvested and the cell number was counted. After baseline measurements, glucose, the oxidative phosphorylation inhibitor oligomycin, and the glycolytic inhibitor 2-DG were sequentially injected into each well at the indicated time points. Data were analysed by Seahorse XFp Wave software. ECAR is reported in mpH/minute. The cells in each well were digested by trypsin digestion (Gibco, United States), and count cell numbers by cell counting chamber. The results were normalized to normalized to cell number in each well.

RNA Immunoprecipitation (RIP)

Cells were rinsed twice with ice-cold PBS and lysed with an equal pellet volume of RIPA-2 buffer. Protein-A Dynabeads (Invitrogen) were incubated with either mouse IgG or FLAG antibody (Abcam, ab205606). Beads coated in antibody were resuspended in NT2 buffer. Thawed and clarified lysates were added and the bead/antibody/lysate mixture was incubated at

4°C overnight rotating end-over-end. Beads were washed with cold NT2 buffer five times. Proteinase K treatment released RNAs from bound proteins and input and bound RNA was isolated with TRIzol (Invitrogen) and reverse transcribed as described above.

Polysome Analysis

Cells were transfected with empty vector or Flag-PCBP3 and incubated with 100 g/ml cycloheximide for 10 min and lysed with polysome extraction buffer containing 20 mM Tris–HCl, pH 7.5, 100 mM KCl, 5 mM MgCl2 and 0.5% NP-40 as previously described (Kim et al., 2015). Cytoplasmic lysates were fractionated by ultracentrifugation through 10–50% linear sucrose gradients and divided into 12 fractions. The total RNA in each fraction was extracted and analyzed by quantitative RT-PCR analysis.

Overexpression Experiments and RNA Interference

The Plasmid vector encoding PCBP3 and the empty vector were purchased from Hanbio (Shanghai, China). Primary mouse lung fibroblasts were cultured in six well plates (105 cells/well) and added with 2.5 μg of target plasmid per well. After 12 h, the transfection medium was changed to normal medium. Effects of overexpression on mRNA and protein levels were examined 36 h later. The siRNA targeting mouse PFKFB3 (PFKFB3 siRNA: 5′-CCUCUUGACCCUGAUAAAUTT-3′) were synthesized by Genepharma Co. (Shanghai, China). Primary mouse lung fibroblasts were cultured in six well plates (105 cells/well) and transfected using Lipofectamine 3,000 (Invitrogen, CA) with PFKFB3 siRNA or negative control siRNA (NC siRNA) for 48 h following the manufacturer's instructions.

Animal Experiments

All experiments were conducted in accordance with protocols approved by the Southern Medical University Institutional Animal Care and Use Committee. Female mice (C57BL/6), 6–8 weeks of age, were purchased from Southern Medical University. The mice were kept on a 12 h light-dark cycle with free access to food and water. For bleomycin administration, the mice were anesthetized with 2, 2, 2-tribromoethanol (Sigma-Aldrich), followed by intratracheal instillation of BLM (5 U/kg, i. t.) in 50 μL phosphate-buffered saline (PBS) or equally volume PBS for 21 days. The mice were administered dimethyl sulfoxide (DMSO) (control group) or anlotinib (1 mg/kg, i. p.) once daily for 21 consecutive days. Further experiments were designed to measure the effects of delayed anlotinib administration. Anlotinib treatment was initiated 1 week after exposure to bleomycin, and the mice were administered with anlotinib (1 or 2 mg/kg/day) for 2 weeks, and the mice were sacrificed at day 21. The lungs were harvested for further analyses.

Pulmonary Function Test

At endpoint, at least 5 mice from each group were anesthetized with 2,2,2-tribromoethanol in saline, tracheotomized below the larynx, and intubated with a tracheal cannula. After the surgery, the mice were placed inside the plethysmographic chamber and the cannula was connected to the machine. Pulmonary function was measured by pulmonary function test system (BUXCO, United States). The system's software automatically records and displays the pulmonary function parameters.

Hydroxyproline Assay

Lung collagen content was measured with a hydroxyproline (HYP) kit (Nanjing Jian Cheng Institute, Nanjing, China). The lung tissues were prepared for hydrolysis, adjusting the PH value to 6.0–6.8. Subsequently, the developing solution was added to the tissues that were incubated at 37°C for 5 min. Absorbance was read at 550 nm using a microplate reader. Data were expressed as micrograms (μg) of HYP per mg of wet lung tissue.

Materials

TGF-β1 were purchased from R&D Systems, Inc. (Minneapolis, MN, United States). Anlotinib dihydrochloride (AL3818, S8726) were purchased from Selleck (Houston, TX, United States).

Statistical Analysis

The results are expressed as the means ± standard deviation (SD). Multigroup comparisons were performed using one-way ANOVA. Student's t-test was used for comparisons between two groups. A p value of less than 0.05 was considered significant. Replicates consisted of at least three independent experiments. Analyses were performed on SPSS version 25.0 (IBM) for Windows and GraphPad Prism version 6.0 (GraphPad Software, CA).

RESULTS

Anlotinib Represses Myofibroblast Activation and the Profibrogenic Phenotype *in vitro*

Given that TGF-β1 is the predominant cytokine that stimulates the differentiation of lung fibroblasts into myofibroblasts and induces ECM production (Sapudom et al., 2015; Huang et al., 2020), we examined the effect of anlotinib (the chemical structure is shown in **Supplementary Figure S1**) on TGF-β1-induced activation of primary mouse lung fibroblasts (MLFs). The CCK-8 assay results showed that anlotinib did not cause significant cytotoxicity at doses of 1 μM (**Figure 1A**). To mimic the inhibitory effect of anlotinib on the progression of lung fibrosis, primary MLFs were pretreated with anlotinib (1 μM) for 3 h and then exposed to TGF-β1 (10 ng/ml) for an additional 24 h. Our results demonstrated that TGF-β1 induced the expression of fibronectin, collagen I, and α-SMA, but anlotinib reversed the expression of these fibrotic markers (**Figures 1B,C**). Immunofluorescence analysis of α-SMA and fibronectin showed similar results (**Figures 1D,E**). We also examined whether anlotinib affected the proliferation and migration of fibroblasts, which have been shown to significantly contribute to many fibrotic pathologies (Jarman et al., 2014; Huang et al., 2020). As shown by the EdU (**Figures 1F,G**) and CCK-8 results (**Figure 1H**), anlotinib treatment prevented the TGF-β1-induced proliferation of

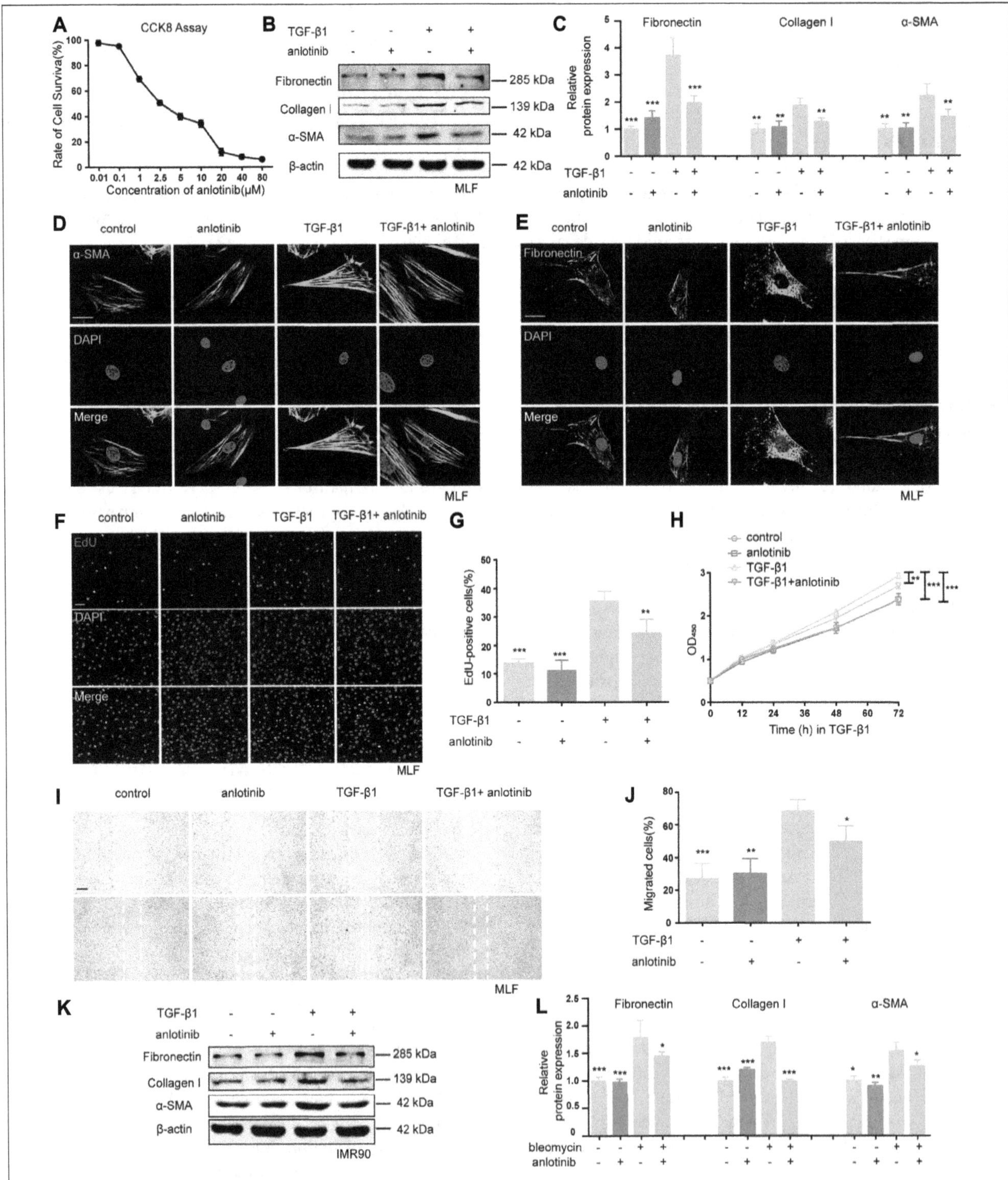

FIGURE 1 | Anlotinib represses myofibroblast activation and the profibrogenic phenotype *in vitro*. **(A)** Dose-dependent cytotoxicity of anlotinib in primary mouse lung fibroblast isolated from healthy mice by CCK-8. **(B)** Western blots analysis of Fibronectin, Collagen I, α-SMA and β-actin in mouse lung fibroblasts treated with anlotinib (1 μM) for 3 h and then exposed to TGF-β1 (10 ng/ml) for 3 h, followed by TGF-β1 for an additional 24 h. **(C)** Quantification for the indicated protein (mean ± SD, n = 3). Immunofluorescence for α-SMA (green) **(D)** and Fibronectin (green) **(E)**. DAPI-stained nuclei (blue). Scale bar, 25 μm. **(F)** An EdU assay was used to observe the proliferative cells. Scale bar, 100 μm. **(G)** The number of EdU-positive cells was recorded (mean ± SD, n = 3). **(H)** A cck8 assay was used to observe the proliferative cells. **(I)** Representative images to show scratch-wound assay. Scale bars, 100 μm. Experiments were performed as in B. Images were taken 0, and 24 h after assay (white lines indicate wound edge). **(J)** Quantitative analysis of migration distance (mean ± SD, n = 3). **(K)** Western blots analysis of Fibronectin, Collagen I, α-SMA and β-actin in IMR90 cells treated with anlotinib (1 μM) for 3 h and then exposed to TGF-β1 (10 ng/ml) for an additional 24 h. **(L)** Quantification for the indicated proteins in IMR90 cells (mean ± SD, n = 3). *$p < 0.05$, **$p < 0.01$, ***$p < 0.001$ VS TGF-β1-treated group (ANOVA).

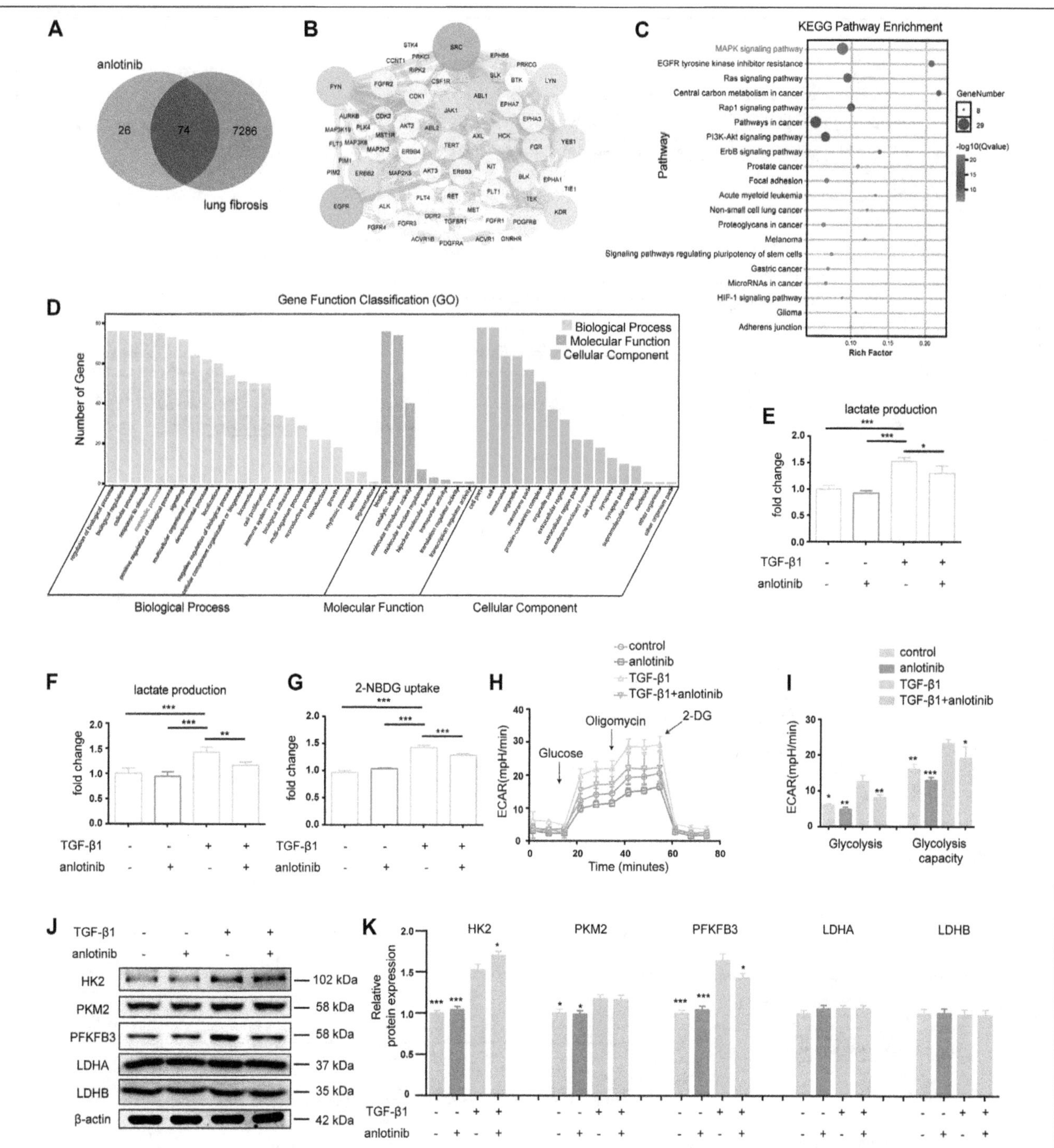

FIGURE 2 | Anlotinib inhibits PFKFB3-driven glycolysis in lung myofibroblasts. **(A)** Venn diagram to show the overlaps between anlotinib targets and lung fibrosis-related targets. **(B)** Protein-protein interaction (PPI) network of common targets between anlotinib and IPF. **(C)** The KEGG enrichment analysis of 74 targets of common targets. **(D)**The GO enrichment for each section listed. The mouse lung fibroblasts were pretreated with anlotinib (1 μM) for 3 h and then exposed to TGF-β1 (10 ng/ml) for an additional 24 h, and then the cells were lysed and lactate contents in the cellular lysates **(E)** and culture media **(F)** were determined. The data are presented as fold change relative to the levels of the untreated control group (mean ± SD, n = 3). **(G)** Glucose uptake detected with 2-NBDG were determined. The data are presented as fold change relative to the levels of the untreated control group (mean ± SD, n = 3). **(H)** Extracellular acidification rate (ECAR) was assessed. **(I)** Glycolysis and glycolysis capacity were quantified and shown as histograms (mean ± SD, n = 3). **(J)** Western blot analysis of HK2、PKM2、PFKFB3、LDHA and LDHB, β-actin was used as a loading control. **(K)** Quantification of HK2、PKM2、PFKFB3、LDHA and LDHB protein levels relative to β-Actin is shown (mean ± SD, n = 3). I, K, $^{*}p < 0.05$, $^{**}p < 0.01$, $^{***}p < 0.001$ VS TGF-β1-treated group by ANOVA.

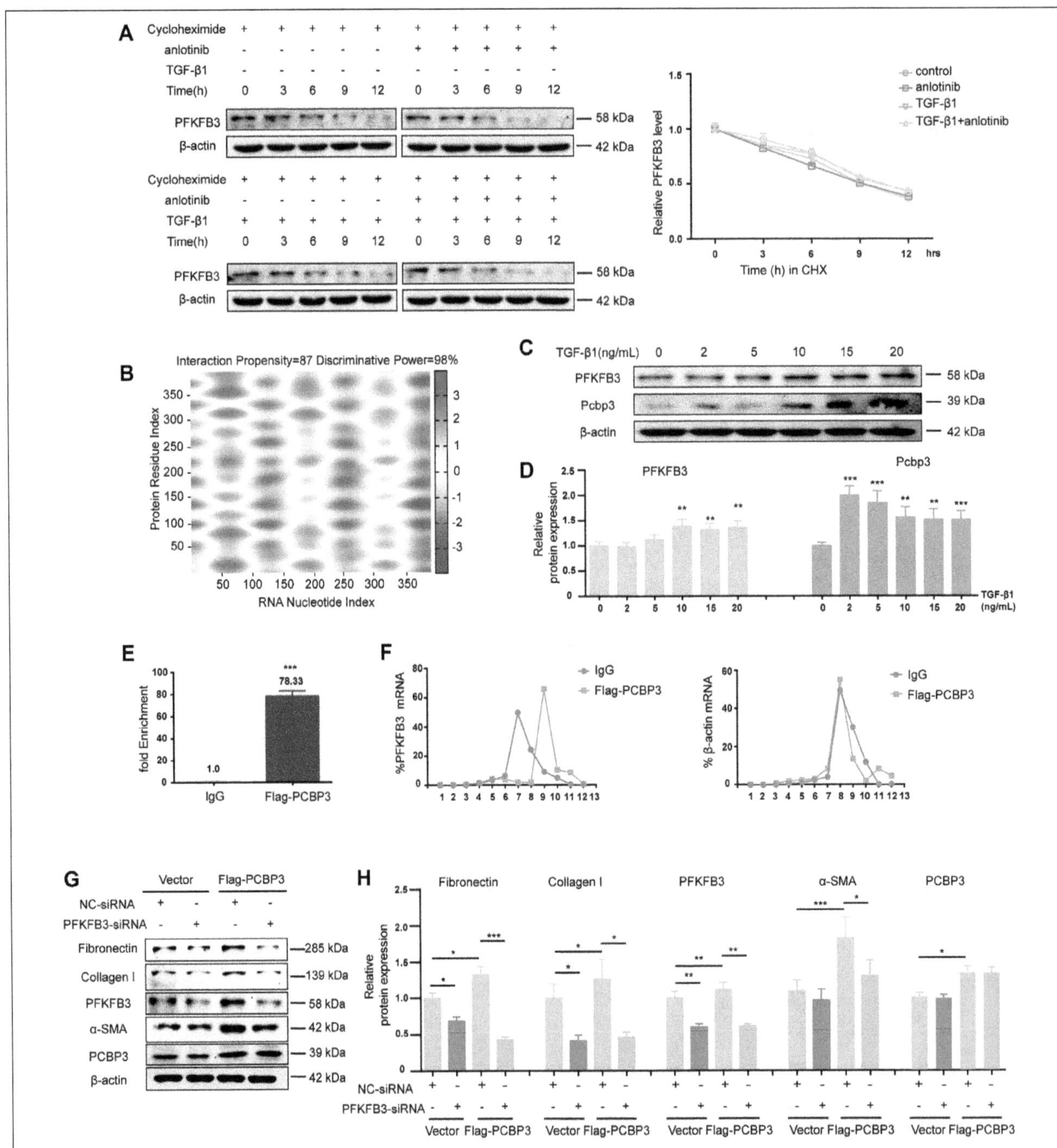

FIGURE 3 | PCBP3 posttranscriptionally increases PFKFB3 expression by promoting its translation during myofibroblast activation.

FIGURE 3 | PCBP3 posttranscriptionally increases PFKFB3 expression by promoting its translation during myofibroblast activation. **(A)** PFKFB3 degradation in mouse lung fibroblasts when protein synthesis was inhibited by 50 μM cycloheximide (mean ± SD, n = 3). **(B)** Prediction of RNA–protein interaction of PFKFB3 mRNA with PCBP3 protein using the catRAPID algorithm. Red represents interaction strength. **(C)** Western blot analysis of PFKFB3 and PCBP3 protein levels in mouse lung fibroblasts stimulated with TGF-β1 for the indicated concentrations. **(D)** Quantification of PFKFB3 and PCBP3 protein levels relative to β-actin is shown (mean ± SD, n = 3, ***p* < 0.01, ****p* < 0.001 compared with 0 by one-way ANOVA). **(E)** Quantitative RT-PCR (qPCR) to show the effect of PCBP3 overexpressing on PFKFB3 RNA immunoprecipitation (RIP) in mouse lung fibroblasts. Values were plotted as mean ± SD from three independent experiments. *p* value was calculated by Student t test. ****p* < 0.001. **(F)** Mouse lung fibroblasts expressing Flag-PCBP3 were fractionated into cytoplasmic extracts through sucrose gradients. The arrow indicates the direction of sedimentation. The distribution of PFKFB3 and β-actin mRNAs was quantified by RT-PCR analysis of RNA isolated from 12 gradient fractions. Statistical analyses were performed using Student t test. ****p* < 0.001. **(G)** Mouse lung fibroblasts were transfected with Flag-PCBP3, and then transfected with PFKFB3-siRNAs or NC-siRNA. The levels of Fibronectin、Collagen I、PFKFB3、α-SMA、PCBP3 and β-actin assessed by western blot. **(H)** Graphical representation of the relative levels of indicated proteins (mean ± SD, n = 3, **p* < 0.05, ***p* < 0.01, ****p* < 0.001 by ANOVA).

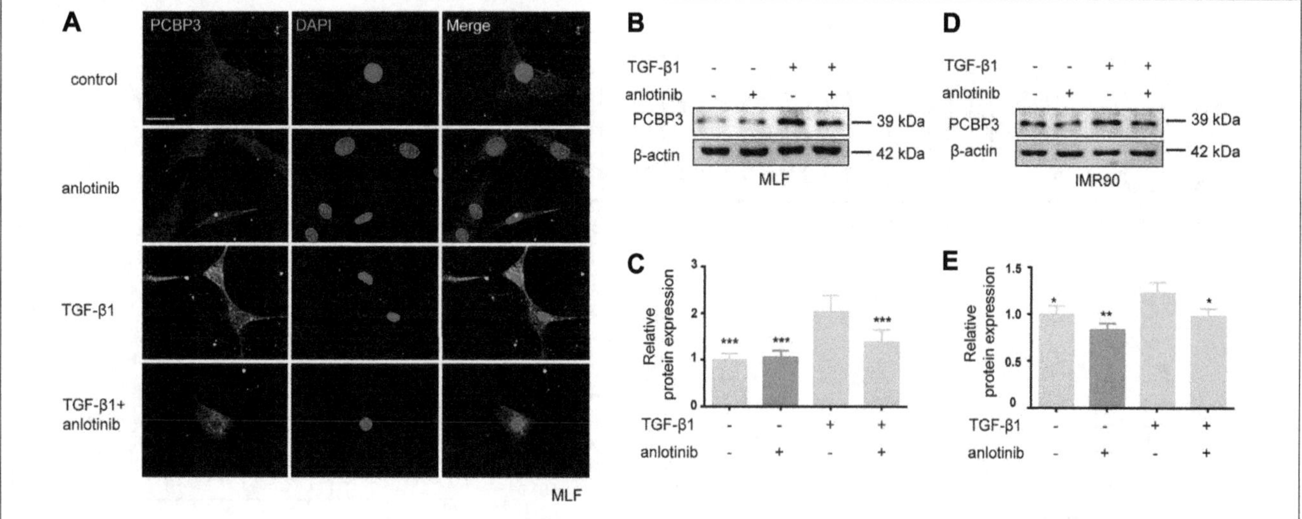

FIGURE 4 | Anlotinib represses PCBP3 expression levels during myofibroblast activation. **(A)** Immunofluorescence for PCBP3 (green) in mouse lung fibroblasts treated with anlotinib for 3 h, followed by TGF-β1 for an additional 24 h. DAPI-stained nuclei (blue). Scale bar, 25 μm. **(B)** Western blots analysis of PCBP3 and β-actin in primary mouse lung fibroblasts. **(C)** Quantification for the indicated proteins (mean ± SD, n = 3). **(D)** The Western blots analysis of PCBP3 and β-actin in IMR90 cells treated with anlotinib for 3 h, followed by TGF-β1 for an additional 24 h. **(E)** Quantification for the indicated proteins (mean ± SD, n = 3). *$p < 0.05$, **$p < 0.01$, ***$p < 0.001$ VS TGF-β1-treated group by ANOVA.

primary MLFs. Moreover, anlotinib inhibited the TGF-β1-induced migration of fibroblasts (**Figures 1I,J**). These results were confirmed in the human IMR90 cell line (**Figures 1K, L** and **Supplementary Figures S2A–D**). These data indicate that anlotinib can repress myofibroblast activation and the profibrogenic phenotype *in vitro*.

Anlotinib Inhibits PFKFB3-Driven Glycolysis in Lung Myofibroblasts

To investigate the potential antifibrotic mechanisms of anlotinib, we estimated the most likely macromolecular targets of anlotinib and obtained 100 potential targets through SwissTargetPrediction (**Table 2**) (Gfeller et al., 2014). A total of 7,360 lung fibrosis-related targets were obtained from the GeneCards database (**Table 3**) (Safran et al., 2002). To clarify the interaction between potential anlotinib targets and lung fibrosis-related targets, the intersection of the targets was mapped by drawing a Venn diagram and constructing a target network (**Figure 2A**). Seventy-four common targets were shared between the potential anlotinib targets and lung fibrosis-related targets (**Table 4**). STRING (version 11.0) was used for protein-protein interaction (PPI) analysis (**Figure 2B**) (Szklarczyk et al., 2019). Bioinformatics analysis data identified mitogen-activated protein kinase (MAPK) signaling pathway-related genes as the top hits among the 74 genes (**Figure 2C**). Given that the MAPK pathway is well recognized as a metabolic regulator and that many of these genes control metabolic processes (**Figure 2D**) (Ho et al., 2004; Papa et al., 2019; Hu et al., 2020; Wang F. et al., 2020), we first confirmed the presence of glycolytic alterations in lung myofibroblasts. We directly measured the levels of lactate and found that both intracellular and extracellular lactate levels in lung myofibroblasts treated with TGF-β1 were significantly increased (**Figures 2E,F**). Consistent with the augmented glycolysis in lung myofibroblasts, these cells also demonstrated increased glucose consumption (**Figure 2G**). However, anlotinib treatment decreased the production and secretion of lactate and reduced the consumption of glucose (**Figures 2E–G**). Accordingly, extracellular acidification rate (ECAR) analysis indicated that treatment with TGF-β1 increased glycolysis and glycolytic activity in primary MLFs, both of which were also reduced by anlotinib (**Figures 2H,I**). To delineate the mechanisms by which anlotinib inhibits the augmented glycolysis observed in lung myofibroblasts, we assessed the expression of key glycolytic enzymes in these cells. We found that PFKFB3 was induced by TGF-β1 in lung fibroblasts and that anlotinib significantly decreased its expression at the protein level (**Figures 2J,K**). PFKFB3 is not a rate-limiting glycolytic enzyme; instead, PFKFB3 catalyzes the conversion of fructose-6-phosphate to fructose-2,6-bisphosphate, which is an allosteric activator of PFK1 and a potent stimulator of glycolysis (Atsumi et al., 2002; De Bock et al., 2013). Taken together, these data suggest that anlotinib can abrogate the PFKFB3-driven increase in glycolysis, participating in myofibroblast activation.

PCBP3 Posttranscriptionally Increases PFKFB3 Expression by Promoting Its Translation During Myofibroblast Activation

Interestingly, the progressive upregulation of PFKFB3 during myofibroblast activation induced by TGF-β1 that was observed at the protein level was not confirmed at the mRNA level, as measured by RT-PCR (**Supplementary Figures S3A, B**). These

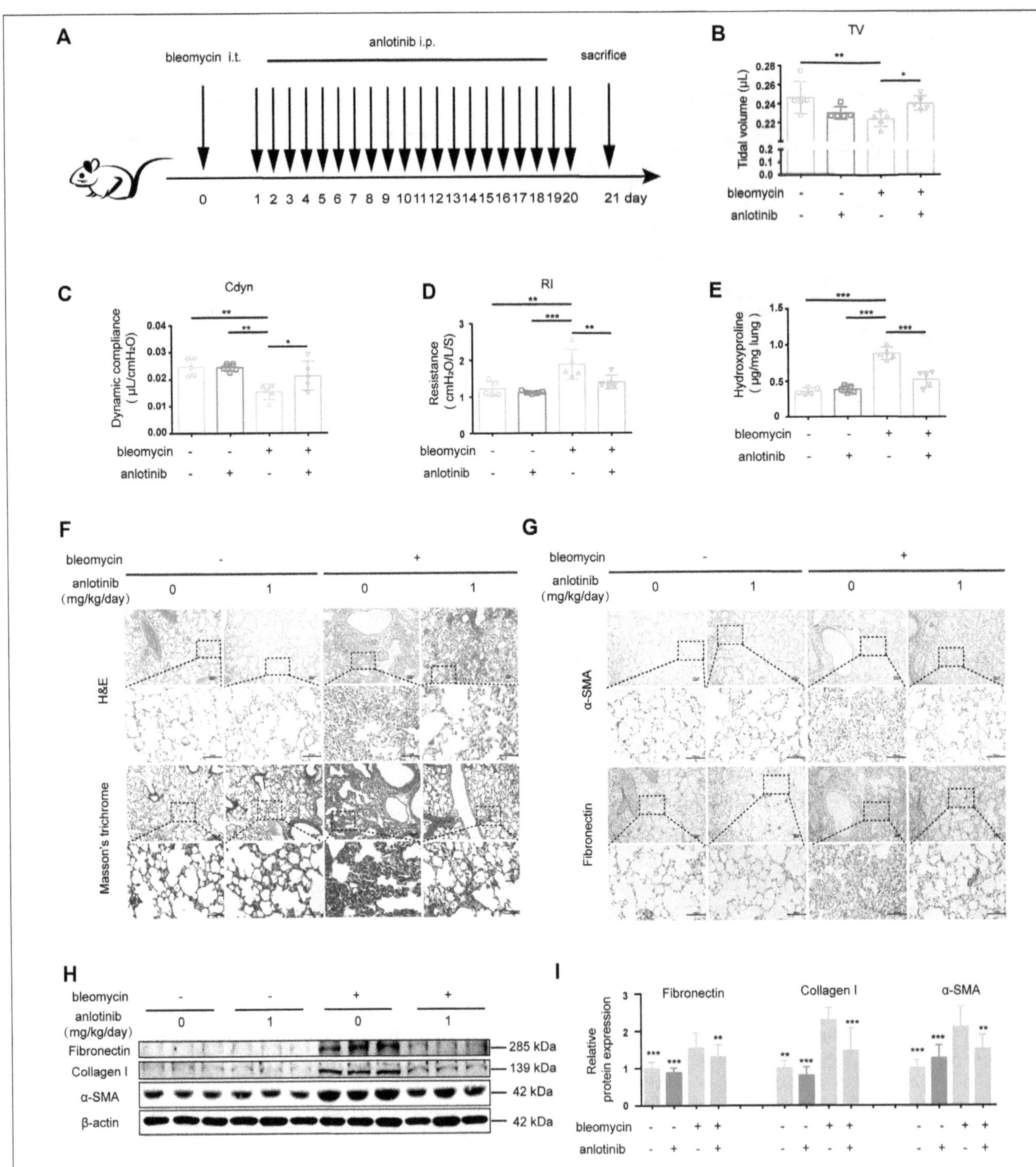

FIGURE 5 | Anlotinib attenuates bleomycin-induced pulmonary fibrosis. **(A)** Intervention dosing regimen of anlotinib in experimental mouse model of fibrosis. C57BL/6 mice were intraperitonealy injuected with 1 mg/kg of anlotinib or vehicle (n = 5-6 per group) daily after bleomycin instillation. Lungs were harvested at 21 days for the following analyses. Analysis of tidal volume (TV) **(B)**, dynamic compliance (Cdyn) **(C)**, and lung resistance (RI) **(D)** (mean ± SD, n = 5). **(E)** Hydroxyproline (HYP) contents in lung tissues from mice (mean ± SD, n = 5). Representative images show haematoxylin and eosin (H&E), Masson's trichrome **(F)**, α-SMA and Fibronectin staining **(G)** of lung sections from the indicated groups of mice. Scale bars, 100 μm. **(H)** Western blot analysis of Fibronectin、Collagen I and α-SMA, β-actin was used as a loading control. **(I)** Quantification of Fibronectin、Collagen I and α-SMA protein levels relative to β-actin is shown (mean ± SD, n = 6). $^{*}p < 0.05$, $^{**}p < 0.01$, $^{***}p < 0.001$ VS BLM-treated group by one-way ANOVA.

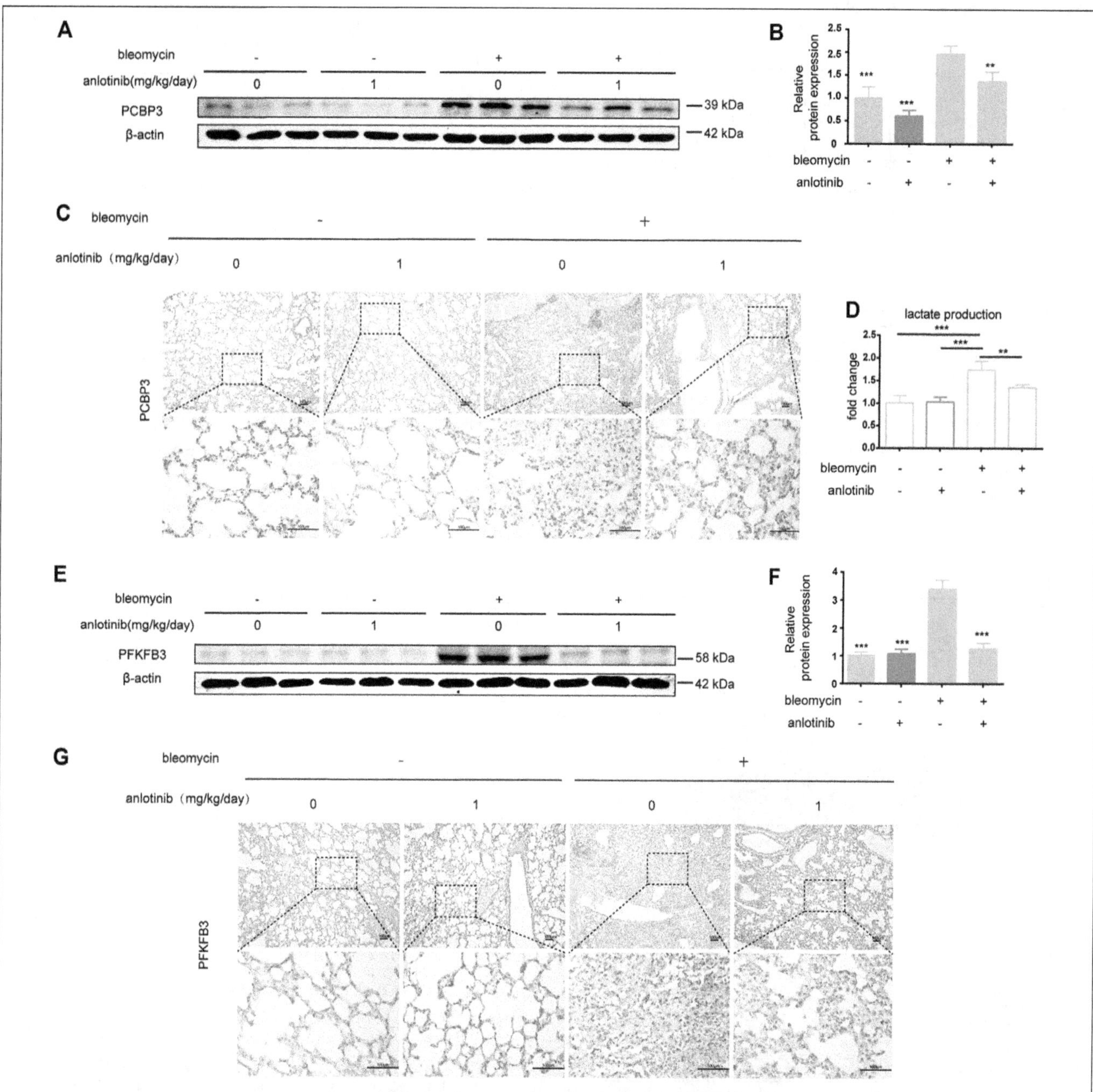

FIGURE 6 | Anlotinib decreases PCBP3 expression and inhibit the PFKFB3-driven glycolysis in fibrotic rodent lungs. **(A)** Intervention dosing regimen of anlotinib in experimental mouse model of fibrosis. C57BL/6 mice were intraperitonealy injuected with 1 mg/kg of anlotinib or vehicle (n = 5-6 per group) daily after bleomycin instillation. Lungs were harvested at 21 days. Western blot analysis of PCBP3, β-actin was used as a loading control (n = 6). **(B)** Quantification of PCBP3 protein levels relative to β-actin is shown (mean ± SD, n = 6). **(C)** Representative images show PCBP3 staining of lung sections from the indicated groups of mice. Scale bars, 100 μm. **(D)** lactate contents in lung tissues from mice (mean ± SD, n = 5). **(E)** Western blot analysis of PFKFB3, β-actin was used as a loading control (n = 6). **(F)** Quantification of PFKFB3 protein levels relative to β-actin is shown (mean ± SD, n = 6). **(G)** Representative images show PFKFB3 staining of lung sections from the indicated groups of mice. Scale bars, 100 μm. $^{**}p < 0.01$, $^{***}p < 0.001$ VS BLM-treated group by one-way ANOVA.

results indicate that TGF-β1-induced overexpression does not require *de novo* transcription of PFKFB3. To further verify these findings, primary MLFs were incubated with cycloheximide to block new protein synthesis, and immunoblotting was used to measure PFKFB3 levels (**Figure 3A**). The half-life of PFKFB3 was not significantly altered, indicating that TGF-β1 does not influence PFKFB3 protein stability. Therefore, we postulated that PFKFB3 upregulation is modulated through posttranscriptional mechanisms in this context. To verify this hypothesis, we used the online tool catRAPID to screen for potential proteins that may interact with PFKFB3 mRNA and identified that PCBP3 (**Table 5**) (Agostini et al., 2013; Livi et al.,

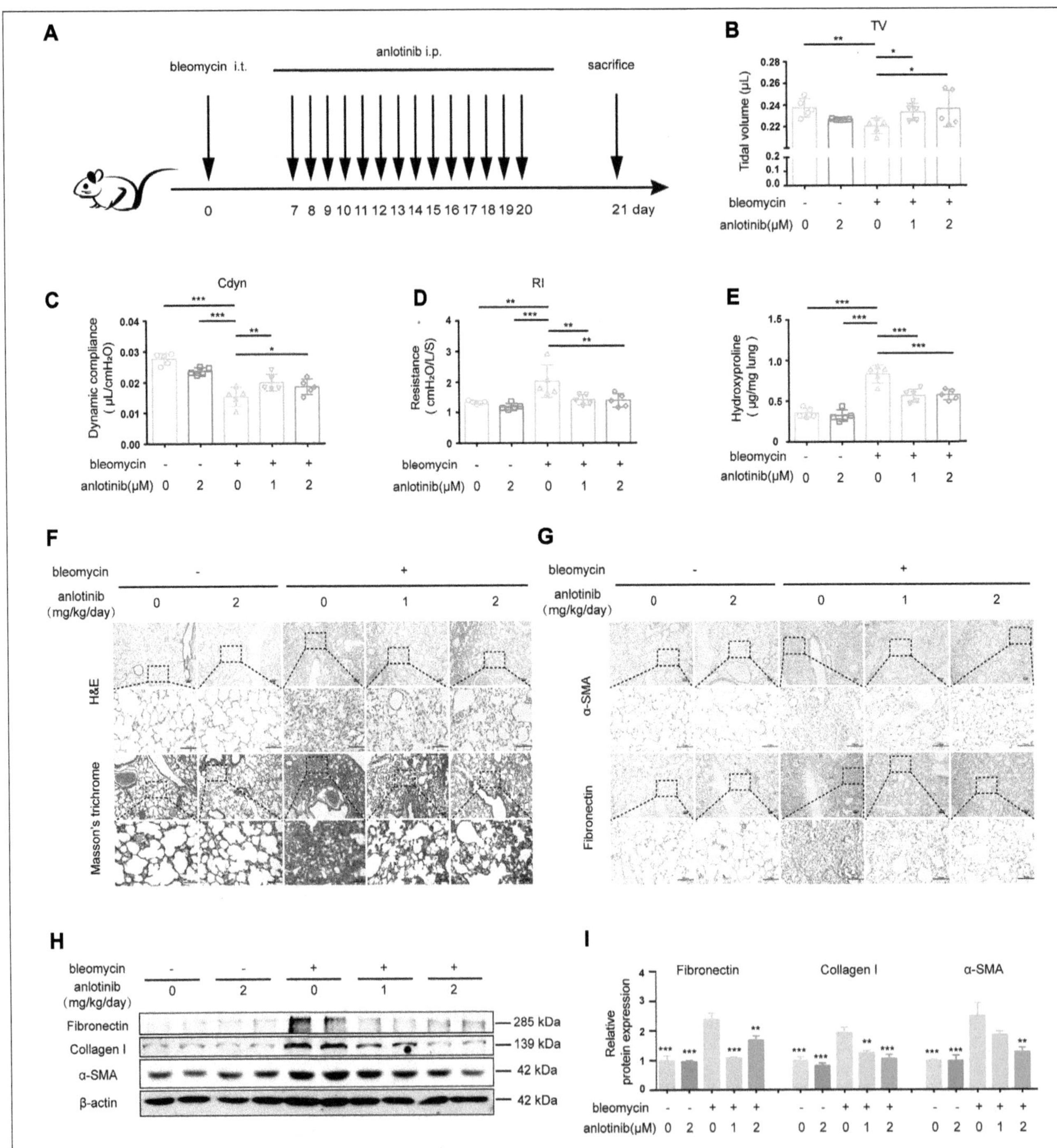

FIGURE 7 | Anlotinib accelerates resolution of bleomycin-induced pulmonary fibrosis. **(A)** Intervention dosing regimen of anlotinib in established pulmonary fibrosis. Bleomycin instillation was used to induce fibrosis and no treatment was given during the first 7 d. Then, mice were intraperitonealy injuected with 1 or 2 mg/kg of anlotinib or vehicle (n = 5-6 per group) daily. Lungs were harvested at 21 days. Tidal volume (TV) **(B)**, dynamic compliance (Cdyn) **(C)**, and lung resistance (RI) **(D)** of mice were measured (mean ± SD, n = 5). **(E)** HYP contents in lung tissues from mice (mean ± SD, n = 5). Representative images show H&E, Masson's trichrome **(F)**, α-SMA and Fibronectin staining **(G)** of lung sections from the indicated groups of mice. Scale bars, 100 μm. **(H)** Western blot analysis of Fibronectin、Collagen I and α-SMA, β-actin was used as a loading control (n = 4). **(I)** Quantification of Fibronectin、Collagen I and α-SMA protein levels relative to β-actin is shown (mean ± SD, n = 5). *p < 0.05, **p < 0.01, ***p < 0.001 VS BLM-treated group by one-way ANOVA.

2016), a member of the PCBP family, has a high probability of directly interacting with PFKFB3 mRNA (**Figure 3B**) (Choi et al., 2007; Kang et al., 2012; Leidgens et al., 2013; Wang J. et al., 2020). We comparatively analyzed the expression of PCBP3 after treatment with different doses of TGF-β1 by immunoblot analysis and found that PCBP3 protein expression was

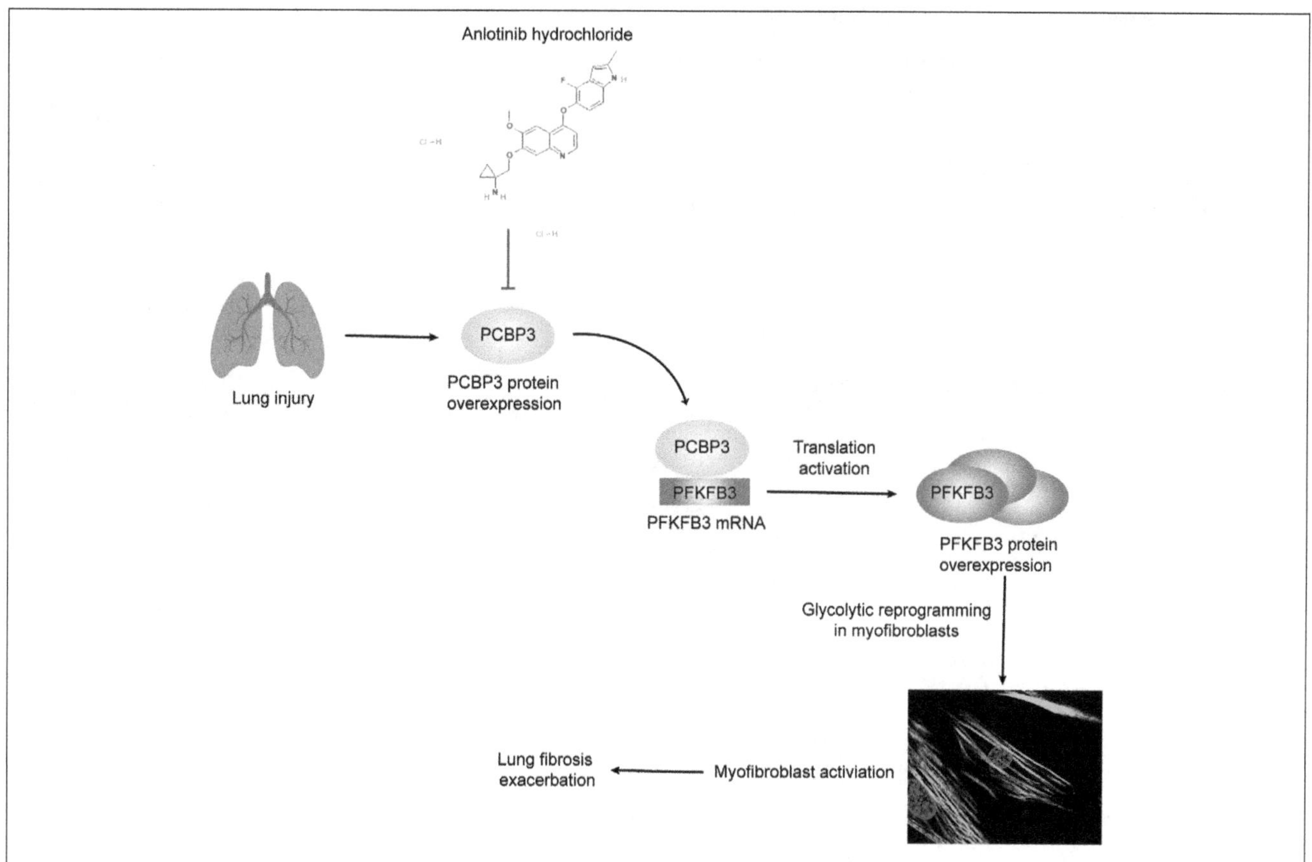

FIGURE 8 | Schematic representation of PCBP3-PFKFB3-dependent glycolysis and the inhibitory effect of anlotinib on this pathway. Lung injury induces PCBP3 expression, which results in an increase in PFKFB3 expression by promoting its translation, resulting in the augmentation of glycolysis in lung fibroblasts. Glycolytic reprogramming participates in myofibroblast activation and furthers lung fibrosis. The tyrosine kinase inhibitor anlotinib inhibits PFKFB3-driven glycolysis by decreasing the expression of PCBP3, thereby suppressing myofibroblast activation and inhibiting the exacerbation of lung fibrosis.

TABLE 1 | List of primer sequences used in this study.

Gene	Species	Forward primer	Reverse primer
β-actin	Mus musculus	GGCTGTATTCCCCTCCATCG	CCAGTTGGTAACAATGCCATGT
PFKFB3	Mus musculus	CCCAGAGCCGGGTACAGAA	GGGGAGTTGGTCAGCTTCG

increased in primary MLFs after TGF-β1 treatment (**Figures 3C,D**), which correlated with PFKFB3 overexpression. To better define the connection between PCBP3 function and PFKFB3, we performed RNA-protein coimmunoprecipitation (RIP) studies in primary MLFs transfected with FLAG-tagged PCBP3 (FLAG-PCBP3). An antibody targeting the FLAG protein was used to immunoprecipitate FLAG-PCBP3 and any interacting molecules from the cell lysates. Reverse transcription followed by PCR was then used to identify individual PFKFB3 mRNAs isolated with FLAG-PCBP3. We found that PFKFB3 transcripts were enriched by PCBP3 coimmunoprecipitation compared to control IgG coimmunoprecipitation (**Figure 3E**), demonstrating that PFKFB3 mRNA is indeed a direct target of PCBP3 in MLFs.

To test the possibility that PCBP3 may influence PFKFB3 translation, we performed polysome analysis in cells transfected with FLAG-PCBP3. Cytoplasmic lysates were fractionated through sucrose gradients to separate ribosomal subunits (40S and 60S), monosomes (80S) and progressively larger polysomes. RNA was extracted from each of the 12 fractions, and the levels of PFKFB3 and β-actin mRNA were quantified by quantitative RT-PCR. While PFKFB3 mRNA levels peaked in fraction 7 in control cells, the distribution of PFKFB3 mRNA shifted rightward when PCBP3 was overexpressed, peaking in fraction 9, indicating that PFKFB3 mRNA formed, on average, larger polysomes after PCBP3 overexpression (**Figure 3F**). The distribution of β-actin mRNA was not affected by PCBP3 overexpression. These results indicated that overexpression of

TABLE 2 | Targets of anlotinib obtained through SwissTargetPrediction.

Target	Common name	Uniprot ID	ChEMBL ID	Target class	Probability*	Known actives (3D/2D)
Tyrosine-protein kinase receptor UFO	AXL	P30530	CHEMBL4895	Kinase	0.106165761464	72/8
Tyrosine-protein kinase receptor TYRO3	TYRO3	Q06418	CHEMBL5314	Kinase	0.106165761464	53/3
Proto-oncogene tyrosine-protein kinase MER	MERTK	Q12866	CHEMBL5331	Kinase	0.106165761464	46/3
Receptor protein-tyrosine kinase erbB-2	ERBB2	P04626	CHEMBL1824	Kinase	0.106165761464	178/5
Tyrosine-protein kinase BRK	PTK6	Q13882	CHEMBL4601	Kinase	0.106165761464	22/2
Serine/threonine-protein kinase Aurora-B	AURKB	Q96GD4	CHEMBL2185	Kinase	0.106165761464	143/14
Vascular endothelial growth factor receptor 1	FLT1	P17948	CHEMBL1868	Kinase	0.106165761464	79/18
Epidermal growth factor receptor erbB1	EGFR	P00533	CHEMBL203	Kinase	0.106165761464	597/31
Vascular endothelial growth factor receptor 2	KDR	P35968	CHEMBL279	Kinase	0.106165761464	485/95
Tyrosine-protein kinase SRC	SRC	P12931	CHEMBL267	Kinase	0.106165761464	448/42
Hepatocyte growth factor receptor	MET	P08581	CHEMBL3717	Kinase	0.106165761464	314/108
Serine/threonine-protein kinase GAK	GAK	O14976	CHEMBL4355	Kinase	0.106165761464	16/2
Kinesin-1 heavy chain/Tyrosine-protein kinase receptor RET	RET	P07949	CHEMBL2041	Kinase	0.106165761464	72/11
ALK tyrosine kinase receptor	ALK	Q9UM73	CHEMBL4247	Kinase	0.106165761464	207/3
Tyrosine-protein kinase ABL	ABL1	P00519	CHEMBL1862	Kinase	0.106165761464	127/11
Stem cell growth factor receptor	KIT	P10721	CHEMBL1936	Kinase	0.106165761464	106/10
Activin receptor type-1	ACVR1	Q04771	CHEMBL5903	Kinase	0.106165761464	29/1
Vascular endothelial growth factor receptor 3	FLT4	P35916	CHEMBL1955	Kinase	0.106165761464	37/8
Tyrosine-protein kinase receptor FLT3	FLT3	P36888	CHEMBL1974	Kinase	0.106165761464	156/14
Platelet-derived growth factor receptor alpha	PDGFRA	P16234	CHEMBL2007	Kinase	0.106165761464	57/14
Fibroblast growth factor receptor 1	FGFR1	P11362	CHEMBL3650	Kinase	0.106165761464	189/9
TGF-beta receptor type I	TGFBR1	P36897	CHEMBL4439	Kinase	0.106165761464	78/4
Tyrosine-protein kinase LCK	LCK	P06239	CHEMBL258	Kinase	0.106165761464	167/19
Tyrosine-protein kinase BTK	BTK	Q06187	CHEMBL5251	Kinase	0.106165761464	67/5
Tyrosine-protein kinase Lyn	LYN	P07948	CHEMBL3905	Kinase	0.106165761464	76/6
Fibroblast growth factor receptor 3	FGFR3	P22607	CHEMBL2742	Kinase	0.106165761464	37/3
Platelet-derived growth factor receptor beta	PDGFRB	P09619	CHEMBL1913	Kinase	0.106165761464	114/8
Tyrosine-protein kinase YES	YES1	P07947	CHEMBL2073	Kinase	0.106165761464	34/3
Fibroblast growth factor receptor 2	FGFR2	P21802	CHEMBL4142	Kinase	0.106165761464	35/27
Tyrosine-protein kinase FGR	FGR	P09769	CHEMBL4454	Kinase	0.106165761464	17/4
Macrophage colony stimulating factor receptor	CSF1R	P07333	CHEMBL1844	Kinase	0.106165761464	149/7
Tyrosine-protein kinase BLK	BLK	P51451	CHEMBL2250	Kinase	0.106165761464	20/4
Serine/threonine-protein kinase PLK4	PLK4	O00444	CHEMBL3788	Kinase	0.106165761464	14/2
Ephrin receptor	EPHB4	P54760	CHEMBL5147	Kinase	0.106165761464	30/3
Tyrosine-protein kinase FYN	FYN	P06241	CHEMBL1841	Kinase	0.106165761464	36/3
Dual specificity mitogen-activated protein kinase kinase 2	MAP2K2	P36507	CHEMBL2964	Kinase	0.106165761464	11/3
Tyrosine-protein kinase HCK	HCK	P08631	CHEMBL3234	Kinase	0.106165761464	30/4
Serine/threonine-protein kinase 10	STK10	O94804	CHEMBL3981	Kinase	0.106165761464	13/4
Tyrosine-protein kinase ABL2	ABL2	P42684	CHEMBL4014	Kinase	0.106165761464	13/4
Tyrosine-protein kinase TIE-2	TEK	Q02763	CHEMBL4128	Kinase	0.106165761464	24/16
Ephrin type-A receptor 8	EPHA8	P29322	CHEMBL4134	Kinase	0.106165761464	9/3
Serine/threonine-protein kinase 2	SLK	Q9H2G2	CHEMBL4202	Kinase	0.106165761464	17/4
Tyrosine-protein kinase FRK	FRK	P42685	CHEMBL4223	Kinase	0.106165761464	15/3
Ephrin type-A receptor 6	EPHA6	Q9UF33	CHEMBL4526	Kinase	0.106165761464	10/4
TRAF2- and NCK-interacting kinase	TNIK	Q9UKE5	CHEMBL4527	Kinase	0.106165761464	20/4
Serine/threonine-protein kinase MST1	STK4	Q13043	CHEMBL4598	Kinase	0.106165761464	11/3
Mitogen-activated protein kinase kinase kinase kinase 5	MAP4K5	Q9Y4K4	CHEMBL4852	Kinase	0.106165761464	12/4
Casein kinase I epsilon	CSNK1E	P49674	CHEMBL4937	Kinase	0.106165761464	12/3
Ephrin type-A receptor 3	EPHA3	P29320	CHEMBL4954	Kinase	0.106165761464	11/3
Tyrosine-protein kinase receptor Tie-1	TIE1	P35590	CHEMBL5274	Kinase	0.106165761464	11/4
Mitogen-activated protein kinase kinase kinase kinase 3	MAP4K3	Q8IVH8	CHEMBL5432	Kinase	0.106165761464	14/3

(Continued on following page)

TABLE 2 | *(Continued)* Targets of anlotinib obtained through SwissTargetPrediction.

Target	Common name	Uniprot ID	ChEMBL ID	Target class	Probability*	Known actives (3D/2D)
Serine/threonine-protein kinase SIK2	SIK2	Q9H0K1	CHEMBL5699	Kinase	0.106165761464	12/3
Mitogen-activated protein kinase kinase kinase kinase 1	MAP4K1	Q92918	CHEMBL5749	Kinase	0.106165761464	14/3
Serine/threonine-protein kinase 33	STK33	Q9BYT3	CHEMBL6005	Kinase	0.106165761464	16/4
Mitogen-activated protein kinase kinase kinase kinase 4	MAP4K4	O95819	CHEMBL6166	Kinase	0.106165761464	17/4
Serine/threonine-protein kinase TAO2	TAOK2	Q9UL54	CHEMBL1075195	Kinase	0.106165761464	7/3
Serine/threonine-protein kinase TAO3	TAOK3	Q9H2K8	CHEMBL5701	Kinase	0.106165761464	12/2
Voltage-gated calcium channel alpha2/ delta subunit 1	CACNA2D1	P54289	CHEMBL1919	Calcium channel auxiliary subunit alpha2delta family	0.106165761464	15/0
Voltage-gated calcium channel alpha2/ delta subunit 2	CACNA2D2	Q9NY47	CHEMBL3896	Calcium channel auxiliary subunit alpha2delta family	0.106165761464	4/0
Receptor protein-tyrosine kinase erbB-4	ERBB4	Q15303	CHEMBL3009	Kinase	0.106165761464	29/3
Mitogen-activated protein kinase kinase kinase 8	MAP3K8	P41279	CHEMBL4899	Kinase	0.106165761464	32/0
Serine/threonine-protein kinase/ endoribonuclease IRE1	ERN1	O75460	CHEMBL1163101	Enzyme	0.106165761464	18/1
Macrophage-stimulating protein receptor	MST1R	Q04912	CHEMBL2689	Kinase	0.106165761464	8/11
Serine/threonine-protein kinase Aurora-C	AURKC	Q9UQB9	CHEMBL3935	Kinase	0.106165761464	15/2
Fibroblast growth factor receptor 4	FGFR4	P22455	CHEMBL3973	Kinase	0.106165761464	15/2
Ephrin type-A receptor 7	EPHA7	Q15375	CHEMBL4602	Kinase	0.106165761464	7/3
Dual specificity mitogen-activated protein kinase kinase 5	MAP2K5	Q13163	CHEMBL4948	Kinase	0.106165761464	11/4
Serine/threonine-protein kinase RIPK2	RIPK2	O43353	CHEMBL5014	Kinase	0.106165761464	6/4
Discoidin domain-containing receptor 2	DDR2	Q16832	CHEMBL5122	Kinase	0.106165761464	13/3
Activin receptor type-1B	ACVR1B	P36896	CHEMBL5310	Kinase	0.106165761464	6/1
Epithelial discoidin domain-containing receptor 1	DDR1	Q08345	CHEMBL5319	Kinase	0.106165761464	14/4
Mitogen-activated protein kinase kinase kinase kinase 2	MAP4K2	Q12851	CHEMBL5330	Kinase	0.106165761464	15/3
Misshapen-like kinase 1	MINK1	Q8N4C8	CHEMBL5518	Kinase	0.106165761464	14/4
Leukocyte tyrosine kinase receptor	LTK	P29376	CHEMBL5627	Kinase	0.106165761464	10/3
Serine/threonine-protein kinase 35	STK35	Q8TDR2	CHEMBL5651	Kinase	0.106165761464	9/4
Ephrin type-A receptor 1	EPHA1	P21709	CHEMBL5810	Kinase	0.106165761464	9/3
Ephrin receptor	EPHB6	O15197	CHEMBL5836	Unclassified protein	0.106165761464	11/4
Receptor tyrosine-protein kinase erbB-3	ERBB3	P21860	CHEMBL5838	Kinase	0.106165761464	4/3
Serine/threonine-protein kinase MST4	STK26	Q9P289	CHEMBL5941	Kinase	0.106165761464	12/2
Eukaryotic translation initiation factor 2-alpha kinase 1	EIF2AK1	Q9BQI3	CHEMBL6029	Kinase	0.106165761464	3/3
SPS1/STE20-related protein kinase YSK4	MAP3K19	Q56UN5	CHEMBL6191	Kinase	0.106165761464	15/4
Serine/threonine-protein kinase AKT2	AKT2	P31751	CHEMBL2431	Kinase	0.106165761464	318/0
Protein kinase C gamma	PRKCG	P05129	CHEMBL2938	Kinase	0.106165761464	38/0
Serine/threonine-protein kinase AKT	AKT3	Q9Y243	CHEMBL4816	Kinase	0.106165761464	73/0
Serine/threonine-protein kinase PIM1	PIM1	P11309	CHEMBL2147	Kinase	0.106165761464	638/0
Serine/threonine-protein kinase PIM2	PIM2	Q9P1W9	CHEMBL4523	Kinase	0.106165761464	448/0
Serine/threonine-protein kinase PIM3	PIM3	Q86V86	CHEMBL5407	Kinase	0.106165761464	331/0
Cyclin-dependent kinase 2/cyclin E1	CCNE1 CDK2	P24864 P24941	CHEMBL1907605	Kinase	0.106165761464	74/0
Tyrosine-protein kinase JAK1	JAK1	P23458	CHEMBL2835	Kinase	0.106165761464	137/0
Dipeptidyl peptidase VIII	DPP8	Q6V1X1	CHEMBL4657	Protease	0.106165761464	346/0
Dipeptidyl peptidase IX	DPP9	Q86TI2	CHEMBL4793	Protease	0.106165761464	239/0
Phosphodiesterase 4B	PDE4B	Q07343	CHEMBL275	Phosphodiesterase	0.106165761464	43/0
Protein kinase C iota	PRKCI	P41743	CHEMBL2598	Kinase	0.106165761464	287/0
Cyclin-dependent kinase 2	CDK2	P24941	CHEMBL301	Kinase	0.106165761464	170/0
Cyclin-dependent kinase 1	CDK1	P06493	CHEMBL308	Kinase	0.106165761464	146/0
Cyclin T1	CCNT1	O60563	CHEMBL2108	Other cytosolic protein	0.106165761464	111/0
Telomerase reverse transcriptase	TERT	O14746	CHEMBL2916	Enzyme	0.106165761464	79/0
Sodium/calcium exchanger 1	SLC8A1	P32418	CHEMBL4076	Electrochemical transporter	0.106165761464	44/0
Gonadotropin-releasing hormone receptor	GNRHR	P30968	CHEMBL1855	Family A G protein-coupled receptor	0.106165761464	431/0
Amine oxidase, copper containing	AOC3	Q16853	CHEMBL3437	Enzyme	0.106165761464	19/0

TABLE 3 | Lung fibrosis-related targets obtained from the GeneCards database.

Number	Gene	Number	Gene	Number	Gene	Number	Gene
1	CFTR	335	PDGFA	669	CPLANE1	1,003	HSPH1
2	TGFB1	336	MIR197	670	MKI67	1,004	MT-ATP6
3	TERT	337	MIRLET7B	671	TBX1	1,005	MIR212
4	TP53	338	MIR195	672	PI3	1,006	CASP10
5	TNF	339	MIR96	673	BMP4	1,007	PDE5A
6	SFTPC	340	CHI3L1	674	PMS2	1,008	SH2D1A
7	EGFR	341	MIRLET7E	675	SLC7A7	1,009	SCN5A
8	IL6	342	MIR16-1	676	E2F1	1,010	RSPH4A
9	MUC5B	343	MIR199A1	677	S100A1	1,011	PIK3R2
10	RTEL1	344	MIR210	678	TKT	1,012	DNAH9
11	IL10	345	MIR20A	679	MYRF	1,013	PSMA7
12	SFTPB	346	MIR378A	680	LAMA5	1,014	KIF3A
13	SFTPA1	347	THBD	681	COL2A1	1,015	CYP3A5
14	ELN	348	DMBT1	682	DEFB1	1,016	LOC111674466
15	ABCA3	349	MIR185	683	RPL5	1,017	ADM
16	CAV1	350	IL9	684	SOD1	1,018	PSMC3
17	IFNG	351	CFM1	685	PLK1	1,019	WDPCP
18	MUC1	352	CD79A	686	SCGB3A2	1,020	MIR101-1
19	SFTPA2	353	DYNC2LI1	687	SLC9A3R1	1,021	PRKCB
20	SERPINA1	354	NEK1	688	IREB2	1,022	IL13RA2
21	STAT3	355	IQCB1	689	LOC113664106	1,023	MYH11
22	TERC	356	MIR204	690	FADD	1,024	PRKG2
23	CCN2	357	HLA-A	691	CYP3A4	1,025	SUFU
24	IL13	358	IGF2	692	HSPB1	1,026	PIK3C2A
25	TLR4	359	FLNA	693	MAPK14	1,027	PSMC5
26	PARN	360	BCL2	694	CTSB	1,028	KCNQ1OT1
27	CTNNB1	361	GSN	695	IGF2R	1,029	MIR133A1
28	CCR6	362	MAP2K2	696	BAP1	1,030	GOPC
29	AKT1	363	BPIFA1	697	GATA2	1,031	TRAF2
30	MIR21	364	MIR15A	698	MMP8	1,032	TNFRSF6B
31	NKX2-1	365	EPHX1	699	ITGAV	1,033	MIR139
32	MMP1	366	HPS5	700	PTX3	1,034	LOC111674470
33	SMAD4	367	TRAF3IP1	701	MSLN	1,035	IGHMBP2
34	ACE	368	CFTR-AS1	702	AFF4	1,036	PSMA3
35	SPP1	369	AP3B1	703	CTCF	1,037	PSMC6
36	CXCL8	370	GAPDH	704	ADA	1,038	GADD45B
37	EGF	371	KRT19	705	KITLG	1,039	FKRP
38	FASLG	372	MIR107	706	ZNF423	1,040	DNAAF2
39	CDH1	373	CP	707	IL12A	1,041	ERCC5
40	KRAS	374	HLA-B	708	PRKCA	1,042	E2F3
41	SERPINE1	375	MMP12	709	EGR1	1,043	PIK3R3
42	BRAF	376	AGER	710	DLL4	1,044	PRF1
43	SMAD3	377	DDR1	711	IFNA1	1,045	IFNAR1
44	PRTN3	378	TNNT2	712	EZR	1,046	PF4
45	PIK3CA	379	CCL18	713	LGALS3	1,047	MIR27B
46	IL1RN	380	MIR148B	714	AFP	1,048	VTN
47	HMOX1	381	MIR141	715	TUBB2B	1,049	DNAJC5
48	IL1B	382	INS	716	EPCAM	1,050	BGLAP
49	HLA-DRB1	383	GLI3	717	APOB	1,051	MIR455
50	FAM13A	384	JAK2	718	SPPL2C	1,052	LOC111674471
51	FAS	385	EVC	719	CDK2	1,053	CSF3R
52	PTEN	386	HPS3	720	GDF2	1,054	VCL
53	SFTPD	387	IL33	721	EPO	1,055	NAGLU
54	ITGAM	388	NOS2	722	VCP	1,056	GUSB
55	DSP	389	SLPI	723	HSPA8	1,057	NEAT1
56	STN1	390	MIR133B	724	ATP4A	1,058	TBX4
57	TGFBR1	391	TCTN3	725	HBB	1,059	PSMD1
58	SRC	392	TLR5	726	SELE	1,060	PSMD12
59	CDKN2A	393	MUC4	727	NAT2	1,061	GAST
60	ERBB2	394	MIR93	728	FGF10	1,062	MIR99A
61	CTLA4	395	MIR18A	729	BMP7	1,063	CREB1
62	NFE2L2	396	SLC11A1	730	ETS1	1,064	TRPC6
63	MMP9	397	PSMA6	731	DEFB4A	1,065	EPAS1
64	MTOR	398	RNASE3	732	PRDM10	1,066	MIR125B1

(Continued on following page)

TABLE 3 | (*Continued*) Lung fibrosis-related targets obtained from the GeneCards database.

Number	Gene	Number	Gene	Number	Gene	Number	Gene
65	HRAS	399	SMAD2	733	GJA1	1,067	IFNGR1
66	TINF2	400	ICAM1	734	RPS6KB1	1,068	PGR
67	FGFR1	401	TGFA	735	JAK3	1,069	TLR1
68	COL1A1	402	RPGR	736	TP63	1,070	CD40
69	NPHP3	403	ANXA5	737	HNF1B	1,071	DLK1
70	F2	404	CXCR1	738	BBS10	1,072	FOS
71	DPP9	405	IL2	739	ITGA2	1,073	DNAL1
72	TGFB2	406	GREM1	740	HOTAIR	1,074	MAD1L1
73	ATP11A	407	CD274	741	SGK1	1,075	PSMD11
74	HFE	408	MIR142	742	DNAAF1	1,076	HBA2
75	PDGFRB	409	GSTP1	743	DNMT1	1,077	RAB11B
76	ITGA3	410	PHOX2A	744	DAB2	1,078	CCKBR
77	MIRLET7D	411	SOS2	745	CDH2	1,079	CLCN3
78	MBL2	412	LMNA	746	HJV	1,080	PPARA
79	NOTCH1	413	ENPP2	747	PRKAA1	1,081	MB
80	MET	414	TOP1	748	HSPA5	1,082	GAS5-AS1
81	TIMP1	415	APEX1	749	CHUK	1,083	LOC111674474
82	SERPINH1	416	CXCL9	750	SKP2	1,084	KCNJ1
83	SCNN1A	417	PLAU	751	ILK	1,085	KIAA0319L
84	MMP2	418	MIRLET7C	752	ADORA2B	1,086	PSMA2
85	ELANE	419	MIR30E	753	SST	1,087	PSMD3
86	VEGFA	420	MIR214	754	CFLAR	1,088	LOC111674473
87	PLG	421	MIR486-1	755	CCNB1	1,089	ABCF2
88	MIR130A	422	KRT7	756	ADCY10	1,090	PSMD8
89	ADRB2	423	TNFRSF13B	757	HDAC9	1,091	MIR590
90	KIT	424	MIR106B	758	ARG1	1,092	PSMD7
91	CC2D2A	425	MIR181A1	759	BAK1	1,093	RNF5
92	TGFBR2	426	MTHFR	760	DICER1	1,094	GLIS3
93	PDGFRA	427	BTNL2	761	IKBKG	1,095	CHAT
94	IL4	428	PTPN11	762	MYH6	1,096	LOC111674476
95	NHP2	429	KDR	763	COL4A3	1,097	MIR23B
96	STK11	430	ELMOD2	764	FGA	1,098	MIR130B
97	NOP10	431	STING1	765	ABL1	1,099	MIR151A
98	ALOX5	432	THY1	766	GJA5	1,100	LOC111674478
99	TMEM67	433	MIR140	767	ARHGAP31	1,101	CD82
100	CCL2	434	VCAM1	768	FCGR3B	1,102	E2F2
101	MIR34C	435	CCR2	769	SLC26A9	1,103	RNF185
102	STAT1	436	CDKN1A	770	LRBA	1,104	MIR423
103	ALB	437	STAT4	771	PMM2	1,105	DEFB103B
104	HGF	438	CEP164	772	ACD	1,106	NFKB2
105	RPGRIP1L	439	MIR128-2	773	CHIT1	1,107	MIR186
106	NPHP1	440	S100A9	774	CDK6	1,108	AFAP1-AS1
107	TSC2	441	TLR3	775	CSF1	1,109	PSMC2
108	MDM2	442	SERPINA3	776	ABCG2	1,110	ERLIN2
109	TTC21B	443	MIR25	777	CASP1	1,111	GADD45G
110	EDN1	444	CD44	778	P2RX7	1,112	CS
111	WDR19	445	MALAT1	779	ASCL1	1,113	CD22
112	CRP	446	COL3A1	780	VWF	1,114	PSMB1
113	CCL11	447	CD28	781	PROM1	1,115	LOC111674479
114	AGT	448	MIR23A	782	PDPN	1,116	LOC111674467
115	CCND1	449	MIR19A	783	PRODH	1,117	SDHB
116	COL1A2	450	HAMP	784	ALG9	1,118	LOC111674465
117	COPA	451	MIR429	785	HOXD13	1,119	PSMD14
118	CASP8	452	MIR335	786	TNFRSF10A	1,120	IFNB1
119	DKC1	453	TTR	787	IL12B	1,121	PLAT
120	ACTC1	454	C2CD3	788	BBS9	1,122	PSMA5
121	FGFR2	455	NR1H4	789	NR3C1	1,123	NEB
122	IL17A	456	G6PD	790	MIR122	1,124	CHGA
123	SCNN1B	457	MIR127	791	ITGB3	1,125	MIR187
124	ATM	458	TNNI3	792	ERF	1,126	LOC113523647
125	MIR155	459	CXCL1	793	CCR5	1,127	HSD3B7
126	SHH	460	MIR424	794	ADIPOQ	1,128	LOC108491823
127	RB1	461	IFT52	795	TF	1,129	IL4R
128	CSF2	462	ZCCHC8	796	RXRA	1,130	PSMB4

(Continued on following page)

TABLE 3 | (*Continued*) Lung fibrosis-related targets obtained from the GeneCards database.

Number	Gene	Number	Gene	Number	Gene	Number	Gene
129	CEP290	463	AGTR2	797	FAT4	1,131	DRC1
130	FCGR2A	464	NSMCE3	798	PSMD4	1,132	MIR361
131	PKHD1	465	TYR	799	UMOD	1,133	COL11A2
132	NPHP4	466	ABCB4	800	TMEM107	1,134	MIR497
133	MIR200B	467	NOS3	801	BLOC1S6	1,135	SBDS
134	MKS1	468	LPAR1	802	MMP14	1,136	TLR6
135	SCNN1G	469	CXCR2	803	PTK2B	1,137	MIR339
136	FAM111B	470	ZIC3	804	PIEZO2	1,138	RECQL4
137	FN1	471	LOC111674475	805	CDK1	1,139	DERL2
138	INVS	472	CCR7	806	SIRT3	1,140	SH2B3
139	STAT6	473	ANKS6	807	IL15	1,141	GUCA2A
140	WRAP53	474	CALR	808	TAP1	1,142	CCDC103
141	FGFR3	475	TCTN1	809	GATA6	1,143	PCNA
142	RET	476	MIR224	810	EPOR	1,144	PSME2
143	NRAS	477	IGF1R	811	PVT1	1,145	NCOR1
144	DDR2	478	XRCC1	812	MUSK	1,146	TTC37
145	FBN1	479	CD34	813	ESR2	1,147	PSMB5
146	OFD1	480	EVC2	814	MAP1B	1,148	PRKG1
147	MAP2K1	481	CEACAM5	815	MT-CYB	1,149	LEPR
148	ENG	482	MIR338	816	TRAF6	1,150	TNC
149	NEK8	483	GATA4	817	PKD1L1	1,151	PTGS1
150	FGF2	484	MIRLET7G	818	RBPJ	1,152	IFNA2
151	MUC5AC	485	SOD2	819	DMD	1,153	DZIP1L
152	NFKB1	486	MIR191	820	FABP4	1,154	MIR296
153	RARB	487	CCR3	821	CD80	1,155	CD86
154	TNFRSF1A	488	CXCL5	822	PSMA4	1,156	MYCL
155	IL5	489	MYLK	823	IGHE	1,157	VPS45
156	APC	490	H2AC18	824	EGFR-AS1	1,158	GBE1
157	SMPD1	491	GPC3	825	DNMT3B	1,159	IL7R
158	MPO	492	TMEM138	826	MIR26A1	1,160	CYP27A1
159	ACTA2	493	MIR377	827	FLT4	1,161	PLA2G7
160	MIR126	494	CCL22	828	CCNA2	1,162	NOTCH2
161	NOD2	495	SLC34A2	829	DNAI2	1,163	CEACAM1
162	MIR17	496	PTPN22	830	TUG1	1,164	MIR485
163	FGF7	497	PKD2	831	IFIH1	1,165	LOC113633876
164	IFT140	498	DNAH5	832	KATNIP	1,166	REG3A
165	KRT18	499	S100A4	833	MMP3	1,167	EPRS1
166	REN	500	BAX	834	KLF6	1,168	LOC113633875
167	PDCD1	501	THPO	835	BLOC1S3	1,169	LOC113604967
168	VEGFC	502	MIR137	836	SERPINB1	1,170	ZEB1
169	IFT80	503	FOXJ1	837	GLA	1,171	FOXM1
170	SCGB1A1	504	BCL2L1	838	LPO	1,172	CASR
171	BRCA2	505	TRPV4	839	F2R	1,173	TALDO1
172	AHI1	506	CCR4	840	BTK	1,174	MIR219A1
173	TCTN2	507	CADM1	841	SOCS3	1,175	CCL26
174	BMPR2	508	TMEM237	842	COL4A2	1,176	LOC113664107
175	RAF1	509	LOC111674463	843	NBAS	1,177	CLCN4
176	CXCR4	510	GBA	844	CEP104	1,178	SNHG1
177	KIAA0586	511	EZH2	845	MAGEA4	1,179	LAMA2
178	HIF1A	512	SOX9	846	DERL1	1,180	TCF7
179	FARSB	513	MIR24-2	847	AKT3	1,181	TFRC
180	TLR2	514	SPARC	848	NPPA	1,182	PLCZ1
181	AGTR1	515	S100A8	849	BCL2L11	1,183	POMC
182	BMP6	516	LTA	850	LAMA1	1,184	ABCC3
183	CDK4	517	MKKS	851	IL3	1,185	CRYAB
184	TMEM216	518	HYDIN	852	ITGA5	1,186	LOC110806263
185	RELA	519	GLI1	853	CYP2D6	1,187	MCM4
186	CSF3	520	BIRC5	854	DOCK6	1,188	TNFSF13B
187	CCL5	521	MAPK3	855	CANX	1,189	MIR149
188	ESR1	522	PSMB8	856	AXIN2	1,190	PLA2G6
189	MIR223	523	AP3D1	857	SCARB2	1,191	KNG1
190	FOXP3	524	MIRLET7A3	858	CDX2	1,192	HOTTIP
191	TTN	525	IDH1	859	SLC9A3	1,193	AR
192	MARS1	526	CYP2E1	860	ICOS	1,194	PSMB2

(Continued on following page)

TABLE 3 | (*Continued*) Lung fibrosis-related targets obtained from the GeneCards database.

Number	Gene	Number	Gene	Number	Gene	Number	Gene
193	MAPK8	527	TNFSF10	861	PTGER4	1,195	LSM1
194	MEG3	528	PRKCD	862	SLC17A5	1,196	NIPBL
195	CCL3	529	MIR181C	863	CXCR5	1,197	PSMA8
196	HPS4	530	CYCS	864	TCTEX1D2	1,198	IL16
197	BRCA1	531	IFT27	865	MXRA5	1,199	CCAT1
198	IL2RA	532	TUBB3	866	FOXP1	1,200	SPRY2
199	HPS1	533	HP	867	MIR138-1	1,201	RIPK1
200	MIR34A	534	ALMS1	868	CLDN1	1,202	PHKG2
201	MIR200C	535	NOX4	869	MIR154	1,203	MIR503
202	B9D1	536	RYR1	870	INSR	1,204	GSTT1
203	Dnase1	537	TSLP	871	UCHL1	1,205	PRKCI
204	TSC1	538	VDAC1	872	DCN	1,206	AGL
205	WDR35	539	U2AF1	873	XPNPEP3	1,207	RAG2
206	WT1	540	CAT	874	KRT13	1,208	HNF1A-AS1
207	INPP5E	541	CALCA	875	COMT	1,209	CCAT2
208	MPL	542	DNAH11	876	EDNRA	1,210	ERLIN1
209	MIR125A	543	NF1	877	CA4	1,211	MIR125B2
210	CSPP1	544	PTK2	878	HLA-DQA1	1,212	MIR15B
211	GRP	545	SP110	879	BBS12	1,213	CREBBP
212	MIR144	546	IL12RB1	880	KRT8	1,214	CTSL
213	RTEL1-TNFRSF6B	547	NQO1	881	CMA1	1,215	NR5A1
214	SERPINC1	548	GAA	882	AKR1B10	1,216	MSR1
215	CD4	549	MIR409	883	LOC113633877	1,217	UTP4
216	DYNC2H1	550	VIP	884	CEP55	1,218	MIR301A
217	MIR145	551	GPT	885	MAP2K4	1,219	MUC7
218	FLT1	552	MIR708	886	CDK5	1,220	CASC2
219	TNFRSF1B	553	NFKBIA	887	P2RY2	1,221	ZNRD1ASP
220	MIR29A	554	KEAP1	888	NLRP3	1,222	PLCG2
221	HLA-DQB1	555	LOC111674477	889	PSMC4	1,223	MIR124-1
222	FHIT	556	CD36	890	HSPA4	1,224	MIR382
223	H19	557	IGFBP3	891	AVPR2	1,225	LAMP1
224	PKD1	558	NKX2-5	892	RPS27A	1,226	CD69
225	SOS1	559	CEP83	893	MIR375	1,227	DANCR
226	SPINK1	560	BDNF	894	MIR33A	1,228	TP53COR1
227	MIR31	561	ABCB11	895	ATF6	1,229	MYL3
228	IFT172	562	FGFR4	896	RXRB	1,230	CYSLTR2
229	MMP7	563	CTSG	897	UBC	1,231	SELL
230	CD8A	564	ITGB1	898	NPC2	1,232	LINC-ROR
231	PDGFB	565	CSF2RA	899	CLCN2	1,233	NOS1
232	SLC2A1	566	DNAI1	900	FOXE1	1,234	IFT20
233	JUN	567	ARL3	901	MIR132	1,235	MIR10B
234	BMP2	568	MECP2	902	HDGF	1,236	CD81
235	HMGB1	569	CDKN1B	903	WNT7B	1,237	ANTXR1
236	ERBB3	570	DNMT3A	904	SLC9A3R2	1,238	PRSS2
237	MIR150	571	VHL	905	H2AX	1,239	SNHG20
238	PRSS1	572	THBS1	906	PRKAG2	1,240	MIR95
239	MIR29C	573	YAP1	907	SERPINB3	1,241	GALC
240	MIR146B	574	TIMP2	908	LRP1B	1,242	DGCR5
241	ABCC1	575	TOLLIP	909	DNAAF3	1,243	HNMT
242	BBS2	576	KCNK3	910	BCL10	1,244	SLCO2A1
243	ABCB1	577	NOTCH3	911	RAG1	1,245	MLH1
244	CXCL10	578	RASSF1	912	LAMA4	1,246	PLA2G2A
245	XIAP	579	SP1	913	HLA-G	1,247	MME
246	KIF21A	580	RHOA	914	PSMB3	1,248	TYMS
247	PIK3R1	581	ABCC2	915	SIRT1	1,249	MIR198
248	BBS1	582	IKBKB	916	MIRLET7A1	1,250	JAK1
249	IRF1	583	GZMB	917	PLA2G1B	1,251	PDE4D
250	IL1A	584	LEP	918	KDM4C	1,252	LAMC2
251	PTPRC	585	BBS5	919	MUC6	1,253	AHR
252	HLA-DPB1	586	APOE	920	TUBB1	1,254	TPM1
253	ERCC6	587	NHLRC2	921	SKIV2L	1,255	MT-CO2
254	STX1A	588	NPPB	922	TPM2	1,256	ASCC1
255	SETD2	589	SYP	923	CCDC40	1,257	EOGT
256	CCL17	590	ACTB	924	TET2	1,258	CCL7

(Continued on following page)

TABLE 3 | *(Continued)* Lung fibrosis-related targets obtained from the GeneCards database.

Number	Gene	Number	Gene	Number	Gene	Number	Gene
257	IDH2	591	PSMA1	925	TRIP11	1,259	TRPM4
258	CXCL12	592	PTCH1	926	ITGA2B	1,260	GPSM2
259	MIR27A	593	LOXL2	927	ENO2	1,261	TARS1
260	GSTM1	594	CEP41	928	EIF2AK3	1,262	TPM3
261	DCTN4	595	MYPN	929	RSPH9	1,263	CD14
262	PRKN	596	CR1	930	MIR193A	1,264	MIR216A
263	CXCR3	597	ERCC1	931	PXN	1,265	CTAG1B
264	MIR200A	598	IGFBP5	932	DNAAF5	1,266	MIR22HG
265	ARL13B	599	MGMT	933	LAT	1,267	MIR10A
266	PTGS2	600	VIM	934	RSPH1	1,268	PCAT1
267	MIR148A	601	ENO1	935	CDKN2B-AS1	1,269	SNHG15
268	MYC	602	NLRC4	936	ADORA1	1,270	BANCR
269	IGF1	603	PIK3CG	937	RAD51	1,271	PSAP
270	IL18	604	MYH7	938	DIABLO	1,272	IL11
271	CYP1A1	605	F13A1	939	TFR2	1,273	MIR362
272	NEK9	606	WNT4	940	RSPO2	1,274	UCA1
273	LOX	607	NME1	941	C4A	1,275	UBE2L3
274	MIR30D	608	CD63	942	IFI27	1,276	FBLN5
275	MIR146A	609	RPGRIP1	943	MIR29B1	1,277	GC
276	IFT122	610	ATP8B1	944	HSPD1	1,278	TP73-AS1
277	B9D2	611	GNAS	945	CCDC39	1,279	PPBP
278	KCNQ1	612	TUBB	946	PDE4A	1,280	LINC00473
279	CYP2A6	613	IFRD1	947	TRIM21	1,281	SOX2-OT
280	MIR483	614	CASP9	948	PLCG1	1,282	MIR181B1
281	MIR183	615	LAMP2	949	IL1RL1	1,283	XIST
282	IL1R1	616	HDAC2	950	BBIP1	1,284	MIR129-1
283	SDCCAG8	617	ANXA1	951	MIR196A1	1,285	PRL
284	PTRH2	618	IFT74	952	BAD	1,286	MIR193B
285	MIR182	619	ROS1	953	MYBPC3	1,287	NR3C2
286	CDKN3	620	CLEC7A	954	ARAF	1,288	MYL1
287	GUCY2C	621	AKT2	955	VDR	1,289	SDC1
288	MIR222	622	WRN	956	MAGEA1	1,290	MIR24-1
289	LOC111674472	623	DTNBP1	957	TAC1	1,291	PHB
290	KIF7	624	CD19	958	IDUA	1,292	MYL2
291	FLNC	625	SMARCA4	959	EPX	1,293	APOA1
292	PPARG	626	ANGPT2	960	ASXL1	1,294	SNHG12
293	XRCC3	627	PARP1	961	MAGEA3	1,295	CEP57
294	SNAI1	628	BBS7	962	RAC1	1,296	IL6R
295	POSTN	629	MIF	963	GATA1	1,297	SERPINF2
296	MIR192	630	SELP	964	GAS5	1,298	CALB2
297	JAG1	631	HSPG2	965	MIR9-1	1,299	MIR152
298	CD40LG	632	ATP12A	966	RYR2	1,300	ADK
299	DYNC2I1	633	HSP90AA1	967	JPH2	1,301	NRG1
300	ACVRL1	634	CHRM3	968	RIOX2	1,302	MIR501
301	MIR221	635	MVP	969	LOC111674464	1,303	GPRC5A
302	IFT43	636	DCDC2	970	TNFAIP3	1,304	LZTR1
303	DES	637	ERCC2	971	PIK3CB	1,305	TLR7
304	MIR22	638	PPP2R1B	972	DHCR7	1,306	POT1
305	TNFRSF10B	639	TYMP	973	C1S	1,307	EP300
306	IRF5	640	CLCA1	974	SNAI2	1,308	FBL
307	ALK	641	OGG1	975	ERBB4	1,309	PLOD2
308	CEP120	642	MCL1	976	ACVR1	1,310	DLL1
309	MIR451A	643	CCN4	977	NPC1	1,311	TOP2A
310	DYNC2I2	644	F3	978	LNX1	1,312	MAGEC2
311	CASP3	645	STAT5B	979	GRB2	1,313	MIR499A
312	CCL4	646	FUZ	980	TFAP2B	1,314	ENSG00000266919
313	HPS6	647	LBR	981	SLC6A4	1,315	TNFRSF11B
314	MIR143	648	CXCL2	982	IFT88	1,316	HOXA11-AS
315	ICOSLG	649	PLAUR	983	NPHS1	1,317	RASGRP1
316	CLCA4	650	ASAH1	984	MAP2K7	1,318	SPRY4-IT1
317	HLA-DPA1	651	BPI	985	PSMD2	1,319	FIP1L1
318	FOXF1	652	NPM1	986	DNAH8	1,320	GSR
319	BIRC3	653	ACTA1	987	B2M	1,321	CST3
320	SMAD7	654	ANGPT1	988	INTU	1,322	LTBP4

(Continued on following page)

TABLE 3 | *(Continued)* Lung fibrosis-related targets obtained from the GeneCards database.

Number	Gene	Number	Gene	Number	Gene	Number	Gene
321	MIR203A	655	GGT1	989	ENTPD1	1,323	ZFAS1
322	MIR30A	656	CAMP	990	PRSS8	1,324	F5
323	MIR324	657	SOD3	991	CCNE1	1,325	STMN1
324	MIR199B	658	F2RL3	992	LRRC56	1,326	AIRE
325	ACP5	659	TEK	993	MAP3K8	1,327	RETN
326	MIR205	660	LTF	994	SHC1	1,328	NTS
327	TP73	661	MT-CO1	995	CCDC114	1,329	KRT5
328	TLR9	662	LIPA	996	ACHE	1,330	F2RL1
329	MAPK1	663	WNT3	997	TBX20	1,331	TNFSF11
330	CLCN5	664	GDF1	998	AURKB	1,332	COL4A5
331	TMEM231	665	SLC40A1	999	ASL	1,333	PIK3CD
332	BBS4	666	GLIS2	1,000	MIR30C1	1,334	FGF9
333	RMRP	667	AREG	1,001	IL2RB	1,335	KRT20
334	TGFB3	668	CDKN2B	1,002	NCF2		

TABLE 4 | Common targets shared between the potential anlotinib targets and lung fibrosis-related targets.

Number	Gene	Number	Gene
1	AXL	38	EPHA3
2	MERTK	39	TIE1
3	ERBB2	40	CACNA2D1
4	AURKB	41	ERBB4
5	FLT1	42	MAP3K8
6	EGFR	43	ERN1
7	KDR	44	MST1R
8	SRC	45	FGFR4
9	MET	46	EPHA7
10	RET	47	MAP2K5
11	ALK	48	RIPK2
12	ABL1	49	DDR2
13	KIT	50	ACVR1B
14	ACVR1	51	DDR1
15	FLT4	52	MAP4K2
16	FLT3	53	EPHA1
17	PDGFRA	54	EPHB6
18	FGFR1	55	ERBB3
19	TGFBR1	56	EIF2AK1
20	BTK	57	MAP3K19
21	LYN	58	AKT2
22	FGFR3	59	PRKCG
23	PDGFRB	60	AKT3
24	YES1	61	PIM1
25	FGFR2	62	PIM2
26	FGR	63	JAK1
27	CSF1R	64	DPP8
28	BLK	65	DPP9
29	PLK4	66	PDE4B
30	FYN	67	PRKCI
31	MAP2K2	68	CDK2
32	HCK	69	CDK1
33	STK10	70	CCNT1
34	ABL2	71	TERT
35	TEK	72	SLC8A1
36	SLK	73	GNRHR
37	STK4	74	AOC3

PCBP3 increases the translation of PFKFB3. Overall, these results suggest that PCBP3 improves PFKFB3 expression levels by increasing its translation rather than by influencing its protein stability.

To determine the functional impact of PCBP3-mediated regulation of PFKFB3 expression in lung fibrosis, we transfected lung fibroblasts with FLAG-PCBP3. Expression of PFKFB3 was significantly increased by PCBP3 overexpression compared to that of the empty vector control. Reliable markers of the phenotypic transformation of fibroblasts into myofibroblasts, fibronectin, collagen I and α-SMA, were markedly increased in FLAG-PCBP3-treated cells at the protein level (**Figures 3G,H**) compared with vector-treated cells. In turn, using small interfering RNA (siRNA) to silence PFKFB3, the FLAG-PCBP3-induced overexpression of fibronectin, collagen I and α-SMA was abolished (**Figures 3G,H**). These findings suggest that PCBP3 protein upregulation is an early and sustained event during fibroblast activation and that the profibrogenic effects of PCBP3 are mediated by PFKFB3 expression. Taken together, these data suggest that PCBP3 posttranscriptionally increases PFKFB3 expression by promoting its translation during myofibroblast activation.

Anlotinib Represses PCBP3 Expression Levels During Myofibroblast Activation

To confirm the regulation of PCBP3 by anlotinib *in vitro*, we evaluated the protein expression of PCBP3 in MLFs and IMR90 cells. We found that TGF-β1 induced the expression of PCBP3 in MLFs and that anlotinib prevented PCBP3 expression by immunofluorescence analysis (**Figure 4A**). Western blot analysis of PCBP3 showed a similar result (**Figures 4B,C**) in MLFs, and these results were confirmed in the human IMR90 cell line (**Figures 4D,E**). Taken together, these data suggest that anlotinib can repress PCBP3 expression levels during myofibroblast activation *in vitro*.

Anlotinib Attenuates Bleomycin-Induced Pulmonary Fibrosis

To investigate the biological effects of anlotinib on pulmonary fibrosis *in vivo*, we established a bleomycin (BLM)-induced mouse model of pulmonary fibrosis. The mice were intraperitoneally injected with 1 mg/kg anlotinib daily after BLM administration (**Figure 5A**). From the first week after bleomycin instillation, the bleomycin-treated mice showed a

TABLE 5 | Potential proteins may interact with PFKFB3 mRNA through the catRAPID algorithm.

#	Protein D	RNA ID	Z score?	Discriminative power (%)?	Interaction strength (%)?	Domain?	Motif?	Ranking?
1	ELAV1_MOUSE_247-308	NC_000068.7:c11_1_5924-6036	−0.13	50	98	yes	yes	HHH
2	ELAV1_MOUSE_247-308	NC_000068.7: c11_1_26816-27008	−0.08	67	99	yes	yes	HHH
3	ELAV1_MOUSE_247-308	NC_000068.7: c11_1_15806-15983	−0.23	40	90	yes	yes	HHH
4	PCBP3_MOUSE_301-351	NC_000068.7: c11_1_41382-41564	−0.69	14	13	yes	yes	HHH
5	ELAV1_MOUSE_247-308	NC_000068.7: c11_1_77223-77340	−0.47	22	74	yes	yes	HHH
6	ELAV1_MOUSE_247-308	NC_000068.7: c11_1_10399-10532	−0.50	20	64	yes	yes	HHH
7	ELAV1_MOUSE_109-176	NC_000068.7:c11_1_5924-6036	−0.14	50	98	yes	yes	HHH
8	ELAV1_MOUSE_109-176	NC_000068.7: c11_1_45706-45815	−0.39	26	85	yes	yes	HHH
9	ELAV1_MOUSE_109-176	NC_000068.7: c11_1_26816-27008	−0.04	63	99	yes	yes	HHH
10	ELAV1_MOUSE_109-176	NC_000068.7: c11_1_15806-15983	−0.24	40	90	yes	yes	HHH
11	ELAV1_MOUSE_109-172	NC_000068.7:c11_1_5924-6036	−0.15	47	97	yes	yes	HHH
12	ELAV1_MOUSE_109-172	NC_000068.7: c11_1_45706-45815	−0.40	26	85	yes	yes	HHH
13	ELAV1_MOUSE_109-172	NC_000068.7: c11_1_15806-15983	−0.26	37	87	yes	yes	HHH
14	PCBP3_MOUSE_301-351	NC_000068.7: c11_1_77461-77636	−0.71	14	9	yes	yes	HHH
15	PCBP3_MOUSE_301-351	NC_000068.7: c11_1_66050-66214	−0.66	14	17	yes	yes	HHH

certain reduction in activity, accompanied by slight shortness of breath. 21 days after bleomycin administration, bleomycin-treated mice showed obvious hyperventilation, accompanied by reduced activity and weight loss, but no similar symptoms were observed in the control group. A single dose of BLM (5 mg/kg) administered by intratracheal instillation successfully induced pulmonary fibrosis in C57BL/6 mice, as evidenced by a decline in pulmonary function, decreased tidal volume (TV, **Figure 5B**) and dynamic compliance (Cdyn, **Figure 5C**), and increased lung resistance (RI, **Figure 5D**). However, treatment with anlotinib significantly reversed bleomycin-induced pulmonary dysfunction. Moreover, we evaluated collagen deposition in the lung tissues by analyzing the hydroxyproline (HYP) content and found that anlotinib treatment reduced the amount of collagen in the lungs of bleomycin-treated mice (**Figure 5E**). Hematoxylin and eosin (H&E) staining indicated that anlotinib-treated mice had decreased lung inflammation and reduced lung architectural damage (**Figure 5F**). Accordingly, Masson's trichrome staining showed decreased collagen deposition in anlotinib-treated mice compared with vehicle-treated mice (**Figure 5F**). Furthermore, attenuated fibrosis was supported by decreased protein levels of fibronectin and α-SMA by immunohistochemical (IHC) staining (**Figure 5G**). We also found that anlotinib treatment reduced fibronectin, collagen I and α-SMA expression by western blotting (**Figures 5H,I**). Taken together, these data show that anlotinib attenuates bleomycin-induced pulmonary fibrosis *in vivo*.

Anlotinib Decreases PCBP3 Expression and Inhibits PFKFB3-Driven Glycolysis in Fibrotic Rodent Lungs

We next examined whether the levels of PCBP3 were regulated by anlotinib *in vivo*. We evaluated the expression of PCBP3 in lung tissues and found that the protein levels of PCBP3 were markedly increased after bleomycin instillation, while anlotinib treatment decreased PCBP3 expression (**Figures 6A,B**). Accordingly, IHC staining showed decreased PCBP3 protein levels in anlotinib-treated mice compared with vehicle-treated mice (**Figure 6C**). In addition, to confirm the regulation of PFKFB3-driven glycolysis by anlotinib *in vivo*, we measured the levels of lactate and the expression of PFKFB3 in the lungs of mice. We found that there were significantly higher levels of lactate in the lungs of bleomycin-treated mice than in the lungs of control mice, and anlotinib decreased lactate levels (**Figure 6D**). Western blot and IHC staining studies revealed that bleomycin-induced PFKFB3 expression in the lungs of mice was prevented by anlotinib (**Figures 6E–G**). Overall, these results suggest that anlotinib decreases PCBP3 expression and inhibits PFKFB3-driven glycolysis in fibrotic rodent lungs.

Anlotinib Accelerates the Resolution of Bleomycin-Induced Lung Fibrosis

We demonstrated that anlotinib treatment could attenuate bleomycin-induced pulmonary fibrosis. In that *in vivo* experiment, anlotinib was administered at approximately the same time as bleomycin instillation. We further examined whether anlotinib could postpone the progression of established fibrosis. Therefore, we performed another *in vivo* experiment in which anlotinib was intraperitoneally injected 7 days after bleomycin instillation (**Figure 7A**). As interventions beginning 7 days post bleomycin were classified as therapeutic (Izbicki et al., 2002; Moeller et al., 2008), we initially treated mice with anlotinib (1 mg/kg/day or 2 mg/kg/day) beginning on day 7 after bleomycin instillation. Pulmonary function tests showed that anlotinib treatment reversed the bleomycin-induced decline in pulmonary function, with increases in TV (**Figure 7B**) and Cdyn (**Figure 7C**) and a decrease in RI (**Figure 7D**). HYP measurements showed that the collagen content was significantly decreased in anlotinib-treated mice compared with vehicle-treated mice (**Figure 7E**). H&E staining and Masson's trichrome staining of lungs collected at day 21 showed enhanced recovery from fibrosis upon anlotinib treatment (**Figure 7F**). Correspondingly, IHC staining showed that anlotinib treatment reduced fibronectin and α-SMA expression in the lungs (**Figure 7G**). Western blot analysis also showed that anlotinib decreased the protein levels of fibronectin, collagen I and α-SMA in the lungs (**Figures 7H,I**). Collectively, these data clearly demonstrate that anlotinib accelerates fibrosis resolution *in vivo* even after the establishment of fibrosis.

DISCUSSION

Despite recent advances in our understanding of IPF pathology, there is still no curative treatment for this disease; indeed, the currently available antifibrotic treatment modalities slow but do not completely stop the progression of the disease (Spagnolo and Maher, 2017). In this study, we demonstrate that anlotinib strongly inhibits fibroblast-to-myofibroblast transdifferentiation and reduces extracellular matrix production in primary MLFs and in the human IMR90 cell line. Accordingly, preventative and therapeutic administration of anlotinib to bleomycin-administered mice resulted in accelerated resolution of fibrosis. No adverse, systemic side effects were observed. Here, we demonstrate a novel mechanism by which anlotinib exerts antifibrotic effects by downregulating PCBP3, reducing PFKFB3 translation and inhibiting glycolysis in myofibroblasts (**Figure 8**).

A previous study revealed that male and female C57BL/6 mice did not differ in terms of their lung fibrotic responses, including cellular infiltration, collagen deposition, and quantifiable morphological changes in the lung architecture, but that the bleomycin-induced decrease in static compliance was significantly greater in males than in females (Voltz et al., 2008). This adverse effect on lung function was found to be due to male sex hormones. So sex differences should be carefully considered when interpreting experimental models of pulmonary fibrosis in mice (Blaauboer et al., 2014). In our study, we used only female mice to avoid the sex differences. We found that anlotinib exerted the preventative effects on bleomycin model of pulmonary fibrosis. Furthermore, anlotinib can also accelerate fibrosis resolution after the establishment of fibrosis.

A recent report showed that anlotinib inhibits the profibrotic effect of TGF-β1 in lung fibroblasts by attenuating inflammation and oxidative stress (Ruan et al., 2020). Our data are in line with that report and reveal an additional mechanism by which anlotinib acts on lung fibroblasts to attenuate fibrosis. There is emerging evidence about the association between metabolic disorders and IPF (Yin et al., 2019; Cho et al., 2020; Hu et al., 2020). Similar to highly proliferative cancer cells, myofibroblasts are highly dependent on glycolysis *in vitro* (Bueno et al., 2020). Furthermore, glycolysis is necessary not only for fibroblast growth and migration but also for the acquisition and maintenance of a myofibroblastic phenotype (Xu et al., 2017; Para et al., 2019). A previous study revealed that inhibition of glycolysis by the PFKFB3 inhibitor 3PO or by genomic disruption of the PFKFB3 gene blunted the differentiation of lung fibroblasts into myofibroblasts and attenuated profibrotic phenotypes in myofibroblasts (Xie et al., 2015). Another study revealed that lung fibroblasts displayed augmented aerobic glycolysis through activation of the PI3K-Akt-mTOR/PFKFB3 pathway in LPS-induced pulmonary fibrosis (Hu et al., 2020). Our data, along with previous studies, demonstrated that glycolytic reprogramming was critical to lung myofibroblast activation and pulmonary fibrosis. Furthermore, we demonstrated that anlotinib could strongly inhibit glycolytic reprogramming *in vitro* and *in vivo*.

The results presented herein provide new insights into the molecular mechanisms of lung fibrogenesis. This work unveils a previously unrecognized posttranscriptional regulation in activated lung fibroblasts composed of the RNA binding protein PCBP3 and the critical glycolytic enzyme PFKFB3, which maintains fibroblasts with higher glycolytic activity in fibrotic lungs compared to normal lung fibroblasts in healthy lungs. PCBP family members perform multiple functions by binding to the poly(C) sequence in both DNA and RNA to modulate mRNA stabilization, translation silencing, or translation enhancement (Blyn et al., 1997; Andino et al., 1999; Ostareck et al., 2001). Our present findings showing that PCBP3 plays an important role in myofibroblast activation and fibrogenesis and significantly extends our previous understanding by identifying an additional node of interaction between PCBP3-mediated posttranscriptional dysregulation and lung disease. We found that PFKFB3 protein overexpression was not accompanied by PFKFB3 mRNA upregulation, indicating that this increase was not transcriptionally derived. Instead, we observed that high PFKFB3 protein levels were maintained during fibroblast transdifferentiation, owing to PCBP3-mediated translational activation. Thus, the PCBP3 protein is upregulated during myofibroblast activation and binds directly to PFKFB3 during transcription. This binding activates PFKFB3 mRNA translation and generates high levels of the glycolysis activator PFKFB3. This mechanism does not exclude additional pathways of regulating PFKFB3 expression. Hence, it is not unusual for key proteins to be regulated at multiple levels, including through transcription, translation, and posttranslational modifications.

Our study is the first to report that anlotinib inhibits PFKFB3-mediated glycolysis in myofibroblasts. Moreover, anlotinib attenuates glycolysis in myofibroblasts by repressing PCBP3 expression levels rather than directly regulating the expression of PFKFB3, as anlotinib treatment does not decrease the mRNA levels of PFKFB3. Our work contributes novel mechanistic insight into the action of anlotinib. However, one of the limitations of this study is that we didn't knock out PCBP3/PFKFB3 in mice to verify their effects in lung fibrosis, which may be explored in the further research. This future direction may be important to better understand how PCBP3 regulates PFKFB3-mediated glycolysis in pulmonary fibrosis. The other one is that this study only used bleomycin mice model for the research. Although the bleomycin model is the most widely used and best-characterized mouse model, the fibrosis of the bleomycin model is self-resolving, which contrasts with the progressive chronic fibrosis typical of human IPF (Liu et al., 2017). Therefore, whether anlotinib could attenuate fibrosis in human IPF still requires *ex vivo* models of pulmonary fibrosis.

In conclusion, our study demonstrated a clear antifibrotic role for anlotinib in the lungs. Its antifibrotic activity is mediated by its ability to decrease PCBP3 expression and attenuate PFKFB3-driven glycolysis, thereby inhibiting myofibroblast activation. Anlotinib might be considered as a potential therapeutic option for IPF patients.

AUTHOR CONTRIBUTIONS

WC, JZ, and WZ performed study concept and design; YL, YL, and ZZ performed development of methodology and writing; HH and XW provided acquisition, analysis and interpretation of data, and statistical analysis; XM and FZ provided technical and material support; SC and HD performed review and revision of the paper.

REFERENCES

Agostini, F., Zanzoni, A., Klus, P., Marchese, D., Cirillo, D., and Tartaglia, G. G. (2013). catRAPID Omics: a Web Server for Large-Scale Prediction of Protein-RNA Interactions. *Bioinformatics* 29 (22), 2928–2930. doi:10.1093/bioinformatics/btt495

Andino, R., Böddeker, N., Silvera, D., and Gamarnik, A. V. (1999). Intracellular Determinants of Picornavirus Replication. *Trends Microbiol.* 7 (2), 76–82. doi:10.1016/s0966-842x(98)01446-2

Atsumi, T., Chesney, J., Metz, C., Leng, L., Donnelly, S., Makita, Z., et al. (2002). High Expression of Inducible 6-Phosphofructo-2-Kinase/fructose-2,6-Bisphosphatase (iPFK-2; PFKFB3) in Human Cancers. *Cancer Res.* 62 (20), 5881–5887. doi:10.2337/diabetes.54.12.3349

Blaauboer, M. E., Boeijen, F. R., Emson, C. L., Turner, S. M., Zandieh-Doulabi, B., Hanemaaijer, R., et al. (2014). Extracellular Matrix Proteins: a Positive Feedback Loop in Lung Fibrosis? *Matrix Biol.* 34, 170–178. doi:10.1016/j.matbio.2013.11.002

Blyn, L. B., Towner, J. S., Semler, B. L., and Ehrenfeld, E. (1997). Requirement of poly(rC) Binding Protein 2 for Translation of Poliovirus RNA. *J. Virol.* 71 (8), 6243–6246. doi:10.1128/jvi.71.8.6243-6246.1997

Bueno, M., Calyeca, J., Rojas, M., and Mora, A. L. (2020). Mitochondria Dysfunction and Metabolic Reprogramming as Drivers of Idiopathic Pulmonary Fibrosis. *Redox Biol.* 33, 101509. doi:10.1016/j.redox.2020.101509

Cao, Y., Zhang, X., Wang, L., Yang, Q., Ma, Q., Xu, J., et al. (2019). PFKFB3-mediated Endothelial Glycolysis Promotes Pulmonary Hypertension. *Proc. Natl. Acad. Sci. U S A.* 116 (27), 13394–13403. doi:10.1073/pnas.1821401116

Chen, Y., Xu, T., Li, M., Li, C., Ma, Y., Chen, G., et al. (2021). Inhibition of SENP2-Mediated Akt deSUMOylation Promotes Cardiac Regeneration via Activating Akt Pathway. *Clin. Sci. (Lond)* 135 (6), 811–828. doi:10.1042/cs20201408

Chen, Z., Liu, M., Li, L., and Chen, L. (2018). Involvement of the Warburg Effect in Non-tumor Diseases Processes. *J. Cel Physiol.* 233 (4), 2839–2849. doi:10.1002/jcp.25998

Cho, S. J., Moon, J. S., Nikahira, K., Yun, H. S., Harris, R., Hong, K. S., et al. (2020). GLUT1-dependent Glycolysis Regulates Exacerbation of Fibrosis via AIM2 Inflammasome Activation. *Thorax* 75 (3), 227–236. doi:10.1136/thoraxjnl-2019-213571

Choi, H. S., Kim, C. S., Hwang, C. K., Song, K. Y., Law, P. Y., Wei, L. N., et al. (2007). Novel Function of the Poly(C)-binding Protein Alpha CP3 as a Transcriptional Repressor of the Mu Opioid Receptor Gene. *FASEB J.* 21 (14), 3963 3973. doi:10.1096/fj.07-8561com

De Bock, K., Georgiadou, M., Schoors, S., Kuchnio, A., Wong, B. W., Cantelmo, A. R., et al. (2013). Role of PFKFB3-Driven Glycolysis in Vessel Sprouting. *Cell* 154 (3), 651–663. doi:10.1016/j.cell.2013.06.037

DeBerardinis, R. J., and Thompson, C. B. (2012). Cellular Metabolism and Disease: what Do Metabolic Outliers Teach Us? *Cell* 148 (6), 1132–1144. doi:10.1016/j.cell.2012.02.032

Gfeller, D., Grosdidier, A., Wirth, M., Daina, A., Michielin, O., and Zoete, V. (2014). SwissTargetPrediction: a Web Server for Target Prediction of Bioactive Small Molecules. *Nucleic Acids Res.* 42, W32–W38. doi:10.1093/nar/gku293

Hinz, B. (2012). Mechanical Aspects of Lung Fibrosis: a Spotlight on the Myofibroblast. *Proc. Am. Thorac. Soc.* 9 (3), 137–147. doi:10.1513/pats.201202-017AW

Hinz, B., Phan, S. H., Thannickal, V. J., Prunotto, M., Desmoulière, A., Varga, J., et al. (2012). Recent Developments in Myofibroblast Biology: Paradigms for Connective Tissue Remodeling. *Am. J. Pathol.* 180 (4), 1340–1355. doi:10.1016/j.ajpath.2012.02.004

Ho, R. C., Alcazar, O., Fujii, N., Hirshman, M. F., and Goodyear, L. J. (2004). p38gamma MAPK Regulation of Glucose Transporter Expression and Glucose Uptake in L6 Myotubes and Mouse Skeletal Muscle. *Am. J. Physiol. Regul. Integr. Comp. Physiol.* 286 (2), R342–R349. doi:10.1152/ajpregu.00563.2003

Hu, X., Xu, Q., Wan, H., Hu, Y., Xing, S., Yang, H., et al. (2020). PI3K-Akt-mTOR/PFKFB3 Pathway Mediated Lung Fibroblast Aerobic Glycolysis and Collagen Synthesis in Lipopolysaccharide-Induced Pulmonary Fibrosis. *Lab. Invest.* 100 (6), 801–811. doi:10.1038/s41374-020-0404-9

Huang, Y., Wang, Y., Wang, X., Lin, L., Wang, P., Sun, J., et al. (2020). The Effects of the Transforming Growth Factor-B1 (TGF-B1) Signaling Pathway on Cell Proliferation and Cell Migration Are Mediated by Ubiquitin Specific Protease 4 (USP4) in Hypertrophic Scar Tissue and Primary Fibroblast Cultures. *Med. Sci. Monit.* 26, e920736. doi:10.12659/msm.920736

Hutchinson, J., Fogarty, A., Hubbard, R., and McKeever, T. (2015). Global Incidence and Mortality of Idiopathic Pulmonary Fibrosis: a Systematic Review. *Eur. Respir. J.* 46 (3), 795–806. doi:10.1183/09031936.00185114

Izbicki, G., Segel, M. J., Christensen, T. G., Conner, M. W., and Breuer, R. (2002). Time Course of Bleomycin-Induced Lung Fibrosis. *Int. J. Exp. Pathol.* 83 (3), 111–119. doi:10.1046/j.1365-2613.2002.00220.x

Jarman, E. R., Khambata, V. S., Cope, C., Jones, P., Roger, J., Ye, L. Y., et al. (2014). An Inhibitor of NADPH Oxidase-4 Attenuates Established Pulmonary Fibrosis in a Rodent Disease Model. *Am. J. Respir. Cel. Mol. Biol.* 50 (1), 158–169. doi:10.1165/rcmb.2013-0174OC

Kang, D. H., Song, K. Y., Choi, H. S., Law, P. Y., Wei, L. N., and Loh, H. H. (2012). Novel Dual-Binding Function of a Poly (C)-binding Protein 3, Transcriptional Factor Which Binds the Double-Strand and Single-Stranded DNA Sequence. *Gene* 501 (1), 33–38. doi:10.1016/j.gene.2012.04.001

Kenyon, N. J., Ward, R. W., McGrew, G., and Last, J. A. (2003). TGF-beta1 Causes Airway Fibrosis and Increased Collagen I and III mRNA in Mice. *Thorax* 58 (9), 772–777. doi:10.1136/thorax.58.9.772

Kim, Y., Noren Hooten, N., Dluzen, D. F., Martindale, J. L., Gorospe, M., and Evans, M. K. (2015). Posttranscriptional Regulation of the Inflammatory Marker C-Reactive Protein by the RNA-Binding Protein HuR and MicroRNA 637. *Mol. Cel. Biol.* 35 (24), 4212–4221. doi:10.1128/mcb.00645-15

Leidgens, S., Bullough, K. Z., Shi, H., Li, F., Shakoury-Elizeh, M., Yabe, T., et al. (2013). Each Member of the poly-R(C)-binding Protein 1 (PCBP) Family Exhibits Iron Chaperone Activity toward Ferritin. *J. Biol. Chem.* 288 (24), 17791–17802. doi:10.1074/jbc.M113.460253

Liang, L., Hui, K., Hu, C., Wen, Y., Yang, S., Zhu, P., et al. (2019). Autophagy Inhibition Potentiates the Anti-angiogenic Property of Multikinase Inhibitor Anlotinib through JAK2/STAT3/VEGFA Signaling in Non-small Cell Lung Cancer Cells. *J. Exp. Clin. Cancer Res.* 38 (1), 71. doi:10.1186/s13046-019-1093-3

Liu, G., Philp, A. M., Corte, T., Travis, M. A., Schilter, H., Hansbro, N. G., et al. (2021). Therapeutic Targets in Lung Tissue Remodelling and Fibrosis. *Pharmacol. Ther.* 225, 107839. doi:10.1016/j.pharmthera.2021.107839

Liu, T., De Los Santos, F. G., and Phan, S. H. (2017). The Bleomycin Model of Pulmonary Fibrosis. *Methods Mol. Biol.* 1627, 27–42. doi:10.1007/978-1-4939-7113-8_2

Livi, C. M., Klus, P., Delli Ponti, R., and Tartaglia, G. G. (2016). catRAPID Signature: Identification of Ribonucleoproteins and RNA-Binding Regions. *Bioinformatics* 32 (5), 773–775. doi:10.1093/bioinformatics/btv629

Meng, Y., Yu, C. H., Li, W., Li, T., Luo, W., Huang, S., et al. (2014). Angiotensin-converting Enzyme 2/angiotensin-(1-7)/Mas axis Protects against Lung Fibrosis by Inhibiting the MAPK/NF-κB Pathway. *Am. J. Respir. Cel. Mol. Biol.* 50 (4), 723–736. doi:10.1165/rcmb.2012-0451OC

Moeller, A., Ask, K., Warburton, D., Gauldie, J., and Kolb, M. (2008). The Bleomycin Animal Model: a Useful Tool to Investigate Treatment Options for Idiopathic Pulmonary Fibrosis? *Int. J. Biochem. Cel. Biol.* 40 (3), 362–382. doi:10.1016/j.biocel.2007.08.011

Nigdelioglu, R., Hamanaka, R. B., Meliton, A. Y., O'Leary, E., Witt, L. J., Cho, T., et al. (2016). Transforming Growth Factor (TGF)-β Promotes De Novo Serine Synthesis for Collagen Production. *J. Biol. Chem.* 291 (53), 27239–27251. doi:10.1074/jbc.M116.756247

Ostareck, D. H., Ostareck-Lederer, A., Shatsky, I. N., and Hentze, M. W. (2001). Lipoxygenase mRNA Silencing in Erythroid Differentiation: The 3'UTR Regulatory Complex Controls 60S Ribosomal Subunit Joining. *Cell* 104 (2), 281–290. doi:10.1016/s0092-8674(01)00212-4

Papa, S., Choy, P. M., and Bubici, C. (2019). The ERK and JNK Pathways in the Regulation of Metabolic Reprogramming. *Oncogene* 38 (13), 2223–2240. doi:10.1038/s41388-018-0582-8

Para, R., Romero, F., George, G., and Summer, R. (2019). Metabolic Reprogramming as a Driver of Fibroblast Activation in PulmonaryFibrosis. *Am. J. Med. Sci.* 357 (5), 394–398. doi:10.1016/j.amjms.2019.02.003

Plantier, L., Cazes, A., Dinh-Xuan, A. T., Bancal, C., Marchand-Adam, S., and Crestani, B. (2018). Physiology of the Lung in Idiopathic Pulmonary Fibrosis. *Eur. Respir. Rev.* 27 (147), 170062. doi:10.1183/16000617.0062-2017

Ruan, H., Lv, Z., Liu, S., Zhang, L., Huang, K., Gao, S., et al. (2020). Anlotinib Attenuated Bleomycin-Induced Pulmonary Fibrosis via the TGF-B1 Signalling Pathway. *J. Pharm. Pharmacol.* 72 (1), 44–55. doi:10.1111/jphp.13183

Safran, M., Solomon, I., Shmueli, O., Lapidot, M., Shen-Orr, S., Adato, A., et al. (2002). GeneCards 2002: towards a Complete, Object-Oriented, Human Gene Compendium. *Bioinformatics* 18 (11), 1542 1543. doi:10.1093/bioinformatics/18.11.1542

Sapudom, J., Rubner, S., Martin, S., Thoenes, S., Anderegg, U., and Pompe, T. (2015). The Interplay of Fibronectin Functionalization and TGF-B1 Presence on Fibroblast Proliferation, Differentiation and Migration in 3D Matrices. *Biomater. Sci.* 3 (9), 1291–1301. doi:10.1039/c5bm00140d

Sato, S., Shinohara, S., Hayashi, S., Morizumi, S., Abe, S., Okazaki, H., et al. (2017). Anti-fibrotic Efficacy of Nintedanib in Pulmonary Fibrosis via the Inhibition of Fibrocyte Activity. *Respir. Res.* 18 (1), 172. doi:10.1186/s12931-017-0654-2

Spagnolo, P., and Maher, T. M. (2017). Clinical Trial Research in Focus: Why Do So many Clinical Trials Fail in IPF? *Lancet Respir. Med.* 5 (5), 372–374. doi:10.1016/s2213-2600(17)30122-4

Sun, Y., Niu, W., Du, F., Du, C., Li, S., Wang, J., et al. (2016). Safety, Pharmacokinetics, and Antitumor Properties of Anlotinib, an Oral Multi-Target Tyrosine Kinase Inhibitor, in Patients with Advanced Refractory Solid Tumors. *J. Hematol. Oncol.* 9 (1), 105. doi:10.1186/s13045-016-0332-8

Szklarczyk, D., Gable, A. L., Lyon, D., Junge, A., Wyder, S., Huerta-Cepas, J., et al. (2019). STRING V11: Protein-Protein Association Networks with Increased Coverage, Supporting Functional Discovery in Genome-wide Experimental Datasets. *Nucleic Acids Res.* 47, D607–D613. doi:10.1093/nar/gky1131

Taniguchi, H., Ebina, M., Kondoh, Y., Ogura, T., Azuma, A., Suga, M., et al. (2010). Pirfenidone in Idiopathic Pulmonary Fibrosis. *Eur. Respir. J.* 35 (4), 821–829. doi:10.1183/09031936.00005209

Taurin, S., Yang, C. H., Reyes, M., Cho, S., Coombs, D. M., Jarboe, E. A., et al. (2018). Endometrial Cancers Harboring Mutated Fibroblast Growth Factor Receptor 2 Protein Are Successfully Treated with a New Small Tyrosine Kinase Inhibitor in an Orthotopic Mouse Model. *Int. J. Gynecol. Cancer* 28 (1), 152–160. doi:10.1097/igc.0000000000001129

Van Schaftingen, E., Lederer, B., Bartrons, R., and Hers, H. G. (1982). A Kinetic Study of Pyrophosphate: Fructose-6-Phosphate Phosphotransferase from Potato Tubers. Application to a Microassay of Fructose 2, 6-bisphosphate. *Eur. J. Biochem.* 129 (1), 191–195. doi:10.1111/j.1432-1033.1982.tb07039.x

Voltz, J. W., Card, J. W., Carey, M. A., Degraff, L. M., Ferguson, C. D., Flake, G. P., et al. (2008). Male Sex Hormones Exacerbate Lung Function Impairment after Bleomycin-Induced Pulmonary Fibrosis. *Am. J. Respir. Cel. Mol. Biol.* 39 (1), 45–52. doi:10.1165/rcmb.2007-0340OC

Wang, F., Qi, X. M., Wertz, R., Mortensen, M., Hagen, C., Evans, J., et al. (2020a). p38γ MAPK Is Essential for Aerobic Glycolysis and Pancreatic Tumorigenesis. *Cancer Res.* 80 (16), 3251–3264. doi:10.1158/0008-5472.CAN-19-3281

Wang, J., Guo, X., Wang, D., and Yang, S. (2020b). Expression Patterns of Pcbp Gene Family Members during Zebrafish Embryogenesis. *Gene Expr. Patterns* 35, 119097. doi:10.1016/j.gep.2020.119097

Wynn, T. A., and Ramalingam, T. R. (2012). Mechanisms of Fibrosis: Therapeutic Translation for Fibrotic Disease. *Nat. Med.* 18 (7), 1028–1040. doi:10.1038/nm.2807

Xie, C., Wan, X., Quan, H., Zheng, M., Fu, L., Li, Y., et al. (2018). Preclinical Characterization of Anlotinib, a Highly Potent and Selective Vascular Endothelial Growth Factor Receptor-2 Inhibitor. *Cancer Sci.* 109 (4), 1207–1219. doi:10.1111/cas.13536

Xie, N., Tan, Z., Banerjee, S., Cui, H., Ge, J., Liu, R. M., et al. (2015). Glycolytic Reprogramming in Myofibroblast Differentiation and Lung Fibrosis. *Am. J. Respir. Crit. Care Med.* 192 (12), 1462–1474. doi:10.1164/rccm.201504-0780OC

Xu, J., Li, J., Yu, Z., Rao, H., Wang, S., and Lan, H. (2017). HMGB1 Promotes HLF-1 Proliferation and ECM Production through Activating HIF1-α-Regulated Aerobic Glycolysis. *Pulm. Pharmacol. Ther.* 45, 136–141. doi:10.1016/j.pupt.2017.05.015

Yin, X., Choudhury, M., Kang, J. H., Schaefbauer, K. J., Jung, M. Y., Andrianifahanana, M., et al. (2019). Hexokinase 2 Couples Glycolysis with the Profibrotic Actions of TGF-β. *Sci. Signal.* 12 (612), eaax4067. doi:10.1126/scisignal.aax4067

11

Idiopathic Pulmonary Fibrosis: An Update on Pathogenesis

Qianru Mei†, Zhe Liu†, He Zuo, Zhenhua Yang and Jing Qu**

School of Basic Medicine, Tongji Medical College, Huazhong University of Science and Technology, Wuhan, China

***Correspondence:**
Zhenhua Yang
zhenhua@hust.edu.cn
Jing Qu
jingqu@hust.edu.cn

†These authors have contributed equally to this work

Idiopathic pulmonary fibrosis (IPF) is a progressive, lethal fibrotic lung disease that occurs primarily in middle-aged and elderly adults. It is a major cause of morbidity and mortality. With an increase in life expectancy, the economic burden of IPF is expected to continuously rise in the near future. Although the exact pathophysiological mechanisms underlying IPF remain not known. Significant progress has been made in our understanding of the pathogenesis of this devastating disease in last decade. The current paradigm assumes that IPF results from sustained or repetitive lung epithelial injury and subsequent activation of fibroblasts and myofibroblast differentiation. Persistent myofibroblast phenotype contributes to excessive deposition of the extracellular matrix (ECM) and aberrant lung repair, leading to tissue scar formation, distortion of the alveolar structure, and irreversible loss of lung function. Treatments of patients with IPF by pirfenidone and nintedanib have shown significant reduction of lung function decline and slowing of disease progression in patients with IPF. However, these drugs do not cure the disease. In this review, we discuss recent advances on the pathogenesis of IPF and highlight the development of novel therapeutic strategies against the disease.

Keywords: idiopathic pulmonary fibrosis, pathogenesis, alveolar epithelial cells, fibroblasts, extracellular matrix

INTRODUCTION

Idiopathic pulmonary fibrosis (IPF) is a chronic and progressive interstitial lung disease of unknown etiology and with a poor prognosis. IPF primarily occurs in middle-aged and elderly adults. In the United States, median age of newly diagnosed patients is 62 years, and 54% of them are male (Mortimer et al., 2020). The epidemiological survey of IPF shows that the global incidence and prevalence of IPF are in the range of 0.09 and 1.30 per 10,000 people and increasing year by year. Compared with other countries studied, the United States, South Korea and Canada have the highest incidence (Schafer et al., 2020; Maher et al., 2021a). Histopathological characteristics of IPF include excessive deposition of the extracellular matrix (ECM), leading to distortion of normal lung architecture and irreversible loss of lung function (Glass et al., 2020). IPF is clinically manifested by progressive dyspnea and a significant decrease in lung compliance (Schafer et al., 2020). In the past decade, significant progress has been made on our understanding of the mechanisms underlying this disease. The development of IPF is thought to be associated with both genetic and environmental factors. It is proposed that repetitive micro-injuries to alveolar epithelial cells trigger abnormal epithelial-fibroblast communication, which eventually results in abnormal ECM accumulation and pathological lung remodeling (Heukels et al., 2019; Martinez et al., 2017; Richeldi et al., 2017).

There is a growing portfolio of treatment options for IPF. Two drugs, nintedanib and pirfenidone, have been approved for treatment of patients with IPF. Nintedanib is a tyrosine kinase inhibitor, while pirfenidone is an oral pyridine that has anti-inflammatory, antioxidant, and anti-fibrotic effects. The two drugs have demonstrated reduction of lung function decline and slowing of disease progression, but they were also associated with some side effects and tolerability issues (Liu et al., 2017). Lung transplantation is the fundamental treatment for IPF. The average survival time of post-transplantation is 4–5 years. However, due to the restricted supply of donor organs and the limitation of chronic allograft rejection, only a few patients can receive this intervention (Kumar et al., 2018). Currently, IPF management is still aim to ameliorate symptoms, improve health status and preserve lung function (Glassberg, 2019). A better understanding of the pathogenesis of IPF will benefit the development of more efficient and safer therapies against IPF. This review will summarize recent advances in the pathogenesis of IPF (**Figure 1**) and highlight promising novel therapeutic strategies against the devastating fibrotic lung disease.

RISK FACTORS

Genetic

Genetic factors play an important role in the development of IPF (**Figure 1**). Genetic susceptibility of IPF includes single nucleotide polymorphisms (SNPs) and the resultant changes in gene expression. Familial interstitial pneumonia (FIP) is an autosomal dominant genetic disease with variable penetrance in which rare genetic variants have been identified (Kropski et al, 2015; Lorenzo-Salazar et al., 2019). These genetic variations involve the maintenance of telomere length (telomerase reverse transcriptase-TERT, telomerase RNA component-TERC, poly (A) -specific ribonuclease-PARN and regulator of telomere elongation helicase-RTEL) (Barros et al., 2019) and epithelial barrier function (desmoplakin-DSP, dipeptidyl peptidase 9-DPP9, AKAP13, CTNNA) (Allen et al., 2017; Fingerlin et al., 2013). Mutations in Toll-interacting protein (TOLLIP) (encoding an inhibitor of transforming growth factor-β (TGF-β) pathway and key regulator of Toll-like receptor-mediated innate immune responses) are associated with decreased expression of TLR mRNA and increased susceptibility to lung infections (Barros et al., 2019).

The genome-wide association studies (GWAS) found that a SNP (rs35705950) in the promoter region of mucin 5B (MUC5B) greatly increases the risk of IPF (Moore et al., 2019). MUC5B contributes to airway mucus production and plays an important role in innate immunity of lungs. Overexpression of MUC5B is related to impaired mucociliary clearance (MCC) and the degree and duration of fibrosis (Hancock et al., 2018; Zhang Q et al., 2019). The rs35705950 minor allele mutation can lead to overexpression of mucin 5B in small airway epithelial cells, and DNA methylation is closely related to genetic susceptibility of MUC5B (Zhang Q et al., 2019). In addition, a study identified a positive feedback bistable ERN2-XBP1S pathway upregulated MUC5B mRNAs in IPF and further regulated mucus secretion, providing an unfolded protein response (UPR)-dependent mechanism with rs35705950 variant (Chen G et al., 2019).

Environmental

Environmental exposure and genetic predisposition may have a synergistic effect in the development of IPF (**Figure 1**). In both sporadic and familial pulmonary fibrosis, environmental exposures to lung epithelium can increase the risk of IPF. Of them, smoking and metal dust are the strongest risk factors (Kc et al., 2018; Pardo and Selman, 2020). Cigarette smoke can cause a variety of cellular changes through epigenetic mechanisms. It also induces miRNA imbalance and ER stress, promoting spontaneous lung injury and differentiation from fibroblast to myofibroblast (Mascaux et al., 2009; Song et al., 2019). Pollutants and ultrafine particles in cigarette smoke contain carbon black (CB) and cadmium (Cd). The content of Cd and CB in IPF lung tissue increased significantly and was directly proportional to the amounts of citrullinated vimentin (Cit-Vim). Under activation of Akt1 and peptidylarginine deiminase 2 (PAD2), Cd/CB can induce Vim citrullination and Cit-Vim secretion, which in turn triggers fibroblasts to infiltrate lung microspheres, promotes increased expression of collagen and α-smooth muscle actin (α-SMA), and induces lung fibrosis (Li et al., 2021).

Microorganisms (viruses, fungi and bacteria) play a potential role in the pathogenesis of IPF (Lipinski et al., 2020). Compared with normal people, IPF patients have an imbalance in the composition of the lung microbiota, which can serve as a persistent stimuli for repetitive alveolar injury (Molyneaux et al., 2017). The inflammatory and fibrotic mediators and immune disorders in the lungs of IPF patients are related to bacterial load. In animal models of pulmonary fibrosis, pulmonary dysbiosis precedes the peak of lung injury and persists throughout the period of fibrosis. After adjusting the relevant clinical and physiological variables, lung bacterial burden can predict disease progression of IPF patients (O'Dwyer et al., 2019). In addition, Epstein-Barr virus (EBV), cytomegalovirus (CMV) and human herpes virus are detected in alveolar epithelial cells of patients with IPF, suggesting a link between viral infection and increased risk of IPF. Although the mechanisms by which viral infection is associated with IPF remains unclear, studies suggest that it may be related to activation of epithelial-mesenchymal transition, promotion of TGF-β expression, and induction of epigenetic reprogramming (Li et al., 2018; Sides et al., 2011). Interestingly, IPF patients expressing MUC5B risk alleles have a significantly lower bacterial burden compared with the patients who do not bear the risk allele (Molyneaux et al., 2014). NEDD4-2 modulates epithelial Na^+ channel (ENaC) through ubiquitination, which is essential for proper mucociliary clearance of inhaled irritants and pathogens. Recent study has shown that expression of NEDD4-2 is reduced in IPF lung tissue. NEDD4-2 promotes fibrosis remodeling through regulating the expression of proSP-C, Smad2/3 and TGF-β signaling pathway (Duerr et al., 2020).

Aging

Aging is a pathological feature of both human IPF and experimental lung fibrosis in animals. The major characteristics of aging lungs include telomere mutations, epigenetic changes, loss of protein homeostasis, mitochondrial dysfunction, and cellular senescence (**Figure 1**). Telomere mutations often result in abnormal DNA repair and genome instability, which serves as a trigger for cell senescence (Lopez-Otin et al., 2013; Barros et al., 2019). In addition to DNA damage, telomere shortening or damage may also promote fibrosis by impairing tissue repair function, activating p53, reducing mitochondrial biosynthesis, and triggering cellular senescence pathways (Sui et al., 2016; Pineiro-Hermida et al., 2020). There is evidence that in IPF, most of the changes related to aging, including shortening of telomeres which mainly occurs in Alveolar epithelial type II cells (AT2) (Selman et al., 2019). F-box and WD repeat domain-containing protein 7 (FBW7) is identified as a driver of pulmonary premature senescence and fibrosis. It is an E3 ubiquitin ligase that facilitates telomere protective protein 1 (TPP1) multisite polyubiquitination and accelerates degradation through binding to TPP1, thereby triggering telomere uncapping, cause cell senescence and tissue fibrosis (Wang L et al., 2020). Studies have shown that expression of core senescence-related markers is significantly elevated in IPF AT2 cells. These markers include CDKN1A/p21, CDKN2A/p16, TP53, MDM2, CCND1 (Barnes et al., 2019; Liu B et al., 2019). In addition, aging may cause dysfunction of stem/progenitor cell renewal, rendering alveolar epithelial cells incapable of repairing and regenerating injured lungs. Aging epithelial cells can produce a variety of pro-inflammatory and pro-fibrotic mediators, such as Interleukin 6 (IL-6), IL-1 and TGF-β, which are part of the senescence-associated secretory phenotype (SASP) (Merkt et al., 2020). In contrast, aging fibroblasts have stronger anti-apoptotic ability to resist environmental stress and can increase extracellular matrix components (Mora et al., 2017; Moore et al., 2019). Metabolic changes, such as glycolytic reprogramming, also play an important role in the pathogenesis of pulmonary fibrosis. Human metabolomics studies have shown that IPF lung tissues displayed increased glycolysis compared with healthy controls (Zhao et al., 2017). Specifically, aging fibroblasts increase glucose utilization and increase resistance to apoptosis (Cho et al., 2017; Selvarajah et al., 2019; Cho and Stout-Delgado, 2020). Studies have suggested that plasminogen activator inhibitor 1 (PAI-1) can protect (myo) fibroblasts from apoptosis in old mice. PAI-1 is the effector molecule of TGF-β, which can induce senescence by inducing p21 (Huang et al., 2015). Aged mice develop nonresolving pulmonary fibrosis following lung injury. Intriguingly, p53 signaling is abnormally activated in aging AT2, and silencing the expression of p53 can inhibit the development of progressive fibrosis (Borok et al., 2020; Yao et al., 2020). Changfu Y et al. determined that senescence rather than AT2 cell depletion is the key link in promoting progressive fibrosis, so genetic intervention for p53 activation and senescence will become a therapeutic target for pulmonary fibrosis in the future (Yao et al., 2020). These findings suggest that targeting aged cells may be effective for the treatment of fibrotic lung disease.

Epigenetic Reprogramming

Increasing evidence demonstrated that under the influence of environmental factors and aging, epigenetic changes play an important role in IPF (Kadel et al., 2019; Yamada, 2020; Yang and Schwartz, 2015). Epigenetic modifications include DNA methylation, histone modifications, and changes in the expression of non-coding RNA (especially microRNA) (Chen et al., 2017). When individuals are exposed to environmental stresses, such as smoke and dust, air pollution can cause epigenetic changes. It has been shown that silica exposure increases expression of DNA methyltransferase 1 (DNMT1) in patients with IPF, leading to the accumulation of collagen and lung fibrosis (Zhang N et al., 2019).

Genome-wide methylation analysis has shown that there are 2130 differentially methylated regions (DMR) in IPF lungs compared with healthy lungs (Yang et al., 2014). Methylation in these DMRs may regulate expression of multiple target genes and miRNAs involved in the development of IPF (Luo et al., 2020). Changes in DNA methylation correspond to altered mRNA expression of a variety of genes, some of which, such as apoptosis regulation and biosynthesis processes, have known roles in IPF (Cisneros et al., 2012; Rabinovich et al., 2012; Sanders et al., 2012). Regulation of DNA methylation has been demonstrated as a key pathogenetic pathway in TGF-β-induced lung fibrosis, through reduction of prostaglandin E2 (PGE2) and stimulation of epithelial-mesenchymal transition (Hu et al., 2010; Huan et al., 2015). Li et al. confirmed that MBD2 is highly expressed in macrophages in fibrotic lung. MBD2 is a member of the methyl-CpG-binding domain (MBD) proteins family. It directly binds to methylated CpG DNA to regulate PI3K/Akt signaling, thereby enhancing macrophage M2 program and promoting TGF-β signaling (Wang et al., 2021). In addition, HMG AT-hook 2 protein (HMGA2), a member of high-mobility group (HMG) proteins family, can regulate the transcription of its target genes by changing the chromatin structure at the promoter and/or enhancers, which can mediate transformation TGF-β1 signaling. Recent studies have found that inhibiting HMGA2-FACT-ATM-pH2A.*X* axis of human lung fibroblasts *in vitro* could reduce fibrotic hallmarks (Dobersch et al., 2021).

Studies of histone modifications of IPF lungs found that when treated with histone modification-related drugs (TSA, SpA, etc.), the level of surfactant protein C (Sp-C), the activation and proliferation of fibroblasts are all significantly affected. Additionally, histone modifications can also affect the anti-apoptotic ability of fibroblasts by inhibiting anti-fibrotic genes such as FAS and caveolin 1 (Cav-1) (Bartczak et al., 2020). Ligresti,G et al. identified that histone methyltransferase G9a/chromobox homolog 5 (CBX5)/methylated lysine 9 residue on histone 3 (H3K9me) were key regulators of fibroblast activation, and determined that by participating in the CBX5/G9a pathway, TGFβ and increased matrix stiffness effectively inhibited PGC1α expression in lung fibroblasts (Ligresti et al., 2019).

miRNA microarray analysis showed that expression of miR-21 and miR-199a-5p was increased in IPF lungs, while expression of miR-31, let-7 and miR-200 was decreased (Yang et al., 2015). Among them, miR-21 can induce epithelial-mesenchymal transition (EMT) by inhibiting Smad7 and promote TGF-β-induced fibrosis (Liu et al., 2010), while Let7 may participate in fibrotic process by targeting HMGA2 (Chirshev et al., 2019). The miR-200 family promote AT2s to restore its ability to transdifferentiate into Alveolar epithelial type I cells (AT1)

(Moimas et al., 2019). The presence of miR-145 can activate TGF-β to induce fibrosis, and it can also induce expression of α-smooth muscle actin (α-SMA), which is a hallmark of fibroblast to myofibroblast differentiation (Yang et al., 2013). MiR-424 targets Smurf2 (TGF-β pathway inhibitor) to promote fibroblast differentiation and promote TGF-β secretion (Xiao et al., 2015). MiR-301a can regulate fibroblast activation induced by TGF-β and IL-6 (Wang J et al., 2020). miR-29 is a main negative regulator of ECM production. Further studies have found that IPF ECM inhibited miR-29 expression upstream at the transcriptional level, and suppressed Dicer1 downstream at the processing steps to maintain the fibrosis progression (Herrera et al., 2018).

CELLS AND REGULATORS

Epithelial Cells Damage

Currently, the prominent initiation of IPF is widely considered to be repeated lung epithelial cell damage and repair dysfunction. Under normal circumstances, the damage of alveolar epithelial cells will lead to recruitment of inflammatory cells, fibrosis and matrix deposition in order to repair the damaged cells. This stage is temporary and then normal pulmonary homeostasis will be restored through activation of apoptotic pathways and phagocytosis of macrophages during the injury repair stage (Desmouliere et al., 1995). However, in IPF lungs, mutations of lung epithelial restriction genes (SFTPC, SFTPA2 and ABCA3) and abnormal expression of genes such as MUC5B cause lung epithelial mucosal barrier dysfunction (Hancock et al., 2018). Repeated stimulation of microorganisms, smoking, gastroesophageal reflux and other factors destroys the integrity of the lung epithelium. In addition, inflammation, excessive production of reactive oxygen species (ROS) and endoplasmic reticulum stress (ERS) in IPF lungs lead to repetitive damage to epithelial cells (Ornatowski et al., 2020).

In the past decades, there has been numerous works to determine the central role of stem cells in epithelial repair, including AT2s and its subsets, basal cells, bronchoalveolar alveolar stem cells (BASC) (Frank et al., 2016; Hewlett et al., 2018). Studies have identified a subset of fibroblasts expressing PDGFRα$^+$ or Lgr5$^+$ can participate in alveolar homeostasis by stimulating Wnt signaling (Axin2+) located in the alveolar compartment. These subset of fibroblasts are involved in promotion of alveolar growth and maturation, and preferentially differentiate into myofibroblasts after lung epithelial injury (Lee et al., 2017; Zepp et al., 2017).

Lung Stem Cells Dysfunction and Exhaustion

In IPF, genetic and environmental factors may cause damage to AT1s, while dysfunction of AT2s makes it difficult to repair the damaged AT1s. AT2s, serve as the predominant epithelial progenitor in alveoli, play an important role in maintaining lung homeostasis (Parimon et al., 2020). Abnormal function of alveolar epithelial cells is associated with activation of signal pathways such as Wnt/β-catenin and Sonic Hedgehog (Stewart et al., 2003; Nabhan et al., 2018; Reyfman et al., 2019). Recent study identified a rare subset of mature AT2 cells with stem cell propertie marked by continuous expression of the Wnt target gene Axin2. Canonical Wnt signaling pathway blocks reprogramming of alveolar stem cells into AT1 cells. When injury occurs in epithelial cells, Wnt signaling pathway is activated and participates in " ancillary" AT2 stem cell progenitor cell activity (Nabhan et al., 2018). Wnt-reactive alveolar epithelial progenitor cells (AEP) in AT2 are a stable lineage during alveolar homeostasis, but rapidly expand to regenerate most of the alveolar epithelium after acute lung injury, showing stronger "stemness". AEPs have a unique transcriptome, epigenome and functional phenotype, and specifically respond to Wnt and Fgf signaling (Zacharias et al., 2018). It has been believed that repetitive micro-injuries are a potential cause of AT2 depletion. However, the reduction of AT2 number in IPF lung supports the idea of stem cell exhaustion. In addition, aging, ERS and mitochondrial dysfunction play an important role in AT2 depletion and impaired self-renewal (Kropski and Blackwell, 2018; Borok et al., 2020; Parimon et al., 2020). Loss of Cdc42 in AT2s results in impaired differentiation, exposing alveolar cells to sustained elevated mechanical tension which activates a TGF-β signaling loop in AT2 cells in a spatially regulated manner, thereby promoting lung fibrosis progression from periphery to center (Wu et al., 2020).

Fibroblasts and Myofibroblasts

In IPF, pro-fibrotic mediators secreted by activated fibroblasts continue to act on fibroblasts to form a positive feedback, which leads to production of ECM and myofibroblast differentiation (Wipff et al., 2007). TGF-β is considered to be the primary factor that promotes fibroblast differentiation into myofibroblasts (Huang et al., 2020). Myofibroblasts secrete more ECM than fibroblasts. They are the main collagen-producing cells in the lung and are characterized by expression of contractile protein α-SMA and fibroblast activation protein (FAP) (Tsukui et al., 2020). FAP is a membrane-spanning protein that is essential for collagen remodeling. As FAP exhibits a low expression state in most healthy cells, it can be used as a molecular marker to exploit for specifically target drugs to fibroblasts that cause fibrosis (Hettiarachchi et al., 2020).

In the normal wound healing process, unwanted fibroblasts are eliminated by activating the apoptotic pathway. The elimination mechanism of fibroblasts limits the ongoing matrix deposition and fibrosis (Desmouliere et al., 1995). In IPF, myofibroblasts were found to resist FAS ligand-induced apoptosis and have stronger proliferation ability when grown on polymerized collagen (Xia et al., 2008; Nho et al., 2011). FasL, Tumor necrosis factor (TNF)-related apoptosis-inducing ligand (TRAIL) and Cav-1 protein expression in these cells decreased, while AKT activity increased (Hohmann et al., 2019). In addition, myofibroblast contraction is irreversible, which contribute to regulate the remodeling of collagen, trigger the spatial structural reorganization of collagen fibrils, increase their mechanical stress, and stiffen the ECM (Zhou et al., 2020). Periostin is highly expressed in IPF lungs. Further studies have found that in lung fibroblasts, periostin/integrin αVβ3 can promote expression of cell cycle-related molecules, including cyclins, cyclin-dependent kinases (CDKs) and E2F families, and transcription factors (such as B-MYB and FOXM1), which play a vital role in the proliferation of lung fibroblasts (Yoshihara et al., 2020).

Basal Cells

An important feature of epithelial cell remodeling in IPF is the expansion of distal basal cells, which can serve as stem/progenitor cells of the pseudostratified epithelium of the lung. In the cellular area of IPF, secretory sensitized basal cells (SPB) are enriched, and the formation and secretion function of its subpopulations are regulated by Notch signal. Specifically, NOTCH2 restricts the differentiation of basal cells, while NOTCH3 can inhibit secretory differentiation (Carraro et al., 2020). In addition, RNA-seq analysis for IPF indicates that expression of LncRNA MEG3 in basal cells increased. MEG3 plays a role in abnormal epithelial cell differentiation in IPF and regulates epithelial cell migration related genes including TP63, STAT3, KRT14, YAP1 and AXL, which together contribute to the restructuring of IPF (Gokey et al., 2018). Milena S et al. confirmed that MMP9 expressed by airway base cells (ABC) in IPF was significantly increased and regulated by TGF-β pathway. When targeting MMP9, the anti-fibrotic effect is related to the reduction of TGF-β activation in a subgroup of IPF patients, which reveals an association with expression of type 1 IFN in ABC-like cells (Espindola et al., 2021).

Growth Factors

There is overwhelming evidence in support of a key role of TGF-β in the pathogenesis of IPF (Huang et al., 2020). TGF-β promotes epithelial-mesenchymal transition, epithelial cell migration, fibroblast proliferation, activation, and differentiation into myofibroblasts (**Figure 1**). TGF-β can also increase the production of other fibrotic mediators and pro-angiogenic mediators (Grimminger et al., 2015; Song et al., 2020). TGF-β is synthesized as a latent complex by binding to the latency-related peptide (LAP), which covalently binds to the ECM protein (Biernacka et al., 2011). Latent TGF-β can be activated by a range of factors, including αvβ6 integrin (John et al., 2020). In IPF, expression of αvβ6 in alveolar epithelial cells is increased, which binds to LAP to induce TGF-β activation (Jenkins et al., 2006). Once activated, TGF-β binds to its receptors and stimulates phosphorylation of transcription factor Smad3. Phospho-Smad3 interacts with Smad4 to form a complex which translocates into the nucleus to induce expression of target genes, including profibrotic genes such as α-SMA, CTGF and ECM major collagen 1A1 (COL1A1) (Biernacka et al., 2011; Massague, 2012). Interestingly, the expression of negative-regulating factor tripartite motif 33 (TRIM33) of TGF-β/SMAD in IPF increased. TRIM33 is an E3 ubiquitin ligase, which can promote SMAD4 ubiquitination and induce SMAD4 to export from the nucleus, thereby inhibiting transcriptional activity of SMADs. However, the combination of TRIM33 and small heat shock protein (HSPBS) weakened its inhibitory activity. The upregulation of TRIM33 may be regarded as a failed attempt to prevent the progression of fibrosis in IPF and lung fibrosis models (Boutanquoi et al., 2020).

CTGF, also known as cellular communication network factor 2 (CCN2), is an important mediator of organ fibrosis in human body (Falke et al., 2020; Wang et al., 2019). It is considered to be a predictor of pulmonary fibrosis disease and a potential target for anti-fibrosis therapy (Leask, 2011). CTGF is secreted and activated under stimulation of TGF-β. CTGF mediates lung matrix deposition and fibroblast differentiation by activating downstream MAP kinase pathway (Duncan et al., 1999; Inui et al., 2021). In addition, CXCL12 can also induce the expression of CTGF in human lung fibroblasts by activating the MEKK1/JNK signaling pathway (Lin et al., 2018). Studies have found that gene promoter of CTGF contains numerous transcription factor binding sites such as NF-κB, signal transducer and activator of transcription (STAT), activator protein-1 (AP-1) and SMAD (Lin et al., 2018), indicating these factors may affect IPF through CTGF.

PDGF is widely expressed in macrophages, platelets, endothelial cells and fibroblasts (Hewlett et al., 2018). Highly expressed PDGF can be detected in BALF of IPF patients and bleomycin-induced IPF model mice (Phan et al., 2021). The abnormal expression and signal transduction of PDGF ligands and receptors have been confirmed to be closely related to IPF. In IPF, TGF-β signaling promotes expression of PDGF-B through regulatory T cells (Tregs), thereby stimulating PDGF-B-mediated fibroblast proliferation and migration (Kanaan and Strange, 2017; Kishi et al., 2018).

Insulin-like growth factor (IGF1) is a key molecule that regulates cellular senescence (Duran-Ortiz et al., 2021). As mentioned above, senescence has been identified as an important reason for the weakened repair function of AT2s in IPF. Under pathological conditions, ATs release IGF1, which activates the surface of adjacent normal ATs. IGF receptor (IGFR-1), and further activate the PI3K/AKT signaling pathway, and participate in ATs senescence and IPF by releasing CTGF, TGF-β1 and MMP9 (Sun et al., 2021).

MOLECULAR MECHANISMS

Extracellular Matrix Deposition

The massive deposition of extracellular matrix in IPF is mainly involved in changes in two families of proteins: MMPs and tissue inhibitors of metalloproteinases (TIMPs) (**Figure 1**). Studies have found that expression levels and localization of MMP and TIMP in IPF lungs undergo substantial changes. The levels of MMP1, MMP2, MMP9 and the four TIMPs are up-regulated. Among them, MMP1 is more common in alveolar macrophages and epithelial cells, while TIMP is highly expressed by myofibroblasts in IPF fibroblastic foci (Betensley et al., 2016). The extracellular matrix of IPF can also change transcriptional profile of lung fibroblasts and affect the translation of ECM proteins, such as COL1A1, COL1A2, COL3A1, COL5A2, COL4A2, MMP2, MMP3, MMP10 and TIMP2 (Zolak and de Andrade, 2012). Together, these findings suggest that there is a positive feedback pathway between fibroblasts and abnormal ECM, in which the fibrotic extracellular matrix is both the cause and the result of fibroblast activation (Guiot et al., 2017).

Matrix Stiffness and Scaffolding

Matrix stiffening is a prominent feature of lung fibrosis. Compared with healthy lung scaffolds, IPF scaffolds increase tissue stiffness, density, ultimate force, and differential expressions of matrisome proteins (**Figure 1**). The collagen, proteoglycan and ECM glycoprotein in the IPF scaffold increased, but specific basement membrane (BM) proteins (such as laminins and collagen IV) were decreased, while nidogen-2 was increased, accompanied by periostin and proteoglycans production were increased (Elowsson Rendin et al., 2019). The increased stiffness of ECM tissue is a result of dysregulated collagen cross-linking, which is related to post-translational modification of collagen involved in lysyl oxidase-like (LOXL) 2 and LOXL3 (Jones et al., 2018). ECM stiffness participates in the pathogenesis of IPF. Accumulating evidence indicates that mechanical interactions between fibroblasts and the stiffened ECM provide a feedforward mechanism that sustains and/or perpetuates pulmonary fibrosis (Zhou et al., 2013).

In previous study, we demonstrated that matrix stiffness regulates the ability of fibrotic lung myofibroblasts to invade the BM, by increasing α6-expression, mediating MMP-2-dependent pericellular proteolysis of BM collagen IV. Genetic ablation of α6 in collagen-expressing mesenchymal cells or pharmacological blockade of matrix stiffness-regulated α6-expression protects mice against bleomycin injury-induced experimental lung fibrosis. Studies found that a mechanotransduction pathway involving Rho/Rho kinase (Rho/ROCK), actin cytoskeletal remodeling, and a mechanosensitive transcription factor, megakaryoblastic leukemia 1 (MKL1), that coordinately regulate myofibroblast differentiation, and pharmacologic disruption of this pathway with the ROCK inhibitor fasudil induced myofibroblast apoptosis through a mechanism involving downregulation of BCL-2 and activation of the intrinsic mitochondrial apoptotic pathway (Zhou et al., 2013). Recently, we have shown that mouse double minute 4 homolog (MDM4) is a matrix stiffness-regulated endogenous inhibitor of p53. MDM4 is highly expressed in the fibrotic lesions of human IPF and experimental pulmonary fibrosis in aged mice. Our studies provides evidence that mechanosensitive MDM4 is a molecular target with promising therapeutic potential against persistent lung fibrosis associated with aging (Qu et al., 2021). Moreover, ECM stiffness is sensitive to exogenous TGF-β stimulation through inhibiting the interaction of inner nuclear membrane protein LEM domain-containing protein 3 (LEMD3) and SMAD2/3. LEMD3 is physically connected to the actin cytoskeleton of cells and inhibits TGF-β signaling (Chambers et al., 2018). At the metabolic level, increased matrix stiffness impairs the synthesis of anti-fibrotic lipid mediator PGE2 and reduces expression of rate-limiting prostaglandin biosynthetic enzyme cyclooxygenase 2 (COX-2) and prostaglandin E synthesis (PTGES) through p38/MAPK signaling pathway (Berhan et al., 2020). Genome-wide association studies (GWASs) have identified DSP (desmoplakin) gene, a type of intercellular junction responsible for maintaining the structural integrity and mechanical stability of the epithelium, as a significant locus associated with IPF (Fingerlin et al., 2013; Mathai et al., 2016; Allen et al., 2017; Tasha E). Our studies demonstrated that matrix stiffness regulates DSP gene expression by an epigenetic mechanism involving alteration of DNA methylation in the DSP promoter. Targeted DNA methylation by CRISPR (clustered regularly interspaced short palindrom2076295ic repeats)/dCas9 (deactivated CRISPR-associated protein-9 nuclease)-mediated epigenome editing effectively reverses stiff matrix-induced DSP overexpression (Qu et al., 2018). We speculate that aberrant DSP expression in IPF may not only represent a robust and persistent epithelial response to chronic/repetitive lung injury but also actively participate in aberrant lung repair and/or the restoration of lung epithelial function (Qu et al., 2018). In addition, studies have identified that rs2076295 (an intron variant in DSP gene) was related to IPF susceptibility and directly regulated DSP expression in human airway epithelial cells. Deletion of DSP enhances expression of extracellular matrix-related genes such as matrix metalloproteinases 7 (MMP7) and MMP9 and promotes cell migration (Hao et al., 2020). For IPF patients with DSP alleles and MUC5B alleles, the mortality rate is lower, and anti-fibrosis drugs are more effective in treatment (Doubkova et al., 2021). These studies indicate that targeting mechanosensitive signaling in myofibroblasts may be an effective approach for treatment of fibrotic disorders.

Endoplasmic Reticulum Stress

Endoplasmic reticulum stress (ERS) occurs when there is an imbalance between cell's demand for protein synthesis and the ability of endoplasmic reticulum to synthesize, process, and package proteins. As ERS occurs, cells activate an UPR, which attempts to restore normal function of the endoplasmic reticulum. When ERS is persisting or severe, it triggers cell apoptosis (Kropski and Blackwell, 2018; Hipp et al., 2019). It has been observed that markers of UPR activation in AT2 in IPF patients are elevated (Kropski and Blackwell, 2018; Baek et al., 2020). ERS may synergize with inflammation and viral infection to induce epithelial cell damage (Chen T et al., 2019). In IPF, UPR stimulates the production of fibrotic mediators, such as TGF-β, PDGF (platelet-derived growth factor), CXCL12 (CXC chemokine 12), CCL2 (chemokine CC ligand 2) (Wolters et al., 2014; Kropski and Blackwell, 2018). The chaperone protein GRP78 (glucose regulatory protein 78) is the main regulator of ER homeostasis and suppresses UPR by interacting with transmembrane ER stress sensors. It is found that the expression of GRP78 in AT2 cells from old mice and IPF lungs decreased, while GRP78 knocked out will induce ERS, apoptosis and lung inflammation to promote fibrosis (Borok et al., 2020). Otherwise, thioredoxin domain containing 5 (TXNDC5), an ER protein enriched in fibroblasts, is highly up-regulated in fibroblasts from IPF lung/BLM-induced mouse and enhances TGF-β signaling by increasing and stabilizing TGF-beta receptor 1 (TGFBR1), while TGF-β promotes TXNDC5 expression via ATF6 ER stress pathway, forming a positive feedback loop (Lee et al., 2020). Mutations in the genes encoding surfactant proteins [surfactant protein C (SFTPC)

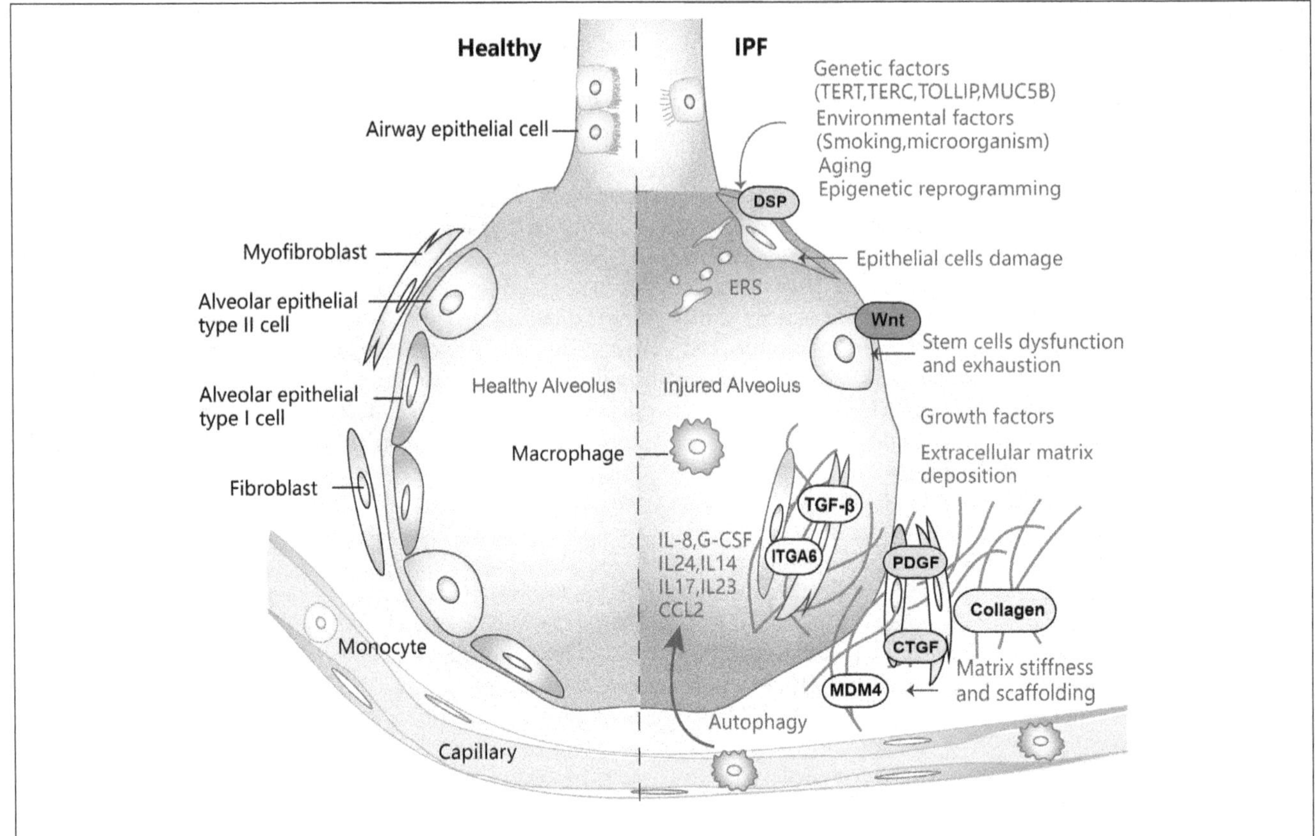

FIGURE 1 | Pathogenesis of idiopathic pulmonary fibrosis. Genetic factors affect the integrity of epithelial cells, environmental factors and aging-related changes will trigger epigenetic reprogramming. The combined action of the three factors will cause epithelial cell damage and trigger the abnormal activation of epithelial cells. Activated epithelial cells secretes a large number of cytokines such as TGF-β which consequently promotes fibroblast migration and proliferation, and also promote fibroblasts to differentiate into myofibroblasts. Myofibroblasts secrete large amounts of ECM, leading to ECM deposition. In addition, epithelial cell damage, disfunction and exhaustion of stem cells, abnormal deposition of extracellular matrix and matrix stiffness play a vital role in progression of abnormal lung fibrosis and remodeling of lung structure.

and A2 (SFTPA2)] can lead to abnormal surfactant folding and ERS, and promote epithelial-mesenchymal transition (Mulugeta et al., 2015; Takezaki et al., 2019).

Inflammation and Immunity

The role of inflammation in the development of IPF remains controversial. In the early stage of alveolar injury, neutrophils are recruited into the injured sites, triggering an immune response by releasing pro-inflammatory cytokines and producing neutrophil elastase (NE) to exacerbate fibrosis (Le Saux and Chapman, 2018). Elevated IL-8 and G-CSF have been found in the bronchoalveolar lavage fluid (BALF) and sputum of IPF patients, suggestive of infiltration and activation of neutrophils (**Figure 1**). IL-8 promotes the development of fibrosis through elastase-mediated activation of TGF-β (Betensley et al., 2016; Guiot et al., 2017; Heukels et al., 2019). IL-24 and IL-4 can synergistically induce M2 program of macrophages, thereby promoting the development of lung fibrosis (Rao et al., 2021). IL17 secreted by Th17 cells can directly promote fibrosis. In acute exacerbation of pulmonary fibrosis, the levels of IL17 and IL23 are increased, and treatment with interleukin-23 antibody can significantly attenuate airway inflammation and fibrosis and reduce IL17 level, suggesting IL23 is essential for the development of acute exacerbation of pulmonary fibrosis (Senoo et al., 2021). Monocyte and macrophages drive fibrosis through excessive repair responses to alveolar cell injury. Compared with normal lungs, the subpopulation of macrophages that highly express SPP1 and MERTK (SPP1hi) and NTN1 (laminin-like protein netrin-1) increased significantly in IPF lungs. The highly proliferated SPP1hi macrophages upregulate the expression of type 1 collagen and MMP2 and contribute to tissue repair and fibrosis (Morse et al., 2019). It has been reported that macrophage-derived NTN1 drive the development of fibrosis through a mechanism involving remodeled adrenergic nerves and their secretory product noradrenaline and α_1 adrenoreceptors (Gao et al., 2021). CCL2 and colony stimulating factor (M-CSF/CSF1) derived from monocytes/macrophages may have a direct fibrotic effect (Coward et al., 2010). Furthermore, recent studies have identified that immune cells in lung tissue predict the severity of IPF and participate in the progress of this disease,

TABLE 1 | Drugs used in the treatment of Idiopathic pulmonary fibrosis (IPF).

Drugs	Mechanism of action	References
Pirfenidone	Anti-fibrotic drug	Nathan et al. (2019)
Nintedanib	Anti-PDGFR, VEGFR, FGFR drug	Flaherty et al. (2019), Makino (2021)
Pamrevlumab	Anti-CTGF antibody	Richeldi et al. (2020)
GSK3008348	αvβ6 antagonist	John et al. (2020)
sildenafil	phosphodiesterase-5 inhibitor	Kang & Song, (2021)
Co-trimoxazole or doxycycline	Antimicrobial drug	Wilson et al. (2020)
Lebrikizumab	Anti-IL13	Maher et al. (2021b)
Carlumab	Anti-CCL2	Raghu et al. (2015)
Simtuzumab	Anti-LOX antibody	Raghu et al. (2017)

which can be used as a reference indicator (Wang Z et al., 2020).

Autophagy

Autophagic pathways (including macroautophagy and mitophagy) in IPF lung epithelial cells and fibroblasts are reduced, aggravating inflammation and fibrosis (Racanelli et al., 2018). Autophagy is involved in the regulation of ECM formation (Lin and Xu, 2020). Studies have shown that increasing autophagy clearance of type 1 collagen in lung fibroblasts can reduce invasiveness of IPF fibroblasts (Surolia et al., 2019). In addition, expression of the autophagy marker LC3B has been found to be significantly reduced in IPF lung fibroblasts (Ghavami et al., 2018). Specifically, the Akt signal pathway directly acts on FoxO3a to reduce its expression, further inhibiting production of autophagy marker LC3B on the collagen matrix, leading to excessive collagen accumulation (Im et al., 2015).

TREATMENTS

Recent research on pathogenesis of IPF has promoted notable advances in pharmacotherapeutic treatment. There are currently two recommended antifibrotic drugs, nintedanib and pirfenidone, have been shown to delay the progression of pulmonary fibrosis and reduce mortality, but there is still no cure for IPF (Cerri et al., 2019; Somogyi et al., 2019). Therefore, new treatment methods and drug targets are needed. Here we summarize some important novel drugs that have been tested in phase II-III trails (**Table 1**). The potential molecular targets of the drugs are also discussed. In addition, strategies of non-pharmacological treatment such as symptomatic support therapy, lung transplantation, comorbidities and management of acute exacerbation of IPF (AE-IPF) are believed to improve symptom control and quality of life (Caminati et al., 2019).

Pirfenidone

Pirfenidone (PFD) is a pharmacological compound for IPF treatment (Flaherty et al., 2019). PFD treatment can reduce all-cause mortality and risk of hospitalization, and benefit patients with advanced pulmonary fibrosis (Nathan et al., 2019). The mechanism of PFD treating IPF is currently unclear. PFD can inhibit TGF-β-mediated fibroblast proliferation and differentiation of fibroblasts into myofibroblasts by attenuating signal transduction induced by TGF- β1/Smad3 (Molina-Molina et al., 2018). In addition, PFD can also inhibit differentiation of myofibroblasts by regulating PDFG, a fibroblast mitogen receptor, but the specific mechanism is still unclear (Ruwanpura et al., 2020). Studies have found that PFD can resist the loss of E-cadherin, the main intermediary protein of A549 cell epithelial cell transformation induced by TGF-β, and pulmonary fibrosis in a rat model of silicosis, indicating that PFD can also inhibit epithelial cell transformation (Zhang Y et al., 2019). The oxidative stress process in lung diseases leads to irreversible oxidative modification of protein and DNA and mitochondrial dysfunction. PFD treatment can improve mitochondrial respiration, possibly by detoxifying mitochondrial peroxidase, such as glutathione peroxidase, thus revealing ability to maintain normal mitochondrial function (Plataki et al., 2019). Therefore, PFD's anti-fibrosis effect may function through reducing the formation of reactive oxygen species and oxidative stress.

Nintedanib

Nintedanib is a triple tyrosine kinase inhibitor with anti-fibrotic effects. In IPF treatment, Nintedanib can reduce the decline of forced vital capacity (FVC) and inhibit progression of pulmonary fibrosis (Flaherty et al., 2019; Makino, 2021). In previous clinical treatments, its safety and tolerability were acceptable. The most common adverse reaction is gastrointestinal infection, manifested as diarrhea and nausea (Bendstrup et al., 2019). Nintedanib can block activation of PDGF receptor, fibroblast growth factor receptor, vascular endothelial growth factor receptor and Src family kinases. Its anti-fibrosis effect is achieved through a variety of mechanisms, including blocking differentiation from fibroblasts into myofibroblasts, inhibiting EMT, inflammation and angiogenesis (Liu F et al., 2019).

Combination Therapies

As mentioned above, pulmonary fibrosis is a complex pathological progression in which pathogenic factors activate complex fibrotic pathways in various cells (Schafer et al., 2020). Therefore, combined treatment of multiple drugs with different targets and mechanisms involved in IPF is of great significance, but adverse effects and tolerance also need attention. It is currently proven that the combination therapy of pirfenidone and nintedanib has controllable safety and tolerability (Vancheri et al., 2018). Although this study has no efficacy evaluation, it still provides a significant research direction for combination therapy of pulmonary fibrosis.

In a recent clinical phase 2b trial, patients with advanced IPF and pulmonary hypertension were treated with pirfenidone plus sildenafil for up to 52 weeks. Unfortunately, there was no therapeutic effect. (Behr et al., 2021). Furthermore, the combination therapy of nintedanib and sildenafil only has pronounced effects on IPF patients who have right heart dysfunction (RHD) (Behr et al., 2019). Combination treatment with inhaled N-acetylcysteine and pirfenidone for 48 weeks may lead to a worse prognosis of IPF (Sakamoto et al., 2021). These clinical trials indicate that combination therapies for pulmonary fibrosis still need to be explored for a long time.

Novel Therapies

Due to adverse effects of currently drugs for IPF and there is no effective cure, IPF research is increasingly focused on developing new molecular targets and treatment options. As mentioned above, CTGF is an important pro-fibrotic growth factor associated with extracellular matrix secretion and abnormal tissue repair (Yanagihara et al., 2021). A recent phase II clinical trial has confirmed that treatment of pamrevlumab, which is a fully human recombinant monoclonal antibody against CTGF, can significantly reduce the decline of FVC and attenuate the progression of IPF. And importantly, it is shown that pamrevlumab has good safety and tolerability which is expected to become a new anti-fibrotic drug (Richeldi et al., 2020). In addition, αvβ6 integrin is the key molecule for activating TGF-β. A selective small molecule RGD-mimetic αvβ6 inhibitor GSK3008348, which can bind to αvβ6 with high affinity in human IPF lung epithelial cells, induces αvβ6 internalization and degradation, and inhibits activation of downstream TGF-β. In the bleomycin-induced mouse lung fibrosis model, significantly reduce lung collagen deposition and serum C3M (a marker of IPF disease progression). At present, inhaled GSK3008348 is safe and well tolerated in phase 1 clinical trials, which may be helpful for development of anti-fibrosis drugs in the future (John et al., 2020).

CONCLUSION AND OUTLOOK

Idiopathic pulmonary fibrosis is an interstitial pulmonary disease with high mortality. It is associated with a large economic and healthcare burden. Genetic and epigenetic changes are important factors in the pathogenesis of IPF, although the definite cause of IPF has yet to be clarified. Our understanding of the pathogenesis of IPF have significantly improved in the past decade. In the last few years, the research progress of idiopathic pulmonary fibrosis has highlighted the important role of stem cell dysfunction and extracellular matrix in mediating lung pathological remodeling and promoting the process of fibrosis (Deng et al., 2020; Wu et al., 2020). Unfortunately, IPF has a very small number of treatments and is still not curable. Nintedanib and pirfenidone can slow the progression of the disease. However, adverse reactions limit their use (Spagnolo et al., 2018). A better understanding of the pathogenesis of IPF and the signal pathways will benefit the development of more effective drug therapies. Gene editing technology provides a promising tool for developing novel treatments for human diseases. CRISPR-mediated genome and epigenome editing may prove to be effective means for correction of abnormal gene expression associated with IPF, thus representing an important direction in the future research. In addition, recent dynamic research activities in IPF pathogenesis have led to the foundation of some novel treatment strategies and identification of therapeutic targets. Several targeted drugs have been further synthesized and developed, and currently under clinical trials. Some of these drugs have been confirmed their effectiveness and safe tolerance. They are expected to become new IPF specific drugs to improve progression of IPF and other fibrosis diseases in the near future.

AUTHOR CONTRIBUTIONS

JQ and ZY guided the scope and research background of the research, and wrote the manuscript. QM wrote the original version of this manuscript. ZL and HZ critically revised the manuscript.

REFERENCES

Allen, R. J., Porte, J., Braybrooke, R., Flores, C., Fingerlin, T. E., Oldham, J. M., et al. (2017). Genetic Variants Associated with Susceptibility to Idiopathic Pulmonary Fibrosis in People of European Ancestry: a Genome-wide Association Study. *Lancet Respir. Med.* 5 (11), 869–880. doi:10.1016/S2213-2600(17)30387-9

Baek, A. R., Hong, J., Song, K. S., Jang, A. S., Kim, D. J., Chin, S. S., et al. (2020). Spermidine Attenuates Bleomycin-Induced Lung Fibrosis by Inducing Autophagy and Inhibiting Endoplasmic Reticulum Stress (ERS)-induced Cell Death in Mice. *Exp. Mol. Med.* 52 (12), 2034–2045. doi:10.1038/s12276-020-00545-z

Barnes, P. J., Baker, J., and Donnelly, L. E. (2019). Cellular Senescence as a Mechanism and Target in Chronic Lung Diseases. *Am. J. Respir. Crit. Care Med.* 200 (5), 556–564. doi:10.1164/rccm.201810-1975TR

Barros, A., Oldham, J., and Noth, I. (2019). Genetics of Idiopathic Pulmonary Fibrosis. *Am. J. Med. Sci.* 357 (5), 379–383. doi:10.1016/j.amjms.2019.02.009

Bartczak, K., Białas, A. J., Kotecki, M. J., Górski, P., and Piotrowski, W. J. (2020). More Than a Genetic Code: Epigenetics of Lung Fibrosis. *Mol. Diagn. Ther.* 24, 665–681. doi:10.1007/s40291-020-00490-7

Behr, J., Kolb, M., Song, J. W., Luppi, F., Schinzel, B., Stowasser, S., et al. (2019). Nintedanib and Sildenafil in Patients with Idiopathic Pulmonary Fibrosis and Right Heart Dysfunction. A Prespecified Subgroup Analysis of a Double-Blind Randomized Clinical Trial (INSTAGE). *Am. J. Respir. Crit. Care Med.* 200 (12), 1505–1512. doi:10.1164/rccm.201903-0488OC

Behr, J., Nathan, S. D., Wuyts, W. A., Mogulkoc Bishop, N., Bouros, D. E., Antoniou, K., et al. (2021). Efficacy and Safety of Sildenafil Added to Pirfenidone in Patients with Advanced Idiopathic Pulmonary Fibrosis and Risk of Pulmonary Hypertension: a Double-Blind, Randomised, Placebo-Controlled, Phase 2b Trial. *Lancet Respir. Med.* 9 (1), 85–95. doi:10.1016/S2213-2600(20)30356-8

Bendstrup, E., Wuyts, W., Alfaro, T., Chaudhuri, N., Cornelissen, R., Kreuter, M., et al. (2019). Nintedanib in Idiopathic Pulmonary Fibrosis: Practical Management Recommendations for Potential Adverse Events. *Respiration* 97 (2), 173–184. doi:10.1159/000495046

Berhan, A., Harris, T., Jaffar, J., Jativa, F., Langenbach, S., Lönnstedt, I., et al. (2020). Cellular Microenvironment Stiffness Regulates Eicosanoid Production and Signaling Pathways. *Am. J. Respir. Cell Mol Biol* 63, 819–830. doi:10.1165/rcmb.2020-0227OC

Betensley, A., Sharif, R., and Karamichos, D. (2016). A Systematic Review of the Role of Dysfunctional Wound Healing in the Pathogenesis and Treatment of Idiopathic Pulmonary Fibrosis. *J. Clin. Med.* 6 (1). doi:10.3390/jcm6010002

Biernacka, A., Dobaczewski, M., and Frangogiannis, N. G. (2011). TGF-β Signaling in Fibrosis. *Growth Factors* 29 (5), 196–202. doi:10.3109/08977194.2011.595714

Borok, Z., Horie, M., Flodby, P., Wang, H., Liu, Y., Ganesh, S., et al. (2020). Grp78 Loss in Epithelial Progenitors Reveals an Age-Linked Role for Endoplasmic Reticulum Stress in Pulmonary Fibrosis. *Am. J. Respir. Crit. Care Med.* 201 (2), 198–211. doi:10.1164/rccm.201902-0451OC

Boutanquoi, P. M., Burgy, O., Beltramo, G., Bellaye, P. S., Dondaine, L., Marcion, G., et al. (2020). TRIM33 Prevents Pulmonary Fibrosis by Impairing TGF-B1 Signalling. *Eur. Respir. J.* 55 (6). doi:10.1183/13993003.01346-2019

Caminati, A., Lonati, C., Cassandro, R., Elia, D., Pelosi, G., Torre, O., et al. (2019). Comorbidities in Idiopathic Pulmonary Fibrosis: an Underestimated Issue. *Eur. Respir. Rev.* 28 (153). doi:10.1183/16000617.0044-2019

Carraro, G., Mulay, A., Yao, C., Mizuno, T., Konda, B., Petrov, M., et al. (2020). Single-Cell Reconstruction of Human Basal Cell Diversity in Normal and Idiopathic Pulmonary Fibrosis Lungs. *Am. J. Respir. Crit. Care Med.* 202, 1540–1550. doi:10.1164/rccm.201904-0792OC

Cerri, S., Monari, M., Guerrieri, A., Donatelli, P., Bassi, I., Garuti, M., et al. (2019). Real-life Comparison of Pirfenidone and Nintedanib in Patients with Idiopathic Pulmonary Fibrosis: A 24-month Assessment. *Respir. Med.* 159, 105803. doi:10.1016/j.rmed.2019.105803

Chambers, D. M., Moretti, L., Zhang, J. J., Cooper, S. W., Chambers, D. M., Santangelo, P. J., et al. (2018). LEM Domain-Containing Protein 3 Antagonizes TGFβ-SMAD2/3 Signaling in a Stiffness-dependent Manner in Both the Nucleus and Cytosol. *J. Biol. Chem.* 293 (41), 15867–15886. doi:10.1074/jbc.RA118.003658

Chen, G., Ribeiro, C. M. P., Sun, L., Okuda, K., Kato, T., Gilmore, R. C., et al. (2019). XBP1S Regulates MUC5B in a Promoter Variant-dependent Pathway in Idiopathic Pulmonary Fibrosis Airway Epithelia. *Am. J. Respir. Crit. Care Med.* 200 (2), 220–234. doi:10.1164/rccm.201810-1972OC

Chen, T., Qiu, H., Zhao, M. M., Chen, S. S., Wu, Q., Zhou, N. Y., et al. (2019). IL-17A Contributes to HSV1 Infection-Induced Acute Lung Injury in a Mouse Model of Pulmonary Fibrosis. *J. Cell Mol Med* 23 (2), 908–919. doi:10.1111/jcmm.13992

Chen, Z., Li, S., Subramaniam, S., Shyy, J. Y., and Chien, S. (2017). Epigenetic Regulation: A New Frontier for Biomedical Engineers. *Annu. Rev. Biomed. Eng.* 19, 195–219. doi:10.1146/annurev-bioeng-071516-044720

Chirshev, E., Oberg, K. C., Ioffe, Y. J., and Unternaehrer, J. J. (2019). Let-7 as Biomarker, Prognostic Indicator, and Therapy for Precision Medicine in Cancer. *Clin. Transl Med.* 8 (1), 24. doi:10.1186/s40169-019-0240-y

Cho, S. J., Moon, J. S., Lee, C. M., Choi, A. M., and Stout-Delgado, H. W. (2017). Glucose Transporter 1-Dependent Glycolysis Is Increased during Aging-Related Lung Fibrosis, and Phloretin Inhibits Lung Fibrosis. *Am. J. Respir. Cell Mol Biol* 56 (4), 521–531. doi:10.1165/rcmb.2016-0225OC

Cho, S. J., and Stout-Delgado, H. W. (2020). Aging and Lung Disease. *Annu. Rev. Physiol.* 82, 433–459. doi:10.1146/annurev-physiol-021119-034610

Cisneros, J., Hagood, J., Checa, M., Ortiz-Quintero, B., Negreros, M., Herrera, I., et al. (2012). Hypermethylation-mediated Silencing of p14(ARF) in Fibroblasts from Idiopathic Pulmonary Fibrosis. *Am. J. Physiol. Lung Cell Mol Physiol* 303 (4), L295–L303. doi:10.1152/ajplung.00332.2011

Coward, W. R., Saini, G., and Jenkins, G. (2010). The Pathogenesis of Idiopathic Pulmonary Fibrosis. *Ther. Adv. Respir. Dis.* 4 (6), 367–388. doi:10.1177/1753465810379801

Deng, Z., Fear, M. W., Suk Choi, Y., Wood, F. M., Allahham, A., Mutsaers, S. E., et al. (2020). The Extracellular Matrix and Mechanotransduction in Pulmonary Fibrosis. *Int. J. Biochem. Cell Biol* 126, 105802. doi:10.1016/j.biocel.2020.105802

Desmoulière, A., Redard, M., Darby, I., and Gabbiani, G. (1995). Apoptosis Mediates the Decrease in Cellularity during the Transition between Granulation Tissue and Scar. *Am. J. Pathol.* 146 (1), 56–66.

Dobersch, S., Rubio, K., Singh, I., Günther, S., Graumann, J., Cordero, J., et al. (2021). Positioning of Nucleosomes Containing γ-H2AX Precedes Active DNA Demethylation and Transcription Initiation. *Nat. Commun.* 12 (1), 1072. doi:10.1038/s41467-021-21227-y

Doubkova, M., Kriegova, E., Littnerova, S., Schneiderova, P., Sterclova, M., Bartos, V., et al. (2021). DSP Rs2076295 Variants Influence Nintedanib and Pirfenidone Outcomes in Idiopathic Pulmonary Fibrosis: a Pilot Study. *Ther. Adv. Respir. Dis.* 15, 17534666211042529. doi:10.1177/17534666211042529

Duerr, J., Leitz, D. H. W., Szczygiel, M., Dvornikov, D., Fraumann, S. G., Kreutz, C., et al. (2020). Conditional Deletion of Nedd4-2 in Lung Epithelial Cells Causes Progressive Pulmonary Fibrosis in Adult Mice. *Nat. Commun.* 11 (1), 2012. doi:10.1038/s41467-020-15743-6

Duncan, M. R., Frazier, K. S., Abramson, S., Williams, S., Klapper, H., Huang, X., et al. (1999). Connective Tissue Growth Factor Mediates Transforming Growth Factor Beta-Induced Collagen Synthesis: Down-Regulation by cAMP. *FASEB J.* 13 (13), 1774–1786. doi:10.1096/fasebj.13.13.1774

Duran-Ortiz, S., List, E. O., Basu, R., and Kopchick, J. J. (2021). Extending Lifespan by Modulating the Growth Hormone/insulin-like Growth Factor-1 axis: Coming of Age. *Pituitary* 24 (3), 438–456. doi:10.1007/s11102-020-01117-0

Elowsson Rendin, L., Löfdahl, A., Åhrman, E., Müller, C., Notermans, T., Michaliková, B., et al. (2019). Matrisome Properties of Scaffolds Direct Fibroblasts in Idiopathic Pulmonary Fibrosis. *Int. J. Mol. Sci.* 20 (16). doi:10.3390/ijms20164013

Espindola, M. S., Habiel, D. M., Coelho, A. L., Stripp, B., Parks, W. C., Oldham, J., et al. (2021). Differential Responses to Targeting Matrix Metalloproteinase 9 in Idiopathic Pulmonary Fibrosis. *Am. J. Respir. Crit. Care Med.* 203 (4), 458–470. doi:10.1164/rccm.201910-1977OC

Falke, L. L., He, N., Chuva de Sousa Lopes, S. M., Broekhuizen, R., Lyons, K., Nguyen, T. Q., et al. (2020). Correction to: FoxD1-Driven CCN2 Deletion Causes Axial Skeletal Deformities, Pulmonary Hypoplasia, and Neonatal Asphyctic Death. *J. Cell Commun Signal* 14 (1), 47–52. doi:10.1007/s12079-020-00559-2

Fingerlin, T. E., Murphy, E., Zhang, W., Peljto, A. L., Brown, K. K., Steele, M. P., et al. (2013). Genome-wide Association Study Identifies Multiple Susceptibility Loci for Pulmonary Fibrosis. *Nat. Genet.* 45 (6), 613–620. doi:10.1038/ng.2609

Flaherty, K. R., Wells, A. U., Cottin, V., Devaraj, A., Walsh, S. L. F., Inoue, Y., et al. (2019). Nintedanib in Progressive Fibrosing Interstitial Lung Diseases. *N. Engl. J. Med.* 381 (18), 1718–1727. doi:10.1056/NEJMoa1908681

Frank, D. B., Peng, T., Zepp, J. A., Snitow, M., Vincent, T. L., Penkala, I. J., et al. (2016). Emergence of a Wave of Wnt Signaling that Regulates Lung Alveologenesis by Controlling Epithelial Self-Renewal and Differentiation. *Cell Rep* 17 (9), 2312–2325. doi:10.1016/j.celrep.2016.11.001

Gao, R., Peng, X., Perry, C., Sun, H., Ntokou, A., Ryu, C., et al. (2021). Macrophage-derived Netrin-1 Drives Adrenergic Nerve-Associated Lung Fibrosis. *J. Clin. Invest.* 131 (1). doi:10.1172/JCI136542

Ghavami, S., Yeganeh, B., Zeki, A. A., Shojaei, S., Kenyon, N. J., Ott, S., et al. (2018). Autophagy and the Unfolded Protein Response Promote Profibrotic Effects of TGF-B1 in Human Lung Fibroblasts. *Am. J. Physiol. Lung Cell Mol Physiol* 314 (3), L493–L504. doi:10.1152/ajplung.00372.2017

Glass, D. S., Grossfeld, D., Renna, H. A., Agarwala, P., Spiegler, P., Kasselman, L. J., et al. (2020). Idiopathic Pulmonary Fibrosis: Molecular Mechanisms and Potential Treatment Approaches. *Respir. Investig.* 58 (5), 320–335. doi:10.1016/j.resinv.2020.04.002

Glassberg, M. K. (2019). Overview of Idiopathic Pulmonary Fibrosis, Evidence-Based Guidelines, and Recent Developments in the Treatment Landscape. *Am. J. Manag. Care* 25 (11 Suppl. l), S195–S203.

Gokey, J. J., Snowball, J., Sridharan, A., Speth, J. P., Black, K. E., Hariri, L. P., et al. (2018). MEG3 Is Increased in Idiopathic Pulmonary Fibrosis and Regulates Epithelial Cell Differentiation. *JCI Insight* 3 (17). doi:10.1172/jci.insight.122490

Grimminger, F., Günther, A., and Vancheri, C. (2015). The Role of Tyrosine Kinases in the Pathogenesis of Idiopathic Pulmonary Fibrosis. *Eur. Respir. J.* 45 (5), 1426–1433. doi:10.1183/09031936.00149614

Guiot, J., Henket, M., Corhay, J. L., Moermans, C., and Louis, R. (2017). Sputum Biomarkers in IPF: Evidence for Raised Gene Expression and Protein Level of IGFBP-2, IL-8 and MMP-7. *PLoS One* 12 (2), e0171344. doi:10.1371/journal.pone.0171344

Hancock, L. A., Hennessy, C. E., Solomon, G. M., Dobrinskikh, E., Estrella, A., Hara, N., et al. (2018). Muc5b Overexpression Causes Mucociliary Dysfunction and Enhances Lung Fibrosis in Mice. *Nat. Commun.* 9 (1), 5363. doi:10.1038/s41467-018-07768-9

Hao, Y., Bates, S., Mou, H., Yun, J. H., Pham, B., Liu, J., et al. (2020). Genome-Wide Association Study: Functional Variant Rs2076295 Regulates Desmoplakin Expression in Airway Epithelial Cells. *Am. J. Respir. Crit. Care Med.* 202 (9), 1225–1236. doi:10.1164/rccm.201910-1958OC

Herrera, J., Beisang, D. J., Peterson, M., Forster, C., Gilbertsen, A., Benyumov, A., et al. (2018). Dicer1 Deficiency in the Idiopathic Pulmonary Fibrosis Fibroblastic Focus Promotes Fibrosis by Suppressing MicroRNA Biogenesis. *Am. J. Respir. Crit. Care Med.* 198 (4), 486–496. doi:10.1164/rccm.201709-1823OC

Hettiarachchi, S. U., Li, Y. H., Roy, J., Zhang, F., Puchulu-Campanella, E., Lindeman, S. D., et al. (2020). Targeted Inhibition of PI3 kinase/mTOR Specifically in Fibrotic Lung Fibroblasts Suppresses Pulmonary Fibrosis in Experimental Models. *Sci. Transl Med.* 12 (567). doi:10.1126/scitranslmed.aay3724

Heukels, P., Moor, C. C., von der Thüsen, J. H., Wijsenbeek, M. S., and Kool, M. (2019). Inflammation and Immunity in IPF Pathogenesis and Treatment. *Respir. Med.* 147, 79–91. doi:10.1016/j.rmed.2018.12.015

Hewlett, J. C., Kropski, J. A., and Blackwell, T. S. (2018). Idiopathic Pulmonary Fibrosis: Epithelial-Mesenchymal Interactions and Emerging Therapeutic Targets. *Matrix Biol.* 71-72, 112–127. doi:10.1016/j.matbio.2018.03.021

Hipp, M. S., Kasturi, P., and Hartl, F. U. (2019). The Proteostasis Network and its Decline in Ageing. *Nat. Rev. Mol. Cell Biol* 20 (7), 421–435. doi:10.1038/s41580-019-0101-y

Hohmann, M. S., Habiel, D. M., Coelho, A. L., Verri, W. A., Jr., and Hogaboam, C. M. (2019). Quercetin Enhances Ligand-Induced Apoptosis in Senescent Idiopathic Pulmonary Fibrosis Fibroblasts and Reduces Lung Fibrosis *In Vivo*. *Am. J. Respir. Cell Mol Biol* 60 (1), 28–40. doi:10.1165/rcmb.2017-0289OC

Hu, B., Gharaee-Kermani, M., Wu, Z., and Phan, S. H. (2010). Epigenetic Regulation of Myofibroblast Differentiation by DNA Methylation. *Am. J. Pathol.* 177 (1), 21–28. doi:10.2353/ajpath.2010.090999

Huan, C., Yang, T., Liang, J., Xie, T., Cheng, L., Liu, N., et al. (2015). Methylation-mediated BMPER Expression in Fibroblast Activation *in vitro* and Lung Fibrosis in Mice *in vivo*. *Sci. Rep.* 5, 14910. doi:10.1038/srep14910

Huang, W. T., Akhter, H., Jiang, C., MacEwen, M., Ding, Q., Antony, V., et al. (2015). Plasminogen Activator Inhibitor 1, Fibroblast Apoptosis Resistance, and Aging-Related Susceptibility to Lung Fibrosis. *Exp. Gerontol.* 61, 62–75. doi:10.1016/j.exger.2014.11.018

Huang, Y., Xie, Y., Abel, P. W., Wei, P., Plowman, J., Toews, M. L., et al. (2020). TGF-β1-induced miR-424 Promotes Pulmonary Myofibroblast Differentiation by Targeting Slit2 Protein Expression. *Biochem. Pharmacol.* 180, 114172. doi:10.1016/j.bcp.2020.114172

Im, J., Hergert, P., and Nho, R. S. (2015). Reduced FoxO3a Expression Causes Low Autophagy in Idiopathic Pulmonary Fibrosis Fibroblasts on Collagen Matrices. *Am. J. Physiol. Lung Cell Mol Physiol* 309 (6), L552–L561. doi:10.1152/ajplung.00079.2015

Inui, N., Sakai, S., and Kitagawa, M. (2021). Molecular Pathogenesis of Pulmonary Fibrosis, with Focus on Pathways Related to TGF-β and the Ubiquitin-Proteasome Pathway. *Int. J. Mol. Sci.* 22 (11). doi:10.3390/ijms22116107

Jenkins, R. G., Su, X., Su, G., Scotton, C. J., Camerer, E., Laurent, G. J., et al. (2006). Ligation of Protease-Activated Receptor 1 Enhances Alpha(v)beta6 Integrin-dependent TGF-Beta Activation and Promotes Acute Lung Injury. *J. Clin. Invest.* 116 (6), 1606–1614. doi:10.1172/JCI27183

John, A. E., Graves, R. H., Pun, K. T., Vitulli, G., Forty, E. J., Mercer, P. F., et al. (2020). Translational Pharmacology of an Inhaled Small Molecule αvβ6 Integrin Inhibitor for Idiopathic Pulmonary Fibrosis. *Nat. Commun.* 11 (1), 4659. doi:10.1038/s41467-020-18397-6

Jones, M. G., Andriotis, O. G., Roberts, J. J., Lunn, K., Tear, V. J., Cao, L., et al. (2018). Nanoscale Dysregulation of Collagen Structure-Function Disrupts Mechano-Homeostasis and Mediates Pulmonary Fibrosis. *Elife* 7. doi:10.7554/eLife.36354

Kadel, D., Zhang, Y., Sun, H. R., Zhao, Y., Dong, Q. Z., and Qin, L. X. (2019). Current Perspectives of Cancer-Associated Fibroblast in Therapeutic Resistance: Potential Mechanism and Future Strategy. *Cell Biol Toxicol* 35 (5), 407–421. doi:10.1007/s10565-019-09461-z

Kanaan, R., and Strange, C. (2017). Use of Multitarget Tyrosine Kinase Inhibitors to Attenuate Platelet-Derived Growth Factor Signalling in Lung Disease. *Eur. Respir. Rev.* 26 (146). doi:10.1183/16000617.0061-2017

Kang, J., and Song, J. W. (2021). Effect of Sildenafil Added to Antifibrotic Treatment in Idiopathic Pulmonary Fibrosis. *Sci. Rep.* 11 (1), 17824. doi:10.1038/s41598-021-97396-z

Kc, R., Shukla, S. D., Gautam, S. S., Hansbro, P. M., and O'Toole, R. F. (2018). The Role of Environmental Exposure to Non-cigarette Smoke in Lung Disease. *Clin. Transl Med.* 7 (1), 39. doi:10.1186/s40169-018-0217-2

Kishi, M., Aono, Y., Sato, S., Koyama, K., Azuma, M., Abe, S., et al. (2018). Blockade of Platelet-Derived Growth Factor Receptor-β, Not Receptor-α Ameliorates Bleomycin-Induced Pulmonary Fibrosis in Mice. *PLoS One* 13 (12), e0209786. doi:10.1371/journal.pone.0209786

Kropski, J. A., and Blackwell, T. S. (2018). Endoplasmic Reticulum Stress in the Pathogenesis of Fibrotic Disease. *J. Clin. Invest.* 128 (1), 64–73. doi:10.1172/JCI93560

Kropski, J. A., Blackwell, T. S., and Loyd, J. E. (2015). The Genetic Basis of Idiopathic Pulmonary Fibrosis. *Eur. Respir. J.* 45 (6), 1717–1727. doi:10.1183/09031936.00163814

Kumar, A., Kapnadak, S. G., Girgis, R. E., and Raghu, G. (2018). Lung Transplantation in Idiopathic Pulmonary Fibrosis. *Expert Rev. Respir. Med.* 12 (5), 375–385. doi:10.1080/17476348.2018.1462704

Le Saux, C. J., and Chapman, H. A. (2018). Idiopathic Pulmonary Fibrosis: Cell Death and Inflammation Revisited. *Am. J. Respir. Cell Mol Biol* 59 (2), 137–138. doi:10.1165/rcmb.2018-0083ED

Leask, A. (2011). Possible Strategies for Anti-fibrotic Drug Intervention in Scleroderma. *J. Cell Commun Signal* 5 (2), 125–129. doi:10.1007/s12079-011-0122-6

Lee, J. H., Tammela, T., Hofree, M., Choi, J., Marjanovic, N. D., Han, S., et al. (2017). Anatomically and Functionally Distinct Lung Mesenchymal Populations Marked by Lgr5 and Lgr6. *Cell* 170 (6), 1149–e12. e1112. doi:10.1016/j.cell.2017.07.028

Lee, T. H., Yeh, C. F., Lee, Y. T., Shih, Y. C., Chen, Y. T., Hung, C. T., et al. (2020). Fibroblast-enriched Endoplasmic Reticulum Protein TXNDC5 Promotes Pulmonary Fibrosis by Augmenting TGFβ Signaling through TGFBR1 Stabilization. *Nat. Commun.* 11 (1), 4254. doi:10.1038/s41467-020-18047-x

Li, F. J., Surolia, R., Li, H., Wang, Z., Liu, G., Kulkarni, T., et al. (2021). Citrullinated Vimentin Mediates Development and Progression of Lung Fibrosis. *Sci. Transl Med.* 13 (585). doi:10.1126/scitranslmed.aba2927

Li, L., Ma, B. B. Y., Chan, A. T. C., Chan, F. K. L., Murray, P., and Tao, Q. (2018). Epstein-Barr Virus-Induced Epigenetic Pathogenesis of Viral-Associated Lymphoepithelioma-like Carcinomas and Natural Killer/T-Cell Lymphomas. *Pathogens* 7 (3). doi:10.3390/pathogens7030063

Ligresti, G., Caporarello, N., Meridew, J. A., Jones, D. L., Tan, Q., Choi, K. M., et al. (2019). CBX5/G9a/H3K9me-mediated Gene Repression Is Essential to Fibroblast Activation during Lung Fibrosis. *JCI Insight* 5. doi:10.1172/jci.insight.127111

Lin, C. H., Shih, C. H., Lin, Y. C., Yang, Y. L., and Chen, B. C. (2018). MEKK1, JNK, and SMAD3 Mediate CXCL12-Stimulated Connective Tissue Growth Factor Expression in Human Lung Fibroblasts. *J. Biomed. Sci.* 25 (1), 19. doi:10.1186/s12929-018-0421-9

Lin, Y., and Xu, Z. (2020). Fibroblast Senescence in Idiopathic Pulmonary Fibrosis. *Front Cell Dev Biol* 8, 593283. doi:10.3389/fcell.2020.593283

Lipinski, J. H., Moore, B. B., and O'Dwyer, D. N. (2020). The Evolving Role of the Lung Microbiome in Pulmonary Fibrosis. *Am. J. Physiol. Lung Cell Mol Physiol* 319 (4), L675–L682. doi:10.1152/ajplung.00258.2020

Liu B, B., Yi, J., Yang, X., Liu, L., Lou, X., Zhang, Z., et al. (2019). MDM2-mediated Degradation of WRN Promotes Cellular Senescence in a P53-independent Manner. *Oncogene* 38 (14), 2501–2515. doi:10.1038/s41388-018-0605-5

Liu F, F., Bayliss, G., and Zhuang, S. (2019). Application of Nintedanib and Other Potential Anti-fibrotic Agents in Fibrotic Diseases. *Clin. Sci. (Lond)* 133 (12), 1309–1320. doi:10.1042/CS20190249

Liu, G., Friggeri, A., Yang, Y., Milosevic, J., Ding, Q., Thannickal, V. J., et al. (2010). miR-21 Mediates Fibrogenic Activation of Pulmonary Fibroblasts and Lung Fibrosis. *J. Exp. Med.* 207 (8), 1589–1597. doi:10.1084/jem.20100035

Liu, Y. M., Nepali, K., and Liou, J. P. (2017). Idiopathic Pulmonary Fibrosis: Current Status, Recent Progress, and Emerging Targets. *J. Med. Chem.* 60 (2), 527–553. doi:10.1021/acs.jmedchem.6b00935

López-Otín, C., Blasco, M. A., Partridge, L., Serrano, M., and Kroemer, G. (2013).

The Hallmarks of Aging. *Cell* 153 (6), 1194–1217. doi:10.1016/j.cell.2013.05.039

Lorenzo-Salazar, J. M., Ma, S. F., Jou, J., Hou, P. C., Guillen-Guio, B., Allen, R. J., et al. (2019). Novel Idiopathic Pulmonary Fibrosis Susceptibility Variants Revealed by Deep Sequencing. *ERJ Open Res.* 5 (2). doi:10.1183/23120541.00071-2019

Luo, Q. K., Zhang, H., and Li, L. (2020). Research Advances on DNA Methylation in Idiopathic Pulmonary Fibrosis. *Adv. Exp. Med. Biol.* 1255, 73–81. doi:10.1007/978-981-15-4494-1_6

Maher, T. M., Bendstrup, E., Dron, L., Langley, J., Smith, G., Khalid, J. M., et al. (2021). Global Incidence and Prevalence of Idiopathic Pulmonary Fibrosis. *Respir. Res.* 22 (1), 197. doi:10.1186/s12931-021-01791-z

Maher, T. M., Costabel, U., Glassberg, M. K., Kondoh, Y., Ogura, T., Scholand, M. B., et al. (2021). Phase 2 Trial to Assess Lebrikizumab in Patients with Idiopathic Pulmonary Fibrosis. *Eur. Respir. J.* 57 (2), 1902442. doi:10.1183/13993003.02442-2019

Makino, S. (2021). Progressive Fibrosing Interstitial Lung Diseases: A New Concept and Indication of Nintedanib. *Mod. Rheumatol.* 31 (1), 13–19. doi:10.1080/14397595.2020.1826665

Martinez, F. J., Collard, H. R., Pardo, A., Raghu, G., Richeldi, L., Selman, M., et al. (2017). Idiopathic Pulmonary Fibrosis. *Nat. Rev. Dis. Primers* 3, 17074. doi:10.1038/nrdp.2017.74

Mascaux, C., Laes, J. F., Anthoine, G., Haller, A., Ninane, V., Burny, A., et al. (2009). Evolution of microRNA Expression during Human Bronchial Squamous Carcinogenesis. *Eur. Respir. J.* 33 (2), 352–359. doi:10.1183/09031936.00084108

Massagué, J. (2012). TGFβ Signalling in Context. *Nat. Rev. Mol. Cell Biol* 13 (10), 616–630. doi:10.1038/nrm3434

Mathai, S. K., Pedersen, B. S., Smith, K., Russell, P., Schwarz, M. I., Brown, K. K., et al. (2016). Desmoplakin Variants Are Associated with Idiopathic Pulmonary Fibrosis. *Am. J. Respir. Crit. Care Med.* 193 (10), 1151–1160. doi:10.1164/rccm.201509-1863OC

Merkt, W., Bueno, M., Mora, A. L., and Lagares, D. (2020). Senotherapeutics: Targeting Senescence in Idiopathic Pulmonary Fibrosis. *Semin. Cell Dev Biol* 101, 104–110. doi:10.1016/j.semcdb.2019.12.008

Moimas, S., Salton, F., Kosmider, B., Ring, N., Volpe, M. C., Bahmed, K., et al. (2019). miR-200 Family Members Reduce Senescence and Restore Idiopathic Pulmonary Fibrosis Type II Alveolar Epithelial Cell Transdifferentiation. *ERJ Open Res.* 5 (4). doi:10.1183/23120541.00138-2019

Molina-Molina, M., Machahua-Huamani, C., Vicens-Zygmunt, V., Llatjós, R., Escobar, I., Sala-Llinas, E., et al. (2018). Anti-fibrotic Effects of Pirfenidone and Rapamycin in Primary IPF Fibroblasts and Human Alveolar Epithelial Cells. *BMC Pulm. Med.* 18 (1), 63. doi:10.1186/s12890-018-0626-4

Molyneaux, P. L., Cox, M. J., Willis-Owen, S. A., Mallia, P., Russell, K. E., Russell, A. M., et al. (2014). The Role of Bacteria in the Pathogenesis and Progression of Idiopathic Pulmonary Fibrosis. *Am. J. Respir. Crit. Care Med.* 190 (8), 906–913. doi:10.1164/rccm.201403-0541OC

Molyneaux, P. L., Willis-Owen, S. A. G., Cox, M. J., James, P., Cowman, S., Loebinger, M., et al. (2017). Host-Microbial Interactions in Idiopathic Pulmonary Fibrosis. *Am. J. Respir. Crit. Care Med.* 195 (12), 1640–1650. doi:10.1164/rccm.201607-1408OC

Moore, C., Blumhagen, R. Z., Yang, I. V., Walts, A., Powers, J., Walker, T., et al. (2019). Resequencing Study Confirms that Host Defense and Cell Senescence Gene Variants Contribute to the Risk of Idiopathic Pulmonary Fibrosis. *Am. J. Respir. Crit. Care Med.* 200 (2), 199–208. doi:10.1164/rccm.201810-1891OC

Mora, A. L., Rojas, M., Pardo, A., and Selman, M. (2017). Emerging Therapies for Idiopathic Pulmonary Fibrosis, a Progressive Age-Related Disease. *Nat. Rev. Drug Discov.* 16 (11), 755–772. doi:10.1038/nrd.2017.22510.1038/nrd.2017.170

Morse, C., Tabib, T., Sembrat, J., Buschur, K. L., Bittar, H. T., Valenzi, E., et al. (2019). Proliferating SPP1/MERTK-Expressing Macrophages in Idiopathic Pulmonary Fibrosis. *Eur. Respir. J.* 54 (2). doi:10.1183/13993003.02441-2018

Mortimer, K. M., Bartels, D. B., Hartmann, N., Capapey, J., Yang, J., Gately, R., et al. (2020). Characterizing Health Outcomes in Idiopathic Pulmonary Fibrosis Using US Health Claims Data. *Respiration* 99 (2), 108–118. doi:10.1159/000504630

Mulugeta, S., Nureki, S., and Beers, M. F. (2015). Lost after Translation: Insights from Pulmonary Surfactant for Understanding the Role of Alveolar Epithelial Dysfunction and Cellular Quality Control in Fibrotic Lung Disease. *Am. J. Physiol. Lung Cell Mol Physiol* 309 (6), L507–L525. doi:10.1152/ajplung.00139.2015

Nabhan, A. N., Brownfield, D. G., Harbury, P. B., Krasnow, M. A., and Desai, T. J. (2018). Single-cell Wnt Signaling Niches Maintain Stemness of Alveolar Type 2 Cells. *Science* 359 (6380), 1118–1123. doi:10.1126/science.aam6603

Nathan, S. D., Costabel, U., Albera, C., Behr, J., Wuyts, W. A., Kirchgaessler, K. U., et al. (2019). Pirfenidone in Patients with Idiopathic Pulmonary Fibrosis and More Advanced Lung Function Impairment. *Respir. Med.* 153, 44–51. doi:10.1016/j.rmed.2019.04.016

Nho, R. S., Hergert, P., Kahm, J., Jessurun, J., and Henke, C. (2011). Pathological Alteration of FoxO3a Activity Promotes Idiopathic Pulmonary Fibrosis Fibroblast Proliferation on Type I Collagen Matrix. *Am. J. Pathol.* 179 (5), 2420–2430. doi:10.1016/j.ajpath.2011.07.020

O'Dwyer, D. N., Ashley, S. L., Gurczynski, S. J., Xia, M., Wilke, C., Falkowski, N. R., et al. (2019). Lung Microbiota Contribute to Pulmonary Inflammation and Disease Progression in Pulmonary Fibrosis. *Am. J. Respir. Crit. Care Med.* 199 (9), 1127–1138. doi:10.1164/rccm.201809-1650OC

Ornatowski, W., Lu, Q., Yegambaram, M., Garcia, A. E., Zemskov, E. A., Maltepe, E., et al. (2020). Complex Interplay between Autophagy and Oxidative Stress in the Development of Pulmonary Disease. *Redox Biol.* 36, 101679. doi:10.1016/j.redox.2020.101679

Pardo, A., and Selman, M. (2021). The Interplay of the Genetic Architecture, Aging, and Environmental Factors in the Pathogenesis of Idiopathic Pulmonary Fibrosis. *Am. J. Respir. Cell Mol Biol* 64, 163–172. doi:10.1165/rcmb.2020-0373PS

Parimon, T., Yao, C., Stripp, B. R., Noble, P. W., and Chen, P. (2020). Alveolar Epithelial Type II Cells as Drivers of Lung Fibrosis in Idiopathic Pulmonary Fibrosis. *Int. J. Mol. Sci.* 21 (7). doi:10.3390/ijms21072269

Phan, T. H. G., Paliogiannis, P., Nasrallah, G. K., Giordo, R., Eid, A. H., Fois, A. G., et al. (2021). Emerging Cellular and Molecular Determinants of Idiopathic Pulmonary Fibrosis. *Cell Mol Life Sci* 78 (5), 2031–2057. doi:10.1007/s00018-020-03693-7

Piñeiro-Hermida, S., Autilio, C., Martínez, P., Bosch, F., Pérez-Gil, J., and Blasco, M. A. (2020). Telomerase Treatment Prevents Lung Profibrotic Pathologies Associated with Physiological Aging. *J. Cell Biol* 219 (10). doi:10.1083/jcb.202002120

Plataki, M., Cho, S. J., Harris, R. M., Huang, H. R., Yun, H. S., Schiffer, K. T., et al. (2019). Mitochondrial Dysfunction in Aged Macrophages and Lung during Primary Streptococcus Pneumoniae Infection Is Improved with Pirfenidone. *Sci. Rep.* 9 (1), 971. doi:10.1038/s41598-018-37438-1

Qu, J., Yang, S. Z., Zhu, Y., Guo, T., Thannickal, V. J., and Zhou, Y. (2021). Targeting Mechanosensitive MDM4 Promotes Lung Fibrosis Resolution in Aged Mice. *J. Exp. Med.* 218 (5). doi:10.1084/jem.20202033

Qu, J., Zhu, L., Zhou, Z., Chen, P., Liu, S., Locy, M. L., et al. (2018). Reversing Mechanoinductive DSP Expression by CRISPR/dCas9-mediated Epigenome Editing. *Am. J. Respir. Crit. Care Med.* 198 (5), 599–609. doi:10.1164/rccm.201711-2242OC

Rabinovich, E. I., Kapetanaki, M. G., Steinfeld, I., Gibson, K. F., Pandit, K. V., Yu, G., et al. (2012). Global Methylation Patterns in Idiopathic Pulmonary Fibrosis. *PLoS One* 7 (4), e33770. doi:10.1371/journal.pone.0033770

Racanelli, A. C., Kikkers, S. A., Choi, A. M. K., and Cloonan, S. M. (2018). Autophagy and Inflammation in Chronic Respiratory Disease. *Autophagy* 14 (2), 221–232. doi:10.1080/15548627.2017.1389823

Raghu, G., Brown, K. K., Collard, H. R., Cottin, V., Gibson, K. F., Kaner, R. J., et al. (2017). Efficacy of Simtuzumab versus Placebo in Patients with Idiopathic Pulmonary Fibrosis: a Randomised, Double-Blind, Controlled, Phase 2 Trial. *Lancet Respir. Med.* 5 (1), 22–32. doi:10.1016/S2213-2600(16)30421-0

Raghu, G., Martinez, F. J., Brown, K. K., Costabel, U., Cottin, V., Wells, A. U., et al. (2015). CC-chemokine Ligand 2 Inhibition in Idiopathic Pulmonary Fibrosis: a Phase 2 Trial of Carlumab. *Eur. Respir. J.* 46 (6), 1740–1750. doi:10.1183/13993003.01558-2014

Rao, L. Z., Wang, Y., Zhang, L., Wu, G., Zhang, L., Wang, F. X., et al. (2021). IL-24 Deficiency Protects Mice against Bleomycin-Induced Pulmonary Fibrosis by Repressing IL-4-induced M2 Program in Macrophages. *Cell Death Differ* 28 (4), 1270–1283. doi:10.1038/s41418-020-00650-6

Reyfman, P. A., Walter, J. M., Joshi, N., Anekalla, K. R., McQuattie-Pimentel, A. C., Chiu, S., et al. (2019). Single-Cell Transcriptomic Analysis of Human Lung Provides Insights into the Pathobiology of Pulmonary Fibrosis. *Am. J. Respir. Crit. Care Med.* 199 (12), 1517–1536. doi:10.1164/rccm.201712-2410OC

Richeldi, L., Collard, H. R., and Jones, M. G. (2017). Idiopathic Pulmonary Fibrosis. *Lancet* 389 (10082), 1941 1952. doi:10.1016/S0140-6736(17)30866-8

Richeldi, L., Fernández Pérez, E. R., Costabel, U., Albera, C., Lederer, D. J., Flaherty, K. R., et al. (2020). Pamrevlumab, an Anti-connective Tissue Growth Factor Therapy, for Idiopathic Pulmonary Fibrosis (PRAISE): a Phase 2, Randomised, Double-Blind, Placebo-Controlled Trial. *Lancet Respir. Med.* 8 (1), 25–33. doi:10.1016/S2213-2600(19)30262-0

Ruwanpura, S. M., Thomas, B. J., and Bardin, P. G. (2020). Pirfenidone: Molecular Mechanisms and Potential Clinical Applications in Lung Disease. *Am. J. Respir. Cell Mol Biol* 62, 413–422. doi:10.1165/rcmb.2019-0328TR

Sakamoto, S., Kataoka, K., Kondoh, Y., Kato, M., Okamoto, M., Mukae, H., et al. (2021). Pirfenidone Plus Inhaled N-Acetylcysteine for Idiopathic Pulmonary Fibrosis: a Randomised Trial. *Eur. Respir. J.* 57 (1). doi:10.1183/13993003.00348-2020

Sanders, Y. Y., Ambalavanan, N., Halloran, B., Zhang, X., Liu, H., Crossman, D. K., et al. (2012). Altered DNA Methylation Profile in Idiopathic Pulmonary Fibrosis. *Am. J. Respir. Crit. Care Med.* 186 (6), 525–535. doi:10.1164/rccm.201201-0077OC

Schäfer, S. C., Funke-Chambour, M., and Berezowska, S. (2020). Idiopathic Pulmonary Fibrosis-Epidemiology, Causes, and Clinical Course. *Pathologe* 41 (1), 46–51. doi:10.1007/s00292-019-00747-x

Selman, M., Martinez, F. J., and Pardo, A. (2019). Why Does an Aging Smoker's Lung Develop Idiopathic Pulmonary Fibrosis and Not Chronic Obstructive Pulmonary Disease? *Am. J. Respir. Crit. Care Med.* 199 (3), 279–285. doi:10.1164/rccm.201806-1166PP

Selvarajah, B., Azuelos, I., Platé, M., Guillotin, D., Forty, E. J., Contento, G., et al. (2019). mTORC1 Amplifies the ATF4-dependent de novo Serine-glycine Pathway to Supply glycine during TGF-B1-Induced Collagen Biosynthesis. *Sci. Signal.* 12 (582). doi:10.1126/scisignal.aav3048

Senoo, S., Taniguchi, A., Itano, J., Oda, N., Morichika, D., Fujii, U., et al. (2021). Essential Role of IL-23 in the Development of Acute Exacerbation of Pulmonary Fibrosis. *Am. J. Physiology-Lung Cell Mol. Physiol.* 321, L925–L940. doi:10.1152/ajplung.00582.2020

Sides, M. D., Klingsberg, R. C., Shan, B., Gordon, K. A., Nguyen, H. T., Lin, Z., et al. (2011). The Epstein-Barr Virus Latent Membrane Protein 1 and Transforming Growth Factor-Bβ1 Synergistically Induce Epithelial-Mmesenchymal Transition in Lung Epithelial Cells. *Am. J. Respir. Cell Mol Biol* 44 (6), 852–862. doi:10.1165/rcmb.2009-0232OC

Somogyi, V., Chaudhuri, N., Torrisi, S. E., Kahn, N., Müller, V., and Kreuter, M. (2019). The Therapy of Idiopathic Pulmonary Fibrosis: what Is Next? *Eur. Respir. Rev.* 28 (153). doi:10.1183/16000617.0021-2019

Song, D., Tang, L., Wang, L., Huang, J., Zeng, T., Fang, H., et al. (2020). Roles of TGFβ1 in the Expression of Phosphoinositide 3-kinase Isoform Genes and Sensitivity and Response of Lung Telocytes to PI3K Inhibitors. *Cell Biol Toxicol* 36 (1), 51–64. doi:10.1007/s10565-019-09487-3

Song, M., Peng, H., Guo, W., Luo, M., Duan, W., Chen, P., et al. (2019). Cigarette Smoke Extract Promotes Human Lung Myofibroblast Differentiation by the Induction of Endoplasmic Reticulum Stress. *Respiration* 98 (4), 347–356. doi:10.1159/000502099

Spagnolo, P., Tzouvelekis, A., and Bonella, F. (2018). The Management of Patients with Idiopathic Pulmonary Fibrosis. *Front. Med. (Lausanne)* 5, 148. doi:10.3389/fmed.2018.00148

Stewart, G. A., Hoyne, G. F., Ahmad, S. A., Jarman, E., Wallace, W. A., Harrison, D. J., et al. (2003). Expression of the Developmental Sonic Hedgehog (Shh) Signalling Pathway Is Up-Regulated in Chronic Lung Fibrosis and the Shh Receptor Patched 1 Is Present in Circulating T Lymphocytes. *J. Pathol.* 199 (4), 488–495. doi:10.1002/path.1295

Sui, B., Hu, C., and Jin, Y. (2016). Mitochondrial Metabolic Failure in Telomere Attrition-Provoked Aging of Bone Marrow Mesenchymal Stem Cells. *Biogerontology* 17 (2), 267–279. doi:10.1007/s10522-015-9609-5

Sun, W., Jing, X., Yang, X., Huang, H., Luo, Q., Xia, S., et al. (2021). Regulation of the IGF1 Signaling Pathway Is Involved in Idiopathic Pulmonary Fibrosis Induced by Alveolar Epithelial Cell Senescence and Core Fucosylation. *Aging (Albany NY)* 13 (14), 18852–18869. doi:10.18632/aging.203335

Surolia, R., Li, F. J., Wang, Z., Li, H., Dsouza, K., Thomas, V., et al. (2019). Vimentin Intermediate Filament Assembly Regulates Fibroblast Invasion in Fibrogenic Lung Injury. *JCI Insight* 4 (7). doi:10.1172/jci.insight.123253

Takezaki, A., Tsukumo, S. I., Setoguchi, Y., Ledford, J. G., Goto, H., Hosomichi, K., et al. (2019). A Homozygous SFTPA1 Mutation Drives Necroptosis of Type II Alveolar Epithelial Cells in Patients with Idiopathic Pulmonary Fibrosis. *J. Exp. Med.* 216 (12), 2724–2735. doi:10.1084/jem.20182351

Tsukui, T., Sun, K. H., Wetter, J. B., Wilson-Kanamori, J. R., Hazelwood, L. A., Henderson, N. C., et al. (2020). Collagen-producing Lung Cell Atlas Identifies Multiple Subsets with Distinct Localization and Relevance to Fibrosis. *Nat. Commun.* 11 (1), 1920. doi:10.1038/s41467-020-15647-5

Vancheri, C., Kreuter, M., Richeldi, L., Ryerson, C. J., Valeyre, D., Grutters, J. C., et al. (2018). Nintedanib with Add-On Pirfenidone in Idiopathic Pulmonary Fibrosis. Results of the INJOURNEY Trial. *Am. J. Respir. Crit. Care Med.* 197 (3), 356–363. doi:10.1164/rccm.201706-1301OC

Wang, J., Li, X., Zhong, M., Wang, Y., Zou, L., Wang, M., et al. (2020). miR-301a Suppression within Fibroblasts Limits the Progression of Fibrosis through the TSC1/mTOR Pathway. *Mol. Ther. Nucleic Acids* 21, 217–228. doi:10.1016/j.omtn.2020.05.027

Wang, L., Chen, R., Li, G., Wang, Z., Liu, J., Liang, Y., et al. (2020). FBW7 Mediates Senescence and Pulmonary Fibrosis through Telomere Uncapping. *Cell Metab* 32 (5), 860–e9. doi:10.1016/j.cmet.2020.10.004

Wang, X., Cui, H., and Wu, S. (2019). CTGF: A Potential Therapeutic Target for Bronchopulmonary Dysplasia. *Eur. J. Pharmacol.* 860, 172588. doi:10.1016/j.ejphar.2019.172588

Wang, Y., Zhang, L., Wu, G.-R., Zhou, Q., Yue, H., Rao, L.-Z., et al. (2021). MBD2 Serves as a Viable Target against Pulmonary Fibrosis by Inhibiting Macrophage M2 Program. *Sci. Adv.* 7 (1). doi:10.1126/sciadv.abb6075

Wang, Z., Qu, S., Zhu, J., Chen, F., and Ma, L. (2020). Comprehensive Analysis of lncRNA-Associated Competing Endogenous RNA Network and Immune Infiltration in Idiopathic Pulmonary Fibrosis. *J. Thorac. Dis.* 12 (5), 1856–1865. doi:10.21037/jtd-19-2842

Wilson, A. M., Clark, A. B., Cahn, T., Chilvers, E. R., Fraser, W., Hammond, M., et al. (2020). Effect of Co-trimoxazole (Trimethoprim-Sulfamethoxazole) vs Placebo on Death, Lung Transplant, or Hospital Admission in Patients with Moderate and Severe Idiopathic Pulmonary Fibrosis: The EME-TIPAC Randomized Clinical Trial. *JAMA* 324 (22), 2282–2291. doi:10.1001/jama.2020.22960

Wipff, P. J., Rifkin, D. B., Meister, J. J., and Hinz, B. (2007). Myofibroblast Contraction Activates Latent TGF-Beta1 from the Extracellular Matrix. *J. Cell Biol* 179 (6), 1311–1323. doi:10.1083/jcb.200704042

Wolters, P. J., Collard, H. R., and Jones, K. D. (2014). Pathogenesis of Idiopathic Pulmonary Fibrosis. *Annu. Rev. Pathol.* 9, 157–179. doi:10.1146/annurev-pathol-012513-104706

Wu, H., Yu, Y., Huang, H., Hu, Y., Fu, S., Wang, Z., et al. (2020). Progressive Pulmonary Fibrosis Is Caused by Elevated Mechanical Tension on Alveolar Stem Cells. *Cell* 180 (1), 107–e17. e117. doi:10.1016/j.cell.2019.11.027

Xia, H., Diebold, D., Nho, R., Perlman, D., Kleidon, J., Kahm, J., et al. (2008). Pathological Integrin Signaling Enhances Proliferation of Primary Lung Fibroblasts from Patients with Idiopathic Pulmonary Fibrosis. *J. Exp. Med.* 205 (7), 1659–1672. doi:10.1084/jem.20080001

Xiao, X., Huang, C., Zhao, C., Gou, X., Senavirathna, L. K., Hinsdale, M., et al. (2015). Regulation of Myofibroblast Differentiation by miR-424 during Epithelial-To-Mesenchymal Transition. *Arch. Biochem. Biophys.* 566, 49–57. doi:10.1016/j.abb.2014.12.007

Yamada, M. (2020). The Roles of MicroRNAs and Extracellular Vesicles in the Pathogeneses of Idiopathic Pulmonary Fibrosis and Acute Respiratory Distress Syndrome. *Tohoku J. Exp. Med.* 251 (4), 313–326. doi:10.1620/tjem.251.313

Yanagihara, T., Tsubouchi, K., Gholiof, M., Chong, S. G., Lipson, K. E., Zhou, Q., et al. (2021). Connective-Tissue Growth Factor (CTGF/CCN2) Contributes to TGF-B1-Induced Lung Fibrosis. *Am. J. Respir. Cell Mol Biol.* doi:10.1165/rcmb.2020-0504OC

Yang, G., Yang, L., Wang, W., Wang, J., Wang, J., and Xu, Z. (2015). Discovery and Validation of Extracellular/circulating microRNAs during Idiopathic Pulmonary Fibrosis Disease Progression. *Gene* 562 (1), 138–144. doi:10.1016/j.gene.2015.02.065

Yang, I. V., Pedersen, B. S., Rabinovich, E., Hennessy, C. E., Davidson, E. J., Murphy, E., et al. (2014). Relationship of DNA Methylation and Gene Expression in Idiopathic Pulmonary Fibrosis. *Am. J. Respir. Crit. Care Med.* 190 (11), 1263–1272. doi:10.1164/rccm.201408-1452OC

Yang, I. V., and Schwartz, D. A. (2015). Epigenetics of Idiopathic Pulmonary Fibrosis. *Transl Res.* 165 (1), 48–60. doi:10.1016/j.trsl.2014.03.011

Yang, S., Cui, H., Xie, N., Icyuz, M., Banerjee, S., Antony, V. B., et al. (2013). miR-145 Regulates Myofibroblast Differentiation and Lung Fibrosis. *FASEB J.* 27 (6), 2382–2391. doi:10.1096/fj.12-219493

Yao, C., Guan, X., Carraro, G., Parimon, T., Liu, X., Huang, G., et al. (2021). Senescence of Alveolar Type 2 Cells Drives Progressive Pulmonary Fibrosis. *Am. J. Respir. Crit. Care Med.* 203, 707–717. doi:10.1164/rccm.202004-1274OC

Yoshihara, T., Nanri, Y., Nunomura, S., Yamaguchi, Y., Feghali-Bostwick, C., Ajito, K., et al. (2020). Periostin Plays a Critical Role in the Cell Cycle in Lung Fibroblasts. *Respir. Res.* 21 (1), 38. doi:10.1186/s12931-020-1299-0

Zacharias, W. J., Frank, D. B., Zepp, J. A., Morley, M. P., Alkhaleel, F. A., Kong, J., et al. (2018). Regeneration of the Lung Alveolus by an Evolutionarily Conserved Epithelial Progenitor. *Nature* 555 (7695), 251–255. doi:10.1038/nature25786

Zepp, J. A., Zacharias, W. J., Frank, D. B., Cavanaugh, C. A., Zhou, S., Morley, M. P., et al. (2017). Distinct Mesenchymal Lineages and Niches Promote Epithelial Self-Renewal and Myofibrogenesis in the Lung. *Cell* 170 (6), 1134–e10. doi:10.1016/j.cell.2017.07.034

Zhang, N., Liu, K., Wang, K., Zhou, C., Wang, H., Che, S., et al. (2019). Dust Induces Lung Fibrosis through Dysregulated DNA Methylation. *Environ. Toxicol.* 34 (6), 728–741. doi:10.1002/tox.22739

Zhang, Q., Wang, Y., Qu, D., Yu, J., and Yang, J. (2019). The Possible Pathogenesis of Idiopathic Pulmonary Fibrosis Considering MUC5B. *Biomed. Res. Int.* 2019, 9712464. doi:10.1155/2019/9712464

Zhang, Y., Jones, K. D., Achtar-Zadeh, N., Green, G., Kukreja, J., Xu, B., et al. (2019). Histopathological and Molecular Analysis of Idiopathic Pulmonary Fibrosis Lungs from Patients Treated with Pirfenidone or Nintedanib. *Histopathology* 74 (2), 341–349. doi:10.1111/his.13745

Zhao, Y. D., Yin, L., Archer, S., Lu, C., Zhao, G., Yao, Y., et al. (2017). Metabolic Heterogeneity of Idiopathic Pulmonary Fibrosis: a Metabolomic Study. *BMJ Open Respir. Res.* 4 (1), e000183. doi:10.1136/bmjresp-2017-000183

Zhou, Y., Huang, X., Hecker, L., Kurundkar, D., Kurundkar, A., Liu, H., et al. (2013). Inhibition of Mechanosensitive Signaling in Myofibroblasts Ameliorates Experimental Pulmonary Fibrosis. *J. Clin. Invest.* 123 (3), 1096–1108. doi:10.1172/JCI66700

Zhou, Z., Qu, J., He, L., Zhu, Y., Yang, S. Z., Zhang, F., et al. (2020). Stiff Matrix Instigates Type I Collagen Biogenesis by Mammalian Cleavage Factor I Complex-Mediated Alternative Polyadenylation. *JCI insight* 5 (3). doi:10.1172/jci.insight.133972

Zolak, J. S., and de Andrade, J. A. (2012). Idiopathic Pulmonary Fibrosis. *Immunol. Allergy Clin. North. Am.* 32 (4), 473–485. doi:10.1016/j.iac.2012.08.006

12

Exploring the Anti-Pulmonary Fibrosis Mechanism of Jingyin Granule by Network Pharmacology Strategy

De-wei Zhu[1†], *Qun Yu*[1†], *Mei-fang Jiang*[2], *Dan-dan Wang*[2] *and Yun-hui Shen*[1*]

[1]*School of Pharmacy, Shanghai University of Traditional Chinese Medicine, Shanghai, China,* [2]*SPH Xing Ling Sci. & Tech. Pharmaceutical Co., Ltd., Shanghai, China*

***Correspondence:**
Yun-hui Shen
bravesyh@163.com

[†]*These authors have contributed equally to this work*

Pulmonary fibrosis (PF) is a clinically common disease caused by many factors, which will lead to lung function decline and even respiratory failure. Jingyin granule has been confirmed to have anti-inflammatory and antiviral effects by former studies, and has been recommended for combating H1N1 influenza A virus (H1N1) infection and Coronavirus disease 2019 (COVID-19) in China. At present, studies have shown that patients with severe COVID-19 infection developed lung fibrotic lesions. Although Jingyin granule can improve symptoms in COVID-19 patients, no study has yet reported whether it can attenuate the process of PF. Here, we explored the underlying mechanism of Jingyin granule against PF by network pharmacology combined with *in vitro* experimental validation. In the present study, the active ingredients as well as the corresponding action targets of Jingyin granule were firstly collected by TCMSP and literature data, and the disease target genes of PF were retrieved by disease database. Then, the common targets were subjected to Gene Ontology (GO) and Kyoto Encyclopedia of Genes and Genomes (KEGG) enrichment analyses, and then a PPI network and an ingredient–target network were constructed. Next, UPLC-MS was used to isolate and identify selected representative components in Jingyin granule. Finally, LPS was used to induce the A549 cell fibrosis model to verify the anti-PF effect of Jingyin granule *in vitro*. Our results indicated that STAT3, JUN, RELA, MAPK3, TNF, MAPK1, IL-6, and AKT1 were core targets of action and bound with good affinity to selected components, and Jingyin granule may alleviate PF progression by Janus kinase 2/signal transducers and activators of transcription (JAK2/STAT3), the mammalian nuclear factor-κB (NF-κB), the phosphatidylinositol 3-kinase (PI3K)/protein kinase B (Akt), tumor necrosis factor (TNF), and the extracellular signal-regulated kinases 1 and 2 (ERK1/2) signaling pathways. Overall, these results provide future therapeutic strategies into the mechanism study of Jingyin granule on PF.

Keywords: pulmonary fibrosis, Jingyin granule, molecular mechanism, UPLC-MS, network pharmacology, signaling pathway analysis

HIGHLIGHTS

1. Jingyin granule has a potential anti-pulmonary fibrosis effect.
2. The representative active components of Jingyin granule may include arctigenin, quercetin, luteolin, kaempferol, rutin, gallic acid, and chlorogenic acid.
3. The UPLC-MS method was used to identify arctigenin, quercetin, luteolin, kaempferol, rutin, gallic acid, and chlorogenic acid in Jingyin granule.
4. Jingyin granule inhibited the expression of AKT1, JAK2, MAPK1, MAPK3, RELA, PI3K, STAT3, TNF, etc.
5. Jingyin granule may mediate pulmonary fibrosis through JAK2/STAT3, NF-κB, PI3K-AKT, TNF, and ERK1/2 signal pathways.

INTRODUCTION

Fibrosis, which may occur in any organ, is the outcome of dysregulated tissue repair responses to multiple types of tissue injury, particularly during chronic inflammatory disease processes. Pulmonary fibrosis (PF) is an excessive reparative response to tissue injury characterized by spontaneous, progressive scarring of the lungs in the absence of infectious or autoimmune etiologies (Cui et al., 2020). During the development of PF, fibroblast proliferation and extracellular matrix massive aggregation were accompanied by epithelial cell inflammation injury, and the injury site was gradually replaced by fibrous connective tissue to form fibrotic foci. As a fatal malignant disease of the lung, idiopathic pulmonary fibrosis (IPF) has an unknown etiology, a very poor prognosis, and a very high mortality rate, even worse than several cancers, and lung transplantation is the only curative treatment (Vancheri et al., 2010). Europe and North America have a higher incidence with 3–9 new cases per 100,000 per year, whereas Asia and South America report a lower incidence with approximately half a million new cases per year in China (Hutchinson et al., 2015). The incidence of IPF is high in the elderly, and the condition gradually deteriorates with age, and importantly, the survival rate varies greatly among different patients (Kim et al., 2015), with a median survival of 3–5 years following diagnosis (Raghu et al., 2018), and a 3-year survival rate of only 50% (Cui et al., 2020).

Halting IPF progression and curing remain a challenge, though some drugs are able to produce a significant reduction in lung function decline. Based on safety and efficacy in clinical trials, pirfenidone and nintedanib were approved for the treatment of IPF by the Food and Drug Administration (FDA) in 2014, a revolutionary act in conditionally recommending treatment in the 2015 ATS/ERS/JRS/ALAT guideline (Saito et al., 2019). However, the current drugs do not reverse the progression of fibrosis and are associated with side effects such as gastrointestinal intolerance and skin reactions (Guo et al., 2019). Currently, lung transplantation is the only available effective treatment strategy of IPF, but is subject to a limited donor organ supply and the wide variability in clinical course (Collard et al., 2016). Thus, the therapy emphasizes the urgent need to develop novel strategies for the prevention and more effective treatment of this refractory respiratory disease.

Since patients with PF mainly present with progressive dyspnea, cough spitting saliva, chest pain, vomiting, dry mouth, shortness of breath, etc., traditional Chinese medicine (TCM) has summarized it as "lung impediment" or "lung wilting" and the earliest descriptions date back to *The Yellow Emperor's Inner Canon (first century C)*, the earliest Chinese medical book. It has been generally accepted that PF is mainly caused by the following key pathogenic factors: six-excess external contraction (Wai gan liu yin), internal damage by the seven affects (Nei shang qi qing), qi deficiency (Qi xu), phlegm-stasis (Tan yu), and blood-stasis (Xue yu). Based on pattern identification as the basis for treatment determination, combined with the application of invigorating the blood circulation and transforming phlegm (Huo xue hua tan), supporting and restoring the normal function (Fu zheng gu ben), and so on, TCM treatment of IPF has obvious advantages in improving symptoms and delaying progression.

Jingyin granule is modified from ancient formula Yinqiao Powder, mainly composed of nine herbs [*Nepeta cataria* Linn. (Jingjie), *Lonicera japonica* Thunb. (Jingyinhua), *Euonymus japonicus* Thunb. (Sijiqing), *Houttuynia cordata* Thunb. (Yuxingcao), *Indigofera tinctoria* Linn. (Daqingye), *Taraxacum mongolicum* Hand. (Pugongying), *Arctium lappa* L. (Niubangzi), *Saposhnikovia divaricata* (Trucz.) Schischk. (Fangfeng), and *Glycyrrhiza uralensis* Fisch. (Gancao)]. Subject to clinical judgment, it has detoxification, analgesic, and anti-inflammatory effects and have been used for pulmonary wind-heat cold, acute bronchitis, and acute pneumonia for more than 40 years. Guidance is provided on the pulmonary syndrome of mild wind-heat (aversion to cold with fever or no fever, red tongue with thin and yellow fur, sore pharynx, cough, scant sputum, etc.) of Coronavirus Disease 2019 (COVID-19) patients by Jingyin granule in "COVID-19 Chinese medicine treatment program (second trial edition) in Shanghai." Jingyin granule has been recommended to the fourth Shanghai's medical assistance team to Wuhan and with good clinical effect on COVID-19 in Raytheon Hospital, Wuhan, Hubei.

A network pharmacology study by Wang et al. identified that Jingyin granule could protect against COVID-19 through 88 target genes, among which NOS2, ADAM17, CDK4, MAPK14, and MAPK1 were the top GO-BP enrichment analysis genes (Wang et al., 2021). As indicated in the Guideline on Diagnosis and Treatment of COVID-19 (Trial Version 7th) that was officially issued by the National Health Commission of the People's Republic of China, interstitial fibrosis of the lung might occur in patients with severe COVID-19 (Zhang et al., 2021). Autopsy on patients who died of COVID-19 also showed disrupted alveolar architecture and fibrosis of the pulmonary interstitium (Huang et al., 2020). Therefore, whether Jingyin granule could prevent PF is worth exploring. The underlying mechanisms should be further explored by pharmacological evaluation, and its potential for the prevention and treatment of PF also needs to be evaluated.

Network pharmacology was first proposed by the UK pharmacologist Andrew L. Hopkins in 2007 (Hopkins, 2007), which integrates several disciplines such as systems biology, network biology, computational biology, multi-target pharmacology, and molecular pharmacology. Network pharmacology is widely used in the research of Chinese medicines as some drugs' potential targets for combating diseases are obtained by utilizing it. Current network pharmacology has made a pivotal contribution to the development of Chinese medicines in the prevention and treatment of PF diseases as well as in the COVID-19 outbreak (Jin et al., 2021).

This study aimed to observe the effects of Jingyin granule on an *in vitro* cell model of PF, determining the protein expression levels of Janus kinase 2/signal transducers and activators of transcription (JAK2/STAT3), the mammalian nuclear factor-κB (NF-κB), the phosphatidylinositol 3-kinase (PI3K)/protein kinase B (Akt), tumor necrosis factor (TNF), and the extracellular signal-regulated kinases 1 and 2 (ERK1/2), and to investigate the anti-fibrotic mechanism in preventing PF.

METHODS

Main Candidate Active Ingredients and Targets of Jingyin Granule

The major components of Jingyin granule were obtained by public database screening and literature review. "Jingjie," "Jinyinhua," "Sijiqing," "Yuxingcao," "Daqingye," "Niubangzi," "Fangfeng," and "Gancao" were respectively retrieved in TCMSP (Traditional Chinese Medicine Systems Pharmacology Database and Analysis Platform, http://tcmspw.com/tcmsp.php), and the active ingredients were selected. The active ingredients of *Taraxacum mongolicum* Hand. (Pugongying) were mainly summarized by searching relevant literatures. The chemical information of main active ingredients was traced back to PubChem database (https://pubchem.ncbi.nlm.nih.gov/). The databases retrieved for potential therapeutic targets of Jingyin granule are the following: TCMSP, SEA (https://sea.bkslab.org/), HitPick (http://mips.helmholtz-muenchen.de/hitpick/), Swiss TargetPrediction (http://www.swisstargetprediction.ch/), and STITCH (http://stitch.embl.de/).

Collection of Pulmonary Fibrosis-Related Targets

The human target genes related to PF were searched from DisGeNET (https://www.disgenet.org/), GeneCards (https://www.genecards.org/), and OMIM (https://www.omim.org/) potential Disease Targets analysis platforms. After data deduplication/integration, intersecting genes were obtained and considered as therapeutic targets relevant to PF. Drug and corresponding target data that have been validated for the treatment of PF were obtained from DrugBank (https://go.drugbank.com/) and TTD (http://db.idrblab.net/ttd/) database.

Drug-Target-Disease Network Construction

The predicted action targets of the compounds in Jingyin granule and PF-related disease targets were imported into the Venn online tool (http://www.bioinformatics.com.cn/) to obtain the common targets and Venn diagram. Then, the intersection targets were confirmed by UniProt (https://www.uniprot.org), and Cytoscape software was used to construct a lung fibrosis target network of the main component actions of Jingyin granule.

Construction of Protein–Protein Interaction Network

To evaluate the importance of the intersection targets, these targets were imported into the STRING database (https://string-db.org/) and Cytoscape software to construct and analyze the PPI network of potential PF targets. The core targets in the PPI network were identified.

Functional Enrichment Analysis of Shared Targets

To explore the biological process of Jingyin granule attenuating PF, the screened 109 targets were subjected to gene ontology (GO) enrichment analysis and Kyoto Encyclopedia of Genes and Genomes (KEGG) pathway enrichment analysis using the clusterProfiler package based on R language with $p < 0.05$, $q < 0.05$ of filtering thresholds.

Molecular Docking of Bioactive Components

To verify the binding ability of key components with key targets and explore their accurate binding modes, molecular docking simulation is usually used with the PDB database (http://www.rcsb.org/), PyMOL (2.0) software (http://www.pymol.org/2/), and AutoDock Vina software (http://vina.scripps.edu/). We selected representative targets as receptors in the PPI network and used the representative therapeutic ingredients as the ligand of molecular docking.

Experiment Validation

Materials and Methods

Chemicals and Instruments

Arctigenin (CAS: 7770-78-7, MW: 372.41, purity ≥98%), quercetin (CAS: 117-39-5, MW: 302.24, purity ≥97%), luteolin (CAS: 491-70-3, MW: 286.24, purity ≥98%), kaempferol (CAS: 520-18-3, MW: 286.24, purity ≥98%), rutin (CAS: 153-18-4, MW: 610.52, purity ≥98%), gallic acid (CAS: 149-91-7, MW: 170.12, purity ≥98%), and chlorogenic acid (CAS: 327-97-9, MW: 354.31, purity ≥98%) were purchased from Shanghai Yuanye Bio-technology Co. Ltd. (Shanghai, China). A Waters Acquity UPLC coupled with a Xevo G2-XS Q-TOF quadrupole mass spectrometer was used (Waters Co., Milford, MA, United States).

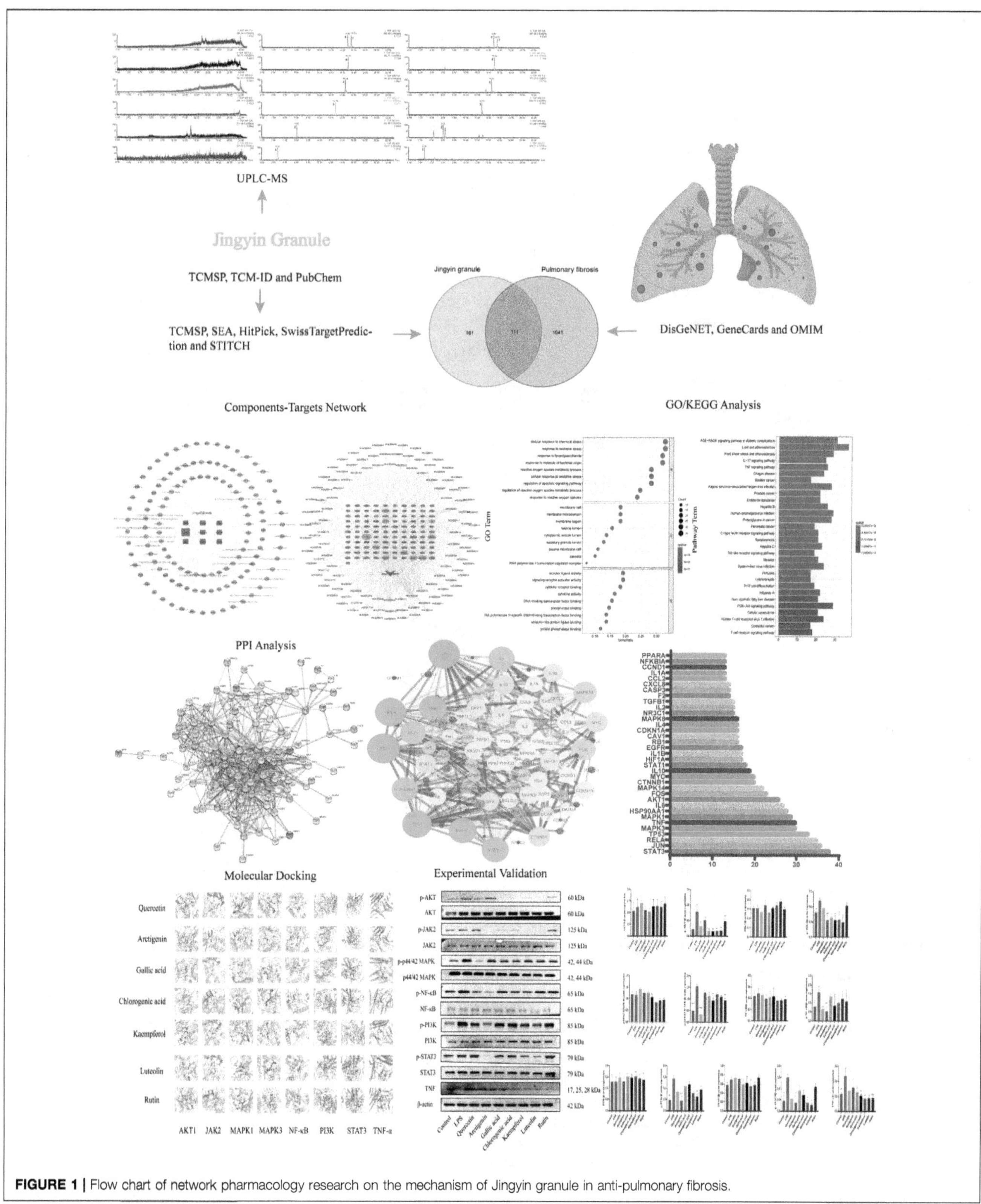

FIGURE 1 | Flow chart of network pharmacology research on the mechanism of Jingyin granule in anti-pulmonary fibrosis.

UPLC Analysis

The Jingyin granule (2 g, lot# 200302) was dissolved with methanol and vortex mixed for 15 s. The solution was in an ultrasonic water for 30 min. Then, the solution was centrifuged at 12,000 rpm for 10 min, and the supernatant was fixed to 25 ml with methanol. Aliquot (1 μl) was injected into UHPLC-MS for

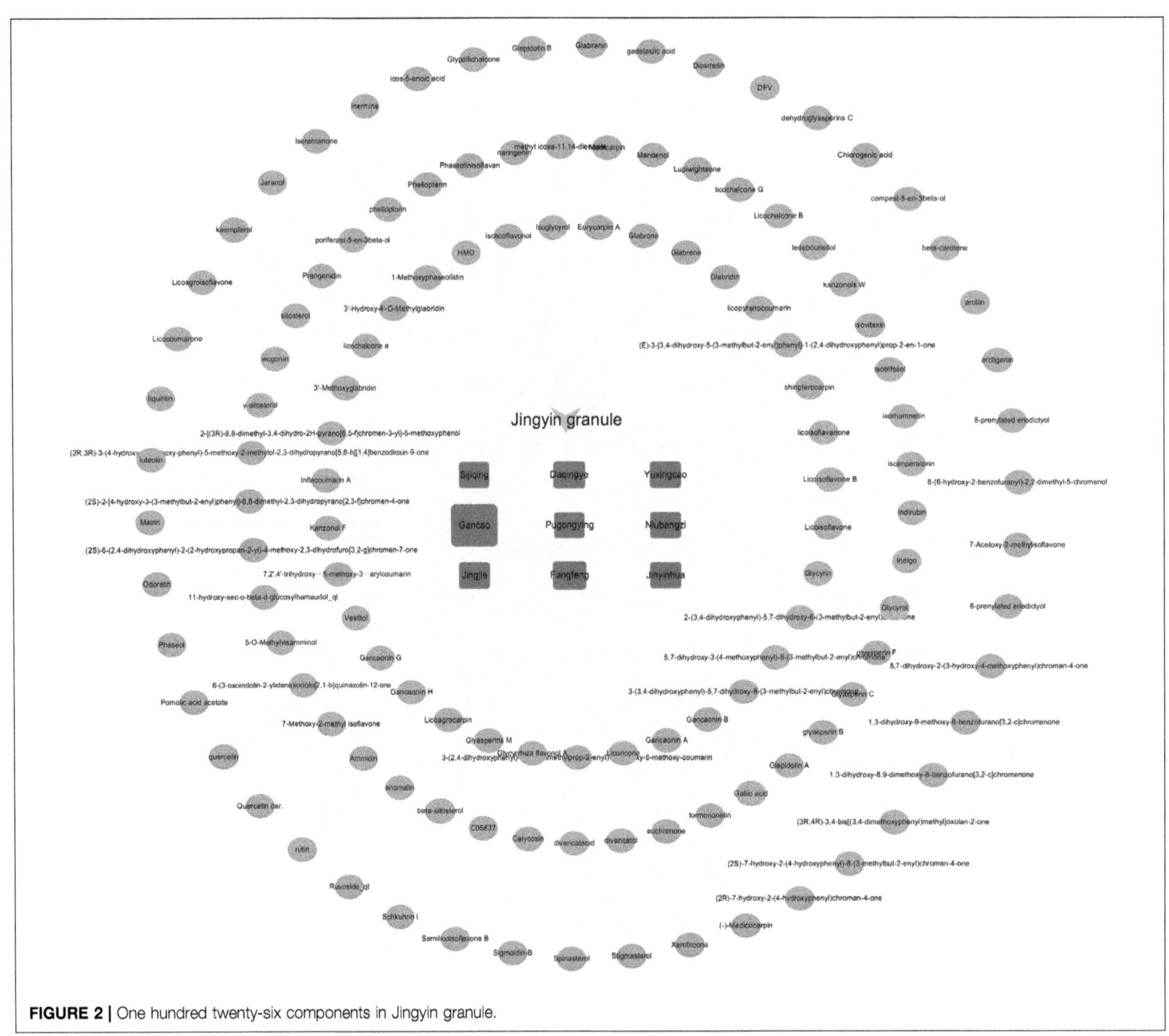

FIGURE 2 | One hundred twenty-six components in Jingyin granule.

TABLE 1 | Information on representative chemical constituents of Jingyin granule.

MOL ID	Mol name	CAS	Smile	Formula	Lipinski	Solubility	Bioavailability	GI absorption
MOL000523	Arctigenin	7770-78-7	COC1 = C(C=C(C=C1)CC2COC(=O)C2CC3 = CC(=C(C=C3)O)OC)OC	$C_{21}H_{24}O_6$	Yes	Moderately soluble	0.55	High
MOL000098	Quercetin	117-39-5	C1 = CC(=C(C=C1C2 = C(C(=O)C3 = C(C=C(C=C3O2)O)O)O)O)O	$C_{15}H_{10}O_7$	Yes	Soluble	0.55	High
MOL000006	Luteolin	491-70-3	C1 = CC(=C(C=C1C2 = CC(=O)C3 = C(C=C(C=C3O2)O)O)O)O	$C_{15}H_{10}O_6$	Yes	Soluble	0.55	High
MOL000415	Rutin	153-18-4	CC1C(C(C(C(O1)OCC2C(C(C(C(O2)OC3 = C(OC4 = CC(=CC(=C4C3 = O)O)O)C5 = CC(=C(C=C5)O)O)O)O)O)O)O)O	$C_{27}H_{30}O_{16}$	No	Soluble	0.17	Low
MOL000513	Gallic acid	149-91-7	C1 = C(C=C(C(=C1O)O)O)C (=O)O	$C_7H_6O_5$	Yes	Very soluble	0.56	High
MOL000422	Kaempferol	520-18-3	C1 = CC(=CC = C1C2 = C(C(=O)C3 = C(C=C(C=C3O2)O)O)O)O	$C_{15}H_{10}O_6$	Yes	Soluble	0.55	High
MOL003871	Chlorogenic acid	327-97-9	C1C(C(C(CC1(C (=O)O)O)OC(=O)C=CC2 = CC(=C(C=C2)O)O)O)O	$C_{16}H_{18}O_9$	Yes	Very soluble	0.11	Low

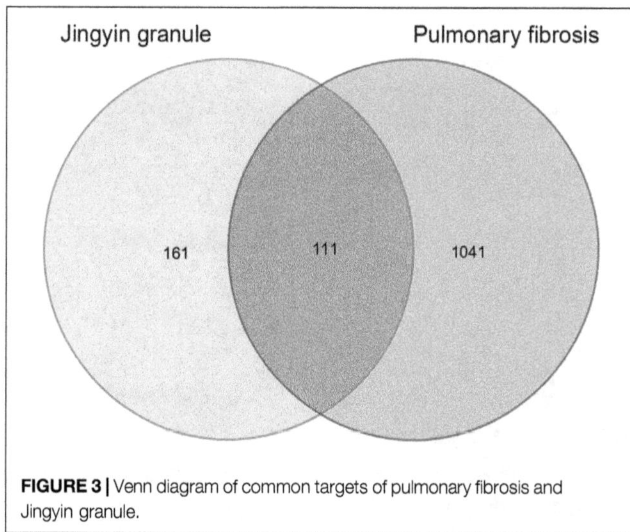

FIGURE 3 | Venn diagram of common targets of pulmonary fibrosis and Jingyin granule.

analysis. All separations of Jingyin granule were performed using a Waters Acquity UPLC T3-C18 column (100 × 2.1 mm, 1.7 μm, Waters Co., Milford, MA). The flow rate was 0.2 ml/min, and the column temperature was 40°C. The mobile phase was 0.1% formic acid water (phase A) and methanol (phase B) with gradient elution, and the elution program was: 0–4 min, 90%–75%A; 4–8 min, 75%–75%A; 8–13 min, 75%–40%A; 13–18 min, 40%–25%A; 18–20 min, 25%–2%A; 20–21 min, 2%–90%A; 21–23 min, 90%–90%A.

Mass spectrometric analysis was performed by both positive and negative ion modes, sensitivity mode (resolution: 30,000). Capillary voltage: 3.0 kV; sample cone voltage: 40 V; source offset voltage: 80 V; source temperature: 120°C; desolvation temperature: 450°C; cone gas: 50 L/h; desolvation gas: 800 L/h; nebulizer pressure: 6.0 bar; mass number correction range: *m/z* 50–800; correction solution: 0.5 mM sodium formate solution; flow rate: 10 μl/min; real-time correction lock spray: 1 ng/UL leucine enkephalin solution, *m/z* 556.2771. Data acquisition was performed using MSE, data types were continuous, energy range was 25–35 V, and scanning time was 0.2 s.

Cell Culture

A549 cells were purchased from the Cell Bank of Chinese Academy of Sciences and cultured at 37°C in a humidified atmosphere of 5% CO_2 and 95% air and in sterile DMEM-H supplemented with 10% fetal bovine serum (Gibco, USA), 100 U/ml penicillin, and 100 ng/ml streptomycin. Cells were seeded in 6-well plates and cultured for 24 h at 37°C. When the A549 cells reached 70%–80% confluence, the culture medium of the cells was replaced with DMEM-H supplemented with 1% fetal bovine serum, 100 U/ml penicillin, and 100 ng/ml streptomycin for 12 h. After that, the cell culture medium was replaced with DMEM-H supplemented with 2% fetal bovine serum, and then treated with 10 μg/ml LPS (from *Escherichia coli* 0111: B4, Sigma-Aldrich, St. Louis, MO, USA) and arctigenin, quercetin, luteolin, kaempferol, rutin, gallic acid, and chlorogenic acid alone or in combination for up to 24 h, respectively.

TABLE 2 | Shared hub targets between pulmonary fibrosis and Jingyin granule.

Number	Gene name	Number	Gene name	Number	Gene name
1	TGFB1	38	CDK4	75	PLAT
2	TNF	39	ALOX5	76	PARP1
3	SLC6A4	40	VCAM1	77	NOS3
4	SCN5A	41	STAT3	78	NFKBIA
5	RELA	42	STAT1	79	NFE2L2
6	PTGS2	43	SOD1	80	MYC
7	PTGS1	44	SLPI	81	MPO
8	PRSS1	45	SELE	82	MMP9
9	PRKACA	46	RB1	83	MMP3
10	PPARG	47	PSMD3	84	MMP2
11	NOS2	48	PPARA	85	MET
12	MAPK14	49	MT-ND6	86	MDM2
13	KDR	50	MAPK8	87	IRF1
14	JUN	51	MAPK3	88	IL2
15	IFNG	52	MAPK10	89	IL1B
16	HSP90AA1	53	MAPK1	90	IL1A
17	F2	54	INSR	91	IL10
18	CYP1A1	55	IL4	92	IGFBP3
19	CHRM3	56	ICAM1	93	IGF2
20	CDKN3	57	HMOX1	94	HIF1A
21	CCL5	58	HMGCR	95	GJA1
22	CASP8	59	GSTM1	96	FOS
23	CASP3	60	GSR	97	F3
24	BCL2	61	CYP3A4	98	ERBB2
25	ADRB2	62	CYP1B1	99	EGFR
26	CCL2	63	APOB	100	CXCL2
27	TP53	64	ADIPOQ	101	CXCL10
28	PRKCD	65	ABCC1	102	CRP
29	NR3C2	66	PTEN	103	CD40LG
30	MMP1	67	CDKN2A	104	CAV1
31	IL6	68	TYR	105	BCL2L1
32	FN1	69	TOP1	106	ALB
33	F10	70	THBD	107	CTNNB1
34	CXCL8	71	SPP1	108	MUC1
35	CDKN1A	72	SERPINE1	109	NR3C1
36	CCND1	73	RAF1	110	INS
37	AKT1	74	PLAU	111	FASLG

Western Blot Analysis

For Western blot analysis, cell lysate was added after the cells were washed three times by PBS. The isolated proteins were quantified and separated on sodium dodecyl sulfate polyacrylamide gel electrophoresis (SDS-PAGE) (10%), transferred onto a PVDF membrane, and blocked with 5% BSA. After blocking, the proteins were incubated with antibodies overnight at 4°C with primary antibody β-actin (1: 3,000, Affinity, USA), Phospho-AKT (1:1,000, Proteintech, USA), AKT (1:1,000, CST, USA), JAK2 (1:1,000, CST, USA), Phospho-JAK2 (1:1,000, CST, USA), p44/42 MAPK (ERK1/2) (1: 1,000, CST, USA), Phospho-p44/42 MAPK (ERK1/2) (1:1,000, CST, USA), STAT3 (1:1,000, CST, USA), Phospho-STAT3 (1: 1,000, CST, USA), NF-κB (1:1,000, CST, USA), Phospho-NF-κB (1:1,000, CST, USA), PI3K (1:1,000, CST, USA), Phospho-PI3K (1:1,000, CST, USA), and TNF-α (1:1,000, CST, USA), followed by horseradish peroxidase (HRP)-linked anti-rabbit (1:2,000, CST, USA) or anti-mouse (1:2,000, CST, USA). The protein bands were analyzed by Tanon 4600SF (Tiangong Technology Co., Ltd., Shanghai, China) with chemiluminescence substrate.

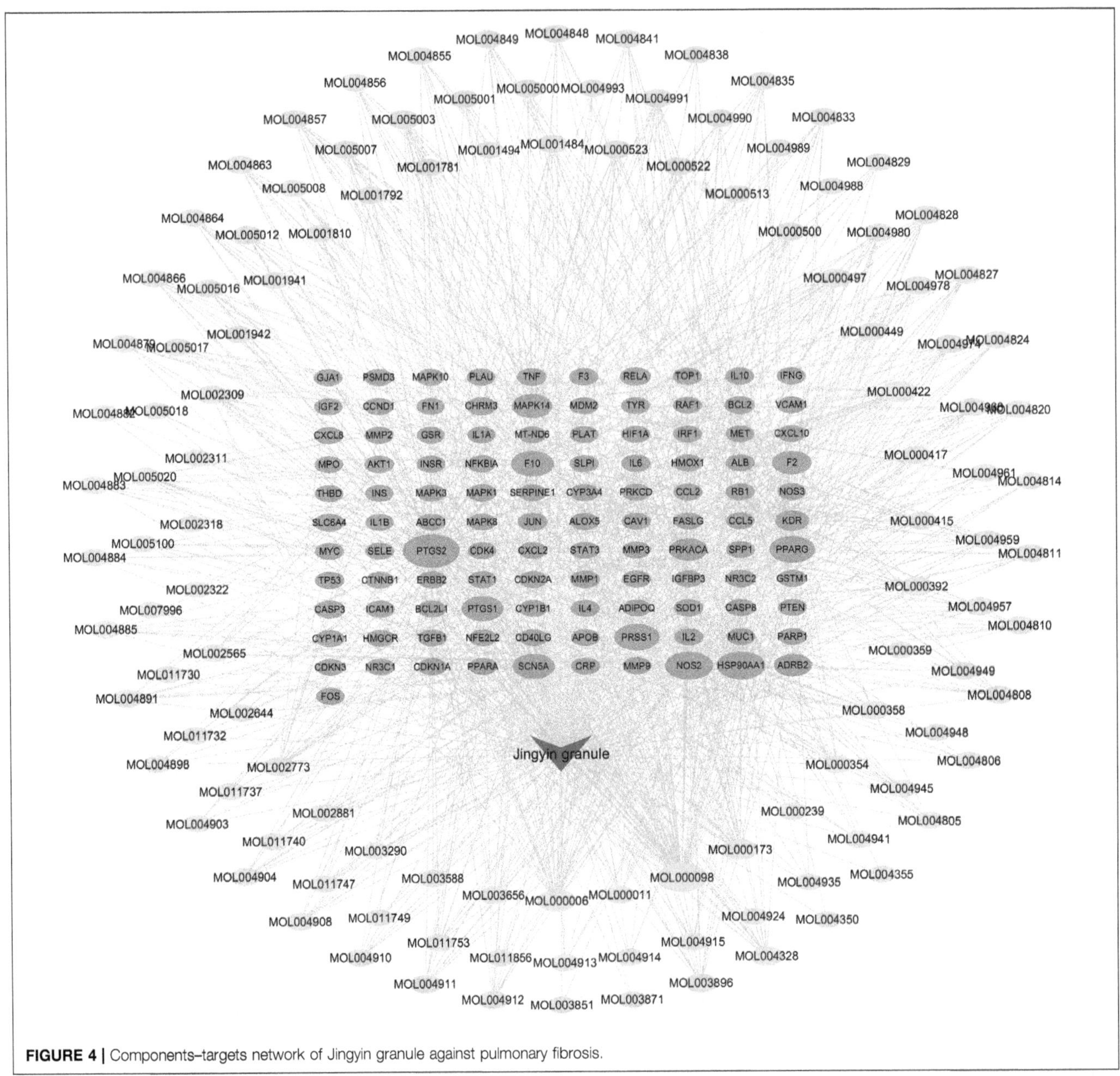

FIGURE 4 | Components–targets network of Jingyin granule against pulmonary fibrosis.

Statistical Analysis

SPSS 25.0 software and GraphPad Prism 8.0.2 software were used for data analysis and processing, and the results were expressed as mean ± standard deviation (SD). One-way analysis of variance (ANOVA) was used for comparisons between groups. Values of $p < 0.05$ were considered statistically significant.

RESULTS

Based on the multi-component, multi-target, and multi-channel function of Chinese medicines, this study found the mechanism of the anti-PF effect of Jingyin granule, which provides a theoretical basis for Jingyin granule in the treatment of PF. This workflow is shown in **Figure 1**.

Active Components and Predicted Therapeutic Targets Results of Jingyin Granule

A total of 126 major chemical constituents of Jingyin granule were obtained from TCMSP public databases combined with literature screening public databases (**Figure 2**). ADMET properties of seven of the active ingredients were evaluated using ACD/labs software and the SwissADME online system (http://www.swissadme.ch/), as shown in **Table 1**. The most relevant targets were selected based on the target information of each database, with TC > 0.4 in SEA,

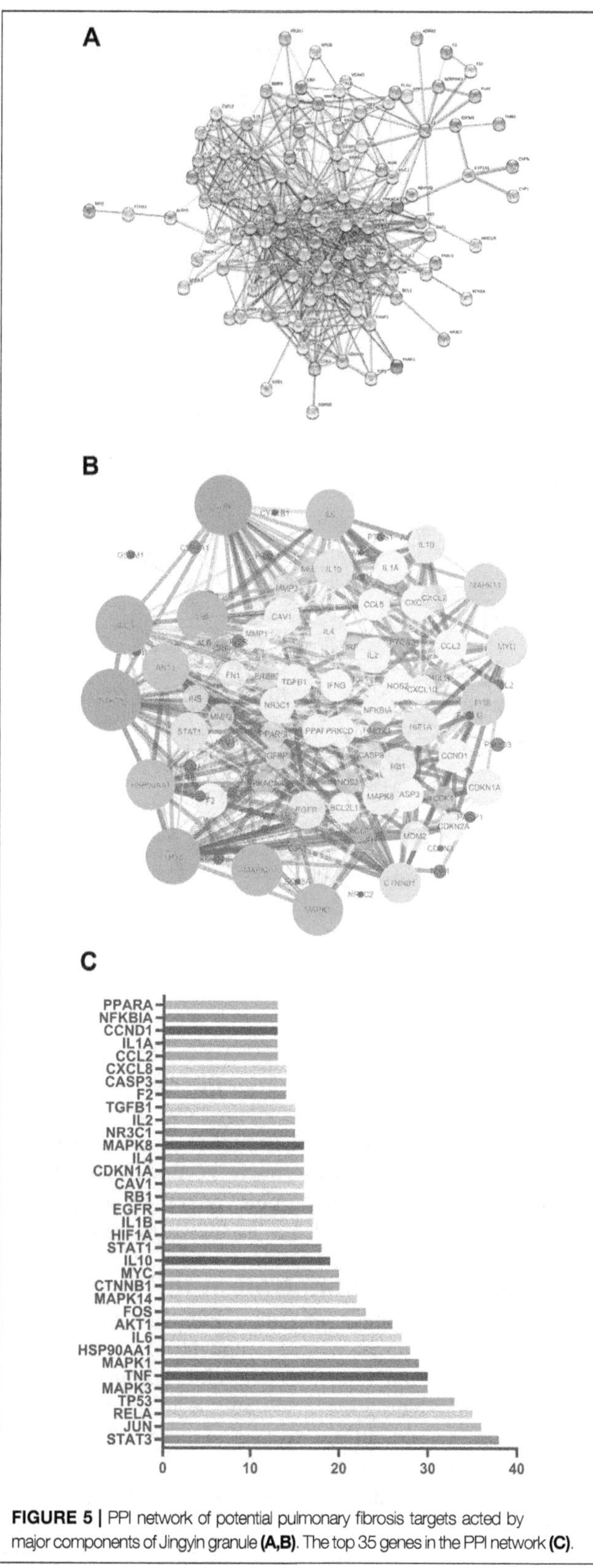

FIGURE 5 | PPI network of potential pulmonary fibrosis targets acted by major components of Jingyin granule **(A,B)**. The top 35 genes in the PPI network **(C)**.

precision >50% in HitPick, the top 15 with the highest scoring value in swisstargetprediction, and stitch based on a score >0.4. A total of 272 potential targets were obtained.

Collection of Disease Targets

PF-related targets were searched in DisGeNET, GeneCards, OMIM, DrugBank, and TTD databases. A total of 1,152 targets were obtained after merging and deleting duplicate values. As shown in **Figure 3**, 111 predicted targets were obtained after the Jingyin granule-related targets were mapped to PF-related targets using the Venn. The details of common target genes are shown in **Table 2**. The 111 targets of intersection were confirmed by UniProt database, and a lung fibrosis–target network of the main components acting on Jingyin granule was constructed by Cytoscape software (**Figure 4**).

PPI Network Analysis Results

A predicted PPI relationship network about 111 predicted targets was constructed in STRING and visualized by Cytoscape (**Figures 5A,B**). The 35 genes in the PPI network have much higher network degree value, betweenness, and closeness centrality compared with the other genes (**Figure 5C**).

GO Analysis and KEGG Pathway Enrichment Analysis of Shared Targets

In order to clarify the biological mechanisms of Jingyin granule against PF, the enrichment analysis of GO and KEGG pathway on 111 targets were performed by the cluster Profiler package based on R language. The GO enrichment analysis annotated the function of key genes from three terms: biological processes (BP), cellular component (CC), and molecular function (MF). A total of 2,709 GO terms were obtained based on *p*-value, and the top 9 items of three parts were selected (**Figure 6**). The BP was related to cellular response to chemical stress (GO: 0062197), response to oxidative stress (GO: 0006979), response to lipopolysaccharide (GO: 0032496), response to molecule of bacterial origin (GO: 0002237), reactive oxygen species metabolic process (GO: 0072593), cellular response to oxidative stress (GO: 0034599), regulation of apoptotic signaling pathway (GO: 2001233), regulation of reactive oxygen species metabolic process (GO: 2000377), and response to reactive oxygen species (GO: 0000302). The MF was related to receptor ligand activity (GO: 0048018), signaling receptor activator activity (GO: 0030546), cytokine receptor binding (GO: 0005126), cytokine activity (GO: 0005125), DNA-binding transcription factor binding (GO: 0140297), phosphatase binding (GO: 0019902), RNA polymerase II-specific DNA-binding transcription factor binding (GO: 0061629), ubiquitin-like protein ligase binding (GO: 0044389), and protein phosphatase binding (GO: 0019903). The CC was related to membrane raft (GO: 0045121), membrane microdomain (GO: 0098857), membrane region (GO: 0098589), vesicle lumen (GO: 0031983), cytoplasmic vesicle lumen (GO: 0060205), secretory granule lumen (GO: 0034774), plasma membrane raft (GO: 0044853), caveola (GO: 0005901), and RNA polymerase II transcription regulator complex (GO: 0090575). A total of 177 KEGG pathways were obtained based on *p*-value, and the top 30 were selected, such as the AGE-RAGE signaling pathway (hsa04933), TNF signaling pathway (hsa04668), Toll-like receptor (TLR) signaling pathway (hsa04620), and PI3K-Akt signaling pathway (hsa04151) (**Figure 7**). Then, a Target

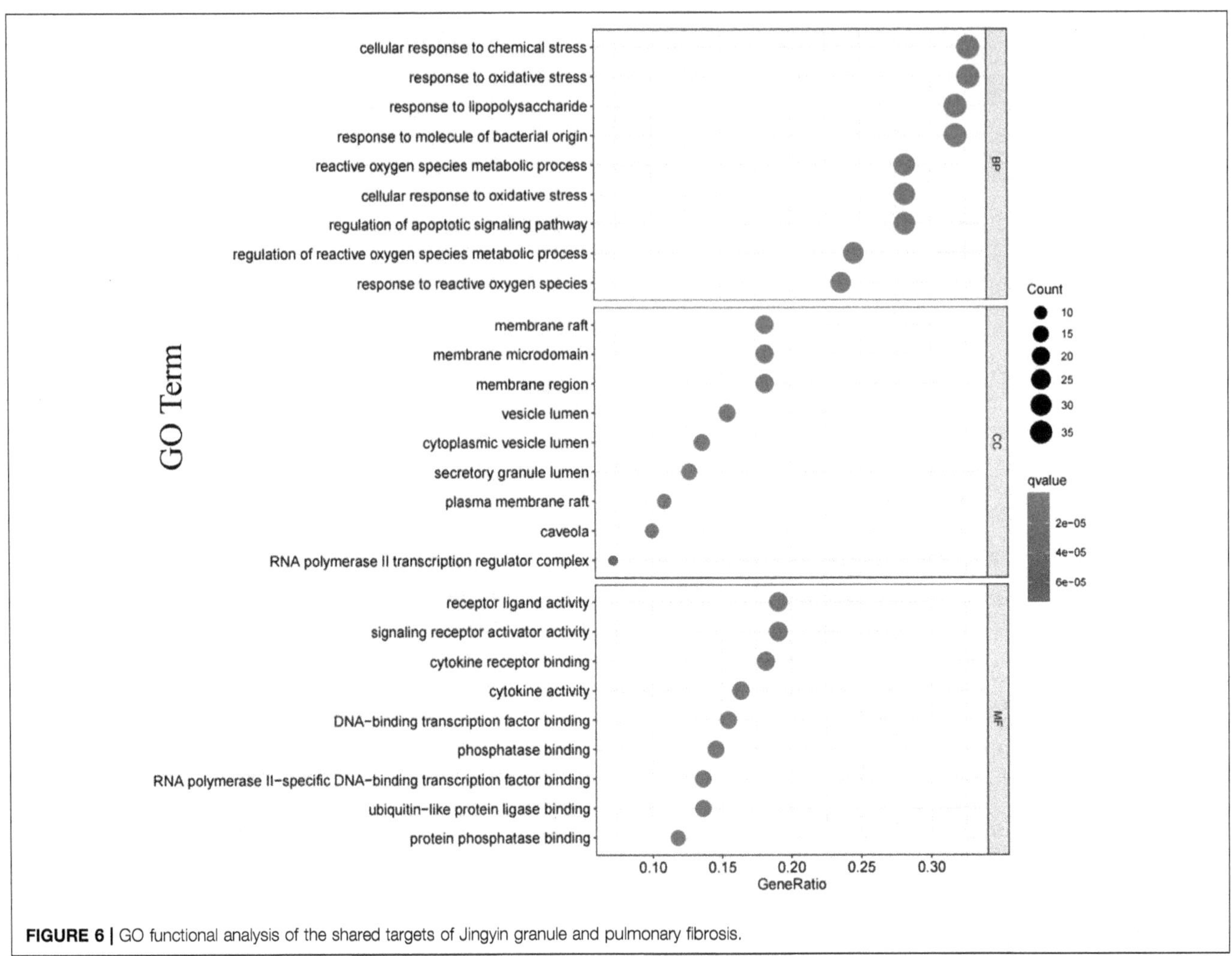

FIGURE 6 | GO functional analysis of the shared targets of Jingyin granule and pulmonary fibrosis.

Genes–Pathways Network was constructed to reveal the relationship between hub targets and pathways intuitively (**Figure 8**).

The Molecular Docking of Representative Components and Core Target Proteins

Seven components were comprehensively selected on the basis of higher degree value in active ingredient–target network, higher content of components in lung, and higher content in Jingyin granule, respectively: arctigenin, quercetin, luteolin, kaempferol, rutin, gallic acid, and chlorogenic acid. The eight core target proteins (AKT1, JAK2, MAPK1, MAPK3, RELA, PI3K, STAT3, and TNF) with high degrees were selected as receptors. The selected compounds showed basically moderate binding potential to receptor proteins with good drug reference values (**Figure 9A**). The docking scores among them are shown in a heatmap (**Figure 9B**).

UPLC-MS Analysis

As a rapid, intelligent, reliable, and accurate technique for identification of chemical constituents, UPLC-MS is widely used in the field of TCM. The UPLC-MS method was used to identify the key components previously selected in Jingyin granule, and the typical chromatograms are shown in **Figure 10**. These seven compounds were identified unambiguously by comparing their accurate masses and retention times with those of pure reference compounds. Molecular weights and details are as shown in **Table 3**.

Experimental Demonstration *In Vitro*

Based on the results of the PPI network, active compounds–disease targets network, and literature data, seven components (arctigenin, quercetin, luteolin, kaempferol, rutin, gallic acid, and chlorogenic acid) and eight targets (AKT1, JAK2, MAPK1, MAPK3, RELA, PI3K, STAT3, and TNF) played crucial roles in anti-PF. To explore the effects of anti-PF, 50 μM quercetin, 200 μM arctigenin, 75 μM gallic acid, 400 μM chlorogenic acid, 50 μM kaempferol, 50 μM luteolin, and 40 μM rutin were used. As per the results obtained, the expression of AKT1, JAK2, MAPK1, MAPK3, RELA, PI3K, STAT3, and TNF was decreased significantly after drug intervention compared with that in the model group ($p < 0.05$ or $p < 0.01$) (**Figures 11A–N**).

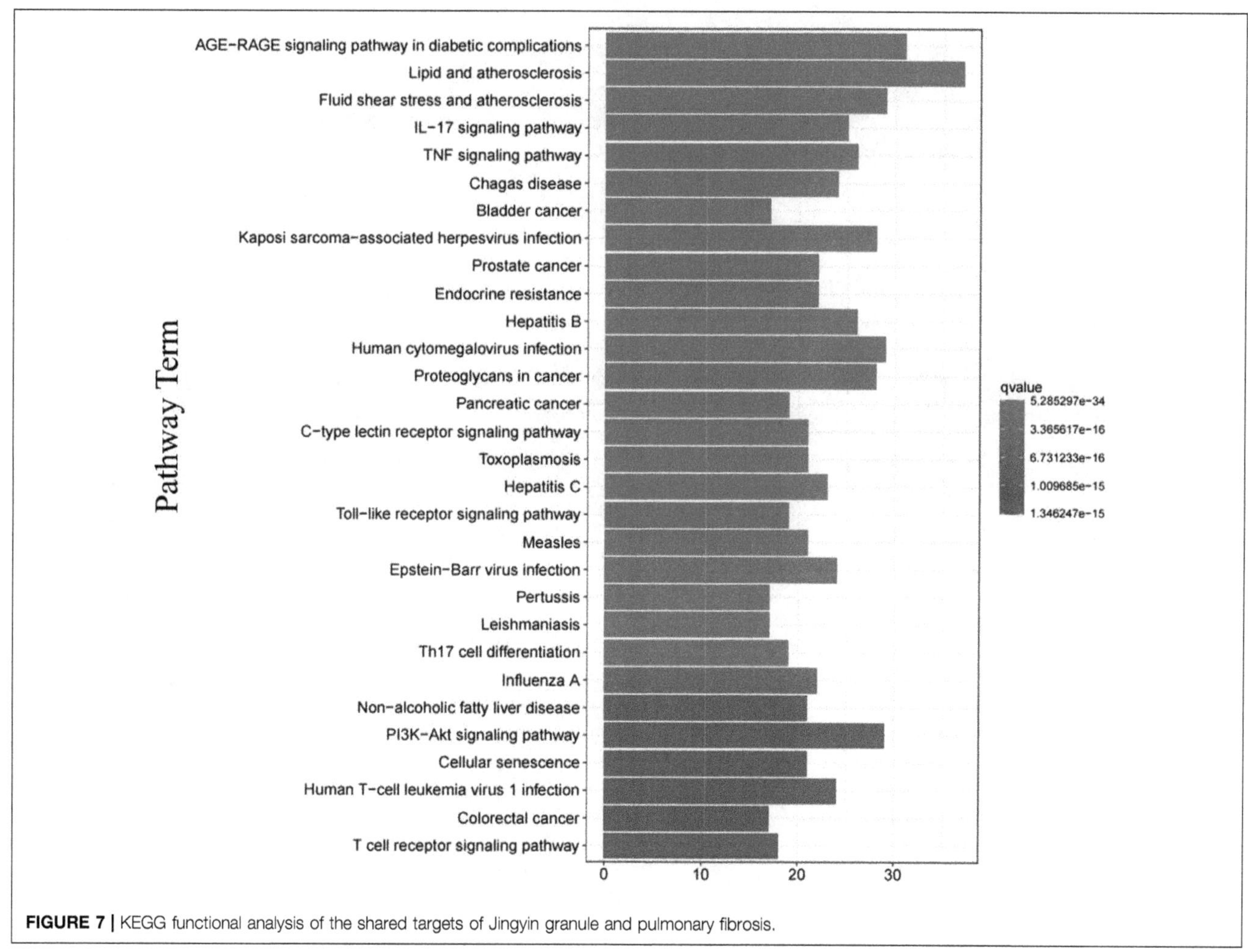

FIGURE 7 | KEGG functional analysis of the shared targets of Jingyin granule and pulmonary fibrosis.

DISCUSSION

The lung has the remarkable ability to repair and recover in response to constant exposure to many injuries, through a cascade of finally synchronized biological processes (Martinez et al., 2017). However, repeated microinjury to alveolar epithelial tissues may result in loss of epithelial integrity and dysregulation of regeneration; excessive repair may predispose the individual to PF. Those external stressors of epithelial damage include environmental and occupational factors such as smoking, viral infections and peripheral lung traction injury, genetic risk, and certain comorbidities (Selman et al., 2001). IPF, as a specific form of chronic, progressive lung disease of unknown cause, is characterized by decline in lung function, worsening quality of life, and early mortality (Cottin et al., 2019), but all currently relevant drugs can only delay lung failure, not reverse the course of PF, and have unavoidable side effects.

Based on syndrome differentiation, IPF is treated through a staged, multi-level dialectical application, and more comprehensive ideas and methods are also being used by TCM, such as staging treatment, prescription treatment, collateral treatment, and acupuncture combined with internal and external treatment (Zhang et al., 2021). Either as monotherapy or in combination with standard Western medical treatment, Chinese medicines usually exert a wider action spectrum in managing the entire medical disorders by the effects of synergism and attenuation (Wang, 2013). Multiple studies have demonstrated that the active agents of single herbs and Chinese medicine formulas, in particular, the flavonoids, terpenes, and alkaloids, have significant therapeutic effects on IPF, the related mechanisms of which appear to involve the regulation of inflammation, oxidant stress, and pro-fibrotic signaling pathways, among others (Li and Kan, 2017).

Jingyin granule obtained new drug approval in China in 2009 as a prescription for anti-atypical pneumonia and is recommended as a reserve medication in Shanghai for the prevention and treatment of H1N1 infection and COVID-19. The prescription of Jingyin granule is complex with many ingredients, some of which have been proven to possess potential benefits in antifibrotic treatment. Miao et al. (2019) demonstrated the protective effects of the water extract of *Lonicera japonica* Thunb. from liver fibrosis in mice treated with carbon tetrachloride (CCl_4), the mechanism of which was inhibition of hepatic stellate cells (HSCs) activation, liver

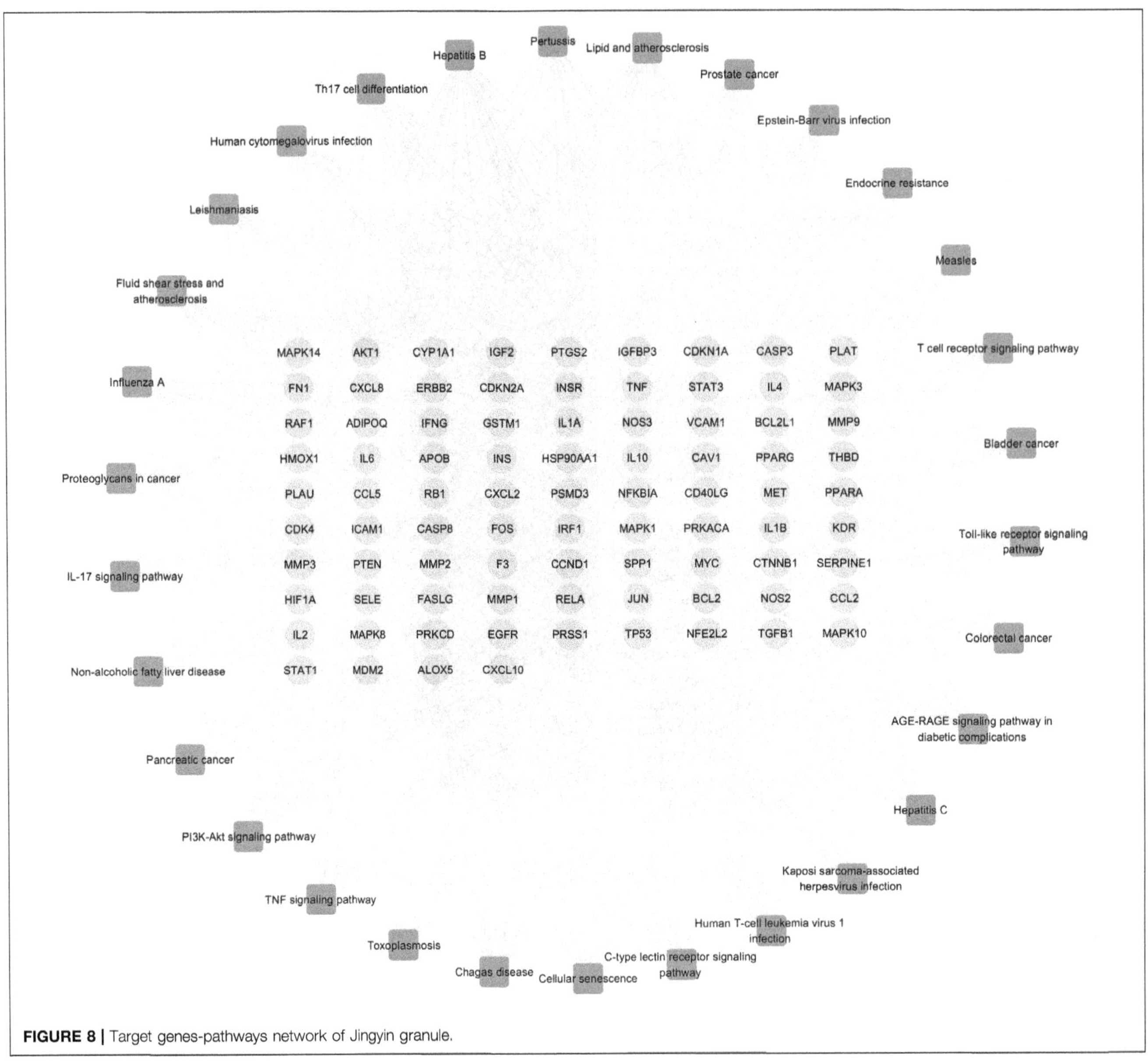

FIGURE 8 | Target genes-pathways network of Jingyin granule.

oxidative stress injury, and the epithelial–mesenchymal transition (EMT) process. The current study found that *H. cordata* Thunb. aqueous extract had obvious antioxidant and protective effects on rats with bleomycin-induced PF (Ng et al., 2007). Our previous network pharmacology study of *H. cordata* Thunb. identified that it may act through multiple signaling pathways to alleviate PF (Zhu et al., 2021). Our *in vivo* experimental study also clarified that sodium houttuyfonate, an adduct compound of houttuynin and sodium bisulfite, may alleviate the degree of fibrosis in bleomycin-induced PF model mice through the transforming growth factor-β (TGF-β)/Smads pathway (Shen et al., 2021). Arctigenin, the main element of *A. lappa* L., has multiple anti-visceral fibrotic functions, such as reversing TGF-β1-induced renal tubular EMT-like changes (Li et al., 2015) and reversing the EMT process in alveolar type II cells in paraquat (PQ)-induced lung fibrosis by the Wnt3a/β-catenin pathway (Gao et al., 2020). In addition, glycyrrhizic acid has been reported to show antifibrosis outcomes in PF and liver fibrosis (Gao et al., 2015; Liang et al., 2015).

We screened out a total of 126 active compounds (after deduplication) from 9 kinds of medicinal herbs in Jingyin granule through TCMSP database and literature search, according to the ADME principle (setting OB $\geq$ 30 and DL $\geq$ 0.18) (Tsaioun et al., 2016). Their corresponding target genes were then retrieved through the database and intersected on PF-related disease targets, resulting in 111 common target genes. The KEGG pathway enrichment analysis revealed the 142 significant ($p < 0.001$) possible pathways against PF including AGE-RAGE, TNF, IL-17, TLR, PI3K/Akt, and MAPK signaling pathway. After that, a PPI predictive relationship network of 111 predicted

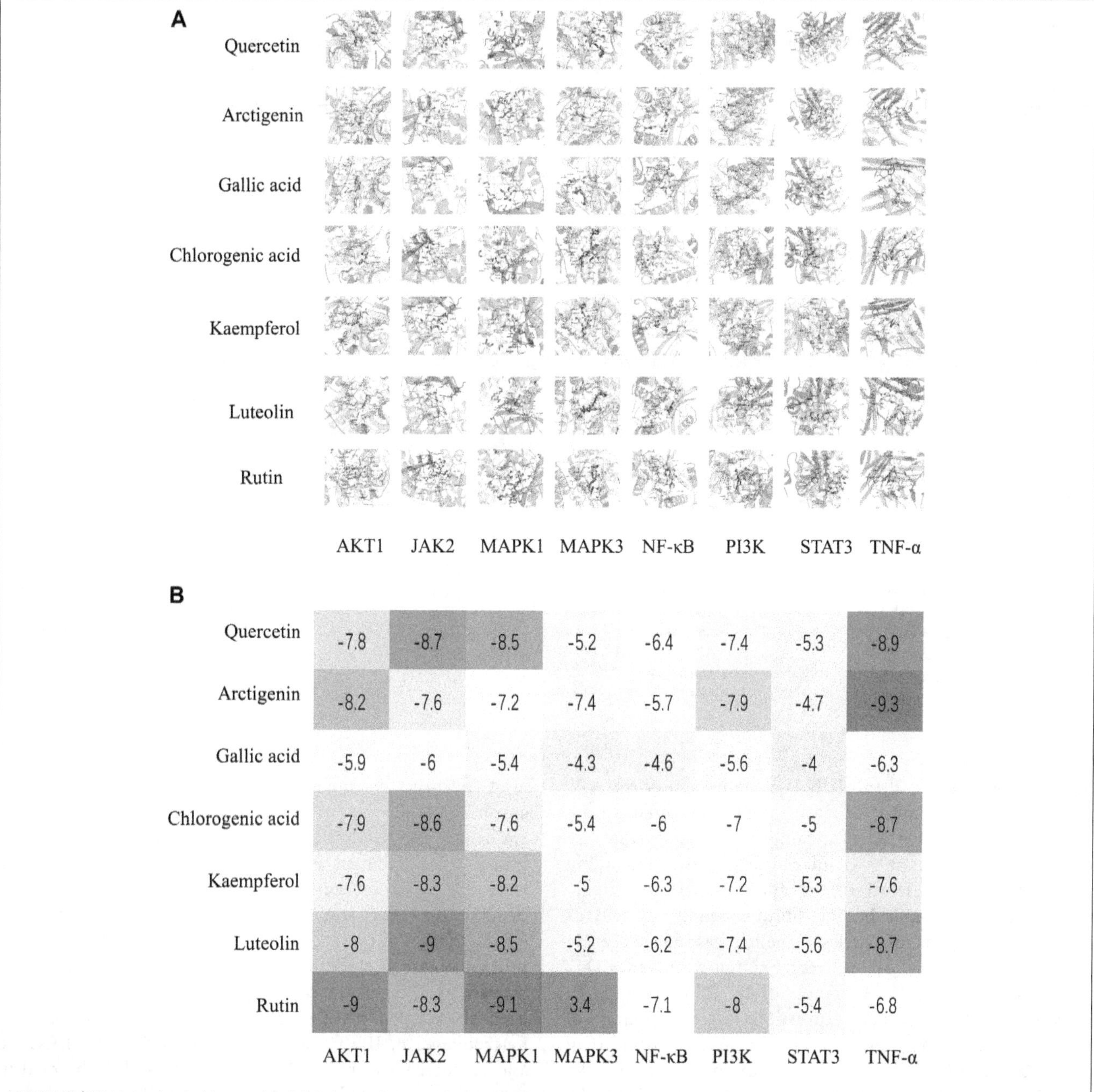

FIGURE 9 | (A) Molecular docking results of Jingyin granule components and selected targets. **(B)** The docking scores of Jingyin granule components and core targets.

targets was constructed and revealed the top 10 hub genes, namely, STAT3, JUN, RELA, TP53, MAPK3, TNF, MAPK1, HSP90AA1, IL6, and AKT1.

IL-6 is a proinflammatory factor that was found to be elevated in the serum of patients with fibrotic diseases (Le et al., 2014). STATs mainly function as transcription factors and have seven member families (STAT1, STAT2, STAT3, STAT4, STAT5A, STAT5b, and STAT6) that regulate several physiological life activities, such as anti-inflammation. STAT3 together with JAK2 and their phosphorylated forms have all been examined in fibrotic lungs from patients with IPF (Milara et al., 2018). The IL-6/STAT3 signaling axis has been shown to play essential roles in the development of inflammatory and fibrotic diseases (O'Donoghue et al., 2012). JAKs are triggered by the activation of members of the IL-6 family that mediates subsequent phosphorylation and activation of STAT3. IL-6-mediated JAK/STAT3 signaling plays a vital role in the airway remodeling of asthma, and its inhibition prevents airway inflammation and remodeling, and blocks Th2 and Th17 cell expansion in a murine asthma

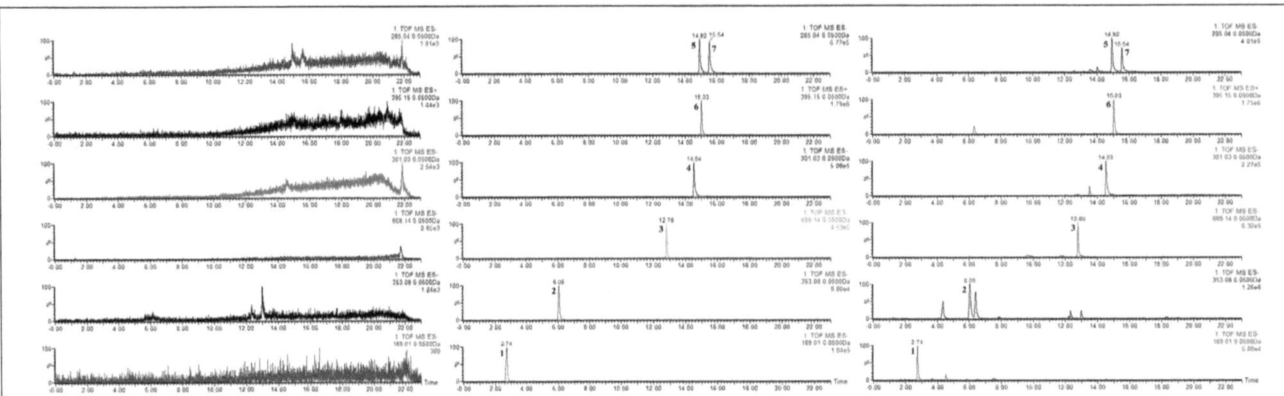

FIGURE 10 | Chromatograms of the seven compounds detected in Jingyin granule. (1: gallic acid, 2: chlorogenic acid, 3: rutin, 4: quercetin, 5: luteolin, 6: arctigenin, 7: kaempferol).

TABLE 3 | Results of qualitative validation for the seven compounds detected in Jingyin granule.

No.	Compound name	CAS	Molecular formula	*m/z*	Retention time
1	Gallic acid	149-91-7	$C_7H_6O_5$	169.0132	2.74
2	Chlorogenic acid	327-97-9	$C_{16}H_{18}O_9$	353.0854	6.05
3	Rutin	153-18-4	$C_{27}H_{30}O_{16}$	609.1447	12.79
4	Quercetin	117-39-5	$C_{15}H_{10}O_7$	301.0337	14.54
5	Luteolin	491-70-3	$C_{15}H_{10}O_6$	285.0381	14.92
6	Arctigenin	7770-78-7	$C_{21}H_{24}O_6$	395.1475	15.03
7	Kaempferol	520-18-3	$C_{15}H_{10}O_6$	285.0381	15.54

model (Gavino et al., 2016). JUN is a component of the AP1 family of transcription factors that coordinates the transcriptional regulation of a multitude of genes that are essential for many cellular processes, including differentiation, proliferation, and apoptosis. JUN is highly expressed in all major human fibrotic conditions and as a downstream gene of MAPK-signaling cascades (Wernig et al., 2017). It has been proved that Jun-mediated CD47 enhancer activation can be amplified by IL-6, resulting in increased CD47 protein expression and induction of profibrotic and immunosuppressive gene expression (Cui et al., 2020). P65-RelA is a subunit of the NF-κB family. NF-κB activation is generally considered central to the innate immune response and will lead to exacerbated chronic inflammation and further reduced lung function. MAPK3 (ERK1) and MAPK1 (ERK2), the earliest identified MAPK pathways, are involved in growth factor signaling and regulate various cellular processes including cell proliferation, differentiation, and apoptosis. ERK1/2 can be activated by the IL-6-type family cytokine (Heinrich et al., 2003). Galuppo et al. (2011) confirmed that inhibition of MEK and ERK1/2 by PD98059, a highly selective inhibitor of MAP/ERK kinase1 (MEK1) activation, reduces lung injury and inflammation in a mouse model of bleomycin-induced PF. Similarly, Madala et al. (2012) demonstrated that selective inhibition of MEK prevents progression of lung fibrosis in the TGF-α-induced model. However, current studies also found that ERK1/2 activation in epithelial and endothelial cells subsides, accompanying progression of fibrosis in IPF, and by the later stage of IPF when fibroblast differentiation predominates, inhibition of ERK1/2 may promote IPF progression instead (Yoshida et al., 2002; Lai et al., 2016). AKT1, also referred to as protein kinase B alpha, is one of the three members of the human AKT serine–threonine protein kinase family. It has been shown that p-AKT1 was increased 3-fold in alveolar macrophages of IPF patients compared with normal tissues, and an increase in p-AKT1 expression was also observed in macrophages isolated from the lungs of BLM injured mice (Larson-Casey et al., 2016). Overexpressed AKT1 can increase mitophagy to increase macrophage-derived TGF-β1 expression and apoptosis resistance, thereby promoting fibrosis progression in mice.

Evidence suggests that lipopolysaccharide (LPS), as one of the pathogens that induce acute lung injury, can increase reactive oxygen species (ROS) and TGF-β production and macrophage infiltration, thereby promoting alveolar epithelial mesenchymal transition (EMT) and lung fibrosis (Qiu et al., 2019; Ding et al., 2020).

In this study, arctigenin, quercetin, luteolin, kaempferol, rutin, gallic acid, and chlorogenic acid in Jingyin granule were used for a functional study due to more connected targets in the

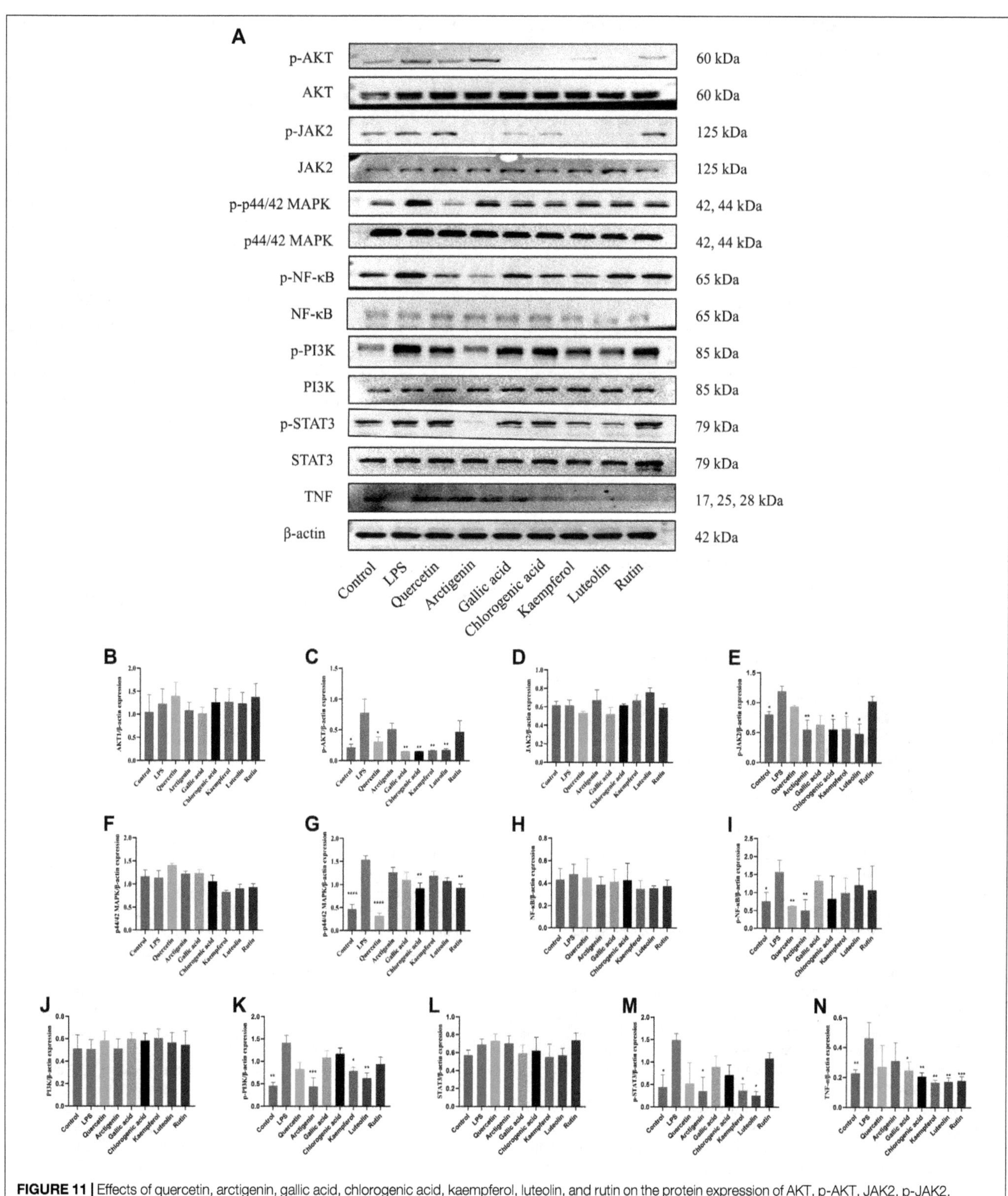

FIGURE 11 | Effects of quercetin, arctigenin, gallic acid, chlorogenic acid, kaempferol, luteolin, and rutin on the protein expression of AKT, p-AKT, JAK2, p-JAK2, p44/42 MAPK (ERK1/2), p-p44/42 MAPK (ERK1/2), NF-κB, p-NF-κB, PI3K, p-PI3K, STAT3, p-STAT3, and TNF-α of LPS-induced A549 cells **(A–N)**. *$p < 0.05$, **$p < 0.01$, compared with the LPS group.

ingredient–target network and more distribution in lung tissue in a pharmacokinetic study. Firstly, Jingyin granule was analyzed by a simple and accurate HPLC method, UPLC-MS, for the simultaneous separation and identification of the seven ingredients for functional evaluation. Molecular docking indicated that the key components combined well with target proteins. *In vitro* cell experiments proved that the important ingredients, arctigenin and luteolin, inhibited the production of fibrosis in LPS-induced A549 cells by suppressing the JAK2/STAT3, NF-κB, PI3K-AKT, TNF, and ERK1/2 signaling pathways. Moreover, we are doing the *in vivo* experiment to provide more mechanism study for the anti-fibrosis effect of Jingyin granule.

CONCLUSION

tIn conclusion, our present study systematically analyzed the related targets and signaling pathways of Jingyin granule against PF and conducted an *in vitro* experiment and demonstrated that Jingyin granule obviously inhibited the activation of JAK2/STAT3, NF-κB, PI3K/AKT, TNF, and ERK1/2 signaling pathways in LPS-induced PF. This underlying mechanism we elucidated may become a theoretical basis for the use of Jingyin granule for the treatment of PF.

AUTHOR CONTRIBUTIONS

Y-HS: Conception and design, Conceptualization, Methodology, Data curation, Visualization, Investigation, Supervision, Validation, Writing—Reviewing and Editing, Project administration, and Funding acquisition. D-WZ: Investigation, Conceptualization, Methodology, Data curation, Data and image processing, Visualization, Validation, Writing—Original draft preparation, and Writing—Reviewing and Editing. QY: Software, Methodology, Data curation, Data and image processing, Visualization, and Validation. M-FJ: Data and image processing, Visualization, and Methodology. D-DW: Investigation, Supervision, and Validation. All authors contributed to and have approved the final manuscript.

REFERENCES

Collard, H. R., Ryerson, C. J., Corte, T. J., Jenkins, G., Kondoh, Y., Lederer, D. J., et al. (2016). Acute Exacerbation of Idiopathic Pulmonary Fibrosis. An International Working Group Report. *Am. J. Respir. Crit. Care Med.* 194 (3), 265–275. doi:10.1164/rccm.201604-0801CI

Cottin, V., Wollin, L., Fischer, A., Quaresma, M., Stowasser, S., and Harari, S. (2019). Fibrosing Interstitial Lung Diseases: Knowns and Unknowns. *Eur. Respir. Rev.* 28 (151), 180100. doi:10.1183/16000617.0100-2018

Cui, L., Chen, S. Y., Lerbs, T., Lee, J. W., Domizi, P., Gordon, S., et al. (2020). Activation of JUN in Fibroblasts Promotes Pro-fibrotic Programme and Modulates Protective Immunity. *Nat. Commun.* 11 (1), 2795. doi:10.1038/s41467-020-16466-4

Ding, Z., Wu, X., Wang, Y., Ji, S., Zhang, W., Kang, J., et al. (2020). Melatonin Prevents LPS-Induced Epithelial-Mesenchymal Transition in Human Alveolar Epithelial Cells via the GSK-3β/Nrf2 Pathway. *Biomed. Pharmacother.* 132, 110827. doi:10.1016/j.biopha.2020.110827

Galuppo, M., Esposito, E., Mazzon, E., Di Paola, R., Paterniti, I., Impellizzeri, D., et al. (2011). MEK Inhibition Suppresses the Development of Lung Fibrosis in the Bleomycin Model. *Naunyn Schmiedebergs Arch. Pharmacol.* 384 (1), 21–37. doi:10.1007/s00210-011-0637-7

Gao, F., Zhang, Y., Yang, Z., Wang, M., Zhou, Z., Zhang, W., et al. (2020). Arctigenin Suppressed Epithelial-Mesenchymal Transition through Wnt3a/β-Catenin Pathway in PQ-Induced Pulmonary Fibrosis. *Front. Pharmacol.* 11, 584098. doi:10.3389/fphar.2020.584098

Gao, L., Tang, H., He, H., Liu, J., Mao, J., Ji, H., et al. (2015). Glycyrrhizic Acid Alleviates Bleomycin-Induced Pulmonary Fibrosis in Rats. *Front. Pharmacol.* 6, 215. doi:10.3389/fphar.2015.00215

Gavino, A. C., Nahmod, K., Bharadwaj, U., Makedonas, G., and Tweardy, D. J. (2016). STAT3 Inhibition Prevents Lung Inflammation, Remodeling, and Accumulation of Th2 and Th17 Cells in a Murine Asthma Model. *Allergy* 71 (12), 1684–1692. doi:10.1111/all.12937

Guo, J., Li, B., Wu, W., Wang, Z., Wang, F., and Guo, T. (2019). Chinese Herbal Medicines Compared with N-Acetylcysteine for the Treatment of Idiopathic Pulmonary Fibrosis: A Systematic Review of Randomized Controlled Trials. *Evid. Based Complement. Alternat Med.* 2019, 5170638. doi:10.1155/2019/5170638

Heinrich, P. C., Behrmann, I., Haan, S., Hermanns, H. M., Müller-Newen, G., and Schaper, F. (2003). Principles of Interleukin (IL)-6-type Cytokine Signalling and its Regulation. *Biochem. J.* 374 (Pt 1), 1–20. doi:10.1042/bj20030407

Hopkins, A. L. (2007). Network Pharmacology. *Nat. Biotechnol.* 25 (10), 1110–1111. doi:10.1038/nbt1007-1110

Huang, Y., Tan, C., Wu, J., Chen, M., Wang, Z., Luo, L., et al. (2020). Impact of Coronavirus Disease 2019 on Pulmonary Function in Early Convalescence Phase. *Respir. Res.* 21 (1), 163. doi:10.1186/s12931-020-01429-6

Hutchinson, J., Fogarty, A., Hubbard, R., and McKeever, T. (2015). Global Incidence and Mortality of Idiopathic Pulmonary Fibrosis: a Systematic Review. *Eur. Respir. J.* 46 (3), 795–806. doi:10.1183/09031936.00185114

Jin, D., An, X., Zhang, Y., Zhao, S., Duan, L., Duan, Y., et al. (2021). Potential Mechanism Prediction of Herbal Medicine for Pulmonary Fibrosis Associated with SARS-CoV-2 Infection Based on Network Analysis and Molecular Docking. *Front. Pharmacol.* 12, 602218. doi:10.3389/fphar.2021.602218

Kim, H. J., Perlman, D., and Tomic, R. (2015). Natural History of Idiopathic Pulmonary Fibrosis. *Respir. Med.* 109 (6), 661–670. doi:10.1016/j.rmed.2015.02.002

Lai, J. M., Zhang, X., Liu, F. F., Yang, R., Li, S. Y., Zhu, L. B., et al. (2016). Redox-sensitive MAPK and Notch3 Regulate Fibroblast Differentiation and Activation: a Dual Role of ERK1/2. *Oncotarget* 7 (28), 43731–43745. doi:10.18632/oncotarget.9667

Larson-Casey, J. L., Deshane, J. S., Ryan, A. J., Thannickal, V. J., and Carter, A. B. (2016). Macrophage Akt1 Kinase-Mediated Mitophagy Modulates Apoptosis Resistance and Pulmonary Fibrosis. *Immunity* 44 (3), 582–596. doi:10.1016/j.immuni.2016.01.001

Le, T. T., Karmouty-Quintana, H., Melicoff, E., Le, T. T., Weng, T., Chen, N. Y., et al. (2014). Blockade of IL-6 Trans Signaling Attenuates Pulmonary Fibrosis. *J. Immunol.* 193 (7), 3755–3768. doi:10.4049/jimmunol.1302470

Li, A., Wang, J., Zhu, D., Zhang, X., Pan, R., and Wang, R. (2015). Arctigenin Suppresses Transforming Growth Factor-B1-Induced Expression of Monocyte Chemoattractant Protein-1 and the Subsequent Epithelial-Mesenchymal Transition through Reactive Oxygen Species-dependent ERK/NF-κB Signaling Pathway in Renal Tubular Epithelial Cells. *Free Radic. Res.* 49 (9), 1095–1113. doi:10.3109/10715762.2015.1038258

Li, L. C., and Kan, L. D. (2017). Traditional Chinese Medicine for Pulmonary Fibrosis Therapy: Progress and Future Prospects. *J. Ethnopharmacol* 198, 45–63. doi:10.1016/j.jep.2016.12.042

Liang, B., Guo, X. L., Jin, J., Ma, Y. C., and Feng, Z. Q. (2015). Glycyrrhizic Acid Inhibits Apoptosis and Fibrosis in Carbon-Tetrachloride-Induced Rat Liver Injury. *World J. Gastroenterol.* 21 (17), 5271–5280. doi:10.3748/wjg.v21.i17.5271

Madala, S. K., Schmidt, S., Davidson, C., Ikegami, M., Wert, S., and Hardie, W. D. (2012). MEK-ERK Pathway Modulation Ameliorates Pulmonary Fibrosis Associated with Epidermal Growth Factor Receptor Activation. *Am. J. Respir. Cel Mol Biol* 46 (3), 380–388. doi:10.1165/rcmb.2011-0237OC

Martinez, F. J., Collard, H. R., Pardo, A., Raghu, G., Richeldi, L., Selman, M., et al. (2017). Idiopathic Pulmonary Fibrosis. *Nat. Rev. Dis. Primers* 3, 17074. doi:10.1038/nrdp.2017.74

Miao, H., Zhang, Y., Huang, Z., Lu, B., and Ji, L. (2019). Lonicera japonica

Attenuates Carbon Tetrachloride-Induced Liver Fibrosis in Mice: Molecular Mechanisms of Action. *Am. J. Chin. Med.* 47 (2), 351–367. doi:10.1142/s0192415x19500174

Milara, J., Hernandez, G., Ballester, B., Morell, A., Roger, I., Montero, P., et al. (2018). The JAK2 Pathway Is Activated in Idiopathic Pulmonary Fibrosis. *Respir. Res.* 19 (1), 24. doi:10.1186/s12931-018-0728-9

Ng, L. T., Yen, F. L., Liao, C. W., and Lin, C. C. (2007). Protective Effect of Houttuynia Cordata Extract on Bleomycin-Induced Pulmonary Fibrosis in Rats. *Am. J. Chin. Med.* 35 (3), 465–475. doi:10.1142/s0192415x07004989

O'Donoghue, R. J., Knight, D. A., Richards, C. D., Prêle, C. M., Lau, H. L., Jarnicki, A. G., et al. (2012). Genetic Partitioning of Interleukin-6 Signalling in Mice Dissociates Stat3 from Smad3-Mediated Lung Fibrosis. *EMBO Mol. Med.* 4 (9), 939–951. doi:10.1002/emmm.201100604

Qiu, P., Liu, Y., and Zhang, J. (2019). Recent Advances in Studies of Molecular Hydrogen against Sepsis. *Int. J. Biol. Sci.* 15 (6), 1261–1275. doi:10.7150/ijbs.30741

Raghu, G., Remy-Jardin, M., Myers, J. L., Richeldi, L., Ryerson, C. J., Lederer, D. J., et al. (2018). Diagnosis of Idiopathic Pulmonary Fibrosis. An Official ATS/ERS/JRS/ALAT Clinical Practice Guideline. *Am. J. Respir. Crit. Care Med.* 198 (5), e44–e68. doi:10.1164/rccm.201807-1255ST

Saito, S., Alkhatib, A., Kolls, J. K., Kondoh, Y., and Lasky, J. A. (2019). Pharmacotherapy and Adjunctive Treatment for Idiopathic Pulmonary Fibrosis (IPF). *J. Thorac. Dis.* 11 (Suppl. 14), S1740–s1754. doi:10.21037/jtd.2019.04.62

Selman, M., King, T. E., and Pardo, A. (2001). Idiopathic Pulmonary Fibrosis: Prevailing and Evolving Hypotheses about its Pathogenesis and Implications for Therapy. *Ann. Intern. Med.* 134 (2), 136–151. doi:10.7326/0003-4819-134-2-200101160-00015

Shen, Y. H., Cheng, M. H., Liu, X. Y., Zhu, D. W., and Gao, J. (2021). Sodium Houttuyfonate Inhibits Bleomycin Induced Pulmonary Fibrosis in Mice. *Front. Pharmacol.* 12, 596492. doi:10.3389/fphar.2021.596492

Tsaioun, K., Blaauboer, B. J., and Hartung, T. (2016). Evidence-based Absorption, Distribution, Metabolism, Excretion (ADME) and its Interplay with Alternative Toxicity Methods. *Altex* 33 (4), 343–358. doi:10.14573/altex.1610101

Vancheri, C., Failla, M., Crimi, N., and Raghu, G. (2010). Idiopathic Pulmonary Fibrosis: a Disease with Similarities and Links to Cancer Biology. *Eur. Respir. J.* 35 (3), 496–504. doi:10.1183/09031936.00077309

Wang, B., Sun, X., Kong, X., and Gao, Y. (2021). Systematic Elucidation of the Mechanism of Jingyin Granule in the Treatment of Novel Coronavirus (COVID-19) Pneumonia via Network Pharmacology. *Int. J. Med. Sci.* 18 (7), 1648–1656. doi:10.7150/ijms.53575

Wang, J. (2013). Treatment of Food Anaphylaxis with Traditional Chinese Herbal Remedies: from Mouse Model to Human Clinical Trials. *Curr. Opin. Allergy Clin. Immunol.* 13 (4), 386–391. doi:10.1097/ACI.0b013e3283615bc4

Wernig, G., Chen, S. Y., Cui, L., Van Neste, C., Tsai, J. M., Kambham, N., et al. (2017). Unifying Mechanism for Different Fibrotic Diseases. *Proc. Natl. Acad. Sci. U S A.* 114 (18), 4757–4762. doi:10.1073/pnas.1621375114

Yoshida, K., Kuwano, K., Hagimoto, N., Watanabe, K., Matsuba, T., Fujita, M., et al. (2002). MAP Kinase Activation and Apoptosis in Lung Tissues from Patients with Idiopathic Pulmonary Fibrosis. *J. Pathol.* 198 (3), 388–396. doi:10.1002/path.1208

Zhang, Y., Lu, P., Qin, H., Zhang, Y., Sun, X., Song, X., et al. (2021). Traditional Chinese Medicine Combined with Pulmonary Drug Delivery System and Idiopathic Pulmonary Fibrosis: Rationale and Therapeutic Potential. *Biomed. Pharmacother.* 133, 111072. doi:10.1016/j.biopha.2020.111072

Zhu, D. W., Yu, Q., Sun, J. J., and Shen, Y. H. (2021). Evaluating the Therapeutic Mechanisms of Selected Active Compounds in Houttuynia Cordata Thunb. In Pulmonary Fibrosis via Network Pharmacology Analysis. *Front. Pharmacol.* 12, 733618. doi:10.3389/fphar.2021.733618

13

Blueberry Juice Attenuates Pulmonary Fibrosis *via* Blocking the TGF-β1/Smad Signaling Pathway

Yali Li[1,2,3], *Liqun Wang*[2], *Qianyu Zhang*[2], *Li Tian*[2], *Cailing Gan*[1], *Hongyao Liu*[1], *Wenya Yin*[2]* *and Tinghong Ye*[1]*

[1]*Sichuan University-University of Oxford Huaxi Joint Centre for Gastrointestinal Cancer, Frontiers Science Center for Disease-Related Molecular Network, State Key Laboratory of Biotherapy, West China Hospital, Sichuan University, Chengdu, China,* [2]*West China School of Public Health and West China Fourth Hospital, Sichuan University, Chengdu, China,* [3]*Prenatal Diagnosis Center, The Third Affiliated Hospital of Zhengzhou University—Maternal and Child Health Hospital of Henan Province, Zhengzhou, China*

***Correspondence:**
Wenya Yin
yinwenya@scu.edu.cn
Tinghong Ye
yeth1309@scu.edu.cn

Idiopathic pulmonary fibrosis (IPF) is a progressive, fatal, and chronic lung disease, lacking a validated and effective therapy. Blueberry has demonstrated multiple pharmacological activities including anti-inflammatory, antioxidant, and anticancer. Therefore, the objective of this study was to investigate whether blueberry juice (BBJ) could ameliorate IPF. Experiments *in vitro* revealed that BBJ could significantly reduce the expressions of TGF-β1 modulated fibrotic protein, which were involved in the cascade of fibrosis in NIH/3T3 cells and human pulmonary fibroblasts. In addition, for rat primary lung fibroblasts (RPLFs), BBJ promoted the cell apoptosis along with reducing the expressions of α-SMA, vimentin, and collagen I, while increasing the E-cadherin level. Furthermore, BBJ could reverse epithelial–mesenchymal transition (EMT) phenotypic changes and inhibit cell migration, along with inducing the upregulation of E-cadherin in A549 cells. Compared with the vehicle group, BBJ treatment alleviated fibrotic pathological changes and collagen deposition in both bleomycin-induced prevention and treatment pulmonary fibrosis models. In fibrotic lung tissues, BBJ remarkably suppressed the expressions of collagen I, α-SMA, and vimentin and improved E-cadherin, which may be related to its inhibition of the TGF-β1/Smad pathway and anti-inflammation efficacy. Taken together, these findings comprehensively proved that BBJ could effectively prevent and attenuate idiopathic pulmonary fibrosis *via* suppressing EMT and the TGF-β1/Smad signaling pathway.

Keywords: blueberry juice, idiopathic pulmonary fibrosis, TGF-β1/Smad signaling pathway, epithelial–mesenchymal transition, reactive oxygen species

INTRODUCTION

Idiopathic pulmonary fibrosis (IPF) is recognized widely as a fatal, chronic, and irreversible devastating interstitial lung disease. And it is characterized by the destruction of the lung parenchyma and fibrotic remodeling of the lung tissue (Wynn, 2007). There are over 150,000 patients in the United States, approximately 5,000 new cases in the United Kingdom, and more than five million people in the world who are suffering from IPF annually (Beers and Morrisey, 2011; Navaratnam et al., 2011; Thannickal et al., 2014). Several studies have uncovered the risk factors, such as aging, cigarette smoking, environmental exposures, and virus infections (Baumgartner et al., 1997; Hubbard, 2001; Taskar and Coultas, 2006; Raghu et al., 2011). The accurate prevalence of IPF in China is still unclear. However, considering these ubiquitous risk factors, there should be more cases than we expected. It is no doubt that IPF is slowly becoming a stumbling block to keeping people healthy worldwide. IPF is associated with poor prognosis, cough, dyspnea, and diminished quality of life. Drug intervention, symptom-oriented therapies, and pulmonary transplantation are the three well-accepted clinical treatments of IPF (Raghu and Richeldi, 2017; Richeldi et al., 2017).

During the pathogenesis of IPF, alveolar epithelial cells undergo repetitive microinjuries. This damage generates the secretions of coagulants, cytokines, and fibrogenic growth factors such as transforming growth factor-beta 1 (TGF-β1) (Horowitz and Thannickal, 2006). TGF-β1 could induce differentiation of fibroblasts, myofibroblast recruitment, mesenchymal cell proliferation, and epithelial–mesenchymal transition (EMT) (Rock et al., 2011; Hung et al., 2013). The myofibroblast abnormal deposit leads to the excess synthesis of extracellular matrix (ECM) proteins such as collagen I in the lung tissue, which in turn promotes the differentiation of fibroblast to myofibroblast (Parker et al., 2014). In the signaling pathway that regulates IPF, the Smad protein family is a downstream molecule in the TGF-β1 signaling pathway. TGF-β1 promotes Smad2/3 to bind to Smad4, and then the Smad complexes are transmitted into the nucleus and regulate the expressions of target proteins related to ECM, EMT, and profibrotic mediators finally (Hu et al., 2018). Therefore, given the effects of the TGF-β1/Smad signaling pathway on collagen synthesis and EMT, blocking this pathway has become a vital therapeutic strategy in the IPF treatment.

The past 30 years have seen a proliferation of studies showing that blueberry has the best health benefits, such as anti-inflammation, reduction in oxidative stress, prevention of cardiovascular diseases, and anticancer. Bioactive components in blueberries include various kinds of anthocyanins (anthocyanidins, or phenolic aglycone, conjugated with sugar), tannins, chlorogenic acid, citric acid, arbutin, myricetin and its glycoside, flavonoids, pterostilbene, resveratrol, and so on (Chen et al., 2010; Yang and Jiang, 2010). Mounting evidences suggested that these phytochemicals, either individually or synergistically, contribute to the health promotion activity of blueberry (Skrovankova et al., 2015). Recently, a few studies have focused on the anti-fibrosis activity of blueberry. In these studies, rats were administrated orally with blueberry juice (BBJ), and it was discovered that BBJ could alleviate hepatic fibrosis or injury through reducing the expressions of NF-κB p65 and TGF-β1 (Lu et al., 2012; Wang et al., 2013; Zhan et al., 2017; Zhang B. F. et al., 2018). However, the therapeutic use of BBJ and its role in IPF have not been investigated yet. Therefore, this study is designed to evaluate the anti-fibrotic activity of BBJ using various fibroblasts *in vitro* and bleomycin-induced pulmonary fibrosis models *in vivo* to further elucidate its potential mechanism.

MATERIALS AND METHODS

Reagents

Bleomycin (BLM) sulfate was purchased from Chengdu Synguider Technology Co., Ltd (Chengdu, China). Nintedanib was from Chengdu Giant Pharmaceutical Technology Co., Ltd (Chengdu, China). TGF-β1 was purchased from Novoprotein (Shanghai, China). Ten micrograms of TGF-β1 was added into 100 μl sterile ddH_2O and mixed well. Then 0.1 g/L TGF-β1 solution was kept at −80°C.

BBJ Extraction

Fresh blueberry fruits produced from Peru were bought in the market, weighed, washed, and wiped with absorbent papers. Then the fruits were juiced by blender (Joyoung, China) and centrifuged at 4,000 rpm for 5 min. After being filtered by 0.22 μm membrane filters, the supernatant was stored separately and protected from light at −80°C. The yield rate was about 0.24 ml/g (fresh weight), and the mass concentration of BBJ is 1.01 g/ml.

LC/MS Analysis

The ingredients of BBJ were detected by the LC/MS system (Thermo Scientific Q Exactive). In the experiment, a CAPCELL PAK-C18 column (100 mm × 2.1 mm, 2.7 μm) was used. Mobile phase A was the solution with 0.1% formic acid. Mobile phase B was acetonitrile. The gradient was as follows: 0–2 min, 5% B; 2–5 min, from 5% to 30% B; 5–7 min, from 50% to 70% B; 7–8.1 min, from 75% to 90% B; 8.1–10 min, from 95% to 5% B. The flow rate was set as 0.3 ml/min. The injection volume of the sample was 10 μl, and the column temperature was kept at 40°C. The data were analyzed by Compound Discoverer 3.3.3.12 and matched with mzVault and mzCloud databases. Results were visualized by Thermo Xcalibur Qual Browser and Origin 2018 software. Before being injected into the column, samples and mobile phases were filtered by 0.22 μm membrane filters and degassed.

Total Phenols and Flavonoid Content Determination

The total phenol content of BBJ was detected according to a previous study with some modifies (Czerwiński et al., 2004). Phenol components in 1 ml BBJ diluted in 9 ml 75% ethanol were extracted in ultrasound for 30 min. The extraction was used to determine total phenols and flavonoids. Total phenols were measured at 765 nm using a Folin reagent with chlorogenic acid as a standard. Total flavonoid content was estimated by $NaNO_2$-$Al(NO_3)_3$-NaOH colorimetric methods, according to previous description (Bao et al., 2015). And rutin was set as standard. These measurements were conducted in triplicate. Results were expressed as μg/g of BBJ and mean ± SD.

Antioxidant Ability Test

To determine the antioxidant ability of BBJ, DPPH, Fenton reactions, and ABTS experiments were performed according to related work (Bao et al., 2015). These measurements were conducted in triplicate. The half maximal inhibitory concentration (IC_{50} value) was calculated by Excel.

DPPH Assay

For DPPH assay, 5 µl BBJ or Vitamin C was incubated with 195 µl of a 0.035 mg/ml DPPH ethanol solution for 30–40 min at room temperature. The absorbance (A_1) was measured at 517 nm. The DPPH radical scavenging activity (C%) was expressed by the following formula:

$$C\% = \left(1 - \frac{A_1 - A_2}{A_0}\right) \times 100\%$$

In the formula, A_2 stands for the OD value of the mixture of BBJ or Vitamin C and ethanol solution; A_0 is the absorbance of the mixture of ddH_2O and DPPH solution.

Fenton Reaction

For the detection of hydroxyl free radical HO scavenging ability, 7.5 mM ferrous sulfate solution, 6 mM salicylic acid ethanol solution, 0.3% H_2O_2, and different concentrations of BBJ or Vitamin C were added into the tubes. Each volume of these solutions was 0.25 ml. After a water bath at 37°C for 30 min, the absorbance of the 200 µl mixed solution was tested at 520 nm (A_1). The hydroxyl free radical HO scavenging ability (C%) was expressed by the formula in Section 2.5.1. In the formula, A_2 stands for the OD value of the mixture of 7.5 mM ferrous sulfate solution, 6 mM salicylic acid ethanol solution, ddH_2O, and different concentrations of BBJ or Vitamin C; A_0 is the absorbance of the mixture of 7.5 mM ferrous sulfate solution, 6 mM salicylic acid ethanol solution, 0.3% H_2O_2, and ddH_2O.

ABTS Assay

In ABTS assay, 7.4 mM ABTS solution and 2.6 mM potassium persulfate aqueous solution were mixed in equal volume and reacted for 12–16 h, avoiding exposure to light, as ABTS stock solution. The ABTS stock solution was diluted by 20 mM sodium acetate aqueous solution for work solution. Ten microliters of BBJ or Vitamin C was added into 195 µl ABTS work solution. After incubation for 5 min, avoiding exposure to light, the absorbance of mixed solution was determined at 734 nm (A_1). The ABTS scavenging ability was calculated by the formula in Section 2.5.1. In the formula, A_2 stands for the OD value of the mixture of 10 µl different doses of BBJ or Vitamin C and 195 µl sodium acetate solution; A_0 is the absorbance of the mixture of 10 µl ddH_2O and 195 µl ABTS work solution.

Rat Primary Lung Fibroblast (RPLF) Isolation and Cell Culture

RPLFs were isolated from 7- to 8-week-old specific pathogen-free (SPF) male Wister rats with lung fibrosis (permit number: 2018091812). The weight of each rat was about 300 g. After being anesthetized by intraperitoneal injection of 1 ml 10% chloral hydrate solution, the rats were injected with 4 mg/kg body weight BLM saline solution through intratracheal infusion. A week later, the rats were sacrificed. The lung tissues were removed and washed with sterilized Hank's solution. After the fascia were cut off, the lung tissues were minced and resuspended in 10 ml 0.25% trypsin for 40 min at 37°C. The suspension was then filtered by 70 µm nylon mesh and centrifuged at 1,500 rpm for 5 min. The precipitates were resuspended with 10 ml DMEM-F12 medium and centrifuged at 500 rpm for 5 min. The supernatant was centrifuged for 5 min at 1,500 rpm. The supernatant was discarded, and the cells were precipitated and cultured in fresh DMEM-F12 medium with 1% antibiotics (penicillin and streptomycin, MP Biomedical LLC) and 10% heat-inactivated fetal bovine serum (GIBCO, NY) in a culture dish at 37°C in a 5% CO_2 humidified incubator.

HPF (human pulmonary fibroblast, from ATCC) cells were cultured by DMEM with 20% FBS and 1% antibiotics. A549 (human lung carcinoma epithelial cells, from ATCC), NIH/3T3 (mouse embryo fibroblasts, from ATCC), and LO2 (human liver cells, from ATCC) were cultured by DMEM with 10% FBS and 1% antibiotics.

MTT Experiment, Apoptosis Assay, Reactive Oxygen Species (ROS), and Mitochondrial Membrane Potential (ΔΨm) Detections

Cells were seeded in 96-well plates with appropriate number. Overnight, various doses (0–100 µl/ml) of BBJ and 200 µl/ml normal saline (NS) or nintedanib (NTB) were added. After 24, 48, and 72 h, cells were incubated with MTT for 3 h, the supernatant was discarded, and 150 µl/well DMSO was added. The OD value was detected at the length of 570 nm.

Cells were seeded in six-well plates. After adhering to the plates, cells were treated with BBJ and/or TGF-β1 for 24 h. For apoptosis assay, apoptotic cells were tested by an apoptosis kit (KeyGen Biotech, Nanjing, China) and analyzed by a NovoCyte™ flow cytometer (ACEA Bioscience, Inc., CA, USA). For intracellular ROS and ΔΨm detections, DCFH-DA and Rh123 were applied as related dyes and determined using flow cytometry.

Wound-Healing Assay and Cell Morphology

A549 cells were seeded into a six-well plate. When the cells grew to about a density of 85%, cells were cultured with the DMEM without FBS for 6 h. Then, wounds were made by a sterile 100 µl pipette tip. We changed the medium into DMEM with 3% FBS, and cells were treated with 0 or 5 ng/ml TGF-β1. After 1 h, cells were treated with 0 or 50 µl/ml BBJ for 24 h, and these four wells were treated with 0 µl/ml BBJ and 0 ng/ml TGF-β1, 50 µl/ml BBJ and 0 ng/ml TGF-β1, 0 µl/ml BBJ and 5 ng/ml TGF-β1, and 50 µl/ml BBJ and 5 ng/ml TGF-β1, separately. The scratches were photographed at 0 and 24 h. The areas of scratches were analyzed by ImageJ software. Wound closure rate was expressed by the ratio of the difference between the wound area at 0 and 24–0 h. The cell morphology was observed by a microscope when A549 cells were treated with BBJ and TGF-β1 for 24 h.

TABLE 1 | The total phenols and flavonoid contents in BBJ.

	Standard curve	R^2	Standard	Content (μg/g)
Total phenols	Y = 0.0022 × x − 0.0032	0.9953	chlorogenic acid	1,219.15 ± 75.26
Total flavonoids	Y = 0.0010 × x + 0.0035	0.9983	rutin	603.89 ± 29.21

Total phenol content was determined by Folin reagent, using chlorogenic acid as standard; total flavonoids in BBJ were detected by $NaNO_2$-$Al(NO_3)_3$-NaOH colorimetric methods with rutin. Results were shown as mean ± SD from replicate determinations.

Immunofluorescence Assay

A549, NIH/3T3, and HPF were seeded into 24-well plates precoated with sterile cell slides. Overnight and after starvation for 6 h, these cells were treated with BBJ and TGF-β1 as expressed in wound-healing assay for 24 h. Cells were washed with cold PBS, fixed with 4% paraformaldehyde for 15 min, permeabilized with 0.5% Triton-100 solution for 20 min, and blocked with PBS containing 0.05% Triton-100 and 5% bovine serum albumin. Next, cells were incubated with α-SMA (1:150, Abcam, Cambridge, MA) and E-cadherin (1:200, Abcam, Cambridge, MA) for 18 h at 4°C. Then cells were washed with PBST and incubated with FITC or PE-conjugated goat anti-rabbit/mouse antibody (1:200, Alexa Fluor 488 or 647, Life Technologies, Waltham, MA) for 1.5 h at room temperature in the dark. The nuclei were stained by DAPI (Roche Molecular Biochemicals, Inc., Pleasanton, CA) for 10 min, protected from light. The fluorescence was detected by a confocal microscope (Zeiss LSM 880, Germany).

Animal Study

All animal experiments were approved and performed in compliance with the Animal Care and Use Committee of Sichuan University in China. To explore the preventive activity of BBJ, male C57BL/6 mice (6–8 weeks old) were obtained from Beijing HFK Bioscience Co., Ltd., and bred in an SPF condition. After being maintained for 1 week, each anesthetized mouse was injected with 60 μl saline that contained BLM sulfate (approximately 2 mg/kg body weight) by intratracheal instillation, while the sham group was injected with normal saline at the same volume. These mice were divided into four groups: the sham group, vehicle group, BBJ-L (5 ml/kg body weight) group, and BBJ-H (10 ml/kg body weight) group. The sham and vehicle groups were treated with normal saline at a dose of 10 ml/kg body weight. Saline and BBJ were administrated by gavage every day for 4 weeks. The mice were sacrificed at the end of the study.

As for the treatment effect of BBJ on IPF, male C57BL/6 mice (6–8 weeks old) were obtained from Beijing HFK Bioscience Co., Ltd., and bred in an SPF condition. When the weights of mice are over 20 g, mice were anesthetized and injected with 100 μl saline that contained BLM sulfate (approximately 1 mg/kg body weight) by intratracheal instillation. The sham group was injected with normal saline at the same volume. After 1 week, these four groups, sham group (10 ml saline/kg body weight), vehicle group (10 ml saline/kg body weight), BBJ group (10 ml BBJ/kg body weight), and NTB group (30 mg/kg body weight, resolved in the solvent in which the proportion of DMSO, PEG400 and saline was 0.5:3.5:6), started to be administrated every day by gavage. This treatment lasted for 3 weeks, and lung tissues from sacrificed mice were kept.

Hematoxylin and Eosin (H&E), Masson, and Immunohistochemistry (IHC) Staining

The left lung tissues, liver, heart, spleen, and kidney were kept in 4% paraformaldehyde. Next, the lung tissues were rinsed with flowing water, dehydrated, embedded with paraffin, and cut into discontinuous sections at a thickness of 3 μm. Through dewaxing and washing, these sections were stained with H&E, and lung sections were stained with Masson's trichrome by standard protocols. For IHC assay, sections were incubated with primary antibodies (α-SMA, collagen I, p-Smad3, and p-Stat3). All pathological sections were scanned by a Pannoramic MIDI II 3DHISTECH digital pathology system, and the pictures were analyzed with the CaseViewer software. We quantified the pulmonary fibrosis according to H&E results by the method of modified Ashcroft scale (Hübner et al., 2008). Collagen volume fraction and IHC score were analyzed by ImageJ software.

IL-10 and IL-17A Contents in Serum

The detection of IL-10 and IL-17 contents in serum was followed with protocols in a Th1/Th2/Th17 CBA kit (BD Pharmingen, USA).

Hydroxyproline Content Detection

Right lung tissues were kept at −80°C. About 30 mg lung tissues were weighed and hydrolyzed by alkaline. The contents of hydroxyproline were measured by the hydroxyproline assay kit (A030-2-1, Nanjing Jiancheng Bioengineering Institute, China).

Western Blotting

Cells or lung tissues were lysed with RIPA buffer containing protease and phosphatase inhibitor cocktail (Selleck Chemicals, Houston, TX, USA). Protein concentrations were detected by the Bradford method. Western blotting was performed as before (Li et al., 2019). The primary antibodies α-SMA, collagen-I, E-cadherin, and vimentin were purchased from Abcam (Cambridge, MA); Stat3, p-Stat3, Smad2/3, and p-Smad2/3 were from Cell Signaling Technology Company; β-actin were bought from ZSJQ-BIO (Beijing, China) and were involved in western blotting.

Statistical Analysis

Results were expressed as mean ± SD. We analyzed numeric data for statistical significance using the independent-sample *t*-test. A *p*-value <0.05 was considered as significant.

TABLE 2 | The antioxidant activity (IC_{50} values) of BBJ and Vitamin C.

	DPPH assay	Fenton reaction	ABTS assay
BBJ (g/100 ml)	46.69 ± 0.33	7.24 ± 0.33	4.01 ± 0.11
Vitamin C (mg/100 ml)	17.21 ± 0.65	20.58 ± 0.69	658.29 ± 3.06

To verify the antioxidant ability of BBJ, Fenton reaction, DPPH, and ABTS assays were applied. Vitamin C was set as the positive control. Half maximal inhibitory concentrations were calculated in Excel. Results were shown as mean ± SD from replicate determinations.

RESULTS

Ingredients, Total Phenol, and Flavonoid Contents in BBJ and Antioxidant Ability

The yield rate of BBJ was about 24% (ml juice/100 g fresh fruit). To figure out the components of BBJ, the LC/MS system was used. After being matched with the mzVault and mzCloud database, 30 possible substances, whose suitability was both over 80 or more than 90 in one database, were displayed in **Supplementary Table S1**. And the total ion chromatography result in determination is shown in **Supplementary Figure S1**. We found carbohydrates, amino acids, liquids, vitamins, and phytochemicals including phenols in BBJ.

According to this result, we used chlorogenic acid as a standard to determine the total phenols in BBJ. As shown in **Table 1**, the contents of total phenols and flavonoids in BBJ were 1,219.15 and 603.89 μg/g, respectively.

According to **Table 2**, IC_{50} values of BBJ in DPPH, Fenton, and ABTS tests were 46.69, 7.24, and 4.01 g/100 ml, respectively. And to eliminate 50% of free radicals in these three assays, 17.21, 20.58, and 658.29 mg/100 ml of Vitamin C were needed, which meant that BBJ's antioxidant ability was weaker than Vitamin C. However, plenty of water in BBJ should be taken into consideration when evaluating the antioxidant ability. Additionally, according to published research, the ABTS method is more suitable than DPPH assay to detect and

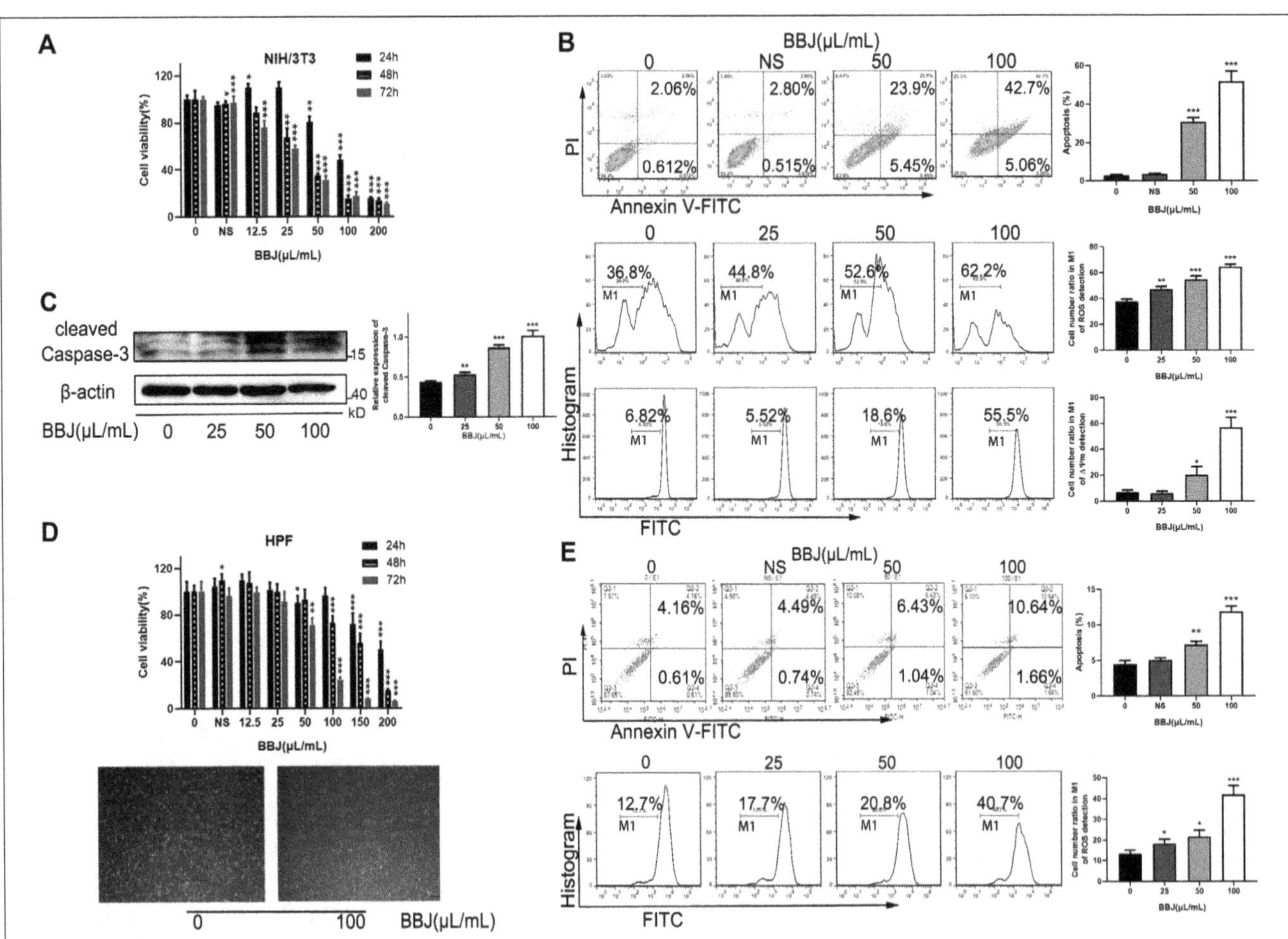

FIGURE 1 | BBJ induced apoptosis in NIH/3T3 and HPF. **(A)** NIH/3T3 was treated with BBJ or NS for 24, 48, and 72 h. The cell viability was disclosed by MTT assay. **(B)** Apoptotic rate, ROS, and ΔΨm of NIH/3T3 treated with BBJ for 24 h were analyzed and expressed as bar histograms. **(C)** Expression of cleaved caspase-3 in NIH/3T3 was detected through a western blot assay and calculated by ImageJ after incubation with BBJ for 24 h. **(D)** Under treatment with various doses of BBJ for 24 h, the viability of HPF was determined by MTT tests, and cell morphology was observed. **(E)** HPF was dealt with BBJ for 24 h, and apoptosis and ROS were analyzed by flow cytometry. *$p < 0.05$; **$p < 0.01$; ***$p < 0.001$ compared with the control group.

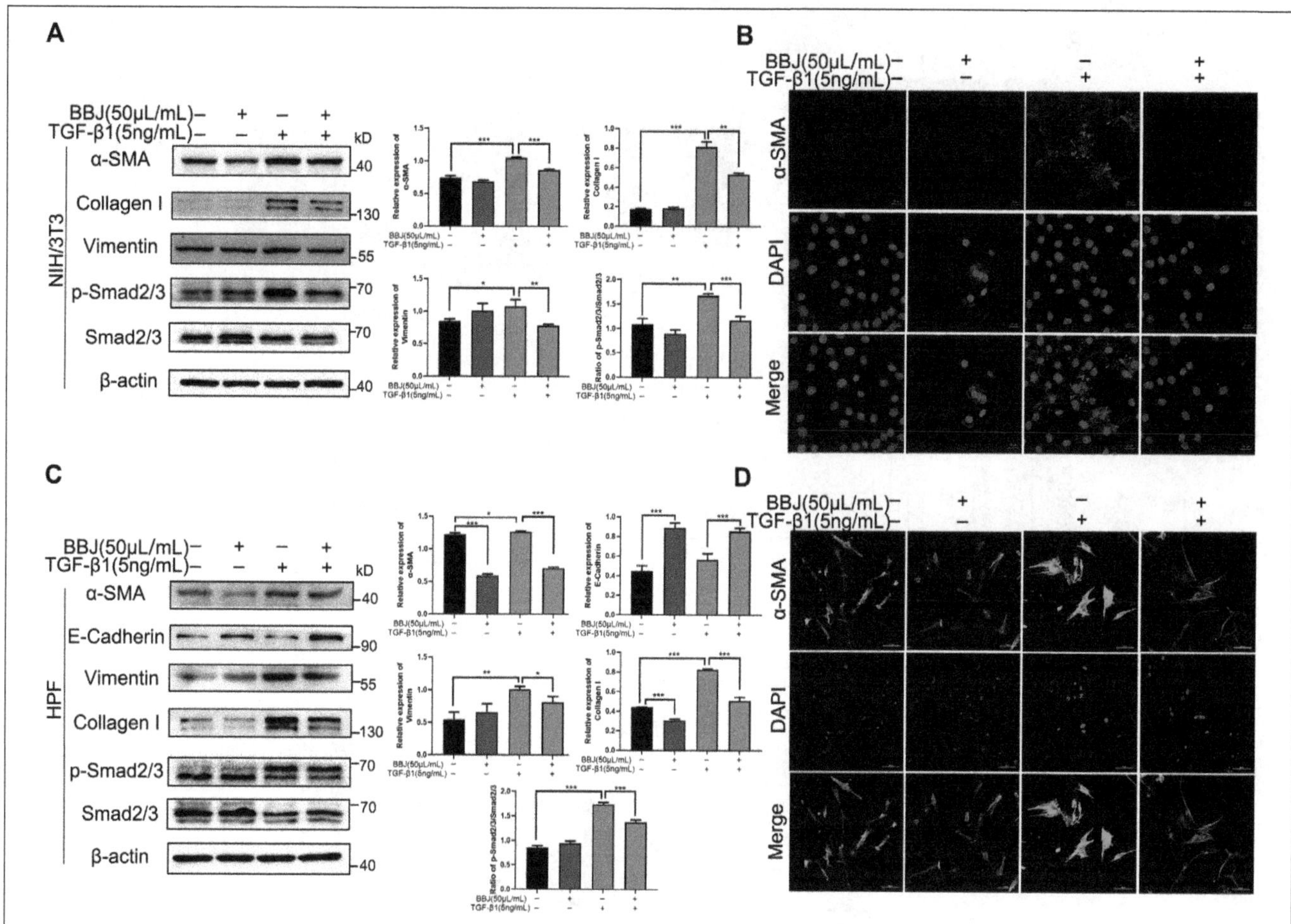

FIGURE 2 | BBJ restrained activation and differentiation of NIH/3T3 and HPF induced by TGF-β1. NIH/3T3 or HPF was planted, starved for 6 h, stimulated by 5 ng/ml TGF-β1 for 1 h, and then incubated with 50 μl/ml BBJ for an extra 24 h. **(A)** Expressions of α-SMA, vimentin, collagen-I, Smad2/3, p-Smad2/3, and β-actin in NIH/3T3 were presented by western blotting. **(B)** The expression of α-SMA in NIH/3T3 was visualized by a confocal microscope (×40). **(C)** Expressions of α-SMA, E-cadherin, vimentin, collagen-I, Smad2/3, p-Smad2/3, and β-actin in HPF were tested by western blotting. **(D)** The expression of α-SMA in HPF was visualized by a confocal microscope (×40). $^*p < 0.05$; $^{**}p < 0.01$; $^{***}p < 0.001$ versus the control group or the TGF-β1 group.

evaluate the antioxidant activity of pigments and hydrophilic antioxidants in blueberries (Mishra et al., 2012; Li et al., 2017).

BBJ-Induced Cell Death and Apoptosis in NIH/3T3 and HPF

We first investigated the antifibrotic activity of BBJ treatment on cell proliferation using NIH/3T3 and HPF. As shown in **Figures 1A,D**, we found that BBJ treatment significantly inhibited cell proliferation in a time- and dose-dependent manner. When intervened with 50 μl/ml BBJ for 24 h, cell viability rates were between 70% and 90% (**Figures 1A,D**). Additionally, compared with the vehicle group, an extra 27.68% apoptotic cells and 15.80% and 11.78% loss of ROS and ΔΨm, respectively, were induced by 50 μl/ml BBJ in NIH/3T3, as shown in **Figure 1B**. BBJ stimulated apoptosis in NIH/3T3 *via* the upregulated cleaved caspase-3 (**Figure 1C**). In HPF, as revealed in **Figure 1E**, an additional 2.80% of apoptotic rate and 8.10% of intracellular ROS loss were induced by 24 h treatment of 50 μl/ml BBJ, compared with the vehicle group. To sum up, these results suggested that the BBJ have potential antioxidant ability and can trigger cell death in NIH/3T3 and HPF *in vitro*.

BBJ Suppressed Differentiation in NIH/3T3 and HPF Through Inhibiting TGF-β1/Smad2/3 Signaling

Numerous studies have shown that TGF-β is an important cytokine in the development of fibrosis and recruits downstream Smad2/3 proteins. To uncover the potential mechanism of BBJ's anti-lung fibrosis in fibroblasts, TGF-β1 was applied to lead fibroblast activation. In NIH/3T3 and HPF cells, TGF-β1 induced upregulation of α-SMA, collagen-I, and vimentin. In other words, TGF-β1 caused fibroblast differentiation successfully. However, the addition of BBJ could suppress this increase, as shown in the results of western blot (**Figures 2A,C**).

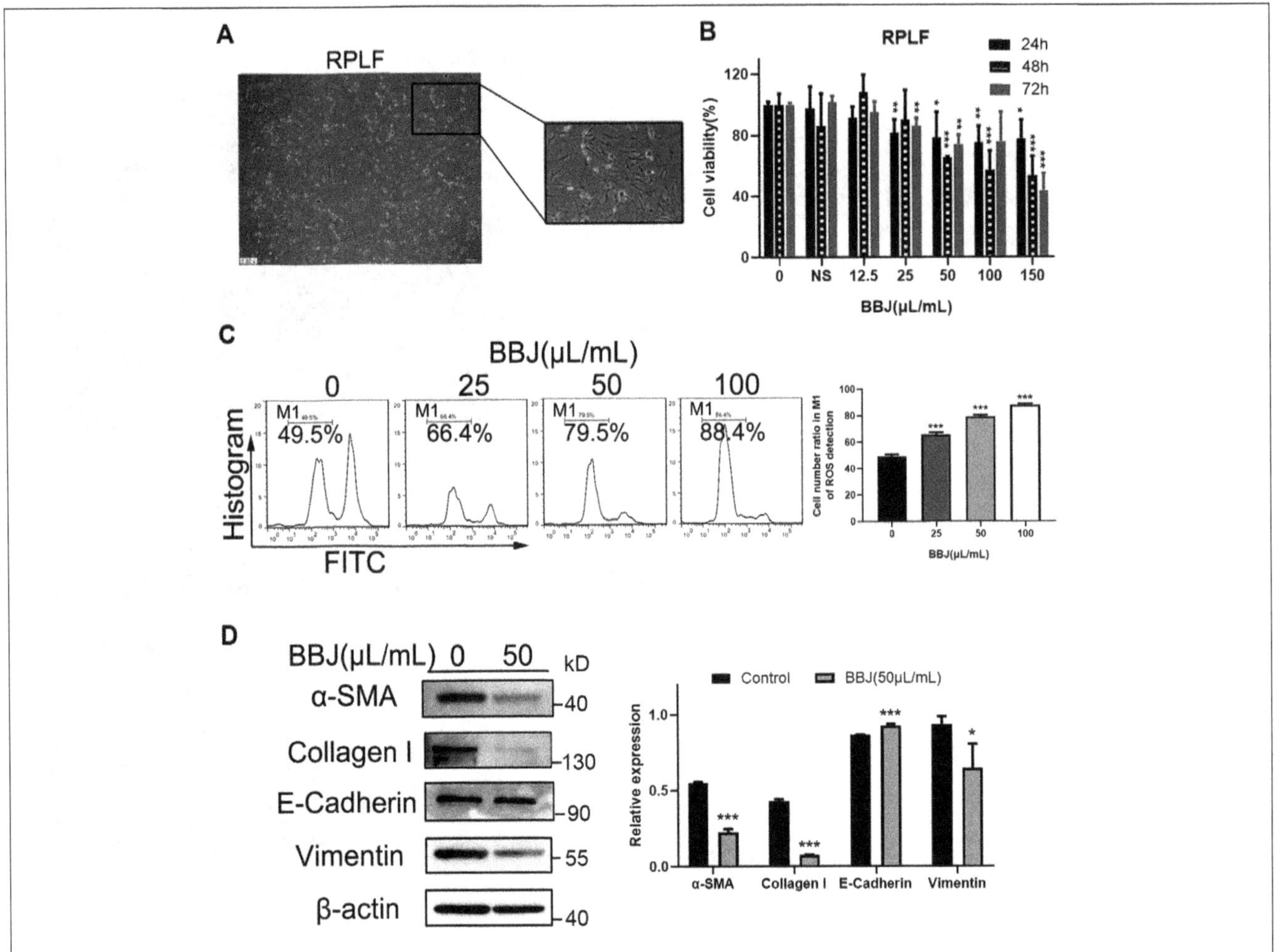

FIGURE 3 | The inhibitory effect of BBJ in RPLF. **(A)** Cell morphology of RPLF was photographed by an inverted microscope (×10). **(B)** RPLFs were treated with BBJ or normal saline for 24, 48, and 72 h. Cell viability was detected by MTT tests. **(C)** ROS in RPLF was analyzed after 24 h treatment of BBJ or NS. **(D)** Expressions of α-SMA, E-cadherin, vimentin, collagen-I, and β-actin in RPLF were determined by western blot assay. Protein expressions were treated statistically by ImageJ. $^{*}p < 0.05$; $^{**}p < 0.01$; $^{***}p < 0.001$ versus the control group.

And immunofluorescence results, as exhibited in **Figures 2B,D**, verified that BBJ restrained the upregulation of α-SMA induced by TGF-β1. More importantly, BBJ decreased the high ratio of p-Smad2/3 to Smad2/3 expression caused by TGF-β1 in NIH/3T3 and HPF. In conclusion, these changes indicated that BBJ could inhibit lung fibrosis through the TGF-β1/Smad2/3 pathway.

BBJ Had an Inhibitory Effect in RPLF

To further illustrate BBJ's disincentive function in fibroblasts, RPLF cells were extracted from the pulmonary fibrosis model, which was built by BLM tracheal infusion in male rats. RPLFs were considered as active fibroblasts. The cell morphology of RPLF was observed under an inverted microscope, presenting a slender fusiform with two to four antennae (**Figure 3A**). When RPLFs were treated with BBJ, their cell viability dropped, as shown in **Figure 3B**. The IC_{50} value of BBJ at 24 h in RPLF was over 200 μl/ml, while that in NIH/3T3 was 95.66 μl/ml and that in HPF was 145.47 μl/ml. As shown in **Figure 3C**, BBJ apparently gave rise to ROS loss in RPLF. BBJ exerted the ability to degrade expressions of α-SMA, collagen-I, and vimentin as well as increase E-cadherin slightly at 50 μl/ml (**Figure 3D**). In summary, these outcomes in RPLF further confirmed that BBJ has antifibrotic effects *in vitro*.

BBJ Could Restrain the EMT Process in A549 Cells

EMT plays an important role in many respiratory diseases, especially in fibrosis. To make explicit the antifibrotic ability of BBJ, A549 cells were used as a model of EMT. Firstly, MTT assay was utilized to determine the cytotoxicity of BBJ. The IC_{50} value at 24 h was 107.63 μl/ml (**Figure 4A**). At a dosage of 50 μl/ml, A549 cell viability was around 90%. Moreover, 50 μl/ml of BBJ had just induced 15.20% more ROS loss than the vehicle group (**Figure 4B**). Hence, in the following tests, A549 cells were treated with 50 μl/ml of BBJ. TGF-β1 induced EMT in A549, including changes of cell morphology, enhanced cell migration,

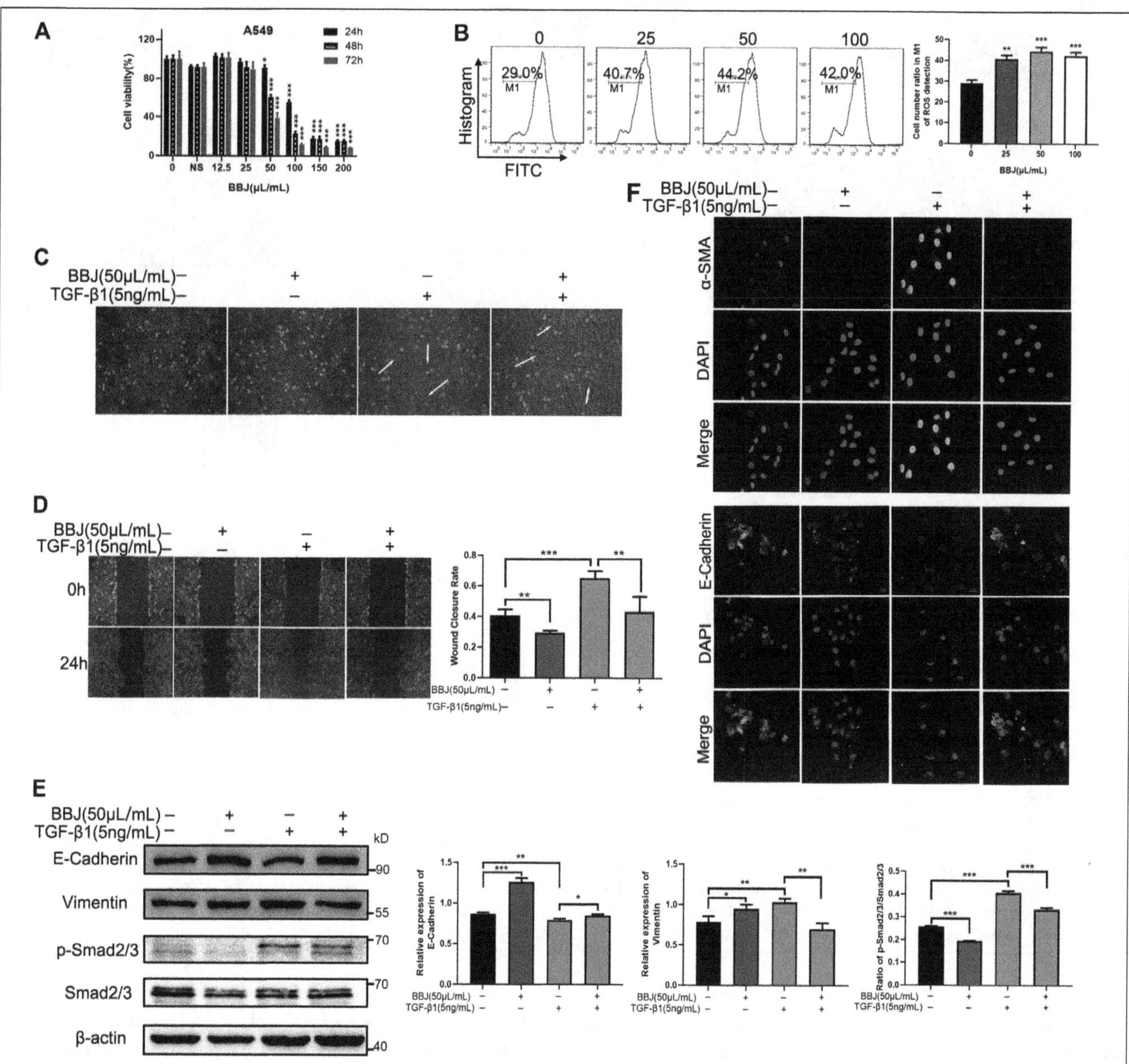

FIGURE 4 | BBJ could reverse EMT progress in A549. **(A)** The cytotoxicity of BBJ on A549 was determined by an MTT test. A549 cells were treated with different doses of BBJ and 200 μl/ml normal saline for 24, 48, and 72 h. Data were presented as mean ± SD from three experiments. **(B)** ROS of A549 treated with BBJ for 24 h were detected by flow cytometry and counted. **(C)** After starvation for 6 h with serum-free medium, fresh medium with 5 ng/ml TGF-β1 was replaced. One hour later, 50 μl/ml BBJ was added. After 24 h, cell morphology of A549 was observed by a microscope (×10). **(D)** A549 cells were seeded in six-well plates for 24 h and starved for 6 h with serum-free medium. Then, a scratch was made by 100 μl pipette tips, and fresh medium with 5 ng/ml TGF-β1 was added. One hour later, 50 μl/ml BBJ was added. The scratches were photographed at 0 and 24 h by an inverted microscope (×10). The scratch areas were treated statistically by ImageJ. **(E)** After incubation with 5 ng/ml TGF-β1 for 1 h and 50 μl/ml BBJ for an extra 24 h, expressions of E-cadherin, vimentin, p-Smad2/3, Smad2/3, and β-actin in A549 were analyzed by western blotting. **(F)** After stimulation by TGF-β1 for 1 h and treatment with BBJ for 24 h, expressions of α-SMA and E-cadherin were visualized by a confocal fluorescence microscope (×40). *$p < 0.05$; **$p < 0.01$; ***$p < 0.001$ versus the control group or TGF-β1 group.

and altered related proteins' expressions. Firstly, we observed the significant increased proportion of elongated cells induced by TGF-β1, which was reversed by BBJ (**Figure 4C** and **Supplementary Figure S2**). As shown in **Figure 4D**, 24 h treatment of 50 μl/ml BBJ could inhibit A549 cell migration stimulated by 5 ng/ml of TGF-β1 apparently. In the meantime,

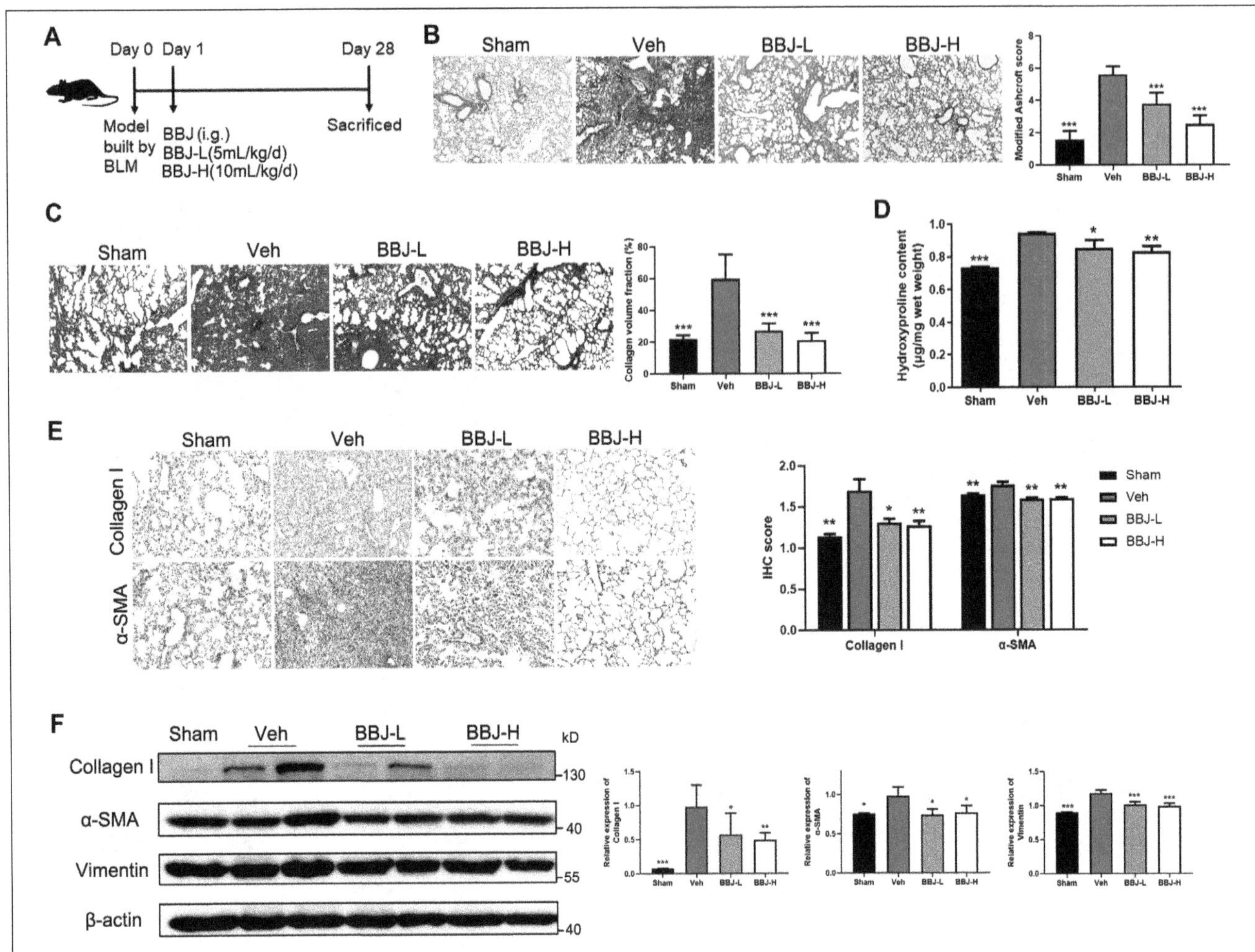

FIGURE 5 | The BBJ could prevent fibrosis formation induced by BLM in mice. **(A)** Arrangement of animal study in the prevention model. The fibrosis model was built by tracheal injection of BLM on day 0. Next day, vehicle and BBJ-fed groups were administrated by saline and BBJ for 4 weeks, respectively. **(B)** Lung sections of each group were stained with H&E (×10). Modified Ashcroft scores were applied to evaluate the degree of pulmonary fibrosis. **(C)** Lung sections of each group were stained by Masson trichrome (×10). Collagen volume fractions were analyzed from the results of Masson-stained lung sections by ImageJ. **(D)** Hydroxyproline contents were tested by the hydroxyproline assay kit. **(E)** The expressions of collagen-I and α-SMA in lung sections were detected by IHC staining, and these proteins' expressions were calculated by ImageJ. **(F)** Expressions of collagen-I, α-SMA, vimentin, and β-actin in lung tissues of each group were analyzed by western blotting. ImageJ software was used to calculate these proteins' expressions. *p < 0.05; **p < 0.01; ***p < 0.001 compared with the vehicle group.

western blotting and immunofluorescence assays were utilized to elucidate mechanisms by which BBJ restrained the EMT process in A549. α-SMA, E-cadherin, and vimentin were involved in the EMT process. TGF-β1 could induce upregulation of α-SMA, p-Smad2/3, and vimentin as well as downregulation of E-cadherin. BBJ reversed these changes significantly, which is expressed in **Figures 4E,F**.

BBJ Could Suppress Formation and Development of Lung Fibrosis *In Vivo*

To determine the antifibrotic ability of BBJ, pulmonary fibrosis models were built through administration of BLM (2 mg/kg for prevention model and 1 mg/kg for treatment model). The sham group was injected with saline. As shown in **Figure 5A**, mice were intragastrically administrated with BBJ or saline every day from day 1 in the prevention model. After 4 weeks, mice were sacrificed, and lung tissues were harvested for histopathology, immunoblot, and hydroxyproline content analyses. As explicated in **Figures 5B,C**, H&E- and Masson-stained results were present. According to the H&E-stained lung sections in the vehicle group, there were variable alveolar septa and large contiguous fibrotic masses (about 40% of the microscopic field). Furthermore, the lung architecture was severely damaged, and part of it was not preserved. After intervention with BBJ, the damage of the lung tissue was reduced. In Masson's trichrome results (**Figure 5C**), collagen fibers were dyed blue. There was no doubt that BBJ could reduce collagen fibers compared to the vehicle group, and the lung sections of the high-dose group tended to be normal. Besides, in the BBJ group, contents of hydroxyproline in the lung tissue were lower than those in the vehicle group, which was treated with saline, as shown in **Figure 5D**. Moreover, contents of

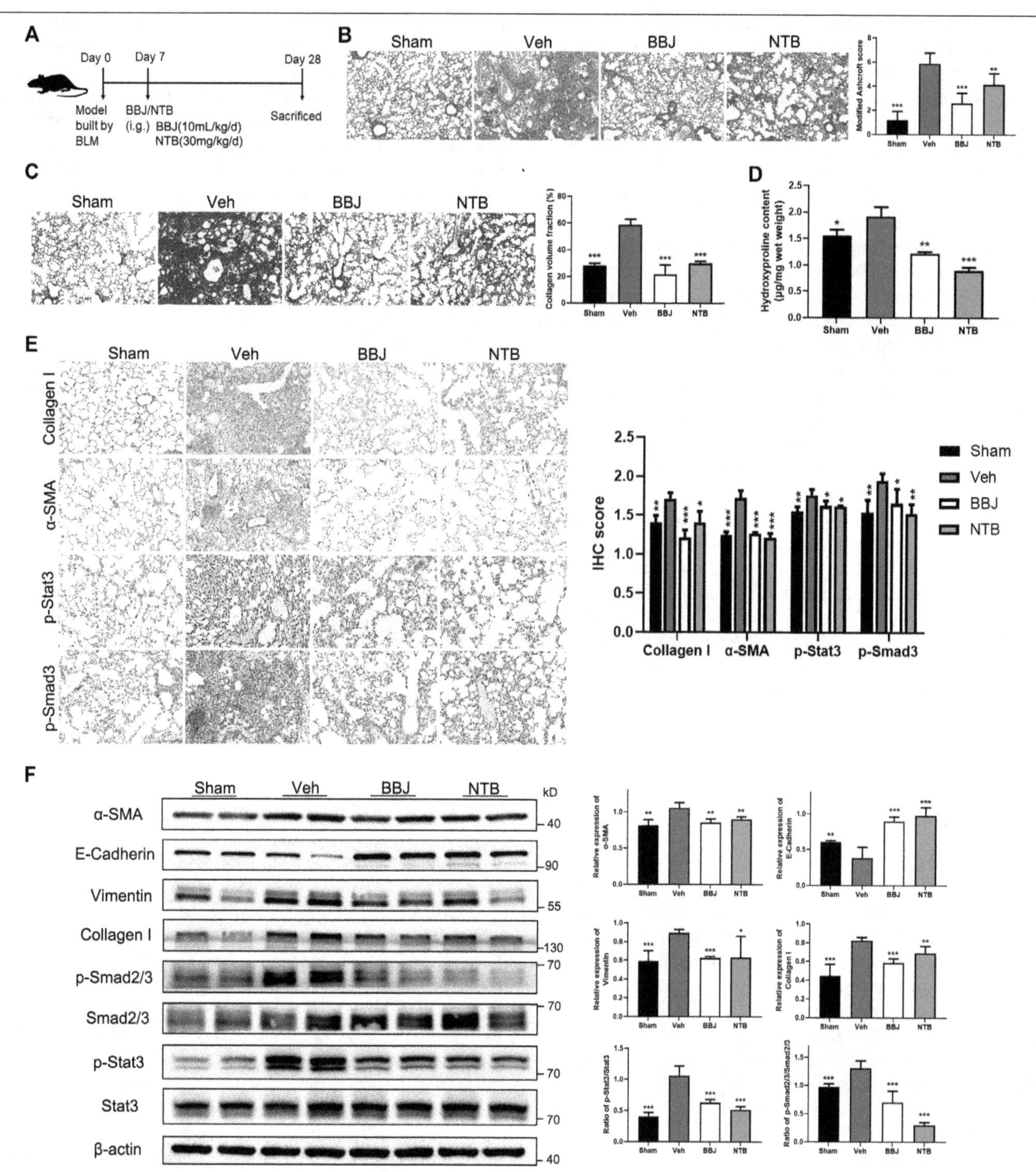

FIGURE 6 | BBJ could alleviate pulmonary fibrosis caused by BLM. **(A)** Arrangement of animal study in the treatment model. The fibrosis model was built by tracheal injection of BLM on day 0. On day 7, vehicle, BBJ-fed, and NTB-fed groups were administrated with saline, BBJ, and NTB for 3 weeks, respectively. **(B)** Lung sections of each group were stained with H&E (×10). Modified Ashcroft scores were applied to evaluate the degree of pulmonary fibrosis. **(C)** Lung sections of each group were stained with Masson trichrome (×10). Collagen volume fractions were analyzed from the results of Masson-stained lung sections by ImageJ. **(D)** Hydroxyproline contents were tested by the hydroxyproline assay kit. **(E)** The expressions of collagen-I, α-SMA, p-Stat3, and p-Smad3 in lung sections were detected by IHC staining, and these proteins' expressions were calculated by ImageJ. **(F)** Expressions of α-SMA, E-cadherin, vimentin, collagen-I, Smad2/3, p-Smad2/3, Stat3, p-Stat3, and β-actin in lung tissues of each group were analyzed by western blotting. ImageJ software was used to calculate these proteins' expressions. *, $p < 0.05$; **, $p < 0.01$; ***, $p < 0.001$ compared with the vehicle group.

IL-10 and IL-17A in serum, which are involved in idiopathic pulmonary fibrosis, were lower in the BBJ group than in the vehicle group, which was explicated in **Supplementary Figure 3A**. To explore the underlying mechanism by which BBJ prevents lung fibrosis *in vivo*, α-SMA and collagen-I in lung tissues were determined by IHC and western blotting. β-Actin served as a reference. In **Figure 5E,F**, the expressions of α-SMA, collagen-I, and vimentin were upregulated evidently in the vehicle group. In contrast with the vehicle group, the BBJ-fed group showed lower expressions of these proteins.

In the treatment model, nintedanib, which was reported to target tyrosine kinases, was used as positive control to verify the inhibitory effect of BBJ on IPF (Liu et al., 2021). Administrations of BBJ or NTB started from 7 days after building the lung fibrosis model and lasted 3 weeks, as displayed in **Figure 6A**. BBJ reduced the fibrotic degree and collagen fibers' deposition in lung tissues, and the results coincided with those in the prevention model. Furthermore, the pulmonary fibrotic degree and deposition of collagen fibers were reduced in the BBJ and NTB groups, as shown in **Figures 6B,C**. We also discovered that the level of hydroxyproline, one of the main amino acids that make up collagen fibers, was decreased in the BBJ and NTB groups (**Figure 6D**). Similar with the prevention model, BBJ could reduce the contents of IL-10 and IL-17A in serum. Only IL-10 levels dropped in the NTB group, as explicated in **Supplementary Figure 3B**. The IHC and western blot results revealed that BLM increased the expressions of α-SMA, collagen-I, vimentin, p-Smad2/3, and p-Stat3 and reduced E-cadherin. Both BBJ and NTB treatment reversed these changes induced by BLM in mice (**Figures 6E,F**). Therefore, in summary, animal studies proved that BBJ could prevent and restrain pulmonary fibrosis *in vivo*.

DISCUSSION

IPF is considered as a progressive respiratory disorder, ultimately causing death within about 3 years after diagnosis (Tzilas et al., 2017). There are only two drugs, nintedanib and pirfenidone, that received regulatory approval from FDA to treat IPF (Karimi-Shah and Chowdhury, 2015). However, the 5-year survival rate still remains less than 50% (Huang et al., 2015). Blueberry is well known as a significant source of nutrition, containing vitamins, fibers, and other phytochemicals with pharmaceutical interest (Miller et al., 2019). The blueberry used in the present study was from Peru, where blueberry production is dominant. Blueberries are rich in anthocyanins, polyphenols, and flavonoids. We detected 30 potential chemicals in BBJ by the method of LC/MS, which is consistent with previous studies (Chen et al., 2010; Yang and Jiang, 2010). Importantly, trehalose, quercetin, rutin, ferulic acid, abscisic acid, and trolox were reported to relieve fibrosis by inhibiting TGF-β (Galicia-Moreno et al., 2008; Bruzzone et al., 2012; Pan et al., 2014; Mu et al., 2018; Liu et al., 2019; Miyake et al., 2020). These phytochemicals were all found in BBJ and may have contributed to the anti-lung fibrosis function of BBJ. Lyophilized BBJ is reported to scavenge superoxide radicals with an IC_{50} value of 7 μg/ml and DPPH radicals with an IC_{50} value of 99 μg/ml (Cásedas et al., 2017). The many biochemicals, especially phenols, may contribute to the antioxidant property of BBJ. In the present study, we found that BBJ reduced ROS production in NIH/3T3, HPF, RPLF, and A549, which proved the antioxidant activity of BBJ. ROS is one of the indicators of the intracellular homeostasis. Accumulation of intracellular ROS could lead to cell death through ferroptosis and the mitochondrial-mediated apoptosis pathway (Li et al., 2016a; Li et al., 2020). Of note, cell death caused by phytochemicals and plant extracts is often accompanied by ROS reduction (Li et al., 2016b; Li et al., 2019). One explanation was that a decreased ROS level may induce changes in cell-cycle regulatory proteins (Qin et al., 2011). Regardless of ROS accumulation increase or decrease, the balance would be destroyed and lead to changes of cellular state, including cell death. Interestingly, there is a growing body of literature that recognizes the health benefits of blueberry, especially antifibrosis activity in rats (Chen et al., 2010; Zhan et al., 2017). Researchers manifested that BBJ could alleviate CCl_4-induced hepatic fibrosis significantly, which was associated with reducing collagen content and α-SMA expression as well as enhancing the antioxidant capability of the liver (Wang et al., 2013). The above evidence suggested that BBJ possesses a potential antifibrosis function.

In IPF, the TGF-β1/Smad signaling pathway is the major mediator. TGF-β1-stimulated phosphorylated Smad2/3 translocates into the nucleus, regulates target gene expressions, and further participates in EMT, fibroblast proliferation, and myofibroblast differentiation, which promotes the pathogenesis of IPF (Lee et al., 2014; Shen et al., 2021). EMT, collagen deposition, and remodeling of the pulmonary interstitium are the dominant features in the pathological changes of IPF (Richeldi et al., 2017; Zhihui Zhang et al., 2018). When alveolar epithelial cells (ACEs) were attacked continuously, inflammatory repair would induce overdeposition of the extracellular matrix, which results in an abnormal lung architecture. In the EMT process, the secretion of TGF-β1 activates this pathology, which also accelerates lung fibrosis. Recently, A549 cells have served as a model of Type II-like ACEs to explore the mechanism of EMT (Foster et al., 1998; Zhang et al., 2019). BBJ induced cell death and downregulated ROS in A549. In the process of EMT, the morphology of A549 underwent a transformation from oval to fusiform once activated by TGF-β1. Meanwhile, the epithelial markers, such as E-cadherin, were downregulated while the mesenchymal markers, including α-SMA and vimentin, were upregulated. Few mesenchymal cells establish tight connections with neighboring cells, and thus, EMT promotes cell metastasis. In the present study, BBJ was proven to inhibit the process of EMT in A549 by suppressing TGF-β1/Smad2/3 signaling.

The myofibroblast differentiation is characterized by altered expressions of α-SMA and proteins involved in ECM, cell migration, and proliferation (Rockey et al., 2015). After tissue injury, the repair process, including differentiation of fibroblasts into proliferating and contractile myofibroblasts, was initiated. When the normal repair process ends, myofibroblasts are regulated to undergo apoptosis; in pathological fibrosis,

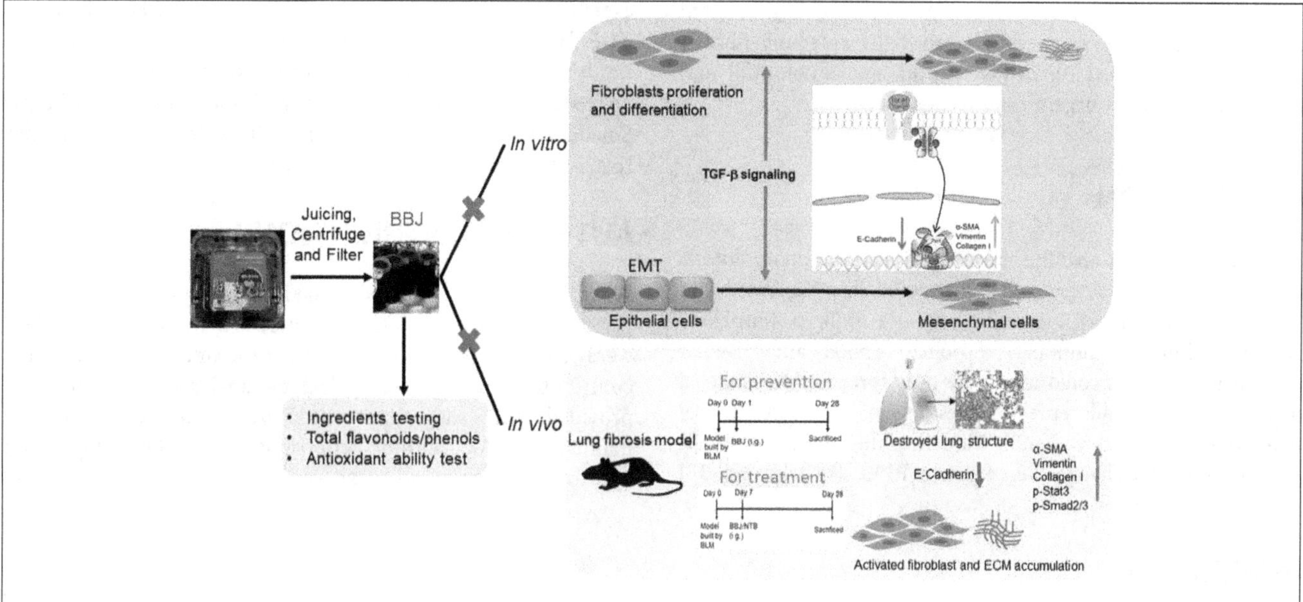

FIGURE 7 | BBJ could inhibit lung fibrosis *in vivo* and *in vitro*. Followed by a series of processing, BBJ was utilized in assays *in vitro* and *in vivo*. BBJ was proven to inhibit EMT in A549. BBJ could also suppress differentiation of fibroblasts to myofibroblasts induced by TGF-β1 proved by the changes of related proteins. In addition, in lung fibrosis, the C57BL/6 mouse model built by BLM, BBJ could prevent and ameliorate lung fibrosis by suppressing the Smad2/3 pathway and Stat3.

myofibroblasts accumulate abnormally in these tissues, increasing the synthesis of extracellular matrix, changing the tissue structure, and finally leading to fibrosis (Darby and Hewitson, 2007). In our study, BBJ could suppress fibroblast proliferation apparently. Fibroblast apoptosis was induced after 24 h intervention with 100 μl/ml BBJ. Furthermore, BBJ curbed differentiation and abnormal recruitment of fibroblasts caused by TGF-β1 by decreasing the upregulated p-Smad2/3 in NIH/3T3 and HPF. High expressions of α-SMA and collagen-I are the typical characteristics of myofibroblasts (Akamatsu et al., 2013). These were also found in RPLF cells, which were activated by BLM. No matter in HPF and NIH/3T3 incubated with TGF-β1 or activated RPLF, BBJ could suppress levels of α-SMA, vimentin, and collagen-I and increase levels of E-cadherin. Additionally, BBJ reversed the high expression of p-Smad2/3 caused by TGF-β1 in NIH/3T3 and HPF. Therefore, BBJ suppressed EMT and activated fibroblasts by blocking the TGF-β1/Smad2/3 signaling pathway.

Our hypothesis of an inhibitory effect of BBJ on pulmonary fibrosis was also supported by the *in vivo* results with BLM-induced lung fibrosis in mice. The BLM-induced lung fibrosis model is a widely used experimental model for lung fibrosis study. In the early phase (7–10 days), an acute inflammatory response is induced by BLM (Chaudhary et al., 2006). In the late phase (21–28 days), the inflammation decreases and fibrotic pathology changes occur and continue (Mouratis and Aidinis, 2011). Therefore, the mice were sacrificed on day 28 to investigate the preventive and inhibitory effects of BBJ on BLM-induced fibrosis, and the dose of BLM was from our preliminary experiments. In the research of anti-hepatic fibrosis activity, rats were gavage-fed daily with BBJ at a dose of 15 g/kg, and hence, we took 5 and 10 ml/kg as the dosages of BBJ to treat the lung fibrotic mice in the prevention model (Wang et al., 2013). And a higher dosage of BBJ was applied in the treatment model. Twenty-eight days after intratracheal injection of BLM, thickening of the lung interstitium, destruction of the alveolar structure, and collagen deposition happened in the lungs. However, continuous daily gavage of BBJ reversed these pathological changes in the dose of 10 ml/kg, whether in the prevention or treatment model. The involved mechanism was similar with altered protein expressions in cells, with remarkable decreased expressions of α-SMA, vimentin, collagen-I, and p-Smad3 and/or p-Smad2/3 as well as upregulated E-cadherin. Besides, collagen deposition was estimated by Masson staining and measuring of hydroxyproline content which decreased in the BBJ group.

Stat3 is a signaling molecule of signal transducers and activators of the transcription family. Our previous studies have elucidated that phytochemicals could suppress tumorigenesis and metastasis by blocking the Stat3 pathway (Li et al., 2019; Zhang et al., 2020). Recently, it is of great interest to manifest the role of Stat3 in fibrosis since abundant activation of Stat3 was confirmed in fibrotic pulmonary IPF patients (O'Donoghue et al., 2012). Also, Stat3 is identified as a positive regular of EMT, the mechanism of which activated Stat3 promotes Smad3 nucleus localization and further accelerates EMT (Junk et al., 2017). Hence, we detected Stat3 expression in the treatment mice model. BBJ and NTB downregulated p-Stat3 expression in fibrotic lung tissue induced by BLM. These results were consistent with previous research that Stat3 was involved in IPF. However, the underlying mechanism needs further study to be elucidated.

Collectively, our present work first revealed that BBJ could prevent and ameliorate IPF by modulating TGF-β1/Smad2/3 signaling. This important discovery not only provides support of dietary guidance for patients with pulmonary fibrosis but also proposes the possibility of juice rich in antioxidants as an accepted therapy for diseases. However, there are still some limitations in the study. One of the limitations in our research is that it is unknown how the ingredients of BBJ exerted antifibrosis activity collectively. Notably, the anti-lung fibrosis activity of BBJ based on evidence from epidemiological and clinical studies is an urgent need to address.

CONCLUSION

Here, we firstly illustrated the effects of BBJ on pulmonary fibrosis *in vitro* and *in vivo*, as expressed in **Figure 7**. When incubated with TGF-β1-stimulated cells, including mouse embryo fibroblasts NIH/3T3, human pulmonary fibroblasts HPF, and alveolar epithelial A549, BBJ could accelerate the expression of epithelial mark E-cadherin and repress expressions of the mesenchymal markers α-SMA and vimentin, hindering the process of EMT. Likewise, the same changes were found in RPLF. Furthermore, BBJ exerted its anti-lung fibrosis effect by preventing cell migration and TGF-β1/Smad2/3 pathway activation. In BLM-induced pulmonary fibrosis mice, BBJ ameliorated the distortion of normal architecture by reducing collagen deposition and inhibiting the TGF-β1/Smad2/3 pathway. All these results indicated comprehensively that BBJ could attenuate lung fibrosis.

AUTHOR CONTRIBUTIONS

WY and TY conceived and designed the experiments. YL and LW performed the experiments and wrote the manuscript. QZ and LT were involved in conducting the experiments. CG and HL contributed reagents/materials/data analysis. TY and WY provided the suggestions for the modification of the manuscript. All authors contributed to the article and approved the submitted manuscript.

REFERENCES

Akamatsu, T., Arai, Y., Kosugi, I., Kawasaki, H., Meguro, S., Sakao, M., et al. (2013). Direct Isolation of Myofibroblasts and Fibroblasts from Bleomycin-Injured Lungs Reveals Their Functional Similarities and Differences. *Fibrog. Tissue Repair* 6 (1), 15. doi:10.1186/1755-1536-6-15

Bao, Y. F., Li, J. Y., Zheng, L. F., and Li, H. Y. (2015). Antioxidant Activities of Cold-Nature Tibetan Herbs Are Signifcantly Greater Than Hot-Nature Ones and Are Associated with Their Levels of Total Phenolic Components. *Chin. J. Nat. Med.* 13 (8), 609–617. doi:10.1016/S1875-5364(15)30057-1

Baumgartner, K. B., Samet, J. M., Stidley, C. A., Colby, T. V., and Waldron, J. A. (1997). Cigarette Smoking: a Risk Factor for Idiopathic Pulmonary Fibrosis. *Am. J. Respir. Crit. Care Med.* 155 (1), 242–248. doi:10.1164/ajrccm.155.1.9001319

Beers, M. F., and Morrisey, E. E. (2011). The Three R's of Lung Health and Disease: Repair, Remodeling, and Regeneration. *J. Clin. Invest.* 121 (6), 2065–2073. doi:10.1172/JCI45961

Bruzzone, S., Battaglia, F., Mannino, E., Parodi, A., Fruscione, F., Basile, G., et al. (2012). Abscisic Acid Ameliorates the Systemic Sclerosis Fibroblast Phenotype *In Vitro*. *Biochem. Biophys. Res. Commun.* 422 (1), 70–74. doi:10.1016/j.bbrc.2012.04.107

Cásedas, G., Les, F., Gómez-Serranillos, M. P., Smith, C., and López, V. (2017). Anthocyanin Profile, Antioxidant Activity and Enzyme Inhibiting Properties of Blueberry and cranberry Juices: a Comparative Study. *Food Funct.* 8 (11), 4187–4193. doi:10.1039/C7FO01205E

Chaudhary, N. I., Schnapp, A., and Park, J. E. (2006). Pharmacologic Differentiation of Inflammation and Fibrosis in the Rat Bleomycin Model. *Am. J. Respir. Crit. Care Med.* 173 (7), 769–776. doi:10.1164/rccm.200505-717OC

Chen, C. F., Li, Y. D., and Xu, Z. (2010). Chemical Principles and Bioactivities of Blueberry. *Yao Xue Xue Bao* 45 (4), 422–429.

Czerwiński, J., Bartnikowska, E., Leontowicz, H., Lange, E., Leontowicz, M., Katrich, E., et al. (2004). Oat (Avena Sativa L.) and Amaranth (Amaranthus Hypochondriacus) Meals Positively Affect Plasma Lipid Profile in Rats Fed Cholesterol-Containing Diets. *J. Nutr. Biochem.* 15 (10), 622–629. doi:10.1016/j.jnutbio.2004.06.002

Darby, I. A., and Hewitson, T. D. (2007). Fibroblast Differentiation in Wound Healing and Fibrosis. *Int. Rev. Cytol.* 257, 143–179. doi:10.1016/S0074-7696(07)57004-X

Foster, K. A., Oster, C. G., Mayer, M. M., Avery, M. L., and Audus, K. L. (1998). Characterization of the A549 Cell Line as a Type II Pulmonary Epithelial Cell Model for Drug Metabolism. *Exp. Cel Res* 243 (2), 359–366. doi:10.1006/excr.1998.4172

Galicia-Moreno, M., Rodríguez-Rivera, A., Reyes-Gordillo, K., Segovia, J., Shibayama, M., Tsutsumi, V., et al. (2008). Trolox Down-Regulates Transforming Growth Factor-Beta and Prevents Experimental Cirrhosis. *Basic Clin. Pharmacol. Toxicol.* 103 (5), 476–481. doi:10.1111/j.1742-7843.2008.00324.x

Horowitz, J. C., and Thannickal, V. J. (2006). Epithelial-Mesenchymal Interactions in Pulmonary Fibrosis. *Semin. Respir. Crit. Care Med.* 27 (6), 600–612. doi:10.1055/s-2006-957332

Hübner, R. H., Gitter, W., El Mokhtari, N. E., Mathiak, M., Both, M., Bolte, H., et al. (2008). Standardized Quantification of Pulmonary Fibrosis in Histological Samples. *BioTechniques* 44 (4), 507–7. doi:10.2144/000112729

Hu, H. H., Chen, D. Q., Wang, Y. N., Feng, Y. L., Cao, G., Vaziri, N. D., et al. (2018). New Insights into TGF-β/Smad Signaling in Tissue Fibrosis. *Chem. Biol. Interact* 292, 76–83. doi:10.1016/j.cbi.2018.07.008

Huang, T. T., Lai, H. C., Ko, Y. F., Ojcius, D. M., Lan, Y. W., Martel, J., et al. (2015). Hirsutella Sinensis Mycelium Attenuates Bleomycin-Induced Pulmonary Inflammation and Fibrosis *In Vivo*. *Sci. Rep.* 5 (1), 15282. doi:10.1038/srep15282

Hubbard, R. (2001). Occupational Dust Exposure and the Aetiology of Cryptogenic Fibrosing Alveolitis. *Eur. Respir. J. Suppl.* 32 (32 Suppl. l), 119s–121s. https://erj.ersjournals.com/content/18/32_suppl/119s

Hung, C., Linn, G., Chow, Y. H., Kobayashi, A., Mittelsteadt, K., Altemeier, W. A., et al. (2013). Role of Lung Pericytes and Resident Fibroblasts in the Pathogenesis of Pulmonary Fibrosis. *Am. J. Respir. Crit. Care Med.* 188 (7), 820–830. doi:10.1164/rccm.201212-2297OC

Junk, D. J., Bryson, B. L., Smigiel, J. M., Parameswaran, N., Bartel, C. A., and Jackson, M. W. (2017). Oncostatin M Promotes Cancer Cell Plasticity through Cooperative STAT3-SMAD3 Signaling. *Oncogene* 36 (28), 4001–4013. doi:10.1038/onc.2017.33

Karimi-Shah, B. A., and Chowdhury, B. A. (2015). Forced Vital Capacity in Idiopathic Pulmonary Fibrosis - FDA Review of Pirfenidone and Nintedanib. *N. Engl. J. Med.* 372 (13), 1189–1191. doi:10.1056/NEJMp1500526

Lee, C.-M., Park, J. W., Cho, W.-K., Zhou, Y., Han, B., Yoon, P. O., et al. (2014). Modifiers of TGF-β1 Effector Function as Novel Therapeutic Targets of Pulmonary Fibrosis. *Korean J. Intern. Med.* 29 (3), 281–290. doi:10.3904/kjim.2014.29.3.281

Li, Y., Liu, B., Yang, F., Yu, Y., Zeng, A., Ye, T., et al. (2016a). Lobaplatin Induces BGC-823 Human Gastric Carcinoma Cell Apoptosis via ROS- Mitochondrial Apoptotic Pathway and Impairs Cell Migration and Invasion. *Biomed. Pharmacother.* 83, 1239–1246. doi:10.1016/j.biopha.2016.08.053

Li, Y., Yang, F., Zheng, W., Hu, M., Wang, J., Ma, S., et al. (2016b). Punica Granatum (Pomegranate) Leaves Extract Induces Apoptosis through Mitochondrial Intrinsic Pathway and Inhibits Migration and Invasion in Non-small Cell Lung Cancer *In Vitro*. *Biomed. Pharmacother.* 80, 227–235. doi:10.1016/j.biopha.2016.03.023

Li, D., Li, B., Ma, Y., Sun, X., Lin, Y., and Meng, X. (2017). Polyphenols, Anthocyanins, and Flavonoids Contents and the Antioxidant Capacity of Various Cultivars of Highbush and Half-High Blueberries. *J. Food Compost. Anal.* 62, 84–93. doi:10.1016/j.jfca.2017.03.006

Li, Y., Gan, C., Zhang, Y., Yu, Y., Fan, C., Deng, Y., et al. (2019). Inhibition of Stat3 Signaling Pathway by Natural Product Pectolinarigenin Attenuates Breast Cancer Metastasis. *Front. Pharmacol.* 10, 1195. doi:10.3389/fphar.2019.01195

Li, J., Cao, F., Yin, H. L., Huang, Z. J., Lin, Z. T., Mao, N., et al. (2020). Ferroptosis: Past, Present and Future. *Cell Death Dis* 11 (2), 88. doi:10.1038/s41419-020-2298-2

Liu, Y., Dai, E., and Yang, J. (2019). Quercetin Suppresses Glomerulosclerosis and TGF-β S-ignaling in a R-at M-odel. *Mol. Med. Rep.* 19 (6), 4589–4596. doi:10.3892/mmr.2019.10118

Liu, H., Wu, X., Gan, C., Wang, L., Wang, G., Yue, L., et al. (2021). A Novel Multikinase Inhibitor SKLB-YTH-60 Ameliorates Inflammation and Fibrosis in Bleomycin-Induced Lung Fibrosis Mouse Models. *Cell Prolif* 54 (7), e13081. doi:10.1111/cpr.13081

Lu, S., Cheng, M.-l., Li, H., Wu, J., and Wang, Y.-p. (2012). Effects of Blueberry on Hepatic Fibrosis and Ultrastructural of Hepatocytes in Rats. *Zhonghua yi xue za zhi* 92, 927–931. doi:10.3760/cma.j.issn.0376-2491.2012.13.015

Miller, K., Feucht, W., and Schmid, M. (2019). Bioactive Compounds of Strawberry and Blueberry and Their Potential Health Effects Based on Human Intervention Studies: A Brief Overview. *Nutrients* 11 (7), 1510. doi:10.3390/nu11071510

Mishra, K., Ojha, H., and Chaudhury, N. K. (2012). Estimation of Antiradical Properties of Antioxidants Using DPPH Assay: A Critical Review and Results. *Food Chem.* 130 (4), 1036–1043. doi:10.1016/j.foodchem.2011.07.127

Miyake, T., Sakai, N., Tamai, A., Sato, K., Kamikawa, Y., Miyagawa, T., et al. (2020). Trehalose Ameliorates Peritoneal Fibrosis by Promoting Snail Degradation and Inhibiting Mesothelial-To-Mesenchymal Transition in Mesothelial Cells. *Sci. Rep.* 10 (1), 14292. doi:10.1038/s41598-020-71230-4

Mouratis, M. A., and Aidinis, V. (2011). Modeling Pulmonary Fibrosis with Bleomycin. *Curr. Opin. Pulm. Med.* 17 (5), 355–361. doi:10.1097/mcp.0b013e328349ac2b

Mu, M., Zuo, S., Wu, R. M., Deng, K. S., Lu, S., Zhu, J. J., et al. (2018). Ferulic Acid Attenuates Liver Fibrosis and Hepatic Stellate Cell Activation via Inhibition of TGF-β/Smad Signaling Pathway. *Drug Des. Devel Ther.* 12, 4107–4115. doi:10.2147/DDDT.S186726

Navaratnam, V., Fleming, K. M., West, J., Smith, C. J., Jenkins, R. G., Fogarty, A., et al. (2011). The Rising Incidence of Idiopathic Pulmonary Fibrosis in the U.K. *Thorax* 66 (6), 462–467. doi:10.1136/thx.2010.148031

O'Donoghue, R. J., Knight, D. A., Richards, C. D., Prêle, C. M., Lau, H. L., Jarnicki, A. G., et al. (2012). Genetic Partitioning of Interleukin-6 Signalling in Mice Dissociates Stat3 from Smad3-Mediated Lung Fibrosis. *EMBO Mol. Med.* 4 (9), 939–951. doi:10.1002/emmm.201100604

Pan, P. H., Lin, S. Y., Wang, Y. Y., Chen, W. Y., Chuang, Y. H., Wu, C. C., et al. (2014). Protective Effects of Rutin on Liver Injury Induced by Biliary Obstruction in Rats. *Free Radic. Biol. Med.* 73, 106–116. doi:10.1016/j.freeradbiomed.2014.05.001

Parker, M. W., Rossi, D., Peterson, M., Smith, K., Sikström, K., White, E. S., et al. (2014). Fibrotic Extracellular Matrix Activates a Profibrotic Positive Feedback Loop. *J. Clin. Invest.* 124 (4), 1622–1635. doi:10.1172/JCI71386

Qin, Y., Pan, X., Tang, T. T., Zhou, L., and Gong, X. G. (2011). Anti-Proliferative Effects of the Novel Squamosamide Derivative (FLZ) on HepG2 Human Hepatoma Cells by Regulating the Cell Cycle-Related Proteins Are Associated with Decreased Ca(2+)/ROS Levels. *Chem. Biol. Interact* 193 (3), 246–253. doi:10.1016/j.cbi.2011.07.004

Raghu, G., and Richeldi, L. (2017). Current Approaches to the Management of Idiopathic Pulmonary Fibrosis. *Respir. Med.* 129, 24–30. doi:10.1016/j.rmed.2017.05.017

Raghu, G., Collard, H. R., Egan, J. J., Martinez, F. J., Behr, J., Brown, K. K., et al. (2011). An Official ATS/ERS/JRS/ALAT Statement: Idiopathic Pulmonary Fibrosis: Evidence-Based Guidelines for Diagnosis and Management. *Am. J. Respir. Crit. Care Med.* 183 (6), 788–824. doi:10.1164/rccm.2009-040GL

Richeldi, L., Collard, H. R., and Jones, M. G. (2017). Idiopathic Pulmonary Fibrosis. *Lancet* 389 (10082), 1941–1952. doi:10.1016/S0140-6736(17)30866-8

Rock, J. R., Barkauskas, C. E., Cronce, M. J., Xue, Y., Harris, J. R., Liang, J., et al. (2011). Multiple Stromal Populations Contribute to Pulmonary Fibrosis without Evidence for Epithelial to Mesenchymal Transition. *Proc. Natl. Acad. Sci. U S A.* 108 (52), E1475–E1483. doi:10.1073/pnas.1117988108

Rockey, D. C., Bell, P. D., and Hill, J. A. (2015). Fibrosis--A Common Pathway to Organ Injury and Failure. *N. Engl. J. Med.* 373 (12), 96–1149. doi:10.1056/NEJMc1504848

Shen, Y. H., Cheng, M. H., Liu, X. Y., Zhu, D. W., and Gao, J. (2021). Sodium Houttuyfonate Inhibits Bleomycin Induced Pulmonary Fibrosis in Mice. *Front. Pharmacol.* 12, 596492. doi:10.3389/fphar.2021.596492

Skrovankova, S., Sumczynski, D., Mlcek, J., Jurikova, T., and Sochor, J. (2015). Bioactive Compounds and Antioxidant Activity in Different Types of Berries. *Int. J. Mol. Sci.* 16 (10), 24673–24706. doi:10.3390/ijms161024673

Taskar, V. S., and Coultas, D. B. (2006). Is Idiopathic Pulmonary Fibrosis an Environmental Disease? *Proc. Am. Thorac. Soc.* 3 (4), 293–298. doi:10.1513/pats.200512-131TK

Thannickal, V. J., Zhou, Y., Gaggar, A., and Duncan, S. R. (2014). Fibrosis: Ultimate and Proximate Causes. *J. Clin. Invest.* 124 (11), 4673–4677. doi:10.1172/JCI74368

Tzilas, V., Bouros, E., Tzouvelekis, A., and Bouros, D. (2017). Guidelines for Idiopathic Pulmonary Fibrosis: Everything Flows. *Respiration* 93 (6), 401–403. doi:10.1159/000473884

Wang, Y., Cheng, M., Zhang, B., Nie, F., and Jiang, H. (2013). Dietary Supplementation of Blueberry Juice Enhances Hepatic Expression of Metallothionein and Attenuates Liver Fibrosis in Rats. *PloS one* 8 (3), e58659. doi:10.1371/journal.pone.0058659

Wynn, T. A. (2007). Common and Unique Mechanisms Regulate Fibrosis in Various Fibroproliferative Diseases. *J. Clin. Invest.* 117 (3), 524–529. doi:10.1172/JCI31487

Yang, H., and Jiang, Y. (2010). Research Progress of Bioactive Constituents, Absorption, Metabolism, and Neuroprotective Effects from Blueberry. *Wei Sheng Yan Jiu* 39 (4), 525–528. doi:10.19813/j.cnki.weishengyanjiu.2010.04.038

Zhan, W., Liao, X., Tian, T., Yu, L., Liu, X., Li, B., et al. (2017). Study on the Effects of Blueberry Treatment on Histone Acetylation Modification of CCl4-Induced Liver Disease in Rats. *Genet. Mol. Res.* 16 (1), 1–10. doi:10.4238/gmr16019188

Zhang, B. F., Cheng, M. L., Wang, Y. P., Zhang, Q., Yu, L., Zhao, X. K., et al. (2018). Effects of Blueberry on Hepatic Fibrosis and Expression of Nuclear Transcription Factor-κB in Rats. *Zhonghua Gan Zang Bing Za Zhi* 26, 590–595. doi:10.3760/cma.j.issn.1007-3418.2018.08.006

Zhang, C., Zhu, X., Hua, Y., Zhao, Q., Wang, K., Zhen, L., et al. (2019). YY1 Mediates TGF-β1-Induced EMT and Pro-fibrogenesis in Alveolar Epithelial Cells. *Respir. Res.* 20 (1), 249. doi:10.1186/s12931-019-1223-7

Zhang, Q., Wang, L., Gan, C., Yu, Y., Li, Y., Deng, Y., et al. (2020). Cryptotanshinone Induces Apoptosis and Inhibits Migration and Invasion in Human Hepatocellular Carcinoma Cells in. *Vitro. Nat. Product. Commun.* 15 (1), 1934578X19899570. doi:10.1177/1934578X19899570

Zhihui Zhang, Z., Qu, J., Zheng, C., Zhang, P., Zhou, W., Cui, W., et al. (2018). Nrf2 Antioxidant Pathway Suppresses Numb-Mediated Epithelial-Mesenchymal Transition during Pulmonary Fibrosis. *Cel Death Dis.* 9 (2), 83. doi:10.1038/s41419-017-0198-x

14

The miR-130a-3p/TGF-βRII Axis Participates in Inhibiting the Differentiation of Fibroblasts Induced by TGF-β1

*Yanhong Liu[1], Yan Ding[1], Yapeng Hou[1], Tong Yu[1], Hongguang Nie[1] and Yong Cui[2]**

[1]Department of Stem Cells and Regenerative Medicine, College of Basic Medical Science, China Medical University, Shenyang, China, [2]Departments of Anesthesiology, The First Hospital of China Medical University, Shenyang, China

***Correspondence:**
Yong Cui
cynhg@cmu.edu.cn

Pulmonary fibrosis (PF) is a chronic progressive interstitial lung disease that has a poor prognosis. Abnormal activation of transforming growth factor-β1 (TGF-β1) plays a crucial role in fibroblast differentiation. Mesenchymal stem cells (MSCs) are currently being considered for the treatment of PF, but the regulatory mechanisms are poorly understood. We co-cultured bone marrow-derived MSCs and mouse lung fibroblasts (MLg) in the presence of TGF-β1, and studied the protein/mRNA expression of fibrosis markers and related signaling pathways. The effects of miR-130a-3p and TGF-β receptor II (TGF-βRII) on the differentiation of MLg induced by TGF-β1 were studied using immunofluorescence assay, Western blot, and quantitative real-time PCR techniques, respectively. Our results showed that MSCs reversed the overexpression of fibrosis markers and TGF-β1/Smad signaling pathway proteins and mRNAs after TGF-β1 treatment and increased the level of miR-130a-3p. TGF-βRII was identified as a target of miR-130a-3p and was evaluated by dual-luciferase reporter assay. The miR-130a-3p/TGF-βRII axis could suppress the differentiation of lung fibroblasts *via* the TGF-β1/Smad signaling pathway, thereby reducing the process of PF.

Keywords: pulmonary fibrosis, mesenchymal stem cells, mouse lung fibroblast, microRNA, TGF-β1

INTRODUCTION

Pulmonary fibrosis (PF) is a chronic lung disease, and its incidence has been rising in recent years (Wu and Xu, 2020; Li et al., 2021). PF usually affects elderly patients, and radiation and mechanical or chemical stimulation have become the main risk factors associated with PF (Froidure et al., 2020; Jin et al., 2020; Yang et al., 2020). The main pathological features of PF are alveolar epithelial cell damage, fibroblast proliferation and activation, excessive collagen deposition, and a large accumulation of extracellular matrix (Sauler et al., 2019; Zhi et al., 2020). Transforming growth factor-β1 (TGF-β1) regulates proliferation and differentiation in a multitude of cell types, and TGF-β1/Smad signaling pathway is associated with fibrosis (Barrett et al., 2017; Liu et al., 2020; Wnuk and Paw, 2020). TGF-β1 binds to TGF-β receptor II (TGF-βRII) on the cell surface, which recruits TGF-βRI. Activation of the latter can phosphorylate Smad2/3 and associates with Smad4, which translocates from the cytoplasm to the nucleus, and regulate gene transcription (Yoshida et al., 2018; Wang et al., 2021).

Abbreviations: miRNAs, microRNAs; MLg, mouse lung fibroblast; MSCs, mesenchymal stem cells; PF, pulmonary fibrosis; qRT-PCR, quantitative real-time PCR; TGF-β1, transforming growth factor-β1; TGF-βRII, TGF-β receptor II.

Mesenchymal stem cells (MSCs) were first discovered and isolated from bone marrow and have multilineage differentiation and self-renewal capacity (Li and Wu, 2020). MSCs are able to promote cell proliferation, repair tissue damage, and improve the microenvironment of the lung tissue *via* extracellular vesicle release to deliver DNA, mRNA, and microRNAs (miRNAs) (Behnke et al., 2020; Kavianpour and Saleh, 2020; Li et al., 2020). Stem cell-derived miRNAs have recently been found to regulate various cellular processes, such as proliferation, apoptosis, stress responses, differentiation, and angiogenesis. Recent literature has shown the potential roles of miRNAs, a type of small noncoding RNA in PF (Dutta et al., 2019; Boateng and Krauss-Etschmann, 2020; Cho et al., 2020), which can regulate target genes or proteins through inflammatory responses related to mRNA degradation or translation inhibition. Among these miRNAs, miR-130a-3p observed in MSCs has been reported to have antitumor effects and has been used for treating neurological diseases (Chen et al., 2010; Glaesel et al., 2020; Zhong et al., 2020). It has also been found that miR-130a-3p could exert cardioprotective effects through the induction of angiogenesis in ischemic hearts after myocardial infarction (Moghaddam, et al., 2019). In the bleomycin-treated mouse PF model, miR-130a-3p mimics significantly reduced the macrophage profibrogenic gene expression (Su et al., 2015). However, studies focused on miR-130a-3p functions in fibroblasts are seldom published. In this study, we investigated bone marrow MSC (BMSC)-derived miR-130a-3p and co-cultured it with mouse lung fibroblasts (MLg) to explore its expression and regulatory mechanism in PF.

By analysis and prediction using TargetScan and miRanda software, we found that miR-130a-3p and TGF-βRII are potential binding partners, the latter of which is important for the TGF-β1 signaling pathway (Kushibiki et al., 2005). We speculate that BMSC-derived miR-130a-3p may participate in the TGF-β1/Smad signaling pathway to inhibit the differentiation of lung fibroblasts, which provides an effective therapeutic approach for PF prevention and treatment by targeting TGF-βRII.

MATERIALS AND METHODS

BMSC Culture and Co-Cultured With MLg

The male C57 mice (weight 9–10 g) were provided by China Medical University, and all experiments were performed with the research protocol approved by the Ethics Committee of China Medical University (No. CMU2019088). According to the method previously reported, BMSCs were isolated and cultured in DMEM/F12 medium with 10% fetal bovine serum (FBS, Gibco, United States), 10 ng/ml recombinant mouse basic fibroblast growth factor (PeproTech, United States), 1% penicillin/streptomycin, and maintained at 37°C in 5% CO_2 (Hou et al., 2020). The medium was changed every 2 days. BMSC characterization has been confirmed in our previously published paper (Zhou et al., 2021). At 80% confluence, the medium of BMSCs was changed with DMEM/F12 medium without FBS. BMSC-CM was collected after 24 h and stored at −80°C. MLg was purchased from American Type Culture Collection (ATCC, United States) and cultured in a 6-well plate with DMEM medium adding 10% fetal bovine serum (FBS, Gibco, United States), and 1% penicillin/streptomycin. For the co-culture mode, the BMSCs were prepared in 6-well Transwell inserts, which were transferred to the 6-well plate with MLg seeded at the bottom after 24 h. The BMSCs co-cultured with MLg were treated with DMEM without FBS for another 24 h, and used for the following experiment.

Cell Transfection

BMSCs or MLg was transfected using Lipofectamine 2000 (GenePharma, CHN) according to the manufacturer's protocol. In brief, 50–60% confluent BMSCs or MLg grown in medium was incubated with Lipofectamine 2000 reagent and TGF-βRII-siRNA (si-TGF-βRII), miR-130a-3p mimic (Mimic), miR-130a-3p inhibitor (Inhibitor), negative control (NC, the negative control of miR-130a-3p mimic or si-TGF-βRII), and inhibitor NC (the negative control of miR-130b inhibitor) for 72 h, respectively. Labeled CY3-miR-130a-3p was also used and its distribution was observed under a fluorescence microscope.

Western Blot Assays

MLg was washed three times with PBS and lysed using a cell lysis reagent. Proteins were analyzed by SDS-PAGE (10% polyacrylamide gels) and transferred to PVDF membranes (Invitrogen, United States). Membranes were blocked with 5% BSA for 1 h and incubated with primary antibodies, which were against α-SMA (Merck, GER; 1:1,000 dilution), FN (Abcam, United States; 1:1,000 dilution), TGF-βRII (Elabscience, CHN; 1:1,000 dilution), SMAD2/3 (Elabscience, CHN; 1:1,000 dilution), p-SMAD2/3 (Elabscience, CHN; 1:1,000 dilution), and β-actin (Santa Cruz, United States; 1:1,000 dilution). The membranes were then washed three times with TBST and incubated with goat anti-rabbit or anti-mouse secondary antibody (ZSGB-BIO, CHN; 1:5,000 dilution) at room temperature for 1 h. The bands of protein were obtained from the same membrane, which were then visualized using an ECL kit on a Tanon-5200 chemiluminescence detection system (Tanon, CHN) and quantified using ImageJ program.

Quantitative Real-Time PCR Analysis

According to the manufacturer's instructions, total RNA was isolated using TRIzol reagent (Invitrogen, United States) and the extracted RNA samples were quantified by NanoDrop 2000C spectrophotometer (Thermo, United States). Total RNA and miRNAs were reverse transcribed into cDNA using synthesis Kit (TaKaRa, Japan). Quantitative real-time PCR (qRT-PCR) reactions were then performed with SYBR Premix Ex Taq II (TaKaRa, Japan) in the ABI 7500 System. Results were calculated using the GAPDH (for mRNAs) or U6 gene (for miRNAs) (Santa Cruz Biotechnology, United States) as internal controls based on the $2^{-\Delta\Delta CT}$ method. All the primers are shown in **Table 1**.

Cell Viability Assay

The effects of miR-130a-3p and si-TGF-βRII on MLg viability were measured by CCK8 assay (Dojindo, CHN) according to the manufacturer's instructions. Briefly, MLg were cultured in a 96-

TABLE 1 | Primer sequences of qRT-PCR.

Gene	Forward primer sequence	Reverse primer sequence
α-SMA	5′-CTA TGA AGG CTA TGC CCT GCC-3′	5′-GCT TCT CCT TGA TGT CTC GCA C-3′
FN	5′-TGT TAT GGA GGA AGC CGA GGT T-3′	5′-CGA TGC AGG TAC AGT CCC AGA-3′
Col III	5′-TGG AAA CTG GGG AAA CAT GC-3′	5′-GGA TTG CCG TAG CTA AAC TGA-3′
TGF-βR I	5′-AAA CTT GCT CTG TCC ACG G-3′	5′-AAT GGC TGG CTT TCC TTG-3′
TGF-βR II	5′-GTA ATA GGA ATG CCC ATC CAC-3′	5′-GAT TTC TGG TTG TCA CAG GTG-3′
SMAD2	5′-AGA ATA TCG GAG GCA GAC AG-3′	5′-GTT ACA GCG AGT CTT TGA TGG-3′
GAPDH	5′-AGA AGG CTG GGG CTC ATT TG-3′	5′-AGG GGC CAT CCA CAG TCT TC-3′
U6	5′-GGA ACG ATA CAG AGA AGA TTA GC-3′	5′-TGG AAC GCT TCA CGA ATT TGC G-3′
miR-130a-3p	5′-CAG UGC AAU GUU AAA AGG GCA U-3′	5′-GCC CUU UUA ACA UUG CAC UGU U-3′

well plate along with NC, miR-130a-3p, or si-TGF-βRII, respectively. After 24 h, TGF-β1 (5 μl) was added to the corresponding well. 48 h after incubation, 10% CCK8 solution was added to each well. After the cells were incubated for additional 2 h, the absorbance was measured at 450 nm wavelength with a microplate reader (Tecan, CH).

Immunofluorescence Staining for α-SMA

MLg was incubated in 6-well plates, and fixed for 30 min with 4% of paraformaldehyde (Sigma, GER). After washing, 0.1% Triton X-100 was used for permeabilization. The cells were then visualized using anti-α-SMA primary antibody (CBL171, Mreck, GER; 1:200 dilution) at 4°C overnight and a labeled secondary antibody for 90 min. The nuclei were stained for DAPI for 15 min in the dark. Finally, the cells were examined using a fluorescence microscope.

Dual Luciferase Reporter Gene Assay

The wild-type (WT) TGF-βRII 3′-untranslated regions (3′-UTR) and mutant-type (MUT) TGF-βRII (3′-UTR) sequences of TGF-βRII were synthesized by GenePharma (CHN). The miR-130a-3p mimic or miR-130a-3p negative control was cotransfected into H441 cells using Lipofectamine 2000. After 48 h, luciferase activities were detected by the Dual Luciferase Reporter Assay Kit (Vazyme, CHN).

Statistical Analysis

All data were processed by Origin 8.0 and presented as the mean ± SE. Normality and homoscedasticity test were done by Levene and Shapiro-Wilk test before applying parametric tests. The differences between two groups was determined by Student's two-tailed *t*-test. When the data did not pass the normality or homoscedasticity test, non-parametric *t*-test (Mann-Whitney *U*-test) was applied. $p < 0.05$ was regarded as statistically significant.

RESULTS

BMSCs Rescues TGF-β1-Induced Myofibroblast Differentiation *In Vitro*

TGF-β1 is involved in the development of PF. Some studies have shown that the inhibition of proliferation and differentiation of fibroblasts are related to the activation of TGF-β1, and the signaling pathways mediated by it play a vital role in lung diseases (Wolters et al., 2014; Aschner and Downey, 2016). The PF model was constructed by treating MLg with 10 ng/mL TGF-β1 for 24 h, which in some case was also added just after MLg was co-cultured with BMSCs. The Western blot assay revealed that the levels of fibrosis markers (α-SMA and FN) in MLg increased after TGF-β1 treatment, whereas the expression levels reduced when co-cultured with BMSCs (**Figures 1A–C**), indicating a successful PF *in vitro* model with TGF-β1-induction. Subsequently, we assessed the expression levels of the above indicators with qRT-PCR, and the result was consistent with that of the Western blot (**Figures 1D–F**). These data suggest that BMSCs significantly rescued TGF-β1-induced myofibroblast differentiation.

Aberrant transcription of signaling pathways might trigger PF, among which TGF-β1 plays a central role (Saito et al., 2018a; Froidure et al., 2020). As expected, TGF-β1/Smad signaling pathway proteins (TGF-βRII, SMAD2/3 and p-SMAD2/3) increased with TGF-β1 treatment, which was reversed after BMSC administration (**Figures 2A–C**), and verified at the mRNA level (**Figures 2D–F**). This observation indicates that the TGF-β1/Smad signaling pathway may participate in the beneficial effect of BMSCs in PF.

BMSCs Enhance the Expression Level of miR-130a-3p After TGF-β1 Induction

It is well known that miRNAs can help MSCs communicate with their surrounding environment (Asgarpour et al., 2020). We hypothesized that the role of BMSCs in TGF-β1-induced fibroblasts may be mediated *via* miRNAs. Based on relevant literature reports and website prediction, we screened out miR-130a-3p that may be beneficial to PF, which was present both in MSCs and MSCs-derived microparticles (Chen et al., 2010; Ferguson, et al., 2018). BMSC-CM is a medium that contains the secretions in BMSCs, such as exosome, miRNAs, etc (Marlina, et al., 2021). We postulated that BMSCs may participate in the protective effects on PF by secreting miR-130a-3p to BMSC-CM and then exert its effects on the receptor cell MLg, and to verify this possibility, we compared the content of miR-130a-3p originating from MLg, BMSC, and BMSC-CM, which showed higher expression levels in BMSC than in BMSC-CM (**Figure 3A**). Moreover, miR-130a-3p significantly decreased after TGF-β1 induction compared with the control group, which was reversed after BMSC administration, suggesting that miR-130a-3p might be related to BMSC treatment of PF (**Figure 3B**).

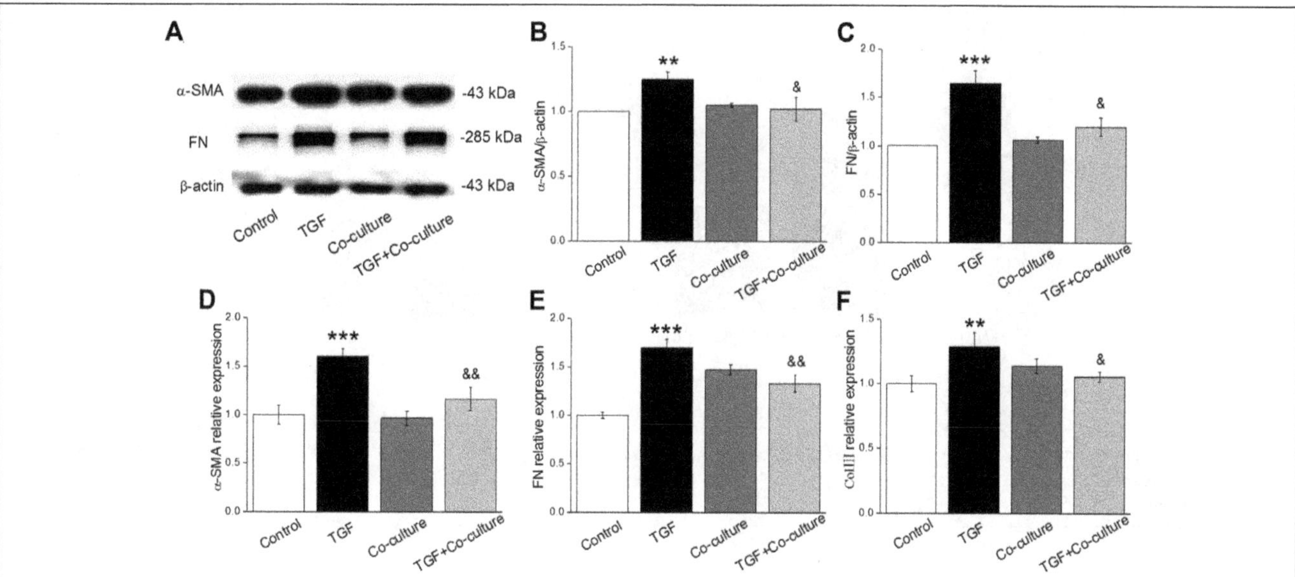

FIGURE 1 | TGF-β1 treatment enhances the level of fibrotic-related protein/mRNAs and BMSCs reverse the above expression in MLg. **(A)** Representative bands of α-SMA and FN protein expression by Western blot in MLg treated with TGF-β1 for 24 h and/or co-cultured with BMSCs for 24 h **(B,C)** Statistical analyses were showed with relative gray values of the protein bands (α-SMA/β-actin and FN/β-actin). **(D-F)** Representative statistical analysis of α-SMA, FN and Col III mRNA by qRT-PCR (α-SMA/GAPDH, FN/GAPDH and Col III/GAPDH). Data were presented as mean ± SE, $^{**}p < 0.01$, $^{***}p < 0.001$, compared with Control group. $^{\&}p < 0.05$, $^{\&\&}p < 0.01$, compared with TGF group. n = 3–6.

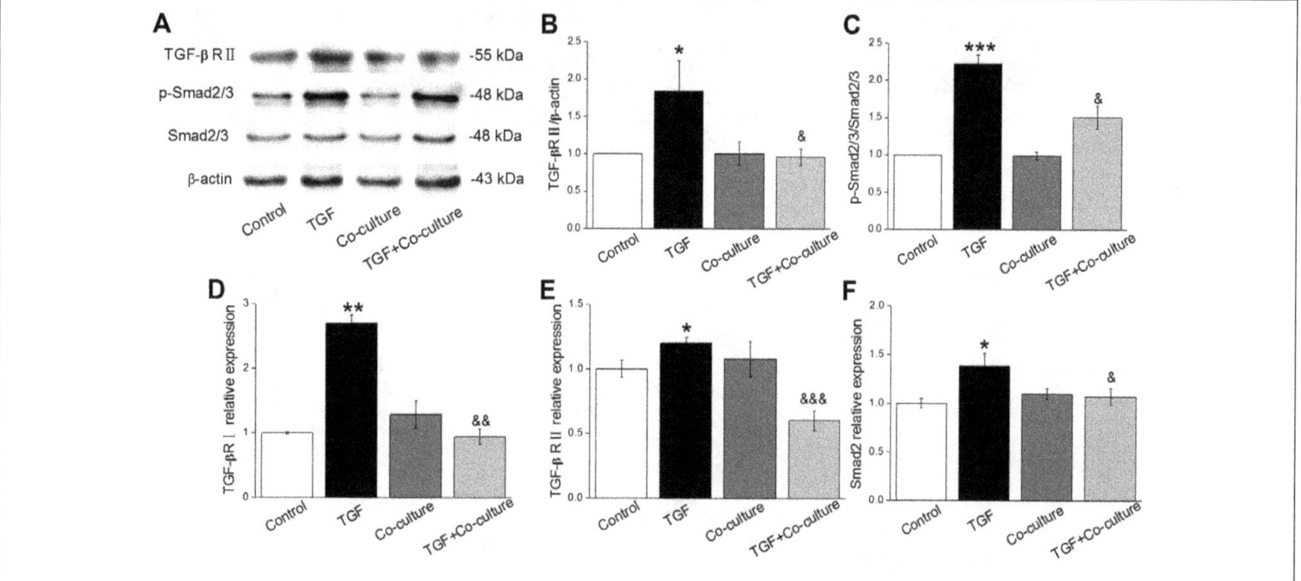

FIGURE 2 | BMSCs decrease the level of TGF-β1/Smad signaling pathway proteins in MLg treated with TGF-β1. **(A)** Representative bands for TGF-βRII, Smad2/3, and p-Smad2/3 protein levels. **(B,C)** Statistical analyses were obtained from relative gray values of the protein bands (TGF-βRII/β-actin and p-Smad2/3/Smad2/3). **(D-F)** Representative statistical analysis of TGF-βRI, TGF-βRII and Smad2 mRNA by qRT-PCR (TGF-βRI/GAPDH, TGF-βRII/GAPDH and Smad2/GAPDH). Data were presented as mean ± SE, $^{*}p < 0.05$, $^{**}p < 0.01$, $^{***}p < 0.001$, compared with Control group. $^{\&}p < 0.05$, $^{\&\&}p < 0.01$, $^{\&\&\&}p < 0.001$, compared with TGF group. n = 3–4.

MiR-130a-3p Inhibits Fibroblast Differentiation

Increasing evidence indicates that both the proliferation and differentiation of fibroblasts contribute to the formation of fibrosis, and TGF-β1 stimulates fibrotic-related α-SMA expression, collagen synthesis, and extracellular matrix deposition (Li et al., 2016; Huang et al., 2017). To confirm the effect of miR-130a-3p, we transfected MLg with the miR-130a-3p mimic and then added TGF-β1 after 48 h. Above all, the CCK8 assay results showed that TGF-β1 significantly promoted the

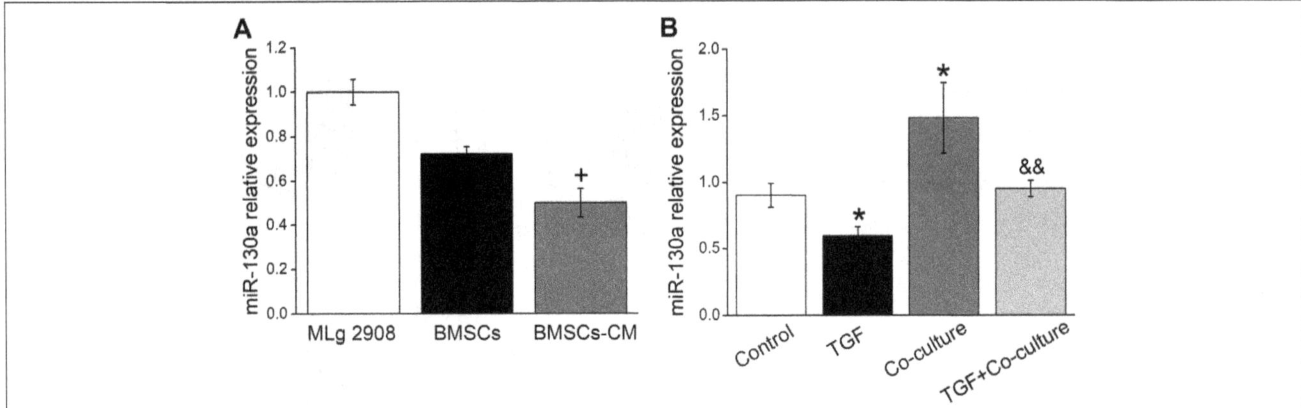

FIGURE 3 | The expression of miR-130a-3p *in vitro*. **(A)** The expression of miR-130a-3p in MLg, BMSCs and BMSCs-CM was detected by qRT-PCR (miR-130a-3p/U6). **(B)** The expression of miR-130a-3p in MLg treated with TGF-β1 for 24 h and/or co-cultured with BMSCs for 24 h $^{+}p < 0.05$, compared with BMSCs group. $^{*}p < 0.05$, compared with Control group. $^{\&\&}p < 0.01$, compared with TGF group. $n = 3$.

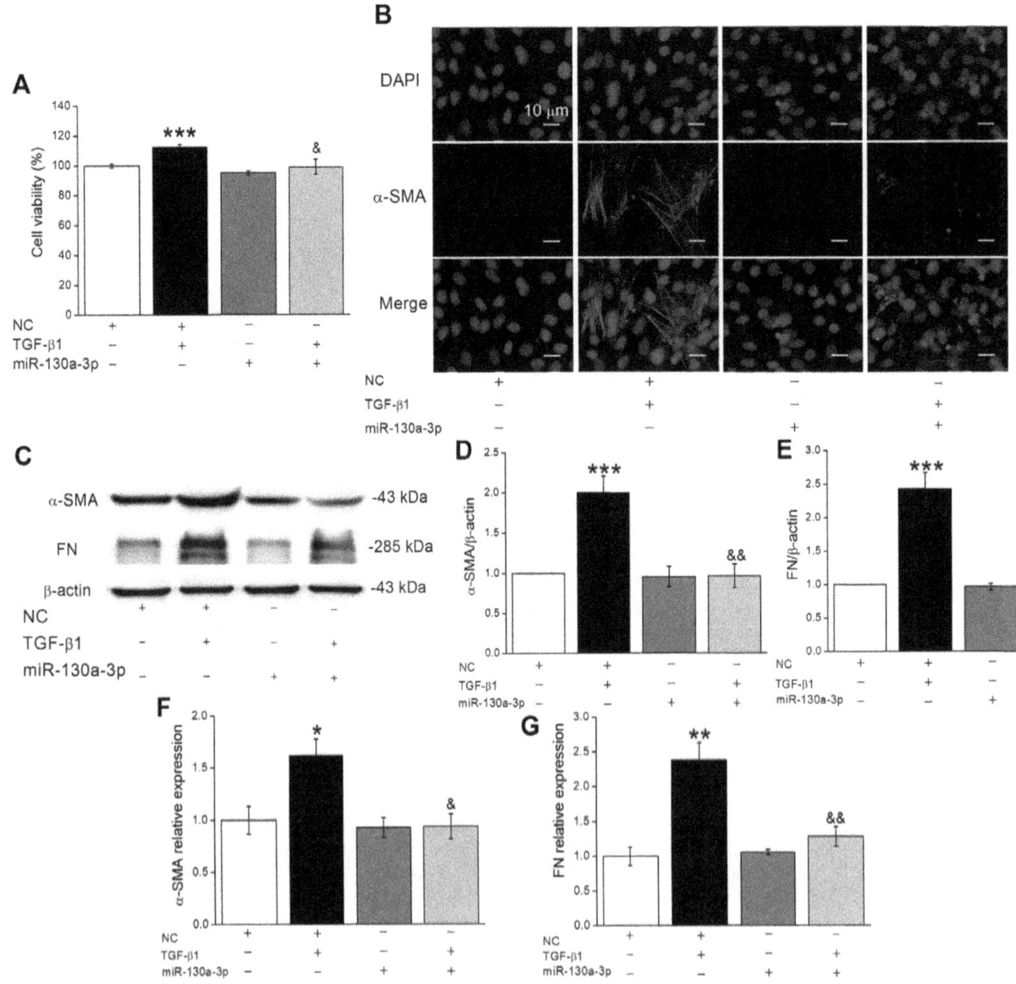

FIGURE 4 | The effect of miR-130a-3p on the differentiation in TGF-β1-induced MLg. **(A)** The relative cell viability was measured in CCK8 assay, and the data for NC group was set to 100%. **(B)** The effect of miR-130a-3p on fibroblast-myofibroblast transition was measured with immunofluorescence. Scale bar = 10 μm. **(C)** Western blot bands of α-SMA and FN protein expression in MLg after transfection of miR-130a-3p. **(D,E)** Statistical analyses were obtained from relative gray values of the protein bands (α-SMA/β-actin and FN/β-actin). **(F,G)** The result of qRT-PCR assay shows the α-SMA and FN mRNA level in MLg (α-SMA/GAPDH, and FN/GAPDH). Data were presented as mean ± SE, $^{*}p < 0.05$, $^{**}p < 0.01$, $^{***}p < 0.001$, compared with NC group. $^{\&}p < 0.05$, $^{\&\&}p < 0.01$, compared with NC + TGF group. $n = 3$–5.

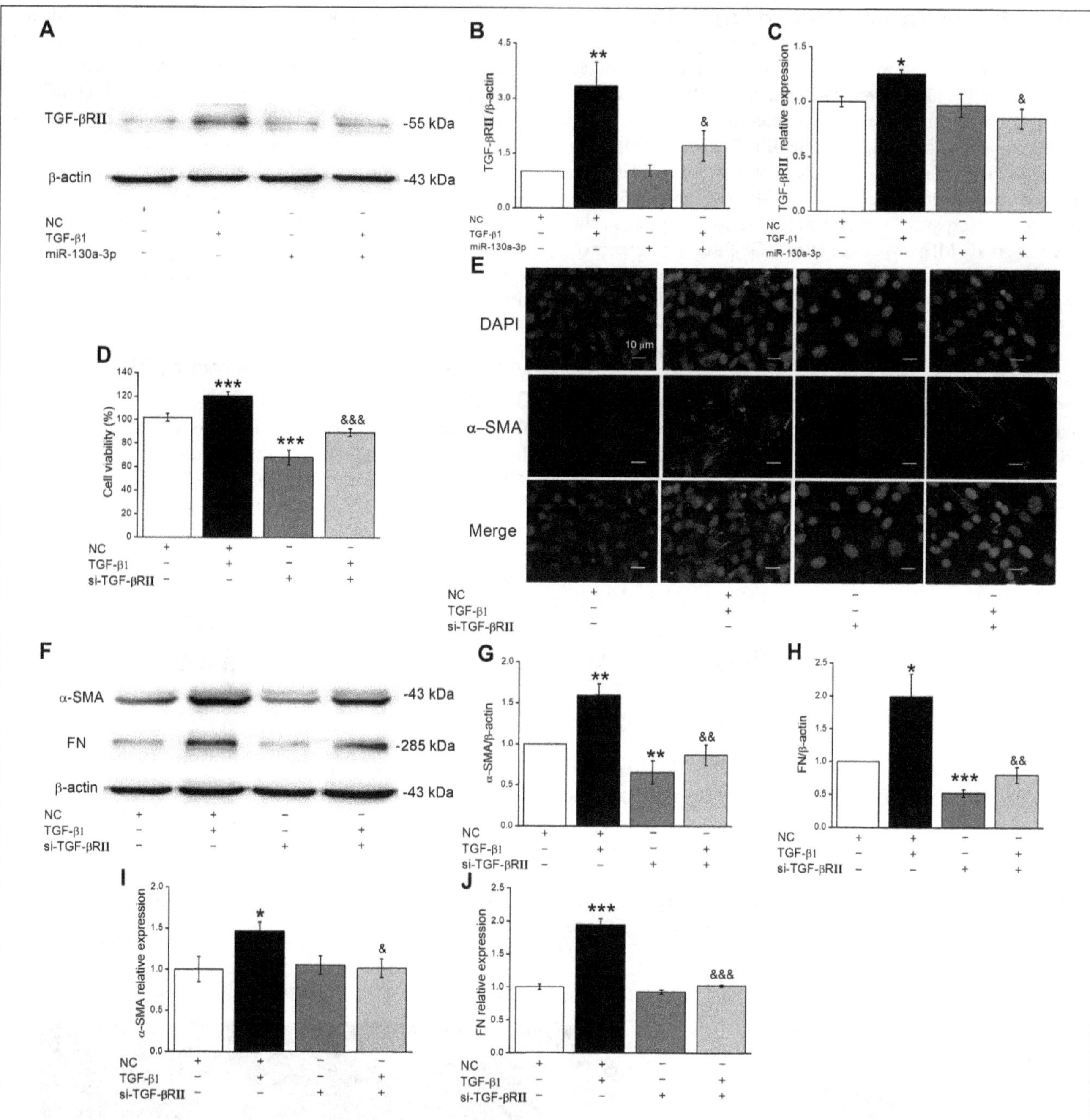

FIGURE 5 | MiR-130a-3p decreases protein level TGF-βRII in MLg and silencing TGF-βRII inhibits TGF-β1-induced MLg differentiation. **(A)** Representative Western blot bands of TGF-βRII protein expression in MLg transfected with miR-130a-3p mimic and treated with TGF-β1 for 24 h. **(B)** Level of TGF-βRII protein was obtained from Western blot analysis. **(C)** Level of TGF-βRII mRNA was analyzed. **(D)** The effect of TGF-βRII knockdown on the inhibition of MLg proliferation. **(E)** Immunofluorescence staining was demonstrated the effect of TGF-βRII silence on MLg differentiation. Scale bar = 10 μm. **(F)** Western blot bands of α-SMA and FN protein expression in MLg after transfection of si-TGF-βRII. **(G,H)** Western blot statistical analyses for α-SMA and FN protein (α-SMA/β-actin and FN/β-actin). **(I,J)** qRT-PCR statistical analyses for α-SMA and FN mRNA (α-SMA/GAPDH and FN/GAPDH). Data were presented as mean ± SE, $^{*}p < 0.05$, $^{**}p < 0.01$, $^{***}p < 0.001$, compared with NC group. $^{\&}p < 0.05$, $^{\&\&}p < 0.01$, $^{\&\&\&}p < 0.001$, compared with NC + TGF group. n = 3–4.

viability in MLg, which was inhibited by miR-130a-3p (**Figure 4A**). Meanwhile, the immunofluorescence results showed that overexpression of miR-130a-3p inhibited the differentiation of MLg, which was enhanced after TGF-β1 stimulation (**Figure 4B**). Consistently, TGF-β1 upregulated the expression of fibrotic-related proteins and mRNAs in MLg, which was reversed by the miR-130a-3p mimic (**Figures 4C–G**). Taken together, these results indicate that miR-130a-3p is involved in the regulation of fibroblast differentiation.

TGF-βRII is a Target Gene of miR-130a-3p

Gene targets of miR-130a-3p were identified using miRNA target prediction databases, and we found that TGF-βRII was a possible target gene of miR-130a-3p. Previous studies showed that the TGF-β1 signaling pathway controls cell proliferation, differentiation, organ development, etc., by combing with TGF-βRII (Shi et al., 2020). First, we examined whether miR-130a-3p downregulated TGF-βRII expression by Western blot and qRT-PCR (**Figures 5A–C**). Moreover, to explore whether miR-130a-3p suppresses the differentiation of MLg by deregulating TGF-βRII, we researched the influence of silencing TGF-βRII on the differentiation of MLg. Using the CCK8 assay, we found that si-TGF-βRII could inhibit the viability of MLg induced by TGF-β1, indicating that TGF-βRII plays an indispensable role in the TGF-β1 signaling pathway (**Figure 5D**). Simultaneously, si-TGF-βRII was further verified to inhibit differentiation in MLg according to an immunofluorescence assay (**Figure 5E**). Finally, as shown in **Figures 5F–J**, fibrosis markers and relative signaling pathways were examined at the protein and mRNA levels, all of which supported that miR-130a-3p could regulate cell differentiation by targeting TGF-βRII.

To further gain evidence regarding miR-130a-3p directly targeted TGF-βRII, we cotransfected NC and the miR-130a-3p mimic (Mimic) into H441 cells with a luciferase reporter system containing the wild-type (WT) or mutated (Mut) 3′-UTR of TGF-βRII (**Figures 6A,B**). The luciferase activity was decreased in H441 cells cotransfected with miR-130a-3p mimic and TGF-βRII-WT (Mimic + WT), compared with H441 cells cotransfected with NC and TGF-βRII-WT (NC + WT). However, the expression of TGF-βRII-Mut (Mimic + Mut) was not suppressed. These data suggest that TGF-βRII is a direct target gene of miR-130a-3p, which could regulate the differentiation of lung fibroblasts by directly interacting with the 3′-UTR of TGF-βRII.

MiR-130a-3p is Transferred to MLg When Co-Cultured With BMSCs

There is increasing evidence that miRNAs secreted by MSCs play their roles by entering into the receptor cells. We transfected miR-130a-3p mimic or NC into BMSCs, then collected BMSCs-CM after 24 h, and verified the expression of miR-130a-3p in BMSCs-CM by

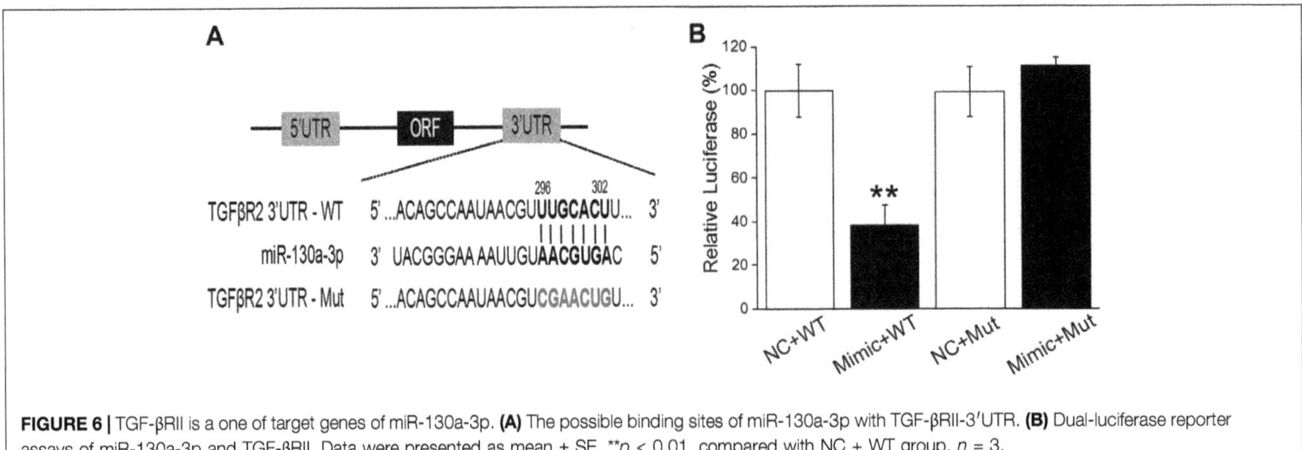

FIGURE 6 | TGF-βRII is a one of target genes of miR-130a-3p. **(A)** The possible binding sites of miR-130a-3p with TGF-βRII-3′UTR. **(B)** Dual-luciferase reporter assays of miR-130a-3p and TGF-βRII. Data were presented as mean ± SE, $^{**}p < 0.01$, compared with NC + WT group. $n = 3$.

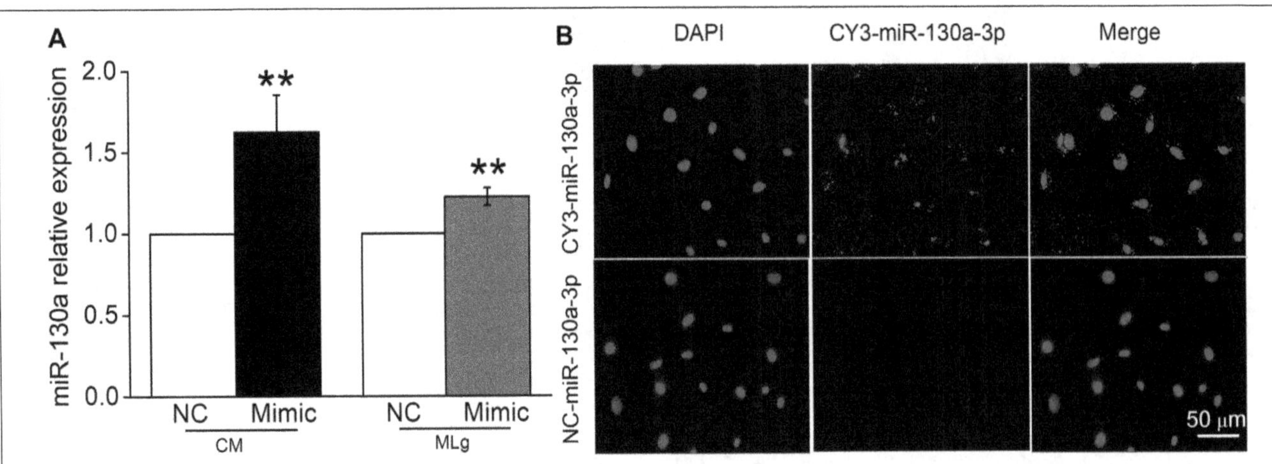

FIGURE 7 | MiR-130a-3p can be transferred to MLg co-cultured with BMSC. **(A)** MiR-130a-3p mimic (Mimic) or negative control (NC) was transfected in BMSCs, and the transfection efficiency was shown in BMSCs-CM (CM) and co-cultured MLg (MLg), respectively. **(B)** BMSCs were transfected with CY3-miR-130a-3p, and co-cultured with MLg for 24 h. The Nuclei were counterstained with DAPI (blue), and a representative CY3-miR-130a-3p stained image was shown in the MLg (red). Scale bar, 50 μm. Data were expressed as mean ± SE, $^{**}p < 0.01$, compared with NC group. $n = 3–6$.

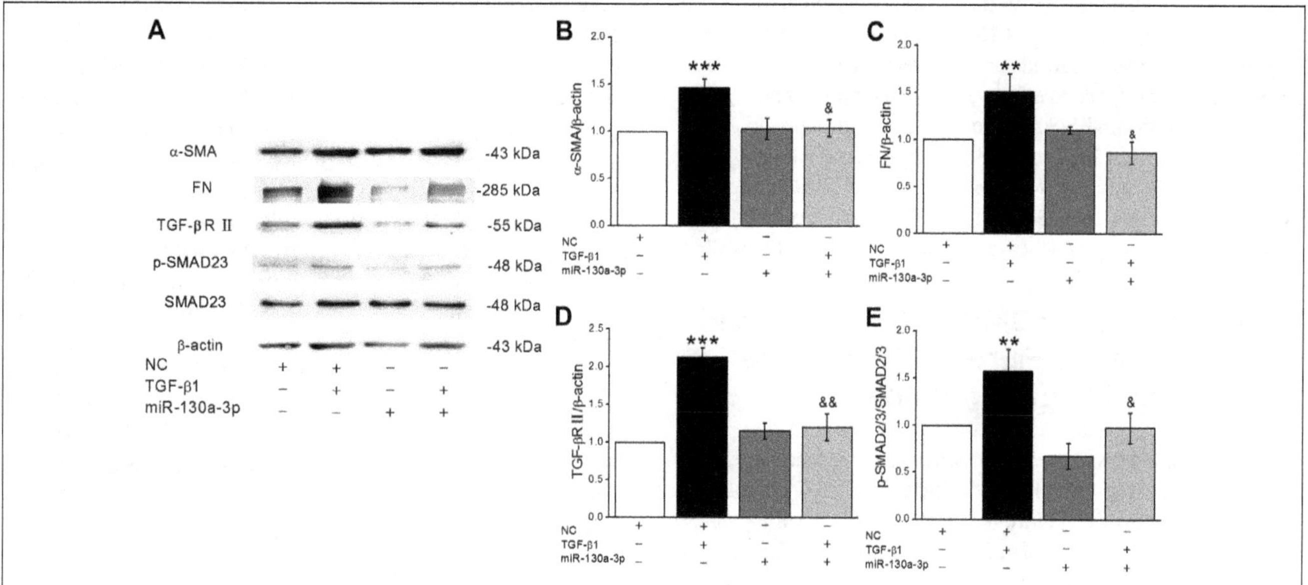

FIGURE 8 | MiR-130a-3p in BMSCs regulates fibrogenesis of MLg induced by TGF-β1 by inhibiting the function of TGF-βRII. **(A)** Representative Western blot bands of α-SMA, FN, TGF-βRII, Smad2/3 and p-Smad2/3 protein expression in BMSCs transfected with NC or miR-130a-3p mimic, followed by co-cultured with MLg. **(B–E)** The statistical analysis of the above-mentioned proteins was obtained from the relative gray values of the protein bands (α-SMA/β-actin, FN/β-actin, TGF-βRII/β-actin, p-Smad2/3/Smad2/3). Data were presented as mean ± SE, $^{**}p < 0.01$, $^{***}p < 0.001$, compared with NC group. $^{\&}p < 0.05$, $^{\&\&}p < 0.01$, compared with NC + TGF group. n = 3–4.

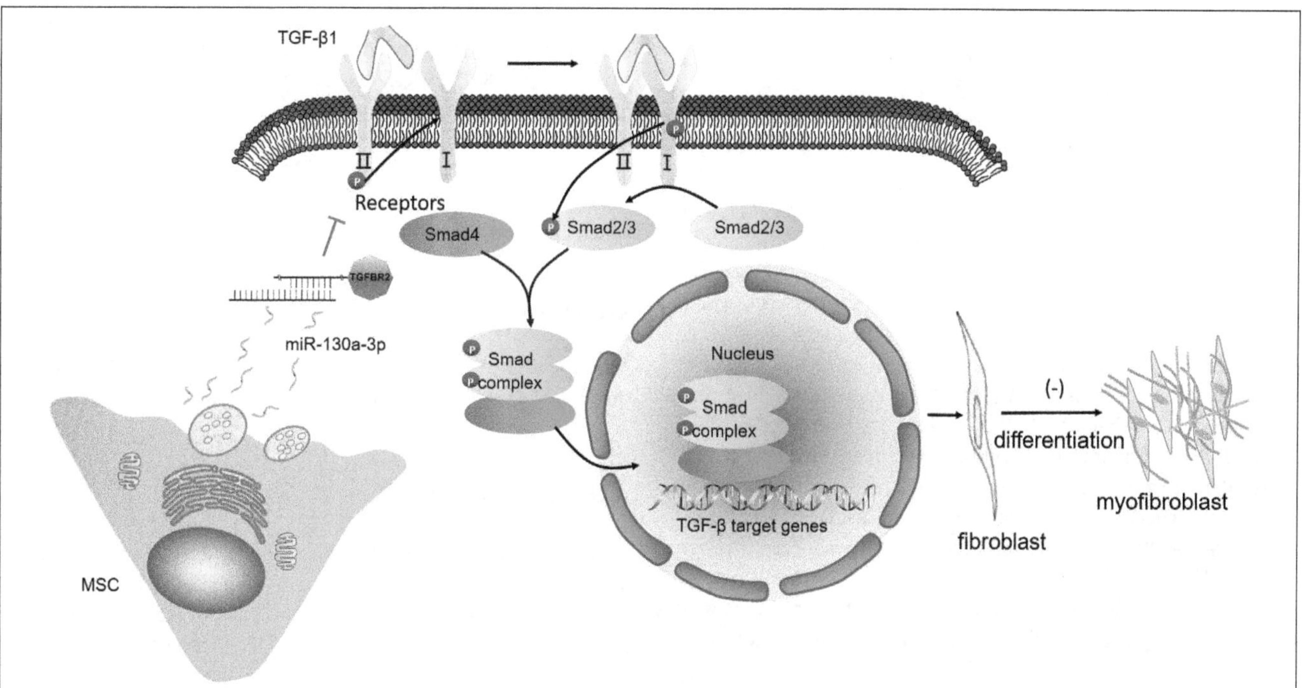

FIGURE 9 | A schematic diagram highlighting the regulation of the cell differentiation by miR-130a-3p in MSCs. The miR-130a-3p secreted by MSCs directly binds to the 3′UTR of TGF-βRII, thereby down-regulating TGF-βRII and inhibiting the recruitment and activation of TGF-βRI, subsequently, phosphorylation of Smad2/3 is inhibited, and unable to form a complex with Smad4, which translocates to the nucleus to regulate gene transcription. MSC, mesenchymal stem cells; TGF-β1, transforming growth factor-β1; TGFBR2, transforming growth factor-β receptor II.

qRT-PCR. Meanwhile, the transfected BMSCs were co-cultured with MLg, and the expression of miR-130a-3p was also detected in MLg (**Figure 7A**). In order to provide direct evidence that miR-130a-3p in BMSCs can be transferred to MLg, we transfected fluorescently labeled CY3-miR-130a-3p into BMSCs and observed its distribution in the co-cultured MLg under a fluorescence microscope. The evidence of CY3-miR-130a-3p appearance in MLg co-cultured with BMSCs, provided us a proof that at least miR-130a-3p from BMSCs could be transferred to the receptor cell MLg, and then exerted its effects on PF (**Figure 7B**).

MiR-130a-3p from BMSCs Participates in the Regulation of Fibrosis Through the TGF-β1/Smad Signaling Pathway

To investigate whether miR-130a-3p from BMSCs could ameliorate the expression of fibrosis markers, we transfected the miR-130a-3p mimic into BMSCs, which were then co-cultured with MLg. As shown in **Figure 8** A-E, MLg treated with TGF-β1 increased expression of α-SMA, FN, TGF-βRII, and p-SMAD2/3, all of which were reversed after administration of miR-130a-3p. The above data suggested that BMSCs may participate in the development of PF through miR-130a-3p, which could regulate the TGF-β1/Smad signaling pathway by targeting TGF-βRII.

DISCUSSION

PF is a progressive interstitial pneumonia characterized by excessive proliferation of fibroblasts and deposition of the extracellular matrix. Currently, the overall prognosis is poor, and effective therapeutic strategies are scarce (Noble et al., 2012; Wang et al., 2016; Chanda et al., 2019). Fibroblasts are regarded as the key effector cells of PF, involved in the key process of pathogenesis (Wuyts et al., 2013). Among them, TGF-β1/Smad signaling participates in the lung epithelium mesenchyme transition, and contributes to the process of PF (Saito et al., 2018b; Liu et al., 2018). In recent years, there has been much enthusiasm regarding MSC therapy for the treatment of lung diseases (Srour and Thébaud, 2015), and there are reports that the beneficial effects of MSCs may be mediated mainly through paracrine action (Willis et al., 2018). In this study, we first demonstrated the impact of BMSCs on MLg with Western Blot and qRT-PCR, and the results showed that compared with the control group, the expression of fibrosis marker and TGF-β1/Smad signaling pathway proteins and mRNAs increased in MLg after using TGF-β1 alone, whereas the effect was opposite after the coadministration of BMSCs. These results confirmed that BMSCs may contribute to alleviating fibrosis formation during PF, the mechanism of which is related to the regulation of the TGF-β1/Smad signaling pathway.

MiRNAs function by binding to the 3′-untranslated regions of mRNA to regulate posttranscriptional processes, thereby controlling various cellular processes (Su et al., 2015; Kang, 2017). We speculate that the above results may also work through miRNAs and evaluate the role of miR-130a-3p, which has been reported to reduce cell senescence and regulate the epithelial-mesenchymal transition (Jiang et al., 2020; Yin et al., 2020). However, it has been relatively seldom studied in TGF-β1-induced lung fibroblasts or PF. First, we confirmed the expression of miR-130a-3p in BMSC-CM and BMSCs by qRT-PCR. In addition, miR-130a-3p was downregulated by treatment with TGF-β1 in MLg, and when co-cultured with BMSCs, the expression level was significantly increased, suggesting that miR-130a-3p derived from BMSCs could influence TGF-β1-induced MLg. Next, overexpression of miR-130a-3p inhibited the cell differentiation phenotype. Future studies are warranted to explore the *in vivo* effects of miR-130a-3p in a bleomycin-induced PF animal model and its translational value as a diagnostic marker and therapeutic target for PF.

Of note, TGF-βRII has been predicted by relevant websites and verified as a potential target of miR-130a-3p using dual-luciferase reporter system in our study. Moreover, TGF-βRII was downregulated after miR-130a-3p overexpression, consistent with the direct targeting role of TGF-βRII for miR-130a-3p. Previous studies have shown that TGF-βRII-deficient mice could effectively resist PF caused by bleomycin (Li et al., 2011), supporting that as a receptor necessary for TGF-β1 signaling, TGF-βRII is essential for the development of PF Li et al., 2011; Zhang et al., 2017). After the induction model was constructed by transfection of TGF-βRII siRNA, we found that cell differentiation were inhibited, and the expression of fibrosis marker proteins and mRNAs was reduced, indicating that silencing TGF-βRII had similar effects on the overexpression of miR-130a-3p in the process of affecting fibroblasts. We also verified that BMSCs transmit miR-130a-3p into TGF-β1-induced MLg to target the TGF-βRII axis, thereby inactivating the TGF-β1/Smad signaling pathway (**Figure 9**), which may provide a future direction for the treatment of PF.

CONCLUSION

MiR-130a-3p in BMSCs inhibits the lung fibroblast differentiation through blocking the activation of TGF-β1/Smad signaling pathway.

AUTHOR CONTRIBUTIONS

Conceived and designed the study: YC and HN. Performed the study: YL and YD. Analyzed the data: YL, YH, and TY. Drafted the manuscript: YL and YC. Revised the draft of manuscript: HN. All authors corrected and approved the final version of the manuscript.

REFERENCES

Aschner, Y., and Downey, G. P. (2016). Transforming Growth Factor-β: Master Regulator of the Respiratory System in Health and Disease. *Am. J. Respir. Cell Mol Biol* 54 (5), 647–655. doi:10.1165/rcmb.2015-0391tr

Asgarpour, K., Shojaei, Z., Amiri, F., Ai, J., Mahjoubin-Tehran, M., Ghasemi, F., et al. (2020). Exosomal microRNAs Derived from Mesenchymal Stem Cells: Cell-To-Cell Messages. *Cell Commun Signal* 18 (1), 149. doi:10.1186/s12964-020-00650-6

Barrett, C. S. X., Millena, A. C., and Khan, S. A. (2017). TGF-β Effects on Prostate Cancer Cell Migration and Invasion Require FosB. *Prostate* 77 (1), 72–81. doi:10.1002/pros.23250

Behnke, J., Kremer, S., Shahzad, T., Chao, C.-M., Böttcher-Friebertshäuser, E., Morty, R. E., et al. (2020). MSC Based Therapies-New Perspectives for the Injured Lung. *J. Clin. Med.* 9 (3), 682. doi:10.3390/jcm9030682

Boateng, E., and Krauss-Etschmann, S. (2020). miRNAs in Lung Development and Diseases. *Int. J. Mol. Sci.* 21 (8), 2765. doi:10.3390/ijms21082765

Chanda, D., Otoupalova, E., Smith, S. R., Volckaert, T., De Langhe, S. P., and Thannickal, V. J. (2019). Developmental Pathways in the Pathogenesis of Lung Fibrosis. *Mol. Aspects Med.* 65, 56–69. doi:10.1016/j.mam.2018.08.004

Chen, T. S., Lai, R. C., Lee, M. M., Choo, A. B. H., Lee, C. N., and Lim, S. K. (2010). Mesenchymal Stem Cell Secretes Microparticles Enriched in Pre-microRNAs. *Nucleic Acids Res.* 38 (1), 215–224. doi:10.1093/nar/gkp857

Cho, S. J., Lee, M., Stout-Delgado, H. W., and Moon, J.-S. (2020). DROSHA-Dependent miRNA and AIM2 Inflammasome Activation in Idiopathic Pulmonary Fibrosis. *Int. J. Mol. Sci.* 21 (5), 1668. doi:10.3390/ijms21051668

Dutta, R. K., Chinnapaiyan, S., and Unwalla, H. (2019). Aberrant microRNAomics in Pulmonary Complications: Implications in Lung Health and Diseases. *Mol. Ther. - Nucleic Acids* 18, 413–431. doi:10.1016/j.omtn.2019.09.007

Ferguson, S. W., Wang, J., Lee, C. J., Liu, M., Neelamegham, S., Canty, J. M., et al. (2018). The microRNA Regulatory Landscape of MSC-Derived Exosomes: a Systems View. *Sci. Rep.* 8 (1), 1419. doi:10.1038/s41598-018-19581-x

Froidure, A., Marchal-Duval, E., Homps-Legrand, M., Ghanem, M., Justet, A., Crestani, B., et al. (2020). Chaotic Activation of Developmental Signalling Pathways Drives Idiopathic Pulmonary Fibrosis. *Eur. Respir. Rev.* 29 (158), 190140. doi:10.1183/16000617.0140-2019

Glaesel, K., May, C., Marcus, K., Matschke, V., Theiss, C., and Theis, V. (2020). miR-129-5p and miR-130a-3p Regulate VEGFR-2 Expression in Sensory and Motor Neurons during Development. *Int. J. Mol. Sci.* 21 (11), 3839. doi:10.3390/ijms21113839

Hou, Y., Zhou, Z., Liu, H., Zhang, H., Ding, Y., Cui, Y., et al. (2020). Mesenchymal Stem Cell-Conditioned Medium Rescues LPS-Impaired ENaC Activity in Mouse Trachea via WNK4 Pathway. *Curr. Pharm. Des.* 26 (29), 3601–3607. doi:10.2174/1381612826666200131141732

Huang, C., Xiao, X., Yang, Y., Mishra, A., Liang, Y., Zeng, X., et al. (2017). MicroRNA-101 Attenuates Pulmonary Fibrosis by Inhibiting Fibroblast Proliferation and Activation. *J. Biol. Chem.* 292 (40), 16420–16439. doi:10.1074/jbc.m117.805747

Jiang, X., Ruan, X. L., Xue, Y. X., Yang, S., Shi, M., and Wang, L. N. (2020). Metformin Reduces the Senescence of Renal Tubular Epithelial Cells in Diabetic Nephropathy via the MBNL1/miR-130a-3p/STAT3 Pathway. *Oxid Med. Cell Longev* 2020, 8708236. doi:10.1155/2020/8708236

Jin, H., Yoo, Y., Kim, Y., Kim, Y., Cho, J., and Lee, Y.-S. (2020). Radiation-Induced Lung Fibrosis: Preclinical Animal Models and Therapeutic Strategies. *Cancers* 12 (6), 1561. doi:10.3390/cancers12061561

Kang, H. (2017). Role of MicroRNAs in TGF-β Signaling Pathway-Mediated Pulmonary Fibrosis. *Int. J. Mol. Sci.* 18 (12), 2527. doi:10.3390/ijms18122527

Kavianpour, M., and Saleh, M. (2020). The Role of Mesenchymal Stromal Cells in Immune Modulation of COVID-19: Focus on Cytokine Storm. *Stem Cell Res Ther* 11 (1), 404. doi:10.1186/s13287-020-01849-7

Kushibiki, T., Nagata-Nakajima, N., Sugai, M., Shimizu, A., and Tabata, Y. (2005). Delivery of Plasmid DNA Expressing Small Interference RNA for TGF-β Type II Receptor by Cationized Gelatin to Prevent Interstitial Renal Fibrosis. *J. Controlled Release* 105 (3), 318–331. doi:10.1016/j.jconrel.2005.02.030

Li, H., Zhao, X., Shan, H., and Liang, H. (2016). MicroRNAs in Idiopathic Pulmonary Fibrosis: Involvement in Pathogenesis and Potential Use in Diagnosis and Therapeutics. *Acta Pharmaceutica Sinica B* 6 (6), 531–539. doi:10.1016/j.apsb.2016.06.010

Li, M., Krishnaveni, M. S., Li, C., Zhou, B., Xing, Y., Banfalvi, A., et al. (2011). Epithelium-specific Deletion of TGF-β Receptor Type II Protects Mice from Bleomycin-Induced Pulmonary Fibrosis. *J. Clin. Invest.* 121 (1), 277–287. doi:10.1172/jci42090

Li, R.-F., Chen, X.-Y., Xu, Y., Feng, F.-C., He, H.-L., and Zhou, X.-M. (2021). Inhibitory Effects of Alkaline Extract from the Pericarp of Citrus Reticulata Blanco on Collagen Behavior in Bleomycin-Induced Pulmonary Fibrosis. *J. Ethnopharmacology* 269, 113761. doi:10.1016/j.jep.2020.113761

Li, S. N., and Wu, J. F. (2020). TGF-β/SMAD Signaling Regulation of Mesenchymal Stem Cells in Adipocyte Commitment. *Stem Cell Res Ther* 11 (1), 41. doi:10.1186/s13287-020-1552-y

Li, Z., Niu, S., Guo, B., Gao, T., Wang, L., Wang, Y., et al. (2020). Stem Cell Therapy for COVID-19, ARDS and Pulmonary Fibrosis. *Cell Prolif* 53 (12), e12939. doi:10.1111/cpr.12939

Liu, Y.-Y., Shi, Y., Liu, Y., Pan, X.-H., and Zhang, K.-X. (2018). Telomere Shortening Activates TGF-β/Smads Signaling in Lungs and Enhances Both Lipopolysaccharide and Bleomycin-Induced Pulmonary Fibrosis. *Acta Pharmacol. Sin* 39 (11), 1735–1745. doi:10.1038/s41401-018-0007-9

Liu, Y. L., Chen, B. Y., Nie, J., Zhao, G. H., Zhuo, J. Y., Yuan, J., et al. (2020). Polydatin Prevents Bleomycin-Induced Pulmonary Fibrosis by Inhibiting the TGF-β/Smad/ERK Signaling Pathway. *Exp. Ther. Med.* 20 (5), 62. doi:10.3892/etm.2020.9190

Marlina, M., Rahmadian, R., Armenia, A., Aviani, J. K., Sholihah, I. A., Kusuma, H. S. W., et al. (2021). Conditioned Medium of IGF1-Induced Synovial Membrane Mesenchymal Stem Cells Increases Chondrogenic and Chondroprotective Markers in Chondrocyte Inflammation. *Biosci. Rep.* 41 (7), BSR20202038. doi:10.1042/bsr20202038

Moghaddam, A. S., Afshari, J. T., Esmaeili, S.-A., Saburi, E., Joneidi, Z., and Momtazi-Borojeni, A. A. (2019). Cardioprotective microRNAs: Lessons from Stem Cell-Derived Exosomal microRNAs to Treat Cardiovascular Disease. *Atherosclerosis* 285, 1–9. doi:10.1016/j.atherosclerosis.2019.03.016

Noble, P. W., Barkauskas, C. E., and Jiang, D. (2012). Pulmonary Fibrosis: Patterns and Perpetrators. *J. Clin. Invest.* 122 (8), 2756–2762. doi:10.1172/jci60323

Saito, A., Horie, M., Micke, P., and Nagase, T. (2018a). The Role of TGF-β Signaling in Lung Cancer Associated with Idiopathic Pulmonary Fibrosis. *Int. J. Mol. Sci.* 19 (11), 3611. doi:10.3390/ijms19113611

Saito, A., Horie, M., and Nagase, T. (2018b). TGF-β Signaling in Lung Health and Disease. *Int. J. Mol. Sci.* 19 (8), 2460. doi:10.3390/ijms19082460

Sauler, M., Bazan, I. S., and Lee, P. J. (2019). Cell Death in the Lung: the Apoptosis-Necroptosis axis. *Annu. Rev. Physiol.* 81, 375–402. doi:10.1146/annurev-physiol-020518-114320

Shi, Q., Wu, H., Li, Y., Shen, L., Tian, X., and Lin, T. (2020). Inhibition of Wilms' Tumor Proliferation and Invasion by Blocking TGF-β Receptor I in the TGF-β/Smad Signaling Pathway. *Biomed. Res. Int.* 2020, 8039840. doi:10.1155/2020/8039840

Srour, N., and Thébaud, B. (2015). Mesenchymal Stromal Cells in Animal Bleomycin Pulmonary Fibrosis Models: a Systematic Review. *Stem Cell Transl Med* 4 (12), 1500–1510. doi:10.5966/sctm.2015-0121

Su, S., Zhao, Q., He, C., Huang, D., Liu, J., Chen, F., et al. (2015). miR-142-5p and miR-130a-3p Are Regulated by IL-4 and IL-13 and Control Profibrogenic Macrophage Program. *Nat. Commun.* 6, 8523. doi:10.1038/ncomms9523

Wang, C., Gu, S., Cao, H., Li, Z., Xiang, Z., Hu, K., et al. (2016). miR-877-3p Targets Smad7 and Is Associated with Myofibroblast Differentiation and Bleomycin-Induced Lung Fibrosis. *Sci. Rep.* 6, 30122. doi:10.1038/srep30122

Wang, X.-M., Liu, X.-M., Wang, Y., and Chen, Z.-Y. (2021). Activating Transcription Factor 3 (ATF3) Regulates Cell Growth, Apoptosis, Invasion and Collagen Synthesis in Keloid Fibroblast through Transforming Growth Factor Beta (TGF-Beta)/SMAD Signaling Pathway. *Bioengineered* 12 (1), 117–126. doi:10.1080/21655979.2020.1860491

Willis, G. R., Fernandez-Gonzalez, A., Anastas, J., Vitali, S. H., Liu, X., Ericsson, M., et al. (2018). Mesenchymal Stromal Cell Exosomes Ameliorate Experimental Bronchopulmonary Dysplasia and Restore Lung Function through Macrophage Immunomodulation. *Am. J. Respir. Crit. Care Med.* 197 (1), 104–116. doi:10.1164/rccm.201705-0925oc

Wnuk, D., and Paw, M. (2020). Enhanced Asthma-Related Fibroblast to Myofibroblast Transition Is the Result of Profibrotic TGF-β/Smad2/3 Pathway Intensification and Antifibrotic TGF-β/Smad1/5/(8)9 Pathway Impairment. *Sci. Rep.* 10 (1), 16492. doi:10.1038/s41598-020-73473-7

Wolters, P. J., Collard, H. R., and Jones, K. D. (2014). Pathogenesis of Idiopathic Pulmonary Fibrosis. *Annu. Rev. Pathol. Mech. Dis.* 9, 157–179. doi:10.1146/annurev-pathol-012513-104706

Wu, Q., and Xu, Y. (2020). A Clinical Model for the Prediction of Acute Exacerbation Risk in Patients with Idiopathic Pulmonary Fibrosis. *Biomed. Res. Int.* 2020, 8848919. doi:10.1155/2020/8848919

Wuyts, W. A., Agostini, C., Antoniou, K. M., Bouros, D., Chambers, R. C., Cottin, V., et al. (2013). The Pathogenesis of Pulmonary Fibrosis: a Moving Target. *Eur. Respir. J.* 41 (5), 1207–1218. doi:10.1183/09031936.00073012

Yang, J., Pan, X., Wang, L., and Yu, G. (2020). Alveolar Cells under Mechanical Stressed Niche: Critical Contributors to Pulmonary Fibrosis. *Mol. Med.* 26 (1), 95. doi:10.1186/s10020-020-00223-w

Yin, J., Ye, Y.-L., Hu, T., Xu, L.-J., Zhang, L.-P., Ji, R.-N., et al. (2020). Hsa_circRNA_102610 Upregulation in Crohn's Disease Promotes Transforming Growth Factor-β1-Induced Epithelial-Mesenchymal Transition via Sponging of Hsa-miR-130a-3p. *World J. Gastroenterol.* 26 (22), 3034–3055. doi:10.3748/wjg.v26.i22.3034

Yoshida, K., Matsuzaki, K., Murata, M., Yamaguchi, T., Suwa, K., and Okazaki, K. (2018). Clinico-Pathological Importance of TGF-β/Phospho-Smad Signaling During Human Hepatic Fibrocarcinogenesis. *Cancers* 10 (6), 183. doi:10.3390/cancers10060183

Zhang, Q., Ye, H., Xiang, F., Song, L.-J., Zhou, L.-L., Cai, P.-C., et al. (2017). miR-18a-5p Inhibits Sub-pleural Pulmonary Fibrosis by Targeting TGF-β Receptor II. *Mol. Ther.* 25 (3), 728–738. doi:10.1016/j.ymthe.2016.12.017

Zhi, N., Mo, Q., Yang, S., Qin, Y. X., Chen, H., Wu, Z. G., et al. (2020). Treatment of Pulmonary Fibrosis in One Convalescent Patient with corona Virus Disease 2019 by Oral Traditional Chinese Medicine Decoction: A Case Report. *J. Integr. Med.* 5, S2095–S4964. doi:10.1016/j.joim.2020.11.005

Zhong, G., Lin, Y., Wang, X., Wang, K., Liu, J., and Wei, W. (2020). H19 Knockdown Suppresses Proliferation and Induces Apoptosis by Regulating miR-130a-3p/SATB1 in Breast Cancer Cells. *Onco Targets Ther.* 13, 12501–12513. doi:10.2147/ott.s280142

Zhou, Z., Hua, Y., Ding, Y., Hou, Y., Yu, T., Cui, Y., et al. (2021). Conditioned Medium of Bone Marrow Mesenchymal Stem Cells Involved in Acute Lung Injury by Regulating Epithelial Sodium Channels via miR-34c. *Front. Bioeng. Biotechnol.* 9, 640116. doi:10.3389/fbioe.2021.640116

15

Azithromycin Attenuates Bleomycin-Induced Pulmonary Fibrosis Partly by Inhibiting the Expression of LOX and LOXL-2

*Xiang Tong, Shijie Zhang, Dongguang Wang, Li Zhang, Jizheng Huang, Tianli Zhang and Hong Fan**

Department of Respiratory Medicine and Critical Care Medicine, West China Hospital/West China School of Medicine, Sichuan University, Chengdu, China

***Correspondence:**
Hong Fan
fanhongfan@qq.com

Pulmonary fibrosis (PF) is a chronic and progressive process of tissue repair. Azithromycin (AZM) may be beneficial for the treatment of PF because AZM has anti-inflammatory and immune regulatory roles and inhibits remodeling, but the mechanism is not entirely clear. In this study, we established a mouse PF model induced by bleomycin (BLM) and primary mouse lung fibroblasts stimulated by transforming growth factor (TGF)-β1 to explore the possible mechanisms of AZM in PF. Results showed that AZM reduces mortality and lung inflammation and attenuates BLM-induced PF in mice. AZM effectively reduced the expression of α-smooth muscle actin (SMA) and type I collagen. Meanwhile, expression of lysyl oxidase (LOX) and lysyl oxidase-like protein (LOXL)-2 in the lung tissue of mice after AZM treatment was significantly lower than in the BLM group. In addition, this study found that AZM significantly inhibits the TGF-β1/Smad and JNK/c-Jun signaling pathways *in vivo*, and expression of a-SMA, type I collagen, LOX and LOXL-2 in the lung tissue of mice treated with AZM was significantly lower than that in the BLM group. *In vitro*, AZM also effectively inhibited type I collagen, LOX, LOXL-2 and JNK-c-Jun signaling pathways in TGF-β1-stimulated primary mouse fibroblasts, and this effect was similar to that of a JNK-specific inhibitor (SP600125). In conclusion, AZM effectively attenuated BLM-induced PF in mice, which may play a role by partially inhibiting the JNK/c-Jun and TGF-β1/Smad signaling pathways and reducing production of LOX and LOXL2.

Keywords: pulmonary fibrosis, azithromycin, LOX, JNK pathway, inflammation

INTRODUCTION

Pulmonary fibrosis (PF) can occur in a variety of clinical conditions and is a chronic and progressive tissue repair response process that leads to irreversible scarring and remodeling of the lung (Noble et al., 2012). Many factors, including respiratory virus infection, connective tissue disease (CTD), environmental and occupational exposure, therapy (such as radiotherapy and immunotherapy), diabetes, gastroesophageal reflux and so on, can cause and maintain fibrosis (Noble et al., 2012; Sgalla et al., 2019). Usually, the type of PF with known etiology is called secondary PF. However, PF can also occur in the absence of any known causes, known as idiopathic pulmonary fibrosis (IPF). Although IPF is considered rare, the incidence rate of IPF is increasing over time, and the prognosis is very poor. In IPF, the median survival time from diagnosis was 2–4 years, which is similar to that of many malignant tumors (Olson et al., 2007; Noble et al., 2012). However, in secondary PF, the prognosis of PF may be different with distinct etiologies. For example, viral pneumonia, including COVID-19 and severe acute respiratory syndrome (SARS), could lead to PF, but most of these patients gradually recover in the later stage (Naik and Moore, 2010; Mineo et al., 2012; George et al., 2020). In contrast, CTD combined with PF may lead to a significant increase in mortality (Cottin et al., 2018; Spagnolo et al., 2021).

The most important part of the pathophysiological mechanism of PF is the accumulation and remodeling of extracellular matrix (ECM) in the lung (Kulkarni et al., 2016; Upagupta et al., 2018). In addition to the abnormal proliferation of fibroblasts and their excessive secretion of ECM, PF is closely related to changes in ECM components or traits caused by posttranslational modifications, such as glycosylation, transglutamination, and cross linking (Upagupta et al., 2018). Previous studies have shown that lysyl oxidase (LOX) and its four lysyl oxidase-like proteins (LOXL1-4) play a key role in cross linking of the ECM (Philp et al., 2018; Chen et al., 2019; Vallet and Ricard-Blum, 2019; Nguyen et al., 2021). The LOX protein family consists of copper amine oxidases characterized by a highly conserved catalytic domain, a lysine tyrosine quinone cofactor and a conserved copper binding site. Its primary function is to catalyze covalent cross-linking of ECM protein collagens and elastin, which can lead to changes in the stiffness and mechanical properties of the ECM (Vallet and Ricard-Blum, 2019). Tjin et al. found that LOXL1 and LOXL2 expression was significantly increased in the lung tissue of IPF, and inhibition of LOX reduced PF (Tjin et al., 2017). Regulation of the LOX protein family involves a series of signaling pathways, including transforming growth factor β (TGF-β), platelet-derived growth factor, epidermal growth factor receptor and inflammatory pathways (Cheng et al., 2014; Laczko and Csiszar, 2020). In recent years, the LOX protein family has been recognized as a potential target for the treatment of PF (Chen et al., 2019).

Azithromycin (AZM) is a broad-spectrum antibacterial macrolide drug that has attracted increasing attention due to its immunomodulatory effect in addition to its antibacterial activity. Macrolide antibiotics have been used as immunomodulatory drugs in chronic obstructive pulmonary disease (COPD), asthma, and bronchiectasis (Yamaya et al., 2012; Tong et al., 2015; Kelly et al., 2018), although their use is still controversial. Wuyts et al. found that AZM attenuated bleomycin (BLM)-induced PF, but the mechanisms whereby this occurred were unclear (Wuyts et al., 2010). Recently, some observational clinical studies have found that AZM reduces the mortality of acute exacerbation and the hospitalization rate in IPF patients (Kawamura et al., 2017; Macaluso et al., 2019). Tsubouchi et al. found that AZM inhibited NADPH oxidase 4 by promoting proteasome degradation, thereby inhibiting myofibroblast differentiation and the development of lung fibrosis (Tsubouchi et al., 2017). Additionally, a recent study showed that AZM promotes the apoptosis of fibroblasts in IPF to exert an antifibrotic effect (Krempaska et al., 2020). In general, these studies suggest that AZM may play a beneficial role in PF, but the specific regulatory mechanisms still need to be further explored.

In addition to the classical TGF-β signaling pathway, the JNK/c-Jun signaling pathway is a member of the mitogen-activated protein kinase (MAPK) superfamily, which is involved in cell proliferation and differentiation, cytoskeleton construction, apoptosis, and inflammation and in the differentiation and apoptosis of fibroblasts (Davis, 2000; Yeap et al., 2010). In our study, we hypothesized that AZM inhibits LOX and LOXL-2 expression partly through the TGF-β1/Smad and JNK/c-Jun signaling pathways, thereby attenuating the degree of PF. We explored this hypothesis through BLM-induced mouse and TGF-β1-stimulated mouse primary fibroblast models.

TABLE 1 | Primers for quantitative RT-PCR.

Primer name	Sequence (5′ to 3′)
M-collagen I-F	AAGAAGCACGTCTGGTTTGGAG
M-collagen I-R	GGTCCATGTAGGCTACGCTGTT
M-α-SMA-F	GTACCACCATGTACCCAGGC
M-α-SMA-R	GAAGGTAGACAGCGAAGCCA
M-LOX-F	ACTTCTTACCAAGCCGCCCT
M-LOX-R	TGGCATCAAGCAGGTCATAGTG
M-LOXL2-F	GGAGCTTTTCTTCTGGGCAACC
M-LOXL2-R	TACTCAGGGTACTGGAGCTGG
M-GAPDH-F	CCTCGTCCCGTAGACAAAATG
M-GAPDH-R	TGAGGTCAATGAAGGGGTCGT

RT-PCR, real-time polymerase chain reaction; SMA, smooth muscle actin; LOX, lysyl oxidase; LOXL2, lysyl oxidase-like protein-2.

MATERIALS AND METHODS

Materials

BLM and the JNK inhibitor (SP600125) were obtained from Selleck China Inc. (Shanghai, China). TGF-β1 was purchased from PeproTech China Inc. (Suzhou, China). Azithromycin was obtained from Sigma-Aldrich Inc. (Shanghai, China). The primary antibodies we used are as follows: anti-vimentin (Proteintech, 60330-1-Ig), anti-alpha-smooth muscle actin (α-SMA) (Proteintech, 14395-1-AP), anti-Collagen 1 (Proteintech, 14695-1-AP), anti-LOX (Proteintech, 17958-1-AP), anti-LOXL2 (Abcam, 96233), anti-TGF-β1 (Proteintech, 21898-1-AP), anti-Smad2 (Cell Signaling Technology, 5339), anti-Smad3 (Cell Signaling Technology, 9523), anti-phospho (P)-smad2 (Cell Signaling Technology, 3108), anti-P-smad3 (Cell Signaling Technology, 9520), anti-JNK (Proteintech, 66210-1-Ig), anti-c-Jun (Proteintech, 66313-1-Ig), anti-P-JNK (Proteintech, 80024-1-RR), anti-P-cJun (Proteintech, 28891-1-AP), anti-α-tubulin (Proteintech, 66031-1-Ig), and anti-GAPDH (Proteintech, 60004-1-Ig). The dilution ratio of all antibodies was 1:1000.

Mouse Models and Treatment

Male C57BL/6 mice (21.3 ± 0.5 g), 7–8 weeks of age, were supplied by Beijing HFK Bioscience Co. Ltd. (Beijing, China). The mouse model of BLM-induced PF was based on previous

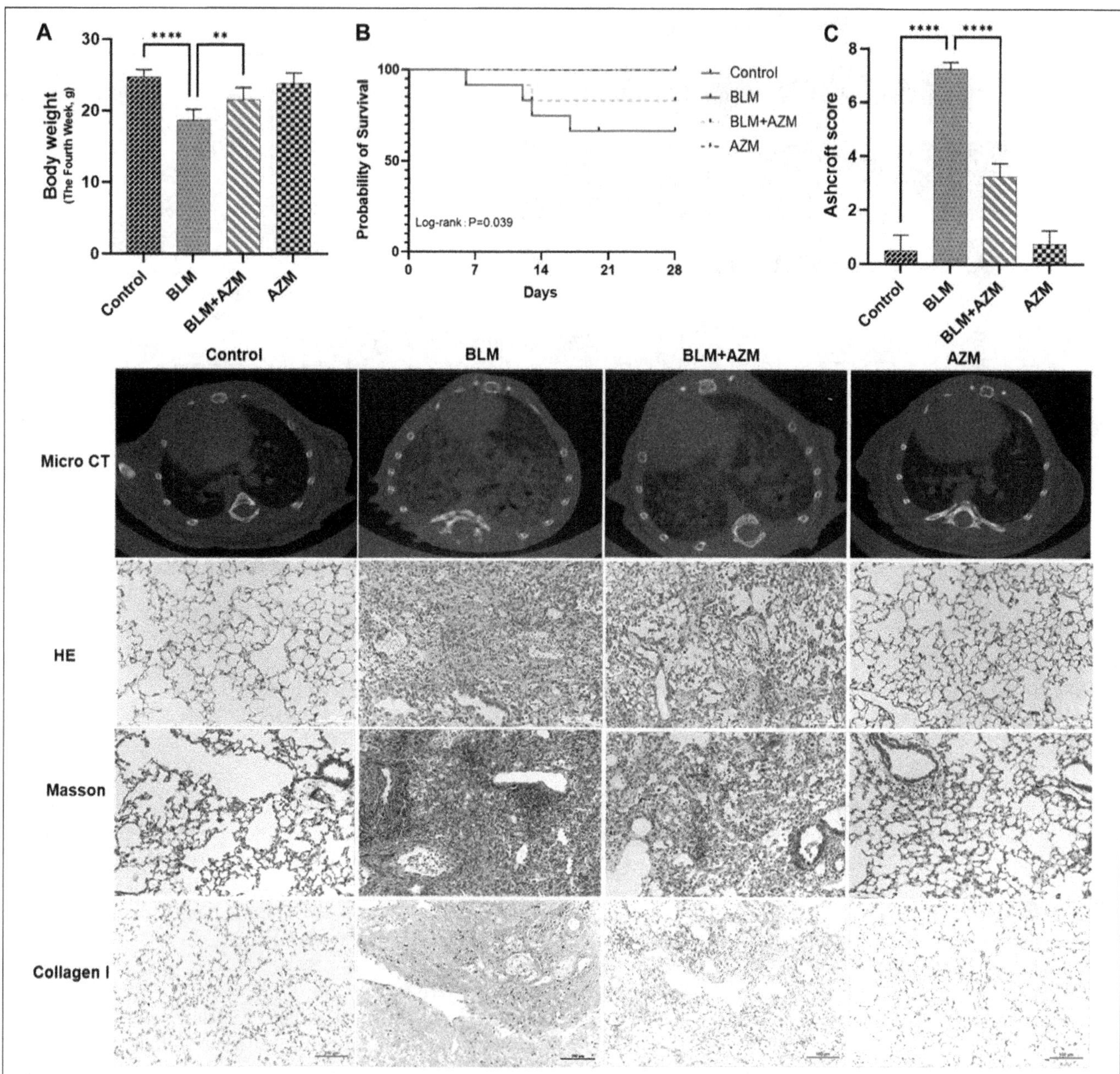

FIGURE 1 | Azithromycin (AZM) attenuated bleomycin (BLM)-induced pulmonary fibrosis in mice. **(A)** Mice body weights were measured in Day 28. **(B)** Survival rate of mice in different groups. **(C)** Ashcroft score for the four groups were based on HE staining. The other images were micro CT results, HE staining, Masson staining, and collagen I staining in different groups (×200 magnification; scale bars = 100 μm). Data were presented as the means ± SD. $^{**}p < 0.01$, $^{****}p < 0.0001$.

literature published by our team (Zhang et al., 2020). AZM was dissolved in ethanol and diluted in normal saline. AZM was administered intraperitoneally at a dose of 50 mg/kg/day (the dose refers to the "toxicology" section of AZM drug instructions, which is equivalent to a dose of 500 mg/day in adults). The dose of AZM used in our study was consistent with that used in a previous asthma study (Beigelman et al., 2009). A total of 48 mice were divided into the following four groups: control: mice were intratracheally atomized with 50 μl of normal saline on day 0 and intraperitoneally injected with 100 μl of normal saline on day 7 for 3 weeks; BLM: mice were intratracheally atomized with 50 μl of BLM on day 0; BLM + AZM: mice were intratracheally atomized with 50 μl of BLM on day 0 and intraperitoneally injected with 100 μl of AZM on day 7 for 3 weeks; and AZM: mice were intratracheally atomized with 50 μl of normal saline on day 0, and intraperitoneal injection of 100 μl AZM was performed on day 7, lasting for 3 weeks. On the 28th day, mice were sacrificed by intraperitoneal injection of excessive sodium pentobarbital. All animals received care in accordance with the recommendations of the National Institutes of Health Guide for Care and Use of Laboratory Animals, and this

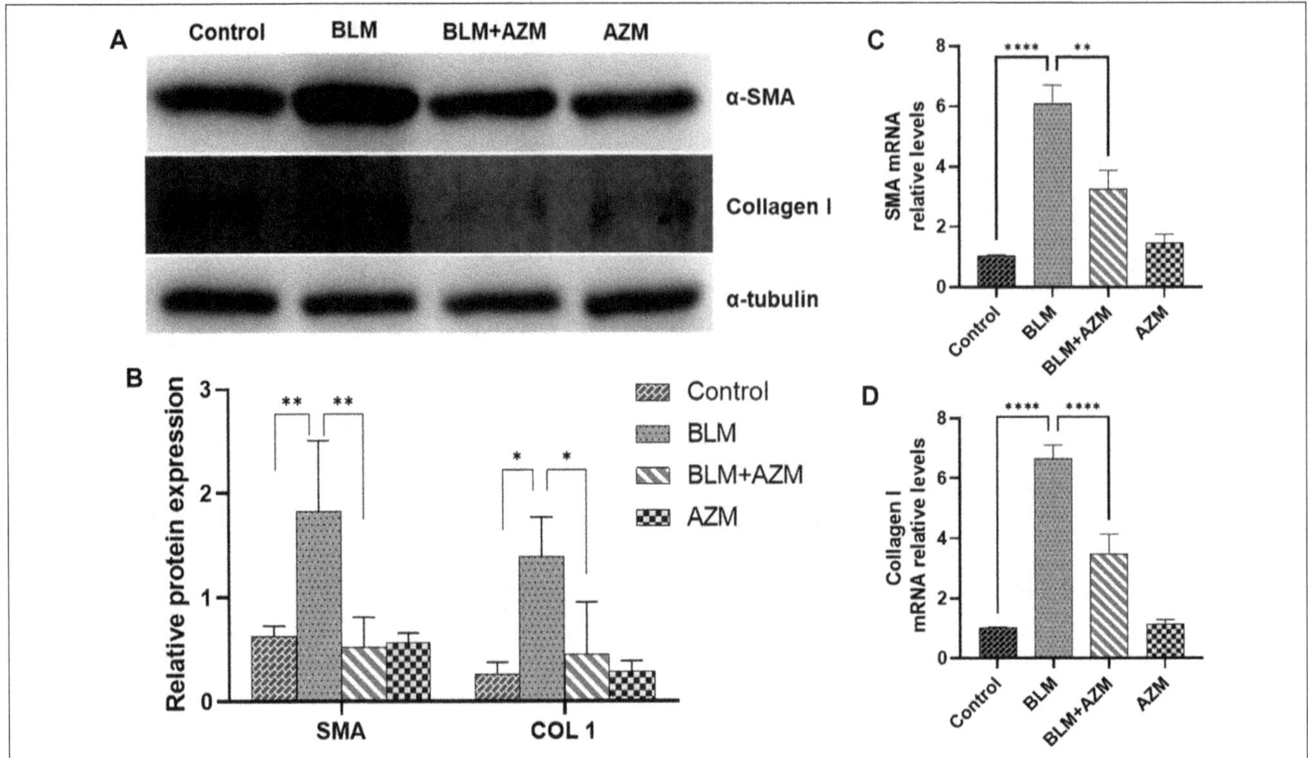

FIGURE 2 | AZM reduced the expression of alpha-smooth muscle actin (α-SMA) and Collagen 1 (COL 1) in lung tissue of mice with pulmonary fibrosis. **(A,B)** The protein expression of α-SMA and COL 1 was measured in each group by Western blot. **(C,D)** The gene expression of α-SMA and COL 1 was measured in each group by RT-PCR. Data were presented as the means ± SD ($n \geq 3$). *$p < 0.05$, **$p < 0.01$, ****$p < 0.0001$.

experimental protocol was approved by the Committee on the Ethics of Animal Experiments of West China Hospital, Sichuan University (No. 2019022A).

Micro-CT Scanning

Referring to the method provided in previous literature (van Deel et al., 2016; Ruscitti et al., 2017), on the 28th day, all mice were scanned by microcomputed tomography (micro-CT). After mice were anesthetized with isoflurane, mouse lung imaging was conducted by a Quantum GX Micro-CT scanner (PerkinElmer, Inc., Waltham, MA) using the cardiorespiratory gated technique (Ruscitti et al., 2017). Images were obtained with an X-ray tube set to 90 kVp and 160 μA, projection radiographs were taken during the whole 360° gantry rotation, and the total scanning time was 4.5 min (Ruscitti et al., 2017).

Histological Analysis and Immunohistochemistry

Lung tissues were fixed in 4% formalin buffer, embedded in paraffin, and cut into 4 μm thick tissue sections. The sections were stained with hematoxylin-eosin (HE) and Masson's trichrome staining. According to previous literature, the Ashcroft scoring system was used to assess the level of fibrosis (Ashcroft et al., 1988). Immunohistochemistry was used to evaluate the expression level of type I collagen in lung tissue. After the sections were dewaxed and rehydrated, endogenous peroxidase activity was inactivated with 3% H_2O_2. The sections were blocked in 5% bovine serum albumin and incubated with the anti-collagen I primary antibody at a dilution of 1:200. Then, the sections were incubated with the secondary antibody at room temperature and developed with diaminobenzidine for observation.

Cell Culture

According to the study published by Edelman et al., primary lung fibroblasts were isolated by the crawl out method (Edelman and Redente, 2018). Purified cells were identified by vimentin immunofluorescence using previously reported methods (Donaldson, 2015). Cells were seeded in Dulbecco's modified Eagle medium (DMEM) containing 10% fetal bovine serum (Gibco, USA) and 1% penicillin-streptomycin (HyClone, USA) and cultured in a 37°C incubator with a humidified 5% CO_2 atmosphere. Cell experiments were divided into 6 groups: control, TGF-β1, TGF-β1+AZM, TGF-β1+JNK inhibitor, AZM, and JNK inhibitor. To establish a cell model, primary lung fibroblasts were stimulated with 5 ng/ml TGF-β1 for 48 h as in the TGF-β1 group. Six hours before stimulation with TGF-β1, 10 μg/ml AZM was added to the culture medium as the intervention group (TGF-β1+AZM group). In addition, to verify whether AZM partially regulated the JNK/c-Jun signaling pathway involved in LOX and LOXL-2 expression, we added a JNK1 inhibitor (20 μM) 6 h before TGF-β1 stimulation (TGF-β1+JNK inhibitor group). Primary cells were used after no more than the fifth generation.

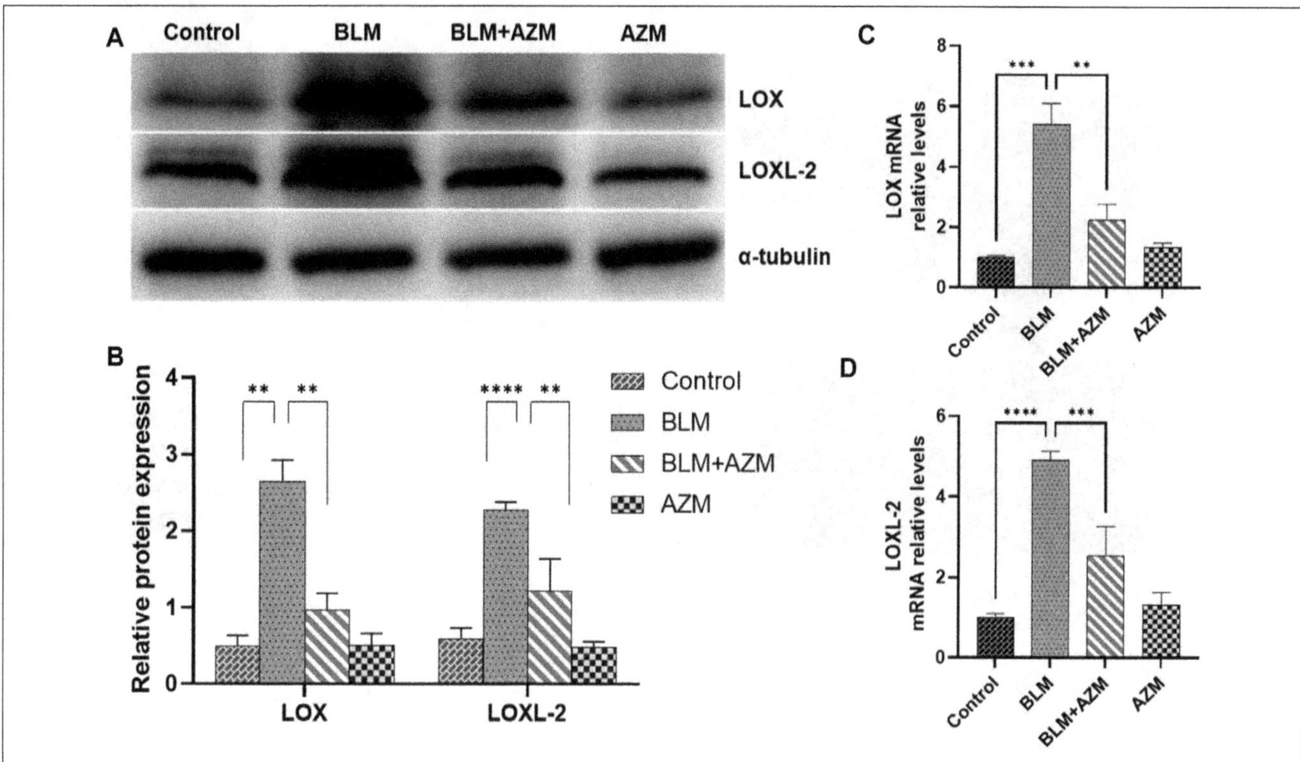

FIGURE 3 | AZM reduced the expression of lysyl oxidase (LOX) and lysyl oxidase-like protein (LOXL2) in lung tissue of mice with pulmonary fibrosis. **(A,B)** The protein relative expression of LOX and LOXL2 was measured in each group by Western blot. **(C,D)** The gene expression of LOX and LOXL2 was measured in each group by RT-PCR. Data were presented as the means ± SD ($n \geq 3$). **$p < 0.01$, ***$p < 0.001$, ****$p < 0.0001$.

Real-Time PCR Analysis

Total RNA was extracted from lung tissue using TRIzol reagent (Invitrogen, USA) and reverse transcribed into complementary DNA (cDNA) according to the instructions of the PrimeScript™ RT reagent kit (Takara, Japan). iTaq Universal SYBR Green Supermix (Bio-Rad, United States) was used for real-time PCR (RT-PCR) to determine mRNA levels of α-SMA, collagen I, LOX, LOXL-2, and GAPDH. **Table 1** shows the primer sequences, relative gene expression levels were normalized to GAPDH and calculated using the $2^{-\Delta\Delta Ct}$ method.

Western Blot Analysis

Lung tissues or cells were fully lysed in RIPA buffer (Beyotime, China) containing a fresh mixture of protease and phosphatase inhibitors (MedChemExpress, United States).

The entire process was performed at 4°C. After centrifugation at 12000 r/min for 20 min, the supernatant was added to 5× protein sample loading buffers (Epizyme, China) and boiled for 10 min. A BCA protein kit (Thermo, USA) was used to determine protein concentrations. Denatured proteins were separated by 10% SDS-PAGE (Epizyme, China) and then transferred onto methanol-activated PVDF membranes (Millipore, USA) at a constant current of 400 mA. After blocking with 5% skim milk for 1 h, membranes were incubated with different primary antibodies overnight at 4°C. After washing the PVDF membrane several times, it was incubated with the appropriate secondary antibody (1:2,000) for 1 h at room temperature. Subsequently, ECL (GE Healthcare, United Kingdom) was used to visualize protein expression, and ImageJ software was used to analyze the band intensities.

Statistical Analysis

Statistical analysis was performed using GraphPad Prism Version 9.0 (GraphPad software, USA). All raw data are shown as the mean ± standard deviation. One-way ANOVA tests were used for analyzing differences, and Tukey's multiple comparison test was used to compare multiple groups. The Kaplan-Meier method was used to draw the survival curve of each group. A p-value less than 0.05 was considered statistically significant.

RESULTS

Azithromycin Attenuates Bleomycin-Induced Pulmonary Fibrosis in Mice

After a single intratracheal atomization of bleomycin (BLM), compared to the control group, the weight of mice in the BLM group was significantly reduced on day 28, and the mortality rate was 41.7% in the BLM group, which was significantly reversed (16.7%) after treatment with AZM (**Figures 1A,B**). There was no significant difference between the control group and the AZM group (**Figures 1A,B**). Microcomputed tomography (micro-CT) results showed that after a single dose of BLM intratracheal

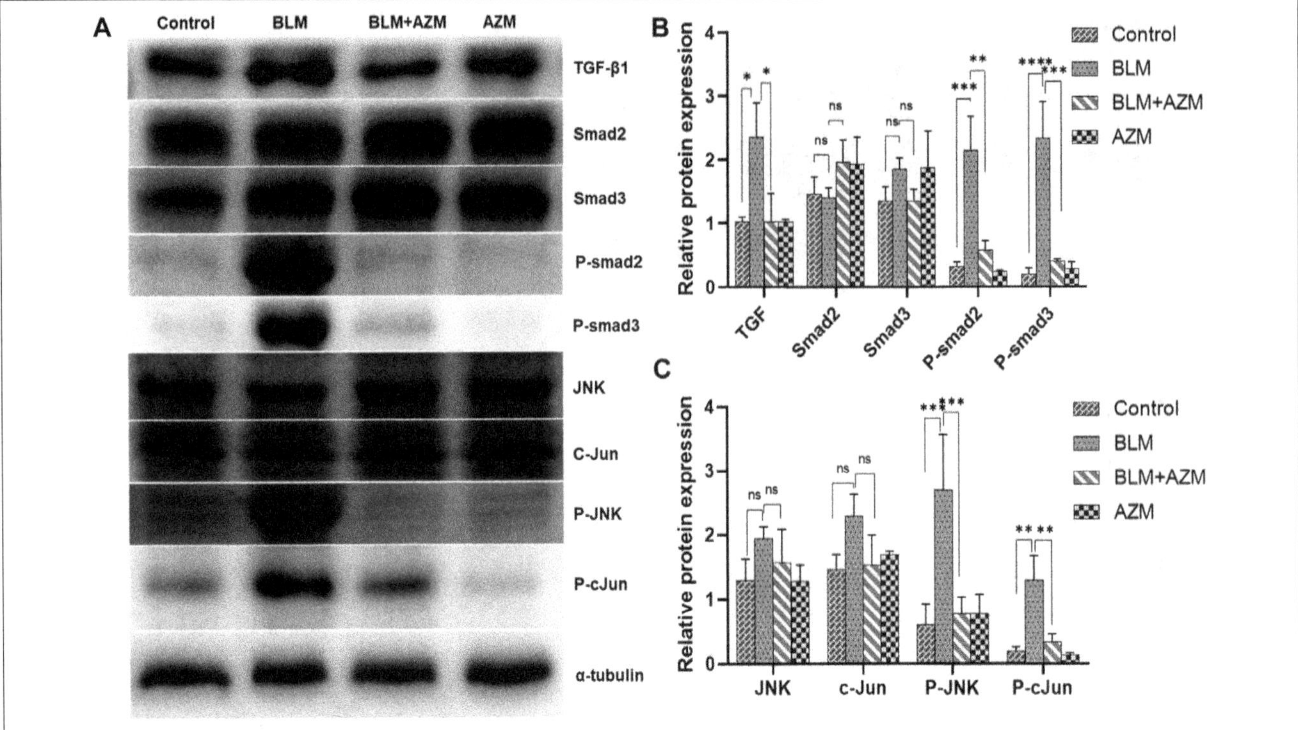

FIGURE 4 | AZM suppressed the TGF-β1/Smad and JNK/c-Jun signaling pathway in BLM-induced mice. **(A)** Western blotting bands of TGF-β1/Smad and JNK/c-Jun pathway proteins in lung tissue of mice in different groups. **(B,C)** The protein relative expression of TGF-β1/Smad and JNK/c-Jun pathway proteins was measured in each group by Western blot. Data were presented as the means ± SD ($n \geq 3$). **$p < 0.01$, ***$p < 0.001$, ****$p < 0.0001$, ns, non-significant.

atomization, the lung structure of mice was destroyed, and imaging features of PF, such as grid shadow, strip shadow, honeycomb lung, and interstitial thickening, appeared in both lungs (**Figure 1**).

As shown in **Figure 1**, hematoxylin-eosin (HE) staining showed that in the BLM group, the alveolar septum was thickened, the alveolar structure was destroyed, and a large number of red blood cells and inflammatory cells infiltrated the alveolar and lung interstitium, while the alveolar structure in the control and AZM groups was normal. Masson staining revealed a large amount of collagen deposition in the lung tissue of the BLM group compared to the control group. AZM treatment significantly reduced inflammatory cell infiltration and collagen deposition and improved alveolar structure.

The fibrosis score of the BLM group was significantly higher than that of the control group, while the fibrosis score of the AZM treatment group was significantly reduced, suggesting that AZM effectively reduces BLM-induced pulmonary fibrosis (**Figure 1C**, $p < 0.001$).

Azithromycin Inhibits Expression of LOX and LOXL-2 in Mice With Bleomycin-Induced Pulmonary Fibrosis

LOX and LOXL-2 were found to be closely related to PF and interacted with the TGF-β and JNK signaling pathways (Sethi et al., 2011; Chien et al., 2014; Wei et al., 2017; Wu et al., 2018). As shown in **Figure 2**, western blot and Real-Time-polymerase chain reaction (RT-PCR) showed that protein and gene expression levels of α-smooth muscle actin (a-SMA) and type I collagen in the BLM group were significantly higher than those in the control group, and AZM effectively reduced expression levels of a-SMA and type I collagen. In addition, expression of LOX and LOXL-2 in the BLM group was significantly upregulated compared to the control group. After AZM intervention, expression of LOX and LOXL-2 in the BLM group was significantly lower than in the BLM group, exhibiting no difference from the control group (**Figure 3**).

Azithromycin Inhibits the Activities of TGF-β/Smad and JNK/C-Jun Signaling Pathways in Mouse Pulmonary Fibrosis

The TGF-β signaling pathway is the most important regulatory pathway in pulmonary fibrosis. The activated TGF-β signaling pathway directly upregulates gene expression of the ECM and stimulates expression of many proinflammatory and fibrosis cytokines, such as interleukin, tumor necrosis factor-α, or platelet-derived growth factor, to further enhance and maintain the fibrotic response (Kang, 2017). The results showed that AZM significantly inhibited expression of TGF-β1 and phosphorylated Smad2 and Smad3 in the lung tissue of BLM-treated mice, while total Smad2 and Smad3 protein levels did not change (**Figure 4**). In addition, the JNK/c-Jun signaling pathway, another important pathway in the regulation of fibrosis, has attracted much attention in recent years (Grynberg et al.,

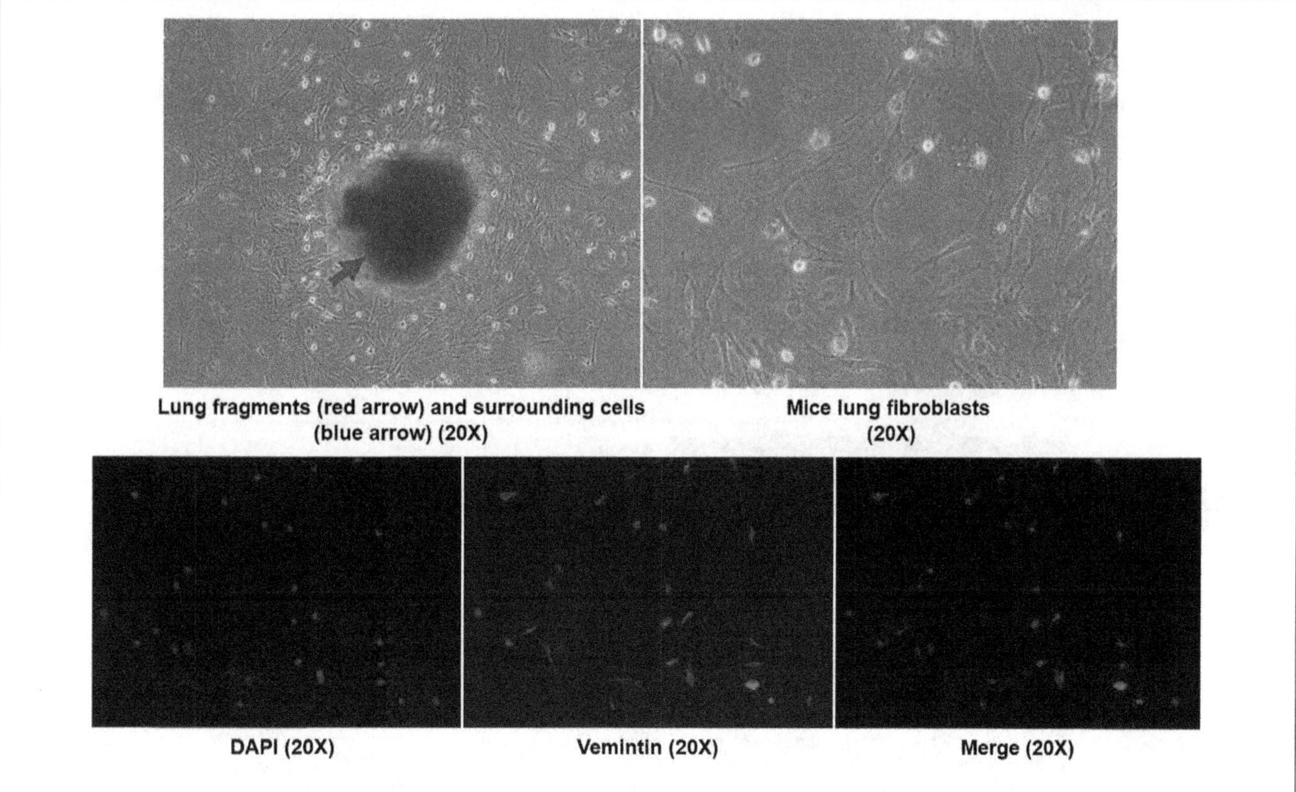

FIGURE 5 | Mice primary lung fibroblasts were isolated by crawl out method, and the immunofluorescence with anti-vimentin antibody was used to identify the cell purity (× 200 magnetization).

2017). The results showed that expression levels of phosphorylated JNK and phosphorylated c-Jun proteins in the BLM group were significantly increased. Total JNK and c-Jun protein levels did not change, but JNK and c-Jun mRNA levels were significantly increased. AZM inhibited expression of phosphorylated JNK and phosphorylated c-Jun in the lung tissues of BLM-treated mice (**Figure 4**).

Azithromycin Attenuates LOX and LOXL-2 Expression in Mouse Lung Fibroblasts by Partially Inhibiting the JNK/ C-Jun Signaling Pathway

As shown in **Figure 5**, we extracted mouse primary lung fibroblasts using previously reported research methods (Edelman and Redente, 2018) and determined the purity of these cells by fluorescence detection of vimentin. The results showed that the purity of primary lung fibroblasts was greater than 90%. According to previous literature, TGF-β1 (5 ng/ml) was used to stimulate fibroblasts to establish a cell model. LOX, LOXL-2, phosphorylated JNK and type I collagen were all significantly increased in response to TGF-β stimulation, while LOX, LOXL-2 and type I collagen levels were decreased and expression of phosphorylated JNK protein decreased simultaneously in response to AZM intervention. After blocking the JNK signaling pathway with SP600125, it was found that it had a similar effect to AZM intervention, and expression of LOX, LOXL-2, type I collagen, total JNK and phosphorylated JNK was significantly reduced (**Figure 6**). Therefore, these results preliminarily suggest that AZM may inhibit expression of LOX and LOXL-2 in fibroblasts, partly through the JNK/c-Jun signaling pathway.

DISCUSSION

Macrolide antibiotics, as anti-inflammatory and immunomodulatory agents, have become potential candidates for the treatment of PF (Krempaska et al., 2020). Our study revealed that AZM effectively reduced expression levels of α-SMA and type I collagen in BLM-induced PF in mice (**Figure 1**). *In vitro*, the study found that AZM also effectively inhibited the expression of type I collagen in mouse lung fibroblasts stimulated by TGF-β1 (**Figure 6**), which is consistent with results previously reported by Wuyts et al. (Wuyts et al., 2010). In addition, AZM could play a key role in reducing tissue remodeling through a variety of mechanisms, such as inhibiting airway epithelial cell apoptosis and epithelial-mesenchymal transition (Liu et al., 2017; Pu et al., 2018). A series of small sample retrospective studies suggested that macrolide antibiotics may improve the prognosis of patients with interstitial lung disease (ILD) (Kawamura et al., 2017; Nagasawa et al., 2021). We conducted a meta-analysis

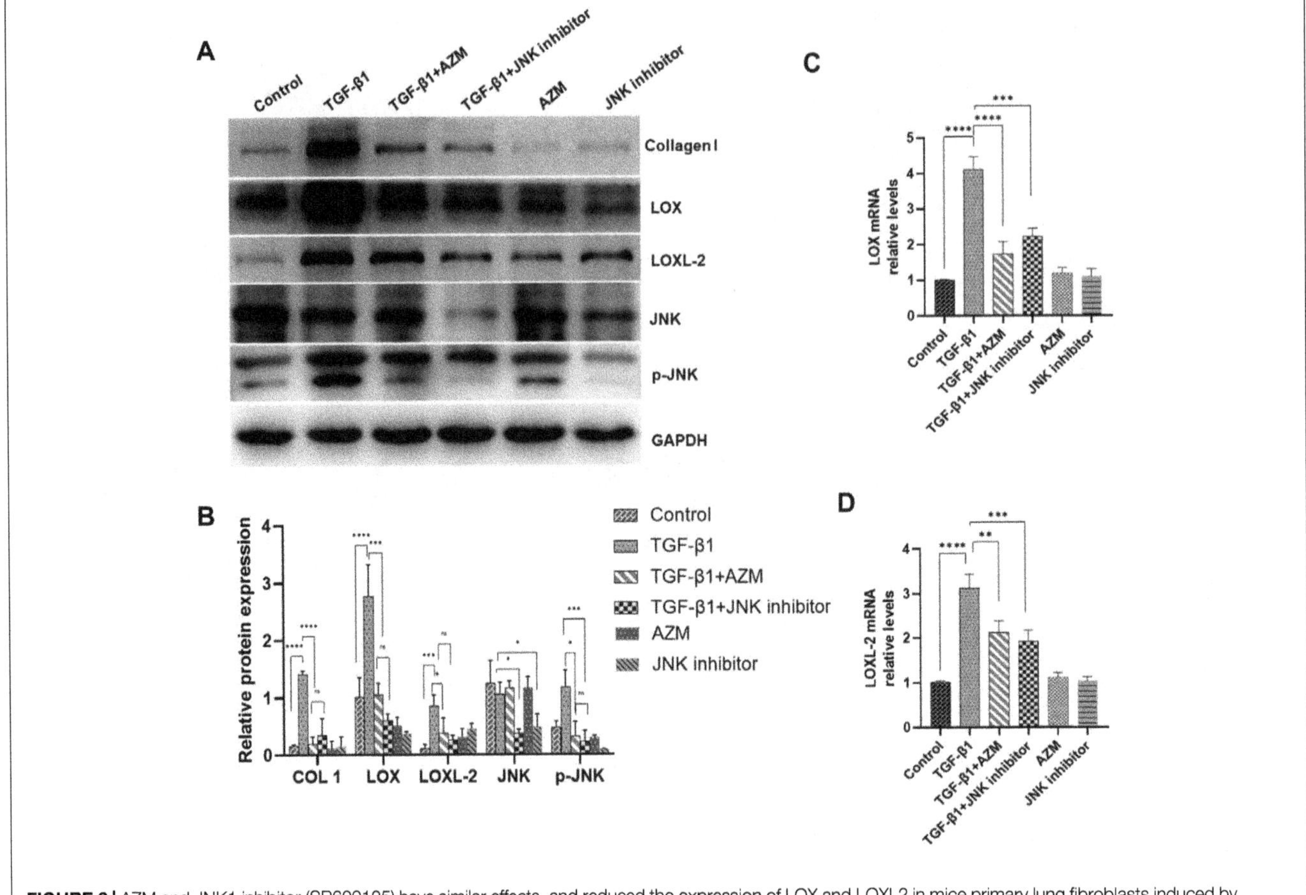

FIGURE 6 | AZM and JNK1 inhibitor (SP600125) have similar effects, and reduced the expression of LOX and LOXL2 in mice primary lung fibroblasts induced by 5 μg/ml TGF-β1. **(A,B)** The protein expression of LOX, LOXL2, COL1, JNK and GAPDH was measured in each group by Western blot. **(C,D)** The gene expression of LOX and LOXL2 was measured in each group by RT-PCR. Data were presented as the means ± SD ($n \geq 3$). *$p < 0.05$, **$p < 0.01$, ***$p < 0.001$, ****$p < 0.0001$, ns, non-significant.

(data unpublished), and found that AZM effectively reduced the mortality of patients with acute exacerbation of ILD, and reduced the incidence of mechanical ventilation in patients.

The LOX protein family, a cross-linked enzyme of the ECM, plays a key role in ECM remodeling and modification, regulating the development of fibrosis (Aumiller et al., 2017; Bellaye et al., 2018; Guo et al., 2020). Our study showed that the expressions of LOX and LOXL-2 were significantly increased in BLM-induced PF in mice (**Figure 3**). To our knowledge, this study was the first time to show that AZM effectively inhibited expression of LOX and LOXL2 in BLM-induced PF in mice. *In vitro*, our study revealed that AZM also inhibited the expression of LOX and LOXL2 in TGF-β1-stimulated mouse primary fibroblasts, and this inhibitory effect is similar to the use of JNK specific inhibitors (**Figure 6**). Aumiller et al. found that expression of LOX and LOXL2 was significantly increased in IPF patients, mouse models and cell models of pulmonary fibrosis (Aumiller et al., 2017). Chien et al. found that higher serum LOXL2 levels was associated with increased risk for IPF disease progression (Chien et al., 2014). In animal study, LOX inhibitors (β-Aminopropiononitrile) could reduce myocardial fibrosis and alleviating myocardial hypertrophy (Martínez-Martínez et al., 2016). Guo et al. (2020) found that triptolide prevents nuclear translocation of NF-κB and DNA binding, effectively reducing the expression of LOX and alleviating the degree of radiation-induced PF in mice. Ikenaga et al. found that selective targeting of LOXL2 inhibits the progression of liver fibrosis and accelerates its reversion (Ikenaga et al., 2017). In a phase II clinical trial (NCT01769196), simtuzumab, a monoclonal antibody against LOXL2, did not improve progression-free survival in IPF patients (Raghu et al., 2017). However, the failure of the clinical trial may be attributed to lack of tissue penetration of the drug in human IPF lung (Meyer, 2017). Since AZM is highly enriched in lung tissues (Parnham et al., 2014), and it could effectively reduce the expression of LOX and LOXL-2, it may have great potential application value for the treatment of PF in the future.

Additionally, our results demonstrated that AZM significantly inhibited the TGF-β signaling pathway (**Figure 4**). In fibrotic disease, the TGF-β signaling pathway is primarily involved in regulating fibroblasts and EMT activation, promoting ECM production, maintaining fibroblast activity, and inhibiting metalloproteinases (Biernacka et al., 2011; Hu et al., 2018). In addition, TGF-β is widely involved in inflammation and immune

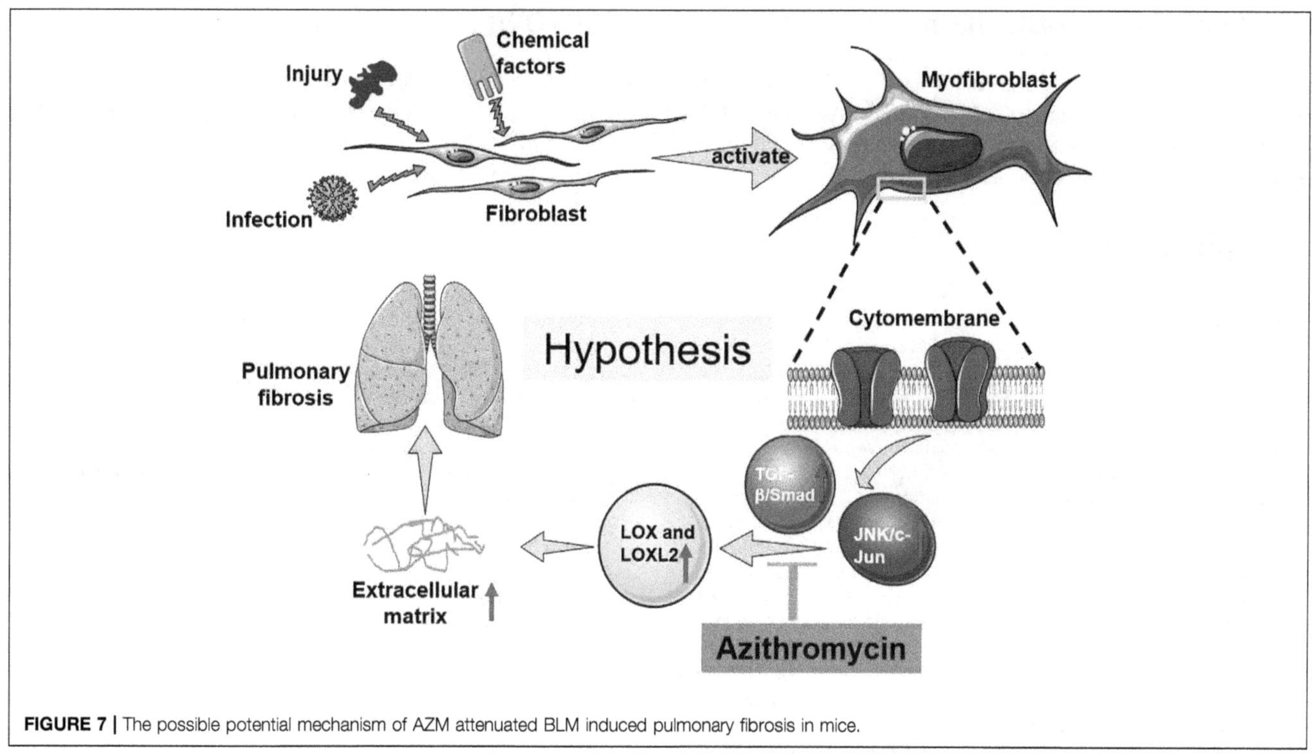

FIGURE 7 | The possible potential mechanism of AZM attenuated BLM induced pulmonary fibrosis in mice.

regulation, which is also a crucial process in fibrosis (Meng et al., 2014; Hu et al., 2018). Ruan et al. found that AZM effectively inhibited TGF-β1 signaling, weaken the activation and differentiation of lung fibroblasts (Ruan et al., 2021). Previous studies have shown that TGF-β1 can significantly upregulate LOX mRNA and protein levels in fibroblasts and epithelial cells during fibrosis (Remst et al., 2014). Other studies have suggested that LOX regulates TGF-β through a feedback loop, which plays a role in skeletal muscle development and IPF (Remst et al., 2014). In addition, direct interaction between LOX and TGF reduced TGF-stimulated Smad3 activation (Remst et al., 2014). Our study suggested that the levels of LOX and LOXL-2 increased in parallel with the level of TGF-β1 in BLM group, and AZM could inhibit the expression of LOX and TGF-β1 (**Figure 4**). Therefore, we speculate that AZM reduces expression of LOX by inhibiting the TGF-β signaling pathway to attenuate the degree of PF (**Figure 7**).

The JNK/c-Jun signaling pathway is a member of the mitogen-activated protein kinase (MAPK) superfamily, which plays an important role in cellular differentiation, apoptosis, stress response, inflammation and the occurrence and development of many human diseases (Bode and Dong, 2007). In a clinical study (NCT01203943), a JNK inhibitor (CC-930) effectively attenuated airway remodeling, reduced the production of pulmonary fibrosis markers, and improved lung function (van der Velden et al., 2016). However, the interaction between the JNK/c-Jun signaling pathway and the LOX protein family is still not well explored in fibrotic diseases. In the current study, we found that AZM effectively inhibited the JNK/c-Jun signaling pathway and simultaneously inhibited expression of LOX and LOXL2 (**Figure 4**). At the same time, we found that JNK pathway-specific inhibitors effectively inhibited expression of LOX and LOXL, attenuating the degree of PF (**Figure 6**). Our results were similar to the previous studies. A recent study suggested that AZM inhibits the MAPK/JNK signaling pathway in a human monocytic cell line (THP-1) induced by LPS (Kuo et al., 2019). Hiwatashi et al. (2011) found that AZM inhibits the proliferation of peripheral blood mononuclear cells by suppressing the activity of JNK and ERK. Based on the above findings, we speculated that AZM partially inhibits the JNK/c-Jun signaling pathway, downregulates expression of LOX and LOXL-2 levels, reduces the production of ECM, and ultimately attenuates PF (**Figure 7**).

Although our study revealed that AZM could attenuate PF by inhibiting the expression of LOX and LOXL-2, the regulatory mechanisms need to be further verified (e.g. using LOX inhibitors or knockdown mice). As we all know, a large number of cells, cytokines, enzymes, and signal pathways are involved in the regulation of ECM, but our study failed to explore other important factors (e.g. matrix metalloproteinases, MMPs) in the regulation of ECM. We will conduct in-depth and comprehensive study on the regulation mechanisms of ECM in the future, such as exploring the interaction between LOX and MMPs. In addition, more rigorous clinical studies or real-world studies need to be designed to accurately evaluate the value of AZM in the treatment of patients with PF.

In summary, AZM effectively attenuated BLM-induced PF in mice, which may occur by partially suppressing the JNK/c-Jun and TGF-β1/Smad signaling pathways and reducing LOX and LOXL2 production (**Figure 7**).

AUTHOR CONTRIBUTIONS

XT and HF conceived the experiment, XT, SZ, DW, LZ, JH, and TZ conducted the experiments, XT, SZ, and DW analyzed the results, XT and SZ contributed to the manuscript writing, HF supervised the study. All of the authors reviewed the manuscript.

ACKNOWLEDGMENTS

We would like to thank Elsevier Language Editing Services for its linguistic assistance during the preparation of this manuscript.

REFERENCES

Ashcroft, T., Simpson, J. M., and Timbrell, V. (1988). Simple Method of Estimating Severity of Pulmonary Fibrosis on a Numerical Scale. *J. Clin. Pathol.* 41 (4), 467–470. doi:10.1136/jcp.41.4.467

Aumiller, V., Strobel, B., Romeike, M., Schuler, M., Stierstorfer, B. E., and Kreuz, S. (2017). Comparative Analysis of Lysyl Oxidase (Like) Family Members in Pulmonary Fibrosis. *Sci. Rep.* 7 (1), 149. doi:10.1038/s41598-017-00270-0

Beigelman, A., Gunsten, S., Mikols, C. L., Vidavsky, I., Cannon, C. L., Brody, S. L., et al. (2009). Azithromycin Attenuates Airway Inflammation in a Noninfectious Mouse Model of Allergic Asthma. *Chest* 136 (2), 498–506. doi:10.1378/chest.08-3056

Bellaye, P. S., Shimbori, C., Upagupta, C., Sato, S., Shi, W., Gauldie, J., et al. (2018). Lysyl Oxidase-like 1 Protein Deficiency Protects Mice from Adenoviral Transforming Growth Factor-B1-Induced Pulmonary Fibrosis. *Am. J. Respir. Cel Mol Biol.* 58 (4), 461–470. doi:10.1165/rcmb.2017-0252OC

Biernacka, A., Dobaczewski, M., and Frangogiannis, N. G. (2011). TGF-β Signaling in Fibrosis. *Growth Factors* 29 (5), 196–202. doi:10.3109/08977194.2011.595714

Bode, A. M., and Dong, Z. (2007). The Functional Contrariety of JNK. *Mol. Carcinog.* 46 (8), 591–598. doi:10.1002/mc.20348

Chen, L., Li, S., and Li, W. (2019). LOX/LOXL in Pulmonary Fibrosis: Potential Therapeutic Targets. *J. Drug Target.* 27 (7), 790–796. doi:10.1080/1061186x.2018.1550649

Cheng, T., Liu, Q., Zhang, R., Zhang, Y., Chen, J., Yu, R., et al. (2014). Lysyl Oxidase Promotes Bleomycin-Induced Lung Fibrosis through Modulating Inflammation. *J. Mol. Cel Biol.* 6 (6), 506–515. doi:10.1093/jmcb/mju039

Chien, J. W., Richards, T. J., Gibson, K. F., Zhang, Y., Lindell, K. O., Shao, L., et al. (2014). Serum Lysyl Oxidase-like 2 Levels and Idiopathic Pulmonary Fibrosis Disease Progression. *Eur. Respir. J.* 43 (5), 1430–1438. doi:10.1183/09031936.00141013

Cottin, V., Hirani, N. A., Hotchkin, D. L., Nambiar, A. M., Ogura, T., Otaola, M., et al. (2018). Presentation, Diagnosis and Clinical Course of the Spectrum of Progressive-Fibrosing Interstitial Lung Diseases. *Eur. Respir. Rev.* 27 (150). doi:10.1183/16000617.0076-2018

Davis, R. J. (2000). Signal Transduction by the JNK Group of MAP Kinases. *Cell* 103 (2), 239–252. doi:10.1016/s0092-8674(00)00116-1

Donaldson, J. G. (2015). Immunofluorescence Staining. *Curr. Protoc. Cel Biol* 69, 41–74. doi:10.1002/0471143030.cb0403s69

Edelman, B. L., and Redente, E. F. (2018). Isolation and Characterization of Mouse Fibroblasts. *Methods Mol. Biol.* 1809, 59–67. doi:10.1007/978-1-4939-8570-8_5

George, P. M., Wells, A. U., and Jenkins, R. G. (2020). Pulmonary Fibrosis and COVID-19: the Potential Role for Antifibrotic Therapy. *Lancet Respir. Med.* 8 (8), 807–815. doi:10.1016/s2213-2600(20)30225-3

Grynberg, K., Ma, F. Y., and Nikolic-Paterson, D. J. (2017). The JNK Signaling Pathway in Renal Fibrosis. *Front. Physiol.* 8, 829. doi:10.3389/fphys.2017.00829

Guo, K., Chen, J., Chen, Z., Luo, G., Yang, S., Zhang, M., et al. (2020). Triptolide Alleviates Radiation-Induced Pulmonary Fibrosis via Inhibiting IKKβ Stimulated LOX Production. *Biochem. Biophys. Res. Commun.* 527 (1), 283–288. doi:10.1016/j.bbrc.2020.04.023

Hiwatashi, Y., Maeda, M., Fukushima, H., Onda, K., Tanaka, S., Utsumi, H., et al. (2011). Azithromycin Suppresses Proliferation, Interleukin Production and Mitogen-Activated Protein Kinases in Human Peripheral-Blood Mononuclear Cells Stimulated with Bacterial Superantigen. *J. Pharm. Pharmacol.* 63 (10), 1320–1326. doi:10.1111/j.2042-7158.2011.01343.x

Hu, H. H., Chen, D. Q., Wang, Y. N., Feng, Y. L., Cao, G., Vaziri, N. D., et al. (2018). New Insights into TGF-β/Smad Signaling in Tissue Fibrosis. *Chem. Biol. Interact* 292, 76–83. doi:10.1016/j.cbi.2018.07.008

Ikenaga, N., Peng, Z. W., Vaid, K. A., Liu, S. B., Yoshida, S., Sverdlov, D. Y., et al. (2017). Selective Targeting of Lysyl Oxidase-like 2 (LOXL2) Suppresses Hepatic Fibrosis Progression and Accelerates its Reversal. *Gut* 66 (9), 1697–1708. doi:10.1136/gutjnl-2016-312473

Kang, H. (2017). Role of MicroRNAs in TGF-β Signaling Pathway-Mediated Pulmonary Fibrosis. *Int. J. Mol. Sci.* 18 (12). doi:10.3390/ijms18122527

Kawamura, K., Ichikado, K., Yasuda, Y., Anan, K., and Suga, M. (2017). Azithromycin for Idiopathic Acute Exacerbation of Idiopathic Pulmonary Fibrosis: a Retrospective Single-center Study. *BMC Pulm. Med.* 17 (1), 94. doi:10.1186/s12890-017-0437-z

Kelly, C., Chalmers, J. D., Crossingham, I., Relph, N., Felix, L. M., Evans, D. J., et al. (2018). Macrolide Antibiotics for Bronchiectasis. *Cochrane Database Syst. Rev.* 3 (3), Cd012406. doi:10.1002/14651858.CD012406.pub2

Krempaska, K., Barnowski, S., Gavini, J., Hobi, N., Ebener, S., Simillion, C., et al. (2020). Azithromycin Has Enhanced Effects on Lung Fibroblasts from Idiopathic Pulmonary Fibrosis (IPF) Patients Compared to Controls [corrected]. *Respir. Res.* 21 (1), 25. doi:10.1186/s12931-020-1275-8

Kulkarni, T., O'Reilly, P., Antony, V. B., Gaggar, A., and Thannickal, V. J. (2016). Matrix Remodeling in Pulmonary Fibrosis and Emphysema. *Am. J. Respir. Cel Mol Biol.* 54 (6), 751–760. doi:10.1165/rcmb.2015-0166PS

Kuo, C. H., Lee, M. S., Kuo, H. F., Lin, Y. C., and Hung, C. H. (2019). Azithromycin Suppresses Th1- and Th2-Related Chemokines IP-10/MDC in Human Monocytic Cell Line. *J. Microbiol. Immunol. Infect.* 52 (6), 872–879. doi:10.1016/j.jmii.2019.10.001

Laczko, R., and Csiszar, K. (2020). Lysyl Oxidase (LOX): Functional Contributions to Signaling Pathways. *Biomolecules* 10 (8), 1093. doi:10.3390/biom10081093

Liu, Y., Pu, Y., Li, D., Zhou, L., and Wan, L. (2017). Azithromycin Ameliorates Airway Remodeling via Inhibiting Airway Epithelium Apoptosis. *Life Sci.* 170, 1–8. doi:10.1016/j.lfs.2016.11.024

Macaluso, C., Maritano Furcada, J., Alzaher, O., Chaube, R., Chua, F., Wells, A. U., et al. (2019). The Potential Impact of Azithromycin in Idiopathic Pulmonary Fibrosis. *Eur. Respir. J.* 53 (2), 1800628. doi:10.1183/13993003.00628-2018

Martínez-Martínez, E., Rodríguez, C., Galán, M., Miana, M., Jurado-López, R., Bartolomé, M. V., et al. (2016). The Lysyl Oxidase Inhibitor (β-Aminopropionitrile) Reduces Leptin Profibrotic Effects and Ameliorates Cardiovascular Remodeling in Diet-Induced Obesity in Rats. *J. Mol. Cel Cardiol.* 92, 96–104. doi:10.1016/j.yjmcc.2016.01.012

Meng, X. M., Nikolic-Paterson, D. J., and Lan, H. Y. (2014). Inflammatory Processes in Renal Fibrosis. *Nat. Rev. Nephrol.* 10 (9), 493–503. doi:10.1038/nrneph.2014.114

Meyer, K. C. (2017). Great Expectations for Simtuzumab in IPF Fall Short. *Lancet Respir. Med.* 5 (1), 2–3. doi:10.1016/s2213-2600(16)30420-9

Mineo, G., Ciccarese, F., Modolon, C., Landini, M. P., Valentino, M., and Zompatori, M. (2012). Post-ARDS Pulmonary Fibrosis in Patients with H1N1 Pneumonia: Role of Follow-Up CT. *Radiol. Med.* 117 (2), 185–200. doi:10.1007/s11547-011-0740-3

Nagasawa, R., Hara, Y., Murohashi, K., Saigusa, Y., Nishikawa, Y., Tanaka, M., et al. (2021). Additional Efficacy of Macrolide for Patients with Acute Deterioration of Interstitial Lung Disease Requiring Corticosteroid Pulse Therapy. *Am. J. Ther.* Publish Ahead of Print. doi:10.1097/mjt.0000000000001321

Naik, P. K., and Moore, B. B. (2010). Viral Infection and Aging as Cofactors for the Development of Pulmonary Fibrosis. *Expert Rev. Respir. Med.* 4 (6), 759–771. doi:10.1586/ers.10.73

Nguyen, X. X., Nishimoto, T., Takihara, T., Mlakar, L., Bradshaw, A. D., and Feghali-Bostwick, C. (2021). Lysyl Oxidase Directly Contributes to Extracellular Matrix Production and Fibrosis in Systemic Sclerosis. *Am. J. Physiol. Lung Cel Mol Physiol.* 320 (1), L29–l40. doi:10.1152/ajplung.00173.2020

Noble, P. W., Barkauskas, C. E., and Jiang, D. (2012). Pulmonary Fibrosis: Patterns and Perpetrators. *J. Clin. Invest.* 122 (8), 2756–2762. doi:10.1172/jci60323

Olson, A. L., Swigris, J. J., Lezotte, D. C., Norris, J. M., Wilson, C. G., and Brown, K. K. (2007). Mortality from Pulmonary Fibrosis Increased in the United States from 1992 to 2003. *Am. J. Respir. Crit. Care Med.* 176 (3), 277–284. doi:10.1164/rccm.200701-044OC

Parnham, M. J., Erakovic Haber, V., Giamarellos-Bourboulis, E. J., Perletti, G., Verleden, G. M., and Vos, R. (2014). Azithromycin: Mechanisms of Action and

Their Relevance for Clinical Applications. *Pharmacol. Ther.* 143 (2), 225–245. doi:10.1016/j.pharmthera.2014.03.003

Philp, C. J., Siebeke, I., Clements, D., Miller, S., Habgood, A., John, A. E., et al. (2018). Extracellular Matrix Cross-Linking Enhances Fibroblast Growth and Protects against Matrix Proteolysis in Lung Fibrosis. *Am. J. Respir. Cel Mol Biol.* 58 (5), 594–603. doi:10.1165/rcmb.2016-0379OC

Pu, Y., Liu, Y., Liao, S., Miao, S., Zhou, L., and Wan, L. (2018). Azithromycin Ameliorates OVA-Induced Airway Remodeling in Balb/c Mice via Suppression of Epithelial-To-Mesenchymal Transition. *Int. Immunopharmacol* 58, 87–93. doi:10.1016/j.intimp.2018.03.016

Raghu, G., Brown, K. K., Collard, H. R., Cottin, V., Gibson, K. F., Kaner, R. J., et al. (2017). Efficacy of Simtuzumab versus Placebo in Patients with Idiopathic Pulmonary Fibrosis: a Randomised, Double-Blind, Controlled, Phase 2 Trial. *Lancet Respir. Med.* 5 (1), 22–32. doi:10.1016/s2213-2600(16)30421-0

Remst, D. F., Blom, A. B., Vitters, E. L., Bank, R. A., van den Berg, W. B., Blaney Davidson, E. N., et al. (2014). Gene Expression Analysis of Murine and Human Osteoarthritis Synovium Reveals Elevation of Transforming Growth Factor β-responsive Genes in Osteoarthritis-Related Fibrosis. *Arthritis Rheumatol.* 66 (3), 647–656. doi:10.1002/art.38266

Ruan, H., Gao, S., Li, S., Luan, J., Jiang, Q., Li, X., et al. (2021). Deglycosylated Azithromycin Attenuates Bleomycin-Induced Pulmonary Fibrosis via the TGF-B1 Signaling Pathway. *Molecules* 26 (9), 2820. doi:10.3390/molecules26092820

Ruscitti, F., Ravanetti, F., Essers, J., Ridwan, Y., Belenkov, S., Vos, W., et al. (2017). Longitudinal Assessment of Bleomycin-Induced Lung Fibrosis by Micro-CT Correlates with Histological Evaluation in Mice. *Multidiscip Respir. Med.* 12, 8. doi:10.1186/s40248-017-0089-0

Sethi, A., Mao, W., Wordinger, R. J., and Clark, A. F. (2011). Transforming Growth Factor-Beta Induces Extracellular Matrix Protein Cross-Linking Lysyl Oxidase (LOX) Genes in Human Trabecular Meshwork Cells. *Invest. Ophthalmol. Vis. Sci.* 52 (8), 5240–5250. doi:10.1167/iovs.11-7287

Sgalla, G., Kulkarni, T., Antin-Ozerkis, D., Thannickal, V. J., and Richeldi, L. (2019). Update in Pulmonary Fibrosis 2018. *Am. J. Respir. Crit. Care Med.* 200 (3), 292–300. doi:10.1164/rccm.201903-0542UP

Spagnolo, P., Distler, O., Ryerson, C. J., Tzouvelekis, A., Lee, J. S., Bonella, F., et al. (2021). Mechanisms of Progressive Fibrosis in Connective Tissue Disease (CTD)-associated Interstitial Lung Diseases (ILDs). *Ann. Rheum. Dis.* 80 (2), 143–150. doi:10.1136/annrheumdis-2020-217230

Tjin, G., White, E. S., Faiz, A., Sicard, D., Tschumperlin, D. J., Mahar, A., et al. (2017). Lysyl Oxidases Regulate Fibrillar Collagen Remodelling in Idiopathic Pulmonary Fibrosis. *Dis. Model. Mech.* 10 (11), 1301–1312. doi:10.1242/dmm.030114

Tong, X., Guo, T., Liu, S., Peng, S., Yan, Z., Yang, X., et al. (2015). Macrolide Antibiotics for Treatment of Asthma in Adults: a Meta-Analysis of 18 Randomized Controlled Clinical Studies. *Pulm. Pharmacol. Ther.* 31, 99–108. doi:10.1016/j.pupt.2014.09.005

Tsubouchi, K., Araya, J., Minagawa, S., Hara, H., Ichikawa, A., Saito, N., et al. (2017). Azithromycin Attenuates Myofibroblast Differentiation and Lung Fibrosis Development through Proteasomal Degradation of NOX4. *Autophagy* 13 (8), 1420–1434. doi:10.1080/15548627.2017.1328348

Upagupta, C., Shimbori, C., Alsilmi, R., and Kolb, M. (2018). Matrix Abnormalities in Pulmonary Fibrosis. *Eur. Respir. Rev.* 27 (148), 180033. doi:10.1183/16000617.0033-2018

Vallet, S. D., and Ricard-Blum, S. (2019). Lysyl Oxidases: from Enzyme Activity to Extracellular Matrix Cross-Links. *Essays Biochem.* 63 (3), 349–364. doi:10.1042/ebc20180050

van Deel, E., Ridwan, Y., van Vliet, J. N., Belenkov, S., and Essers, J. (2016). *In Vivo* Quantitative Assessment of Myocardial Structure, Function, Perfusion and Viability Using Cardiac Micro-computed Tomography. *J. Vis. Exp.* 108, 53603. doi:10.3791/53603

van der Velden, J. L., Ye, Y., Nolin, J. D., Hoffman, S. M., Chapman, D. G., Lahue, K. G., et al. (2016). JNK Inhibition Reduces Lung Remodeling and Pulmonary Fibrotic Systemic Markers. *Clin. Transl Med.* 5 (1), 36. doi:10.1186/s40169-016-0117-2

Wei, Y., Kim, T. J., Peng, D. H., Duan, D., Gibbons, D. L., Yamauchi, M., et al. (2017). Fibroblast-specific Inhibition of TGF-B1 Signaling Attenuates Lung and Tumor Fibrosis. *J. Clin. Invest.* 127 (10), 3675–3688. doi:10.1172/jci94624

Wu, S., Zheng, Q., Xing, X., Dong, Y., Wang, Y., You, Y., et al. (2018). Matrix Stiffness-Upregulated LOXL2 Promotes Fibronectin Production, MMP9 and CXCL12 Expression and BMDCs Recruitment to Assist Pre-metastatic Niche Formation. *J. Exp. Clin. Cancer Res.* 37 (1), 99. doi:10.1186/s13046-018-0761-z

Wuyts, W. A., Willems, S., Vos, R., Vanaudenaerde, B. M., De Vleeschauwer, S. I., Rinaldi, M., et al. (2010). Azithromycin Reduces Pulmonary Fibrosis in a Bleomycin Mouse Model. *Exp. Lung Res.* 36 (10), 602–614. doi:10.3109/01902148.2010.492895

Yamaya, M., Azuma, A., Takizawa, H., Kadota, J., Tamaoki, J., and Kudoh, S. (2012). Macrolide Effects on the Prevention of COPD Exacerbations. *Eur. Respir. J.* 40 (2), 485–494. doi:10.1183/09031936.00208011

Yeap, Y. Y., Ng, I. H., Badrian, B., Nguyen, T. V., Yip, Y. Y., Dhillon, A. S., et al. (2010). c-Jun N-Terminal Kinase/c-Jun Inhibits Fibroblast Proliferation by Negatively Regulating the Levels of Stathmin/oncoprotein 18. *Biochem. J.* 430 (2), 345–354. doi:10.1042/bj20100425

Zhang, L., Tong, X., Huang, J., Wu, M., Zhang, S., Wang, D., et al. (2020). Fisetin Alleviated Bleomycin-Induced Pulmonary Fibrosis Partly by Rescuing Alveolar Epithelial Cells from Senescence. *Front. Pharmacol.* 11, 553690. doi:10.3389/fphar.2020.553690

ACPA Alleviates Bleomycin-Induced Pulmonary Fibrosis by Inhibiting TGF-β-Smad2/3 Signaling-Mediated Lung Fibroblast Activation

Dongxin Chen[1], *Huirong Tang*[1], *Hongchao Jiang*[1], *Lei Sun*[1], *Wenjuan Zhao*[1]* and *Feng Qian*[1,2]*

[1]*Engineering Research Center of Cell and Therapeutic Antibody, Ministry of Education, School of Pharmacy, Shanghai Jiao Tong University, Shanghai, China,* [2]*Anhui Province Key Laboratory of Translational Cancer Research, Bengbu Medical College, Bengbu, China*

Correspondence:
Feng Qian
fengqian@sjtu.edu.cn
Wenjuan Zhao
zhaowj@sjtu.edu.cn

Pulmonary fibrosis is a group of life-threatening diseases with limited therapeutic options. The involvement of cannabinoid type 1 receptors (CB_1R) has been indicated in fibrotic diseases, but whether or not the activation of CB_1R can be a benefit for fibrosis treatment is controversial. In this study, we investigated the effects of arachidonoylcyclopropylamide (ACPA), as a selective CB_1R agonist, on bleomycin (BLM)-induced pulmonary fibrosis. We showed that ACPA treatment significantly improved the survival rate of BLM-treated mice, alleviated BLM-induced pulmonary fibrosis, and inhibited the expressions of extracellular matrix (ECM) markers, such as collagen, fibronectin, and α-SMA. The enhanced expressions of ECM markers in transforming growth factor-beta (TGF-β)-challenged primary lung fibroblasts isolated from mouse lung tissues were inhibited by ACPA treatment in a dose-dependent manner, and the fibroblast migration triggered by TGF-β was dose-dependently diminished after ACPA administration. Moreover, the increased mRNA levels of CB_1R were observed in both lung fibroblasts of BLM-induced fibrotic mice *in vivo* and TGF-β-challenged primary lung fibroblasts *in vitro*. CB_1R-specific agonist ACPA significantly diminished the activation of TGF-β–Smad2/3 signaling, i.e., the levels of p-Smad2 and p-Smad3, and decreased the expressions of downstream effector proteins including slug and snail, which regulate ECM production, in TGF-β-challenged primary lung fibroblasts. Collectively, these findings demonstrated that CB_1R-specific agonist ACPA exhibited antifibrotic efficacy in both *in vitro* and *in vivo* models of pulmonary fibrosis, revealing a novel anti-fibrosis approach to fibroblast-selective inhibition of TGF-β-Smad2/3 signaling by targeting CB_1R.

Keywords: arachidonoylcyclopropylamide, cannabinoid type 1 receptor, fibroblast, idiopathic pulmonary fibrosis, transforming growth factor-beta

INTRODUCTION

Pulmonary fibrosis is a group of chronic, progressive, and usually lethal lung diseases that can be idiopathic or secondary to various diseases, characterized by excessive production and massive deposition of extracellular matrix (ECM) in lung interstitium (Barratt et al., 2018). Idiopathic pulmonary fibrosis (IPF) is a severe type of pulmonary fibrosis with unknown etiology and high mortality. However, available therapeutic options for pulmonary fibrosis, including two FDA-approved IPF drugs (nintedanib and pirfenidone) that slow the progression of the disease, have barely improved the outcomes of patients (Trachalaki et al., 2021). Currently, the prognosis for patients with pulmonary fibrosis remains poor, and it is urgent to identify therapeutic targets and to search novel therapies to slow down or even halt the progression of the disease.

Fibroblasts are the primary cells that build and maintain the ECM. In the pathogenesis of pulmonary fibrosis, lung fibroblasts are activated under the stimulation of profibrotic cytokines and exhibit a series of cell behavior changes, such as proliferation, migration, and ECM production, which is associated with severity of the disease in patients with pulmonary fibrosis and mouse models of pulmonary fibrosis (Xia et al., 2014; DePianto et al., 2015; Kasam et al., 2020). TGF-β family proteins, especially TGF-β1, released by injured lung epitheliums, immune cells, and fibrocytes during pulmonary fibrosis, are considered the principal profibrotic cytokines that drives fibrotic responses (Fernandez and Eickelberg, 2012; Martinez et al., 2017; Aschner et al., 2020; Lee et al., 2020). TGF-β signals are generally transduced through TGF-β type I and type II receptors (TβRI and TβRII) and Smads, and ancillary proteins as well (Aschner et al., 2020; Lee et al., 2020). Although TGF-β signals are attractive targets for lung fibrosis, genetic and pharmacological studies have indicated that broad targeting of general TGF-β signaling pathways might be problematic for treating fibrotic disease due to the pleiotropic roles of TGF-β (Mora et al., 2017; Saito et al., 2018). Therefore, the indirect modulation of TGF-β signals might be an alternative option for therapy of pulmonary fibrosis.

The endocannabinoid system (ECS) plays a critical homeostatic role in the regulation of various cellular and physiological processes through the activation of cannabinoid receptors, and its dysregulation is implicated to contribute to several highly prevalent diseases and disorders (Pacher and Kunos, 2013; Iannotti et al., 2016; Zhou et al., 2021). ECS has demonstrated anti-fibrotic effects in an avalanche of experimental studies, and cannabinoids are considered to be promising for the treatment of fibrosis (Correia-Sá et al., 2020a; Correia-Sá et al., 2020b). However, there is some controversy regarding the cannabinoid system's effects on fibrosis, especially regarding the cannabinoid type 1 receptors (CB_1R), a most well-researched cannabinoid receptor that has been reported overexpressed and activated widely in multiple fibrotic processes (Garcia-Gonzalez et al., 2009; Lecru et al., 2015; Cinar et al., 2017). CB_1R has been found to be associated with multiple pathologic processes in fibrosis, such as promoting/suppressing inflammatory responses, e.g., leukocyte infiltration, microphage activation and cytokine production, in addition to promoting/alleviating fibroblast activation and collagen accumulation in fibrosis (Garcia-Gonzalez et al., 2009; Marquart et al., 2010; Lazzerini et al., 2012; Bronova et al., 2015; Lecru et al., 2015; Chiurchiù et al., 2016; Cinar et al., 2017; Correia-Sá et al., 2020a; Correia-Sá et al., 2020b). Although Cinar R et al. found that the overactivity of CB1 contributed to the pathogenesis of IPF (Cinar et al., 2017), the CB_1R inhibitor rimonabant had no significant efficacy in stopping progression of fibrosis or reversing established fibrosis (Cinar et al., 2016), the pathology of liver fibrosis was still evident in CB_1R knockout mice as well (Teixeira-Clerc et al., 2006; Cinar et al., 2016). Similarly, Wang S et al. recently demonstrated that specific deletion of CB_1R in hepatic stellate cells did not protect mice from fibrosis (Wang et al., 2021). Instead, cannabinoids, such as Δ^9-tetrahydrocannabinol (THC), cannabidiol, cannabichromene, cannabinol, Cesamet (nabilone; Meda Pharmaceuticals, Somerset, NJ, United States), Marinol (dronabinol; THC; AbbVie, Inc., North Chicago, IL, USA), and Sativex (Cannabis extract; GW Pharmaceuticals, Cambridge, USA) were considered useful for the treatment of chronic inflammation and fibrosis (Zurier and Burstein, 2016). Therefore, the role of CB1 signaling in the development of fibrosis, including IPF, has not yet been identified. It is necessary to clarify whether the activation of CB_1R is beneficial or harmful and how it affects the development of pulmonary fibrosis for the pharmaceutical development of CB_1R agonists or antagonists and their potential therapeutic uses in pulmonary fibrosis.

Arachidonoylcyclopropylamide (ACPA) is a selective CB_1R agonist, which is a close analog of endocannabinoid anandamide and binds to the CB_1R with a strong affinity and high selectivity (Hillard et al., 1999). In this work, we explored the efficacy of CB_1R-specific agonist ACPA on bleomycin (BLM)-induced pulmonary fibrosis mouse models and ECM production in TGF-β1-challenged lung fibroblasts. We also revealed the role of CB_1R in fibroblast activation in the progression of pulmonary fibrosis, which might be a druggable target for pulmonary fibrosis therapy.

MATERIALS AND METHODS

Reagents

ACPA (N-cyclopropyl-5Z, 8Z, 11Z, 14Z-eicosatetraenamide; C23H37NO; CAS: 229021-64-1; MW: 343.6, purity ≥98%) was obtained from Cayman Chemical Company. BLM (#RB003) was purchased from BioTang (Lexington, MA, USA). Recombinant TGF-β1 protein (#240-B) was manufactured by R&D Systems (Minneapolis, MN, USA). Primary antibodies against α-smooth muscle actin (α-SMA, #19245), Collagen (#72026), Smad2 (#5339), phospho-Smad2 (Ser465/Ser467, #18338), Smad3 (#9523), phospho-Smad3 (Ser423/425, #9520), Slug (#9585), Snail (#3879), and β-actin (#3700) were purchased from Cell Signaling Technology (Danvers, MA, USA). Primary antibodies against CB_1R (#ab23703), TGF-β receptor II, and Fibronectin (#ab2413) were purchased from Abcam Company (Cambridge, MA, USA). Primary antibody against CB_2R (#sc293188) was from Santa Cruz Biotechnology (Santa Cruz, CA, USA). Anti-rabbit IgG (Alexa Fluor 488 Conjugate) (#4412) was purchased from Cell Signaling Technology (Danvers, MA, USA). DAPI (#C1002), Forskolin (#S1612), Hematoxylin and Eosin (H&E) staining kit (#C0105), and BeyoClick™ EdU Cell Proliferation Kit were purchased from Beyotime (Shanghai, China). Masson staining Kit (#D026-1-3) was obtained from NanJing JianCheng (China). Reverse transcription kit and SYBR Green Real-Time PCR kit were purchased from Toyobo (Osaka, Japan). MTT was purchased from Sigma Chemical Co. (St. Louis, MO, USA).

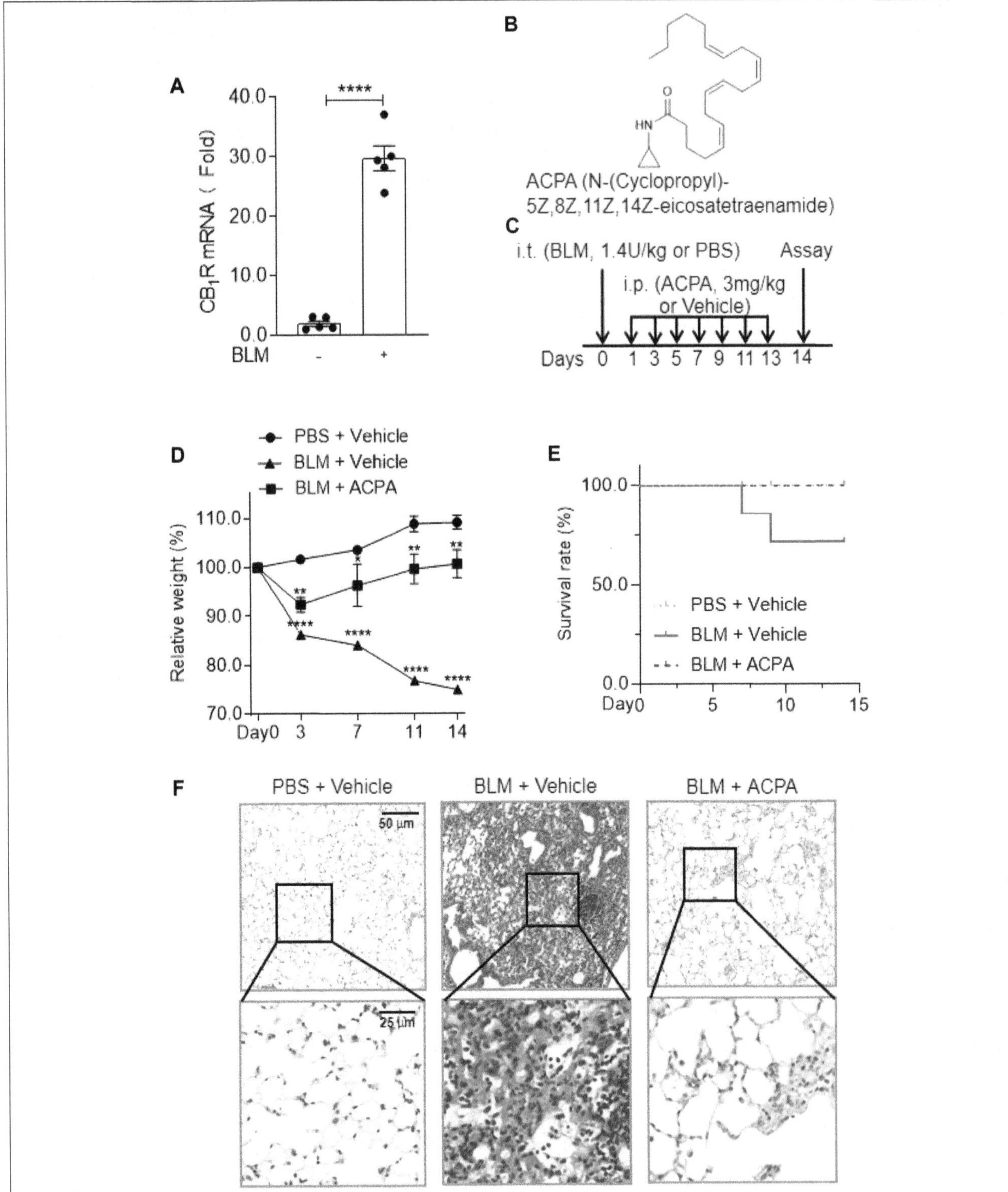

FIGURE 1 | The expression and activation of CB_1R was beneficial to the mice with bleomycin (BLM)-induced pulmonary fibrosis. **(A)** The mRNA levels of cannabinoid type 1 receptors (CB_1R) in lung tissues. **(B)** The chemical structure of the selective CB_1R agonist arachidonoylcyclopropylamide (ACPA). **(C)** The schematic timeline shows the process of BLM model establishment and ACPA administration. C57BL/6 mice were i.t. injected with BLM (1.4 U/kg) or PBS before i.p. injection with ACPA (3 mg/kg) or vehicle, and the mice were sacrificed on day 14. **(D)** Body weight changes in the mice during the experiment. The body weights of the mice were measured at indicated times, and the relative weight was compared with the weight on day 0. **(E)** The survival rate of the mice. **(F)** Representative sections of lung sections performed by hematoxylin and eosin (H&E) staining showing the pathological changes (e.g., infiltration of inflammatory cells and pulmonary lesions). Values are presented as mean ± SEM, n = 5–7 mice per group. $^{*}p < 0.05$, $^{**}p < 0.01$, and $^{***}p < 0.001$.

Animals and Treatments

Six- to eight-week-old C57BL/6 mice were purchased from the Laboratory Animal Center Shanghai Laboratory Animal Center (SLAC, Shanghai, China). Mice were maintained in a climate-controlled room (25°C, 55% humidity, and 12 h light/darkness cycles), and all procedures were conducted with the use of protocols approved by the Institutional Animal Care and Use Committee at Shanghai Jiao Tong University.

C57BL/6 male mice were randomly divided into three groups: the control (PBS + Vehicle) group, BLM (BLM + Vehicle) group, and ACPA (BLM + ACPA) group. ACPA was dissolved in a vehicle (1:1 mixture of PBS and ethanol). For the experiments (**Figure 1C**), the mice received an intratracheal injection (*i.t.*) of BLM (1.4 U/kg) or PBS at a volume of 20 μl per mouse after anesthetized with pentobarbital sodium (50 mg/kg) by intraperitoneal injection (i.p.). From the next day after BLM injection, the mice in the ACPA group were subjected to ACPA (3 mg/kg, i.p.), and the mice in the control and BLM groups received intraperitoneal injection of vehicle solution (1:1 mixture of PBS and ethanol) at a volume of 10 μl/g per body weight every other day (day 0–13). Animals (n = 7 in each group) were inspected daily in survival study, and death was recorded for each animal. Every animal found dead was necropsied. Surviving animals (n = 7 in control group; n = 5 in BLM group; n = 7 in ACPA group) were euthanized at day 14 to collect tissues. The left lungs from three mice of each group were fixed with polyoxymethylene for histological analysis. The remaining right lungs and lungs from other mice were collected for mRNA, protein, and hydroxyproline (HYP) measurements.

Tissue Analysis

The left lungs from three mice of each group were fixed with 4 ml of 4% polyoxymethylene for 48 h, followed by dehydration in graded alcohol and embedding in paraffin. Then the paraffin-embedded sections were sliced into 5-μm sections and stained with H&E kit (Beyotime, Shanghai, China) or Masson staining kit (Nanjing Jiancheng Bioengineering Institute, Nanjing, China) according to the instructions of the manufacturer. Stained sections were photographed with an Olympus BX51 microscope (Tokyo, Japan).

Isolation of Primary Mouse Lung Fibroblasts and Cell Culture

The lungs of the euthanized C57BL/6 mice (6–8 weeks old) were perfused with 10 ml of normal saline, removed immediately into ice-cold Hanks' balanced salt solutions, chopped finely with scissors, and digested with 2 mg/ml of collagenase IV (Sigma-Aldrich, St. Louis, MO, USA) for 0.5 h. Then after washing with PBS three times, the extracted fibroblasts were cultured in Dulbecco's modified Eagle's medium (DMEM, Gibco, MA, USA) supplemented with 10% fetal bovine serum (Sijiqing, Shanghai, China), 1% penicillin and streptomycin (Yishen, Shanghai, China) at 37°C in a 5% CO_2 incubator for 5 days. The medium was changed every 2 days. For the study of the effects of ACPA on the lung fibroblast *in vitro*, the cultured lung fibroblasts were incubated with serum-free medium containing PBS or TGF-β1 (20 ng/ml) for 24 h, and treated with vehicle or ACPA 0.5 h before TGF-β1 stimulation.

Hydroxyproline Assay

The collagen contents in lung tissues were evaluated by HYP assay using an HYP assay kit (Nanjing Jiancheng, Nanjing, China). According to the instructions of the manufacturer, the lung tissues were homogenized in 1 ml of hydrolysate and heated in 1 ml of hydrolysate at 95°C for 20 min, and pH was adjusted from 6.0 to 6.8. The hydroxyproline was detected by incubation with chloramine T and *p*-dimethylaminobenzaldehyde, and the absorbance was measured at 550 nm by a Biotek ELx800 (Winooski, VT, USA).

RNA Extraction and Quantitative Real Time PCR

RNA samples from lung tissues or cells were extracted using Trizol (Sigma-Aldrich, St Louis, MO, United States). cDNA was produced using qPCR RT Master Mix (TOYOBO, Osaka, Japan) according to the protocol of the manufacturer and used in subsequent real-time qPCR reactions. Quantitative real-time PCR was carried out to determine relative gene expression using the SYBR Green Real-time PCR Master Mix (Toyobo, Osaka, Japan) on StepOne Plus (Thermo Fisher Scientific, Waltham, MA, USA) as specified by the manufacturer. The quantification of target genes was identified by comparing Ct values of each sample normalized with Ct value of glyceraldehyde-3-phosphate dehydrogenase (GAPDH), and reaction specificity was verified by melting curve analysis. The primer sequences for target genes in real-time PCR assay were obtained from HuaGene Company (Shanghai, China) as shown below: the primers GAPDH forward 5′-CATCACTGCCACCCA GAAGACTG-3′ and reverse 5′-ATGCCAGTGAGCTTCCCG TTCAG-3′, α-SMA forward 5′-TGCTGACAGAGGCACCAC TGAA-3′ and reverse 5′-CAGTTGTACGTCCAGAGGCAT AG-3′, collagen forward 5′-CCTCAGGGTATTGCTGGACAA C-3′ and reverse 5′- CAGAAGGACCTTGTTTGCCAGG-3′, fibronectin forward 5′-CCCTATCTCTGATACCGTTGTCC-3′ and reverse 5′-TGCCGCAACTACTGTGATTCGG-3 ′, CB_1R forward 5′-ATCGGAGTCACCAGTGTGCTGT-3′ and reverse 5′-CCTTGCCATCTTCTGAGGTGTG-3′.

Western Blot

Protein samples from lung tissues or cultured cells were lysed and extracted with loading buffer containing protease inhibitor cocktail (Sigma-Aldrich, St. Louis, MO, USA) and phosphatase inhibitor cocktail (Roche Applied Science, USA). Protein concentration was measured using BCA Protein Assay kit (Beyotime, Shanghai, China) according to the protocol of the manufacturer. Protein samples were separated in sodium dodecyl sulfate–polyacrylamide gel electrophoresis (SDS-PAGE) and transferred onto nitrocellulose membranes. The membranes were blocked in 10% bovine serum albumin solution for 2 h at room temperature. Then the membranes were incubated with the appropriate primary antibodies overnight at 4°C, followed by the incubation with conjugated secondary antibodies at room temperature for 2 h. To visualize immune complexes, the membranes were stained using chemiluminescent substrate and imaged by a ChemiDoc MP System (Bio-Rad, MA, USA). The intensity of the protein band was quantified by ImageJ software and normalized to β-actin.

Scratch Wound Migration Assay

Scratch wound migration assay and Transwell chamber migration assay were performed to detect the migration of primary lung fibroblasts. In scratch wound migration assay, lung fibroblasts were inoculated on six-well plates (1×10^6 cells per well) and cultured with complete culture medium overnight until the cells adhere to the wall. Then the cells were washed three times with PBS and cultured in serum-free medium. A 200-µl pipet tip was used for scraping the cell monolayer in two straight lines as a cross. The cells were washed three times with serum-free medium to ensure that no cell debris remained in the scratch areas, and the cells were grown in serum-free medium with PBS + Vehicle, TGF-β1 (20 ng/ml) + Vehicle, or TGF-β1 (20 ng/ml) + ACPA (0, 10, 30 µM) for 24 h. Images were captured with a phase-contrast microscope (Olympus, Tokyo, Japan) and analyzed with ImageJ software.

Transwell Chamber Migration Assay

Lung fibroblasts (50,000 cells in 200 µl serum-free medium PBS + Vehicle, TGF-β1 (20 ng/ml) + Vehicle, or TGF-β1 (20 ng/ml) + ACPA (0, 10, 30 µM) were transferred to the upper chambers, and 600 µl of DMEM supplemented with 10% fetal bovine serum was added to the lower chambers. After 24 h of incubation, the medium in the upper chambers was discarded, and the cells that traversed to the reverse face were carefully washed with PBS three times, fixed with the pre-prepared fixative (methanol: acetic acid = 2:1), and then stained with 0.1% crystal violet for 20 min. Pictures were taken with a microscope (Olympus, Tokyo, Japan).

MTT Cell Viability Assay

Lung fibroblasts (1×10^4 cells per well) plated on 96-well plates were treated with vehicle or ACPA (0, 10, 30, and 100 µM) for 24 h. Then 20 µl MTT solution (5 mg/ml) was added into the wells and incubated for 4 h. The culture supernatant was discarded, and 100 µl of DMSO was added into each well. OD absorbance at 490 nm was measured by a microplate reader (BioTek, Vermont, USA).

EdU Cell Proliferation Assay

The EdU Cell Proliferation Kit was used to measure cell proliferation. Lung fibroblasts (5×10^5 cells per well) were seeded on 12-well plates and cultured with complete culture medium overnight with the cells adhering to the wall. The cells were pretreated with different concentrations of ACPA (0, 30, 100 µM) for 30 min and then stimulated with TGF-β1 (20 ng/ml) for 24 h. According to the instructions of the manufacturer, fresh DMEM containing EdU (10 µM) was added to the wells. After a 2-h incubation, the EdU medium was discarded, and the fibroblasts were fixed with 4% paraformaldehyde for 15 min and permeabilized with 0.3% Triton X-100 for 15 min. Next, the cells were incubated with Click Reaction solution for 30 min and stained with Hoechst for 10 min. Finally, images were captured using the microscope (Olympus, Tokyo, Japan).

Immunocytochemistry

Fibroblasts were plated in 12-well plates (3×10^5 cells per well) overnight. The cells were treated with ACPA (30 µM) for 30 min before being challenged with 20 ng/ml of TGF-β1 for 24 h. The cells were fixed with 4% PFA for 15 min, permeabilized with 0.3% Triton X-100 for 15 min, and blocked with 5% BSA for 1 h. Then the cells were incubated with TGF-β receptor II primary antibody overnight at 4°C. After washing with PBS three times, cells were incubated with Alexa 488-labeled secondary antibody for 2 h at room temperature, and then cells were stained with DAPI (5 µg/ml) to visualize the cell nuclei. Immunofluorescence images were recorded by a laser-scanning confocal fluorescence microscope (Leica Microsystem, Wetzlar, Germany).

Statistics Analysis

Statistical analysis was performed using the Prism software (ver. 8.3; GraphPad, San Diego, CA, USA). Comparisons between different groups were analyzed by one-way analysis of variance (ANOVA) followed by Tukey's test, and Student's t-test was used to compare differences between two groups. All experiment results were presented as the mean ± SEM. The referred experiment was performed independently for at least three times. Statistical significance was defined as $^{*}p < 0.05$, $^{**}p < 0.01$, $^{***}p < 0.001$, $^{****}p < 0.0001$.

RESULTS

Cannabinoid Type 1 Receptors Overexpression and Activation Brought About Beneficial Effects on Mice With Bleomycin-Induced Pulmonary Fibrosis

CB_1R has been found to be linked to multiple pathologic processes in fibrosis, including pulmonary fibrosis (Garcia-Gonzalez et al., 2009; Marquart et al., 2010; Lazzerini et al., 2012; Bronova et al., 2015; Lecru et al., 2015; Chiurchiù et al., 2016; Cinar et al., 2017; Correia-Sá et al., 2020a; Correia-Sá et al., 2020b), but the actual function of CB_1R activation in pulmonary fibrosis remains controversial. In the present study, we first examined the expression of CB_1R in the lung tissues of a murine pulmonary fibrosis model by i.t. injection of BLM (1.4 U/kg). We found that the mRNA levels of CB_1R significantly increased in the lung tissues of mice with pulmonary fibrosis compared with normal mice (**Figure 1A**), which indicated that overexpressed CB_1R might play certain role in the pathologic processes of pulmonary fibrosis. Then we observed the influences of CB_1R activation on mice with BLM-induced pulmonary fibrosis using the highly selective CB_1R agonist ACPA (**Figure 1B**) to stimulate CB_1R. The murine model of pulmonary fibrosis was established by i.t. injection of BLM, and the function of ACPA for pulmonary fibrosis was evaluated by i.p. injection (**Figure 1C**). Compared with the mice in normal control group, the pulmonary fibrosis mice subjected to BLM i.t. injection exhibited significantly diminished body weight, an important indicator of pathological severity following BLM challenge, while ACPA treatment largely rescued the weight loss of pulmonary fibrosis mice (**Figure 1D**). Similarly, the survivorship curve also manifested that ACPA treatment improved the survival rate of pulmonary fibrosis mice (**Figure 1E**). In addition, HE staining demonstrated extensive inflammatory cell infiltration and severe pulmonary lesions in lung tissues of mice with BLM-induced pulmonary fibrosis, which were apparently reduced by ACPA administration (**Figure 1F**). Collectively, these data showed that CB_1R overexpression in lung tissues and activation stimulated by ACPA would help to mitigate pathological changes and improve survival of pulmonary fibrosis mice.

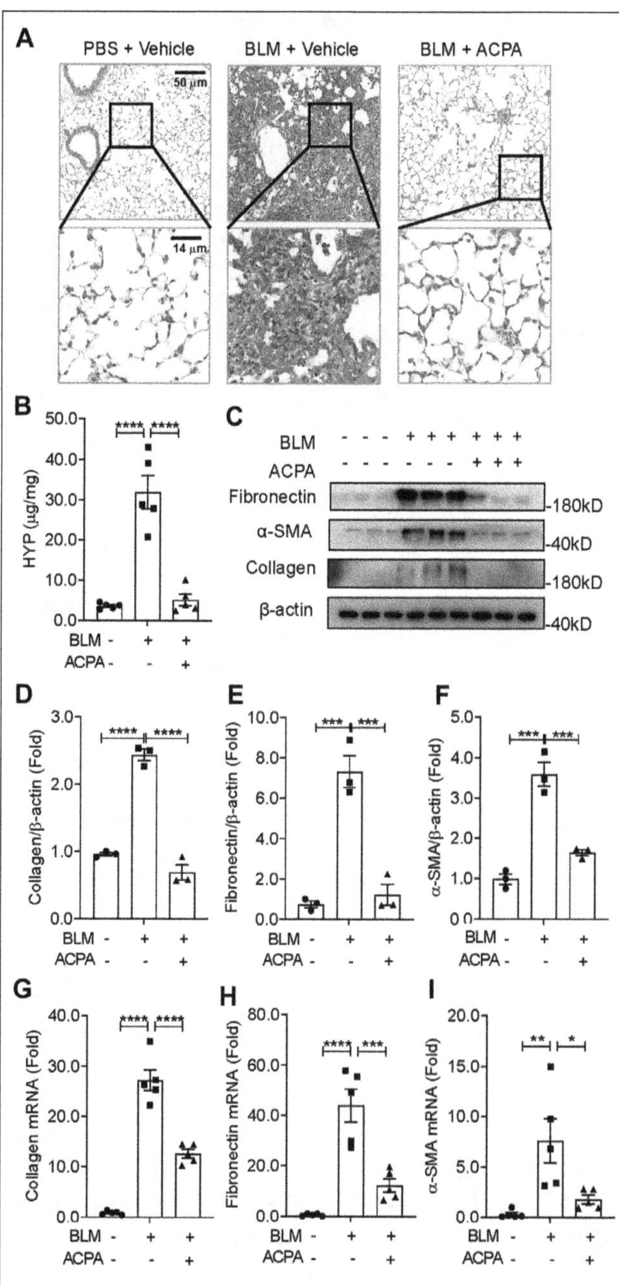

FIGURE 2 | ACPA attenuated BLM-induced pulmonary fibrosis in mice. **(A)** Representative images of lung sections visualized by Masson staining demonstrated collagen deposition, indicative of fibrosis. **(B)** Hydroxyproline (HYP) analysis of lung tissues from mice treated with PBS + Vehicle, BLM + Vehicle, and BLM + ACPA injection. **(C)** Western blots for extracellular matrix (ECM) protein collagen, fibronectin, and α-smooth muscle actin (α-SMA) in lung tissues of mice from each group. Quantification of collagen **(D)**, fibronectin **(E)**, and α-SMA **(F)** proteins normalized to β-actin were analyzed by ImageJ software. Relative mRNA levels of fibrosis markers collagen **(G)**, fibronectin **(H)**, and α-SMA **(I)** in lung tissues of mice from each group were quantified by real-time PCR. Data are presented as means ± SEM, n = 3 per group in **(D–F)** and n = 5 per group in **(B)** and **(G–I)**. *$p < 0.05$, **$p < 0.01$, and ***$p < 0.001$.

Arachidonoylcyclopropylamide Ameliorated Bleomycin-Induced Pulmonary Fibrosis *in Vivo*

Pulmonary fibrosis is a group of lethal disease characterized by deposition of a pathological ECM, we further evaluated the efficacy of CB_1R-selective agonist ACPA on collagen deposition and the expression of fibrotic makers in BLM-induced experimental pulmonary fibrosis *in vivo* (**Figure 2**). Histologic assay of Masson staining demonstrated a dramatic collagen accumulation, the indicative of fibrosis, in BLM-stimulated mice, while ACPA treatment strongly attenuated deposition of pulmonary collagen (**Figure 2A**). Consistently, HYP, the main component of collagen, was also significantly reduced by treatment compared with that in the BLM group (**Figure 2B**). In line with the results of Masson staining and HYP assay, the productions (protein levels) of ECM, e.g., collagen, fibronectin, and α-SMA, which are biomarkers for fibrotic levels, remarkably decreased in ACPA group (**Figures 2C–F**). Similarly, the transcription (mRNA levels) of collagen, fibronectin, and α-SMA were also downregulated by ACPA (**Figures 2G–I**). Collectively, these results showed that CB_1R-selective agonist ACPA protected pulmonary fibrosis mice against BLM-induced pulmonary fibrosis with the inhibition of ECM production.

Arachidonoylcyclopropylamide Reduced the Expression of extracellular Matrix Proteins in TGF-β1-Challenged Lung Fibroblasts *in Vitro*

Fibroblasts are the primary cells that build and maintain the ECM. Increased activation of lung fibroblast is central for the initiation and maintenance of unremitting deposition of ECM and fibrotic lesions in pulmonary fibrosis (Xia et al., 2014; DePianto et al., 2015; Kasam et al., 2020). In this study, we investigated the expression of CB_1R in lung fibroblasts isolated from BLM-challenged mice and found that

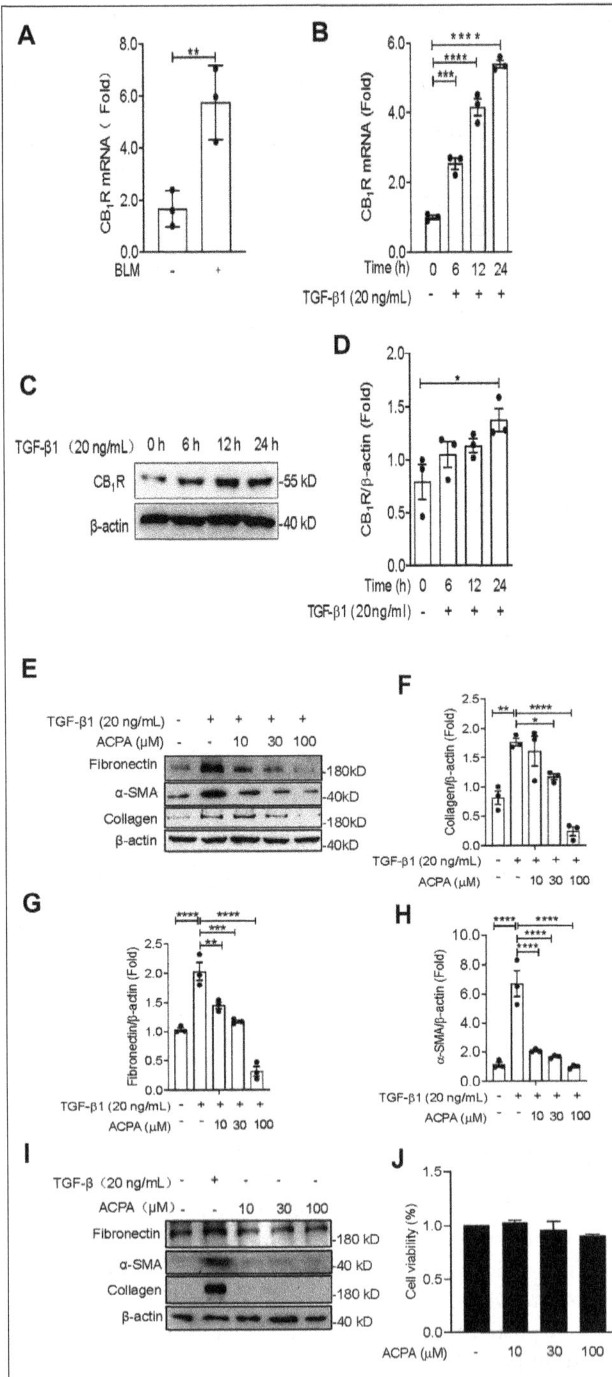

FIGURE 3 | ACPA inhibited the expression of ECM proteins in TGF-β1-challenged primary lung fibroblasts. **(A)** The mRNA levels of CB_1R in lung fibroblasts from normal control mice or the pulmonary fibrosis model mice treated with BLM (1.4 U/kg, i.t.). **(B)** The mRNA levels of CB_1R in primary mouse lung fibroblasts pretreated with TGF-β1 (20 ng/ml). **(C)** Western blots for CB_1R protein in primary mouse lung fibroblasts pretreated with TGF-β1 (20 ng/ml). **(D)** Quantification of CB_1R proteins normalized to β-actin. **(E)** Western blots for ECM protein collagen, fibronectin, and α-SMA in TGF-β1-challenged primary lung fibroblasts. Primary mouse lung fibroblasts were treated with vehicle or ACPA (10, 30, 100 μM) followed by TGF-β1 stimulation for 24 h. Quantification of collagen **(F)**, fibronectin **(G)**, and α-SMA **(H)** proteins normalized to β-actin were analyzed by ImageJ software. **(I)** Western blots for *(Continued)*

FIGURE 3 | ECM protein collagen, fibronectin, and α-SMA in primary lung fibroblasts treated with ACPA (10, 30, 100 μM) alone for 24 h. **(J)** The viability of fibroblasts after treatment with ACPA (10, 30, and 100 μM) alone for 24 h in MTT Cell viability assay. Data shown are mean ± SEM from three independent experiments. $^*p < 0.05$, $^{**}p < 0.01$, and $^{***}p < 0.001$.

CB_1R mRNA levels were significantly increased in the isolated lung fibroblasts from mice with BLM-induced pulmonary fibrosis compared with control mice (**Figure 3A**), which is in accordance with the increased CB_1R mRNA levels in lung tissues of pulmonary fibrosis mice (**Figure 1A**). TGF-β1 is one of the most potent and well-studied profibrotic inducers of pulmonary fibrosis that triggers and greatly enhances the fibrogenic activity of lung fibroblasts (Fernandez and Eickelberg, 2012; Martinez et al., 2017; Aschner et al., 2020; Lee et al., 2020). We isolated primary mouse lung fibroblasts to examine the expression of CB_1R and ECM proteins induced by TGF-β1. Primary mouse lung fibroblasts were incubated with PBS or TGF-β1 for 24 h after pretreated with vehicle or ACPA with different concentrations. As shown in **Figures 3B–D,** both mRNA and protein levels of CB_1R in primary mouse lung fibroblasts demonstrated a time-dependent augmentation with the stimulation of TGF-β1, suggesting that TGF-β1 promotes CB_1R expression in lung fibroblasts. By contrast, CB_2R expression was much lower in lung fibroblasts and its level was not observably changed by TGF-β1 or ACPA treatment (**Supplementary Figures S1A–E**). Consistent with BLM-induced pulmonary fibrosis, the expression of ECM protein collagen, fibronectin, and α-SMA in primary fibroblasts also increased enormously in response to TGF-β1 stimulation. Although ACPA (10, 30 μM) alone did not affect the expression of ECM proteins (**Figure 3I**) or exhibit obvious cytotoxicity to fibroblasts (**Figure 3J**), when administrated with TGF-β1, it significantly reduced the augmentation of ECM proteins induced by TGF-β1, which are also considered as fibrosis markers, in a dose-dependent manner (**Figures 3E–H**). Taken together, these results revealed that lung fibroblasts expressed CB_1R when stimulated by TGF-β1 and CB_1R activation, in turn, inhibiting the excessive expression of ECM proteins in TGF-β-challenged lung fibroblasts.

Arachidonoylcyclopropylamide Subdued the Migration and Motility of Primary Lung Fibroblasts Triggered by TGF-β1

The migratory capacity of fibroblasts by responding to cytokines and chemokines, e.g., TGF-β1, is important for the progression of pulmonary fibrosis (Kasam et al., 2020). To ascertain whether CB_1R activation participates in modulating TGF-β1-triggered cell migration of primary lung fibroblasts, we conducted scratch wound migration assay and Transwell migration assay on primary lung fibroblasts. Primary fibroblasts were pretreated with CB_1R-selective agonist ACPA (0, 10, 30 μM) before stimulating with TGF-β1 for 24 h. In EdU cell proliferation assay, TGF-β1 significantly stimulate the proliferation of fibroblasts, as obviously increased EdU-positive cells were seen in TGF-β1 group than those in the control group, and it was reduced by ACPA (10, 30 μM) treatment (**Figures 4A, D**). Consistently, TGF-β1

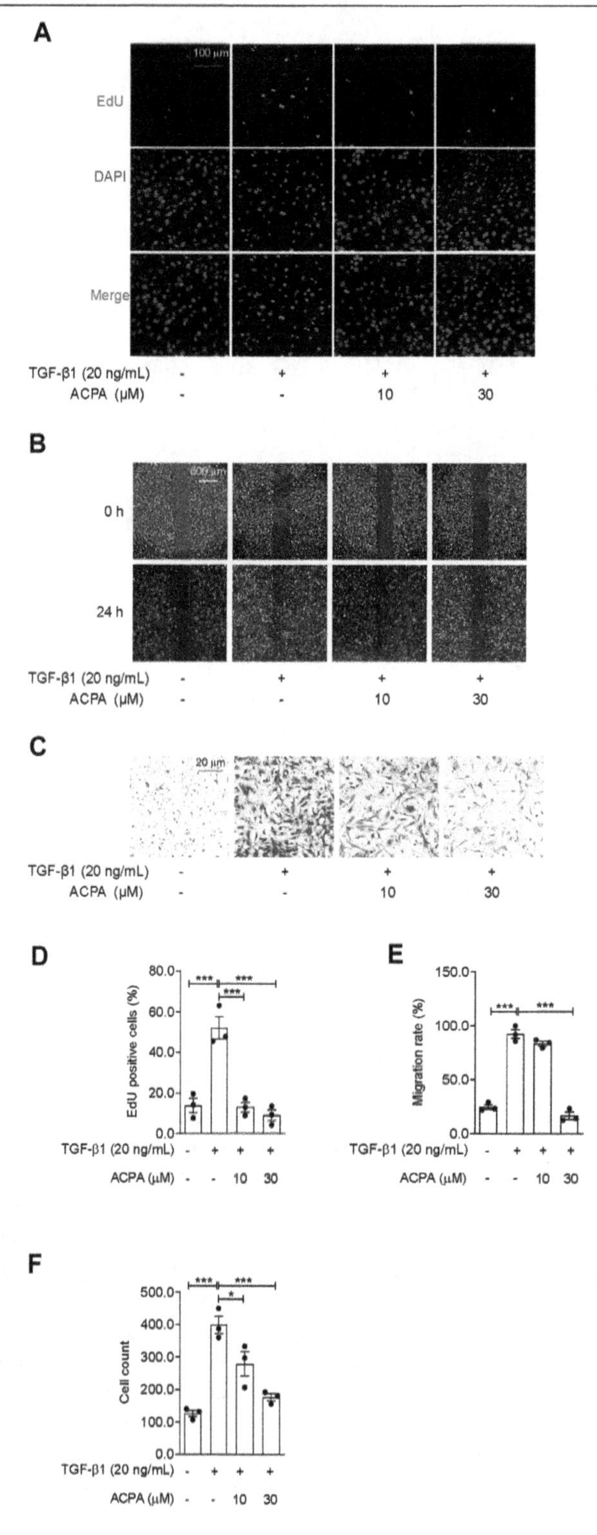

FIGURE 4 | ACPA subdued the cell proliferation and migration of primary lung fibroblasts triggered by TGF-β1. The cell proliferation, migration, and motility of TGF-β1-challenged fibroblasts were detected by EdU cell proliferation assay, scratch wound migration assay, and Transwell migration assay, respectively. Primary mouse lung fibroblasts were pretreated with vehicle or ACPA (10, 30 μM) 0.5 h before TGF-β1 stimulation. **(A)** Representative fluorescence images of EdU staining, nuclei: DAPI (blue), and proliferating cell: EdU + (red). **(B)** Representative images of scratch wounds taken at 24 h after scratch injury in scratch wound migration assay. **(C)** Representative images of the migrated fibroblasts in Transwell migration assay. **(D)** The ratio of proliferating positive cells in EdU cell proliferation assay. **(E)** Quantification of cell migration by measuring the area of the injured region compared with TGF-β1-challenged fibroblasts. **(F)** Cell counting of the migrated fibroblasts in Transwell migration assay. Values are mean ± SEM from three independent experiments; $^{*}p < 0.05$, $^{**}p < 0.01$, and $^{***}p < 0.001$.

significantly spurred fibroblasts to migrate to the scratch guidelines in scratch wound healing assay, while ACPA alleviated the fibroblast migration with the high concentration (30 μM) of ACPA showing a nearly radical inhibition (**Figures 4B, E**). Moreover, numbers of transmigrating fibroblasts were much higher among TGF-β1-challenged fibroblasts than controls, while ACPA (30 μM) obviously decreased the migration of the lung fibroblasts toward fetal bovine serum (**Figures 4C, F**). Thus, we concluded that CB_1R-selective agonist ACPA restrained cell proliferation, migration, and motility of lung fibroblasts triggered by TGF-β1.

Arachidonoylcyclopropylamide Downregulated TGF-β-Smad2/3 Signaling and the Expression of Snail and Slug in TGF-β1-Challenged Lung Fibroblasts

In the present study, we revealed that CB_1R-selective agonist ACPA substantially suppressed ECM production both in the lung tissues of mice with pulmonary fibrosis and in TGF-β-challenged lung fibroblasts, indicating that CB_1R activation downregulated TGF-β signaling mediated the expression of ECM proteins in pulmonary fibrosis. To manifest this, we investigated the activation of canonical TGF-β-Smad2/3 signaling and the levels of its downstream effectors in TGF-β1-challenged primary lung fibroblasts with ACPA treatment. Western blot showing that TGF-β1 stimulation resulted in the activation of canonical TGF-β-Smad2/3 signaling, assessed by the elevated p-Smad2 and p-Smad3 (**Figures 5A–C**), followed by the expression of downstream transcription factors Snail and Slug (**Figures 5A, D, E**), key regulators that mediated TGF-β-Smad signaling triggered the overexpression and excessive production of ECM proteins in pulmonary fibrosis. However, CB_1R-selective agonist ACPA exerted a notable inhibition on elevated p-Smad2, p-Smad3, snail, and slug in lung fibroblasts spurred by TGF-β1 (**Figure 5**). These data indicate that CB_1R activation acted as a negative regulation of canonical TGF-β-Smad2/3 signaling, downregulated TGF-β triggered Snail and Slug expression, and subsequent overexpression of ECM proteins in lung fibroblasts.

DISCUSSION

Pulmonary fibrosis is a life-threatening disease characterized by massive deposition of ECM in the lungs with hardly any therapeutic options. Using both *in vitro* and *in vivo* models of pulmonary fibrosis, we demonstrated that the expression of CB_1R increased in lung fibroblasts in response to pulmonary fibrosis, and the

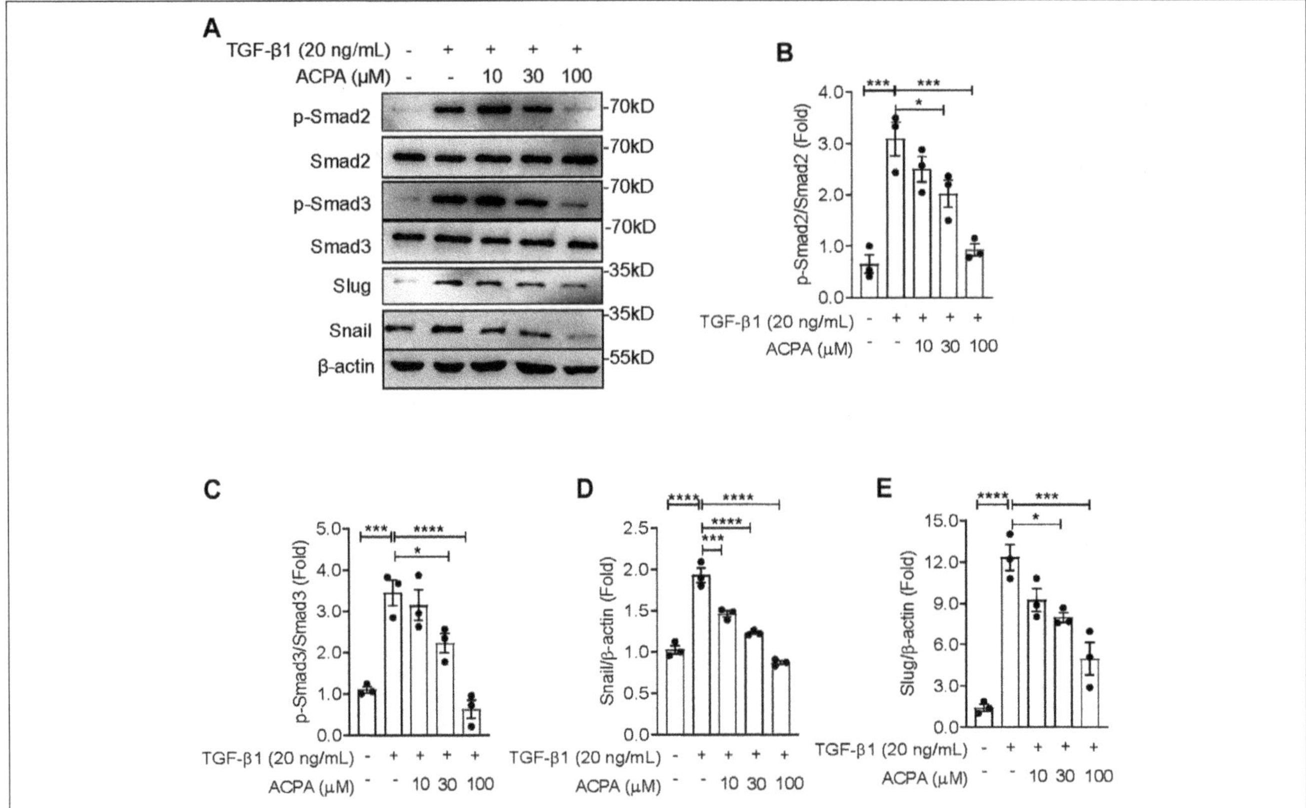

FIGURE 5 | ACPA downregulated the activation of TGF-β-Smad2/3 signaling and the expression of downstream effectors snail and slug in TGF-β1-stimulated lung fibroblasts. **(A)** Western blots for p-Smad2, Smad2, p-Smad3, Smad3, slug, and snail in TGF-β1-challenged lung fibroblasts. Primary mouse lung fibroblasts were treated with vehicle or ACPA (10, 30, 100 μM) followed by TGF-β1 stimulation for 24 h. Quantification of p-Smad2 to Smad2 **(B)**, p-Smad3 to Smad3 **(C)**, snail **(D)**, and slug **(E)** bands normalized to β-actin was pooled from three independent experiments. Data are represented as mean ± SEM. *$p < 0.05$, **$p < 0.01$, and ***$p < 0.001$.

pharmacologic activation of CB_1R with its specific agonist ACPA protected against BLM-induced pulmonary fibrosis, significantly decreasing lung fibroblast migration and the excessive expression of ECM proteins (collagen, fibronectin, and α-SMA) stimulated by BLM *in vivo* or TGF-β1 *in vitro*, rather than the basal expression of ECM proteins in normal control lung fibroblasts. Moreover, we demonstrated that CB_1R-selective agonist ACPA dose-dependently downregulated the activation of TGF-β-Smad2/3 signaling (reduced p-Smad2 and p-Smad3 levels) and the levels of its downstream effectors snail and slug, which are the transcription factors to regulate the expression of ECM proteins. These findings provided the first evidence that CB_1R acted as a negative regulator for TGF-β1-Smad2/3 signaling and its associated fibroblast activation in pulmonary fibrosis (**Figure 6**), and thus, the overexpression of CB_1R on fibroblasts might be a druggable target for the therapy of pulmonary fibrosis.

ECS is an evolutionarily conserved network of signaling systems comprising receptors (such as CB1, CB2, or TRPV-1), their endogenous lipid ligands, or endocannabinoids and synthetic and metabolizing enzymes, present nearly everywhere in the human body. ECS is deeply involved in the maintenance of bodily homeostasis by modulating a wide variety of physiological/pathological processes all over the body (Pacher and Kunos, 2013; Iannotti et al., 2016; Zhou et al., 2021). This is achieved through a negative feedback loop, which works by the activation of synthesis and release of endocannabinoids as they target cannabinoid receptors (Iannotti et al., 2016; Zhou et al., 2021). Increased activity of the endocannabinoid/CB_1R system was also reported to be parallel with the pathogenesis of pulmonary fibrosis and associated with the increased tissue levels of interferon regulatory factor-5, and the pathogenesis of pulmonary fibrosis, while CB_1R inhibition, especially the combined CB_1R/iNOS inhibition, has antifibrotic efficacy in bleomycin-induced pulmonary fibrosis (Cinar et al., 2017). Numerous evidence have demonstrated that CB_1R was increased and got involved in the progression of multiple organ fibrosis, including the liver (Patsenker et al., 2011), kidneys (Lecru et al., 2015), heart (Slavic et al., 2013), skin (Lazzerini et al., 2012; Garcia-Gonzalez et al., 2016; Cinar et al., 2017), and pulmonary fibrosis as well (Bronova et al., 2015; Cinar et al., 2017). Although the CB_1R was consistently found highly activated in the pathogenesis of pulmonary fibrosis, the role of activated CB_1R in fibrosis is controversial. Correia-Sá et al. found that CB_1R agonist ACEA increases, and antagonist AM251 reduces, collagen deposition induced by TGF-β in the fibroblasts obtained from abdominal human skin (Correia-Sá et al., 2021). However, it has been recently proposed that cannabinoids, natural CB_1R

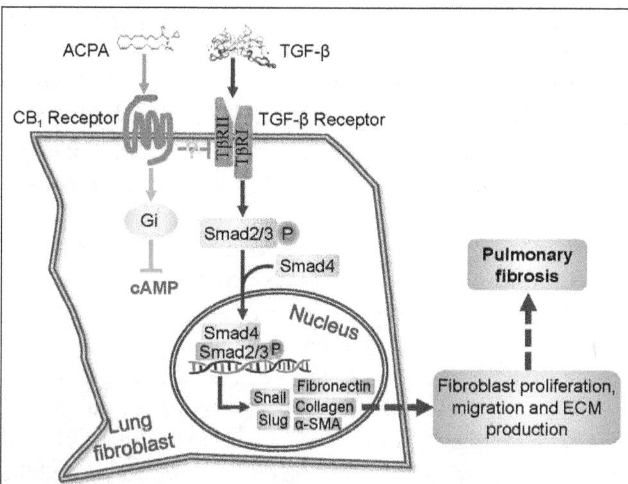

FIGURE 6 | Schematic representation of the possible mechanism by which ACPA inhibits pulmonary fibrosis *via* TGF-β-Smad2/3 signaling-mediated lung fibroblast activation. TGF-β signals are transduced by TGF-β receptor, a TβRI, and TβRII heterodimeric receptor. TGF-β binding to and activating the TGF-β receptor results in the phosphorylation of transcription factors Smad2 and Smad3. The phosphorylated Smad2 and Smad3 then combine with Smad4 in the cytoplasm, and translocate to the nucleus to induce gene transcription, including transcription factor snail and slug and the subsequent unremitting expression of ECM proteins. ACPA selectively binds to and activates CB_1R of lung fibroblasts, which downregulates TGF-β–Smad2/3 signaling and lead to blockage of ECM production/deposition triggered by TGF-β, by an unknown Gi signaling-independent way.

agonists, may manifest as profibrotic or antifibrotic agents in skin fibrosis (Pryimak et al., 2021). Moreover, CB_1R inhibitor rimonabant or the deletion of CB_1R did not prevent, limit, or reverse fibrosis in a substantial body of studies (Teixeira-Clerc et al., 2006; Cinar et al., 2016; Wang et al., 2021). Although the overactivity of CB_1R was found contributing to the pathogenesis of pulmonary fibrosis, the pharmaceutical development of CB_1R antagonist and their potential therapeutic uses in fibrosis was halted (Cinar et al., 2016). On the other hand, the phytocannabinoids (THC, cannabidiol, cannabichromene, and cannabinol) and synthetic preparations (Cesamet, Marinol, and Sativex) are candidates for development as anti-inflammatory and antifibrotic agents (Zurier and Burstein, 2016). In the present study, we found that CB_1R expression dramatically increased in lung tissues and fibroblasts in response to experimental pulmonary fibrosis, but showed that its selective agonist ACPA exhibited marked antifibrotic effect both *in vitro* and *in vivo* models of pulmonary fibrosis, which was inconsistent with CB_1R inhibition that ameliorated fibrosis (Bronova et al., 2015; Cinar et al., 2017; Correia-Sá et al., 2021). This inconsistency is due to different tissues (lungs, liver, kidneys, or skin), cell types (macrophages *vs.* fibroblasts), pathologic stages of fibrotic diseases (inflammatory stage *vs.* fibrosis stage), and various types of G-protein signaling triggered by CB_1R. Previous studies have paid close attention to inflammation period and macrophage functions in pulmonary fibrosis, and the inhibition of CB_1R exhibited anti-inflammatory properties (Cinar et al., 2017). While CB_2R is expressed primarily in spleen and immune system cells, it had been demonstrated that CB_2R agonists can be used to treat inflammation-related diseases. In the supplemental experiments, we showed that CB_2R expression was much lower in lung fibroblasts, and its level was not observably changed by TGF-β1 or ACPA treatment, and the CB_2R mRNA levels in lung fibroblasts from BLM-challenged mice were increased but with no significant differences, indicating that CB_2R in lung fibroblasts might not be involved in the inhibition of ACPA on TGF-β1-stimulated fibroblast activation. However, fibroblasts are responsible for mediating the synthesis and deposition of ECM and deteriorating fibrosis in pulmonary fibrosis. It was shown that CB_1R in mononuclear cells was involved in inflammation, while CB_1R in fibroblastic cells contributed to wound healing (Zhao et al., 2010). So, the modulation of fibroblast CB_1R on ECM production might have more impact on fibrosis.

CB_1R primarily activates Gi/o proteins, which cause downstream inhibition of cAMP accumulation mediated *via* the pertussis toxin-sensitive Gi α-subunit inhibition of adenylyl cyclase. In the supplemental experiments, we used forskolin, a potent adenylate cyclase activator to generate the second messenger, cAMP, to detect the involvement of PKA/cAMP signaling pathway in ACPA-induced downregulation on TGF-β-induced fibroblast activation and found that forskolin did not reverse the inhibition of ACPA on TGF-β1-stimulated ECM production (collagen and α-SMA) of fibroblast (**Supplementary Figures S2A, B**). Although, the activation of Gi subunit triggered by CB_1R was shown to have some limit on uncontrolled fibrosis processes (Garcia-Gonzalez et al., 2009), our results suggest that it might not *via* PKA/cAMP signaling pathway and that ACPA downregulates TGF-β1 signaling and inhibits ECM production by fibroblasts (**Figure 6**). In addition to Gi/o proteins, CB_1R can also couple to Gs, Gq, and G12/13 α-subunits and Gi βγ-subunit depending on the cellular/protein context, which should not be ruled out. Different agonists can also elicit different patterns of G-protein coupling, e.g., WIN55212-2, but not Δ9-THC and ACEA, is able to stimulate G12/13 in mouse cortex (Diez-Alarcia et al., 2016). Like many other GPCRs, CB_1R is internalized, which generally occurs as a result of intensive stimulation by an agonist, subsequent receptor phosphorylation, and β-arrestin binding, followed by clathrin-mediated endocytosis (Fletcher-Jones et al., 2020). Binding of β-arrestin 2 to the type III TGF-β receptor (TβRIII) was also triggered by phosphorylation of the receptor mediated by the type II TGF-β receptor (TβRII), which is itself a kinase like GRK, and leads to internalization of both receptors and downregulation of TGF-β signaling (Chen et al., 2003). Thus, the internalization of ACPA-activated CB_1R and TGF-β1-activated TGF-β receptors might be intertwined, and ACPA might downregulate TGF-β signaling by promoting the endocytosis of TGF-β receptors. This was partly supported by our immunofluorescence analysis on TGF-β receptors located on the cell membrane surface. Our preliminary results showed that TβRII was present predominantly on the cell surface in TGF-β1 (20 ng/ml)-stimulated fibroblasts, and it significantly decreased with ACPA (30 μM) administration together with TGF-β1 (**Supplementary Figure S3**). Nevertheless, direct evidence that CB_1R regulated the endocytosis of TGF-β receptors is needed.

The unclear mechanism and etiology render the current therapy, targeting the pulmonary fibrosis, hardly receiving positive feedback among patients. The activation of lung fibroblasts and their accumulation of excessive ECM proteins is essential to develop pulmonary fibrosis and associated with severity of the disease in patients with pulmonary fibrosis (Kasam et al., 2020). Thus, the profibrotic factors in lung fibroblasts is considered an important therapeutic target to develop novel and effective therapies against pulmonary fibrosis. Actually, nintedanib, one of the two approved drugs for fibrotic disease, has been shown to impact signaling pathways of fibroblast activation by inhibiting multiple tyrosine kinases (Wollin et al., 2015), suggesting that therapeutic approaches targeting fibroblasts are effective to prevent/reverse fibrosis and alleviate pulmonary fibrosis. TGF-β is of greatest interest, as it strongly activates fibroblasts and facilitates ECM production to induce progressive fibrosis in numerous fibrotic diseases (Aschner et al., 2020; Khalil et al., 2017; Derynck and Zhang, 2003). However, TGF-β blockade (e.g., fresolimumab and metelimumab) has major side effects, such as carcinogenesis, systemic autoimmunity, etc.,. due to the pleiotropic roles of TGF-β (Henderson et al., 2020). Thus, strategies to avoid these deleterious effects could involve inhibiting TGF-β signaling selectively in excessive activated lung fibroblasts, as TGF-β-triggered Smad2/3 signaling is pivotal in the induction of pulmonary fibrosis in animal models (**Figure 6**) (Aschner et al., 2020). In this work, we analyzed the effects of CB_1R-selective agonist ACPA on TGF-β1-challenged lung fibroblasts and found that ACPA markedly suppressed TGF-β1-stimulated activation of TGF-β-Smad2/3 signaling with decreased phosphorylation levels of Smad2 and Smad3 in lung fibroblasts, in addition to reducing the expression of ECM proteins and the transcription factors snail and slug, but hardly having an impact on the expression of ECM proteins in lung fibroblasts under normal conditions. In addition, slug and snail are markers of the epithelial–mesenchymal transition (EMT), which is a process whereby part of the lung epithelial cells, mainly type II alveolar epithelial cells (AT2), transition into cells of the mesenchymal phenotype, such as fibroblasts, or myofibroblasts, and it has been shown to be a critical stage during the development of fibrosis (Nieto et al., 2016). As ACPA inhibited TGF-β1-induced expression of EMT-related transcription factors, slug and snail, and CB_1R is also found in epithelial cells, including AT2 cells (Cinar et al., 2017), it might be possible that the activation of CB_1R in the pathogenesis of pulmonary fibrosis also prevented EMT derived from AT2 cells and the ECM it generated. These results revealed that CB_1R activation, which acted as a negative regulation of canonical TGF-β-Smad2/3 signaling, downregulated TGF-β-triggered overexpression of ECM proteins in lung fibroblasts, but did not affect normal ECM production, and CB_1R agonist was proven useful as a potential therapeutic option for pulmonary fibrosis. ACPA itself, however, is unlikely to be used in clinical practice because of a short half-life and its lipophilic characteristic to easily enter the central nervous system, while the fibroblast-selective CB_1R agonist like ACPA nanoparticles and agonistic antibodies to CB_1R would be promising therapeutic drugs for pulmonary fibrosis that might be used clinically.

In summary, our study showed ACPA, a selective agonist of CB_1R, which expression increased in pulmonary fibrosis, exhibited antifibrotic efficacy in both *in vitro* and *in vivo* models of pulmonary fibrosis, inhibited TGF-β1-stimulated lung fibroblast activation and fibrotic ECM production *via* downregulating TGF-β1-Smad2/3 signaling, revealing a novel anti-fibrosis approach to fibroblast-selective negative regulation of TGF-β-Smad2/3 signaling by targeting CB_1R. New candidates selectively targeted to activate CB_1R on lung fibroblasts might be effective clinical agents for the treatment of pulmonary fibrosis.

AUTHOR CONTRIBUTIONS

LS, WZ, and FQ conceived the study. DC, HT, and HJ designed, performed, and interpreted the experimental data. WZ, HT, and FQ wrote the manuscript. All authors read and approved the submitted manuscript.

REFERENCES

Aschner, Y., Nelson, M., Brenner, M., Roybal, H., Beke, K., Meador, C., et al. (2020). Protein Tyrosine Phosphatase-α Amplifies Transforming Growth Factor-β-dependent Profibrotic Signaling in Lung Fibroblasts. *Am. J. Physiol. Lung Cel Mol Physiol* 319 (2), L294–L311. doi:10.1152/ajplung.00235.2019

Barratt, S. L., Creamer, A., Hayton, C., and Chaudhuri, N. (2018). Idiopathic Pulmonary Fibrosis (IPF): An Overview. *J. Clin. Med.* 7 (8), 201. doi:10.3390/jcm7080201

Bronova, I., Smith, B., Aydogan, B., Weichselbaum, R. R., Vemuri, K., Erdelyi, K., et al. (2015). Protection from Radiation-Induced Pulmonary Fibrosis by Peripheral Targeting of Cannabinoid Receptor-1. *Am. J. Respir. Cel Mol Biol* 53 (4), 555–562. doi:10.1165/rcmb.2014-0331OC

Chen, W., Kirkbride, K. C., How, T., Nelson, C. D., Mo, J., Frederick, J. P., et al. (2003). Beta-arrestin 2 Mediates Endocytosis of Type III TGF-Beta Receptor and Down-Regulation of its Signaling. *Science* 301 (5638), 1394–1397. doi:10.1126/science.1083195

Chiurchiù, V., Rapino, C., Talamonti, E., Leuti, A., Lanuti, M., Gueniche, A., et al. (2016). Anandamide Suppresses Proinflammatory T Cell Responses *In Vitro* through Type-1 Cannabinoid Receptor-Mediated mTOR Inhibition in Human Keratinocytes. *J. Immunol.* 197 (9), 3545–3553. doi:10.4049/jimmunol.1500546

Cinar, R., Gochuico, B. R., Iyer, M. R., Jourdan, T., Yokoyama, T., Park, J. K., et al. (2017). Cannabinoid CB1 Receptor Overactivity Contributes to the Pathogenesis of Idiopathic Pulmonary Fibrosis. *JCI Insight* 2 (8), e92281. doi:10.1172/jci.insight.92281

Cinar, R., Iyer, M. R., Liu, Z., Cao, Z., Jourdan, T., Erdelyi, K., et al. (2016). Hybrid Inhibitor of Peripheral Cannabinoid-1 Receptors and Inducible Nitric Oxide Synthase Mitigates Liver Fibrosis. *JCI Insight* 1 (11), e87336. doi:10.1172/jci.insight.87336

Correia-Sá, I., Paiva, A., Carvalho, C. M., and Vieira-Coelho, M. A. (2020). Cutaneous Endocannabinoid System: Does it Have a Role on Skin Wound

Healing Bearing Fibrosis? *Pharmacol. Res.* 159, 104862. doi:10.1016/j.phrs.2020.104862

Correia-Sá, I. B., Carvalho, C. M., Serrão, P. V., Loureiro, A. I., Fernandes-Lopes, C., Marques, M., et al. (2020). A New Role for Anandamide: Defective Link between the Systemic and Skin Endocannabinoid Systems in Hypertrophic Human Wound Healing. *Sci. Rep.* 10 (1), 11134. doi:10.1038/s41598-020-68058-3

Correia-Sá, I. B., Carvalho, C. M., Serrão, P. V., Machado, V. A., Carvalho, S. O., Marques, M., et al. (2021). AM251, a Cannabinoid Receptor 1 Antagonist, Prevents Human Fibroblasts Differentiation and Collagen Deposition Induced by TGF-β - an *In Vitro* Study. *Eur. J. Pharmacol.* 892, 173738.

DePianto, D. J., Chandriani, S., Abbas, A. R., Jia, G., N'Diaye, E. N., Caplazi, P., et al. (2015). Heterogeneous Gene Expression Signatures Correspond to Distinct Lung Pathologies and Biomarkers of Disease Severity in Idiopathic Pulmonary Fibrosis. *Thorax* 70 (1), 48–56. doi:10.1136/thoraxjnl-2013-204596

Derynck, R., and Zhang, Y. E. (2003). Smad-dependent and Smad-independent Pathways in TGF-Beta Family Signalling. *Nature* 425 (6958), 577–584. doi:10.1038/nature02006

Diez-Alarcia, R., Ibarra-Lecue, I., Lopez-Cardona, Á. P., Meana, J., Gutierrez-Adán, A., Callado, L. F., et al. (2016). Biased Agonism of Three Different Cannabinoid Receptor Agonists in Mouse Brain Cortex. *Front. Pharmacol.* 7, 415. doi:10.3389/fphar.2016.00415

Fernandez, I. E., and Eickelberg, O. (2012). The Impact of TGF-β on Lung Fibrosis: from Targeting to Biomarkers. *Proc. Am. Thorac. Soc.* 9 (3), 111–116. doi:10.1513/pats.201203-023AW

Fletcher-Jones, A., Hildick, K. L., Evans, A. J., Nakamura, Y., Henley, J. M., and Wilkinson, K. A. (2020). Protein Interactors and Trafficking Pathways that Regulate the Cannabinoid Type 1 Receptor (CB_1R). *Front. Mol. Neurosci.* 13, 108. doi:10.3389/fnmol.2020.00108

Garcia-Gonzalez, E., Galeazzi, M., and Selvi, E. (2016). Can Cannabinoids Modulate Fibrotic Progression in Systemic Sclerosis? *Isr. Med. Assoc. J.* 18 (3-4), 156–158.

Garcia-Gonzalez, E., Selvi, E., Balistreri, E., Lorenzini, S., Maggio, R., Natale, M. R., et al. (2009). Cannabinoids Inhibit Fibrogenesis in Diffuse Systemic Sclerosis Fibroblasts. *Rheumatology (Oxford)* 48 (9), 1050–1056. doi:10.1093/rheumatology/kep189

Henderson, N. C., Rieder, F., and Wynn, T. A. (2020). Fibrosis: from Mechanisms to Medicines. *Nature* 587 (7835), 555–566. doi:10.1038/s41586-020-2938-9

Hillard, C. J., Manna, S., Greenberg, M. J., DiCamelli, R., Ross, R. A., Stevenson, L. A., et al. (1999). Synthesis and Characterization of Potent and Selective Agonists of the Neuronal Cannabinoid Receptor (CB1). *J. Pharmacol. Exp. Ther.* 289 (3), 1427–1433.

Iannotti, F. A., Di Marzo, V., and Petrosino, S. (2016). Endocannabinoids and Endocannabinoid-Related Mediators: Targets, Metabolism and Role in Neurological Disorders. *Prog. Lipid Res.* 62, 107–128. doi:10.1016/j.plipres.2016.02.002

Kasam, R. K., Ghandikota, S., Soundararajan, D., Reddy, G. B., Huang, S. K., Jegga, A. G., et al. (2020). Inhibition of Aurora Kinase B Attenuates Fibroblast Activation and Pulmonary Fibrosis. *EMBO Mol. Med.* 12 (9), e12131. doi:10.15252/emmm.202012131

Khalil, H., Kanisicak, O., Prasad, V., Correll, R. N., Fu, X., Schips, T., et al. (2017). Fibroblast-specific TGF-β-Smad2/3 Signaling Underlies Cardiac Fibrosis. *J. Clin. Invest.* 127 (10), 3770–3783. doi:10.1172/JCI94753

Lazzerini, P. E., Natale, M., Gianchecchi, E., Capecchi, P. L., Montilli, C., Zimbone, S., et al. (2012). Adenosine A2A Receptor Activation Stimulates Collagen Production in Sclerodermic Dermal Fibroblasts Either Directly and through a Cross-Talk with the Cannabinoid System. *J. Mol. Med. (Berl)* 90 (3), 331–342. doi:10.1007/s00109-011-0824-5

Lecru, L., Desterke, C., Grassin-Delyle, S., Chatziantoniou, C., Vandermeersch, S., Devocelle, A., et al. (2015). Cannabinoid Receptor 1 Is a Major Mediator of Renal Fibrosis. *Kidney Int.* 88 (1), 72–84. doi:10.1038/ki.2015.63

Lee, T. H., Yeh, C. F., Lee, Y. T., Shih, Y. C., Chen, Y. T., Hung, C. T., et al. (2020). Fibroblast-enriched Endoplasmic Reticulum Protein TXNDC5 Promotes Pulmonary Fibrosis by Augmenting TGFβ Signaling through TGFBR1 Stabilization. *Nat. Commun.* 11 (1), 4254. doi:10.1038/s41467-020-18047-x

Marquart, S., Zerr, P., Akhmetshina, A., Palumbo, K., Reich, N., Tomcik, M., et al. (2010). Inactivation of the Cannabinoid Receptor CB1 Prevents Leukocyte Infiltration and Experimental Fibrosis. *Arthritis Rheum.* 62 (11), 3467–3476. doi:10.1002/art.27642

Martinez, F. J., Collard, H. R., Pardo, A., Raghu, G., Richeldi, L., Selman, M., et al. (2017). Idiopathic Pulmonary Fibrosis. *Nat. Rev. Dis. Primers* 3, 17074. doi:10.1038/nrdp.2017.74

Mora, A. L., Rojas, M., Pardo, A., and Selman, M. (2017). Emerging Therapies for Idiopathic Pulmonary Fibrosis, a Progressive Age-Related Disease. *Nat. Rev. Drug Discov.* 16 (11), 755–772. doi:10.1038/nrd.2017.170

Nieto, M. A., Huang, R. Y., Jackson, R. A., and Thiery, J. P. (2016). EMT: 2016. *Cell* 166 (1), 21–45. doi:10.1016/j.cell.2016.06.028

Pacher, P., and Kunos, G. (2013). Modulating the Endocannabinoid System in Human Health and Disease-Ssuccesses and Failures. *FEBS J.* 280 (9), 1918–1943. doi:10.1111/febs.12260

Patsenker, E., Stoll, M., Millonig, G., Agaimy, A., Wissniowski, T., Schneider, V., et al. (2011). Cannabinoid Receptor Type I Modulates Alcohol-Induced Liver Fibrosis. *Mol. Med.* 17 (11-12), 1285–1294. doi:10.2119/molmed.2011.00149

Pryimak, N., Zaiachuk, M., Kovalchuk, O., and Kovalchuk, I. (2021). The Potential Use of Cannabis in Tissue Fibrosis. *Front Cel Dev Biol* 9, 715380. doi:10.3389/fcell.2021.715380

Saito, A., Horie, M., and Nagase, T. (2018). TGF-β Signaling in Lung Health and Disease. *Int. J. Mol. Sci.* 19 (8), 2460. doi:10.3390/ijms19082460

Slavic, S., Lauer, D., Sommerfeld, M., Kemnitz, U. R., Grzesiak, A., Trappiel, M., et al. (2013). Cannabinoid Receptor 1 Inhibition Improves Cardiac Function and Remodelling after Myocardial Infarction and in Experimental Metabolic Syndrome. *J. Mol. Med. (Berl)* 91 (7), 811–823. doi:10.1007/s00109-013-1034-0

Teixeira-Clerc, F., Julien, B., Grenard, P., Tran Van Nhieu, J., Deveaux, V., Li, L., et al. (2006). CB1 Cannabinoid Receptor Antagonism: a New Strategy for the Treatment of Liver Fibrosis. *Nat. Med.* 12 (6), 671–676. doi:10.1038/nm1421

Trachalaki, A., Irfan, M., and Wells, A. U. (2021). Pharmacological Management of Idiopathic Pulmonary Fibrosis: Current and Emerging Options. *Expert Opin. Pharmacother.* 22 (2), 191–204. doi:10.1080/14656566.2020.1822326

Wang, S., Zhu, Q., Liang, G., Franks, T., Boucher, M., Bence, K. K., et al. (2021). Cannabinoid Receptor 1 Signaling in Hepatocytes and Stellate Cells Does Not Contribute to NAFLD. *J. Clin. Invest.* 131 (22), 1. doi:10.1172/JCI152242

Wollin, L., Wex, E., Pautsch, A., Schnapp, G., Hostettler, K. E., Stowasser, S., et al. (2015). Mode of Action of Nintedanib in the Treatment of Idiopathic Pulmonary Fibrosis. *Eur. Respir. J.* 45 (5), 1434–1445. doi:10.1183/09031936.00174914

Xia, H., Bodempudi, V., Benyumov, A., Hergert, P., Tank, D., Herrera, J., et al. (2014). Identification of a Cell-Of-Origin for Fibroblasts Comprising the Fibrotic Reticulum in Idiopathic Pulmonary Fibrosis. *Am. J. Pathol.* 184 (5), 1369–1383. doi:10.1016/j.ajpath.2014.01.012

Zhao, Z. B., Guan, D. W., Liu, W. W., Wang, T., Fan, Y. Y., Cheng, Z. H., et al. (2010). Expression of Cannabinoid Receptor I during Mice Skin Incised Wound Healing Course. *Fa Yi Xue Za Zhi* 26 (4), 241–245.

Zhou, S., Wu, Q., Lin, X., Ling, X., Miao, J., Liu, X., et al. (2021). Cannabinoid Receptor Type 2 Promotes Kidney Fibrosis through Orchestrating Î²-Catenin Signaling. *Kidney Int.* 99 (2), 364–381. doi:10.1016/j.kint.2020.09.025

Zurier, R. B., and Burstein, S. H. (2016). Cannabinoids, Inflammation, and Fibrosis. *FASEB J.* 30 (11), 3682–3689. doi:10.1096/fj.201600646R

17

Predictors of Mortality in Progressive Fibrosing Interstitial Lung Diseases

*Xianqiu Chen[1], Jian Guo[2], Dong Yu[3], Bing Jie[3] and Ying Zhou[4]**

[1]*Department of Respiratory Medicine, Shanghai Pulmonary Hospital, Tongji University School of Medicine, Shanghai, China,* [2]*Department of Pulmonary Function Test, Shanghai Pulmonary Hospital, Tongji University School of Medicine, Shanghai, China,* [3]*Department of Radiology, Shanghai Pulmonary Hospital, Tongji University School of Medicine, Shanghai, China,* [4]*Department of Respiratory Medicine and Clinical Research Center, Shanghai Pulmonary Hospital, Tongji University School of Medicine, Shanghai, China*

Correspondence:
Ying Zhou
happyying79550@sina.com

Background: Progressive fibrosing interstitial lung disease (PF-ILD) and idiopathic pulmonary fibrosis (IPF) share similar progression phenotype but with different pathophysiological mechanism. The purpose of this study was to assess clinical characteristics and outcomes of patients with PF-ILD in a single-center cohort.

Methods: Patients with PF-ILD treated in Shanghai Pulmonary Hospital from Jan. 2013 to Dec. 2014 were retrospectively analyzed. Baseline characteristics and clinical outcomes were collected for survival analysis to identifying clinical predictors of mortality.

Results: Among 608 patients with ILD, 132 patients met the diagnostic criteria for PF-ILD. In this single-center cohort, there were 51 (38.6%) cases with connective tissue disease-associated interstitial lung disease (CTD-ILD) and 45 (34.1%) with unclassifiable ILDs. During follow-up, 83 patients (62.9%) either died (N = 79, 59.8%) or underwent lung transplantations (N = 4, 3.0%) with a median duration follow-up time of 53.7 months. Kaplan-Meier survival curves revealed that the 1, 3 and 5-years survival of PF-ILD were 90.9, 58.8 and 48.1%, respectively. In addition, the prognosis of patients with PF-ILD was similar to those with IPF, while it was worse than non-PF-ILD ones. Multivariate Cox regression analysis demonstrated that high-resolution computed tomography (HRCT) scores (HR 1.684, 95% CI 1.017–2.788, $p = 0.043$) and systolic pulmonary artery pressure (SPAP) > 36.5 mmHg (HR 3.619, 95%CI 1.170–11.194, $p = 0.026$) were independent risk factors for the mortality of PF-ILD.

Conclusion: Extent of fibrotic changes on HRCT and pulmonary hypertension were predictors of mortality in patients with PF-ILD.

Keywords: progressive fibrosing interstitial lung disease, predictor of mortality, fibrotic changes, high-resolution computed tomography, pulmonary arterial hypertension

INTRODUCTION

Progressive fibrosing interstitial lung disease (PF-ILD) is a terminology recently used to describe a subset of patients who have inexorable progression of pulmonary fibrosis despite treatment, and the underlying pathogenetic mechanism and clinical behaviors of which are similar to those of idiopathic pulmonary fibrosis (IPF) (Wells et al., 2018; Brown et al., 2020). The proportion of interstitial lung disease (ILD) patients with progressive fibrosing phenotype has been estimated up to 18–32% by physicians (Wijsenbeek et al., 2019). ILDs associated with a progressive fibrosing phenotype include non-specific interstitial pneumonia (NSIP) (Kim et al., 2010), unclassifiable idiopathic interstitial pneumonia (IIP) (Guler et al., 2018a), hypersensitivity pneumonitis (HP) (De Sadeleer et al., 2019), autoimmune ILDs (Doyle and Dellaripa, 2017; Guler et al., 2018b), sarcoidosis (Walsh et al., 2014a) and occupation-associated lung disease (Khalil et al., 2007). PF-ILD has a distinct clinical phenotype regardless of cause. Patients with PF-ILD suffer from worsening respiratory symptoms, declines of physiological functions, increased mortality even by conventional treatment and significantly impaired quality of life (Wells et al., 2018).

Several factors have been identified as predictors of mortality in patients with PF-ILD. Decline in forced vital capacity (FVC) was associated with an increased risk of death in patients with PF-ILD (Gimenez et al., 2018; Olson et al., 2018) as evidenced by studies including autoimmune ILDs (Solomon et al., 2016; Zamora-Legoff et al., 2017) and chronic HP (Mooney et al., 2013). Usual interstitial pneumonitis (UIP) pattern on high-resolution computed tomography (HRCT) was reported to be associated with worse prognosis in autoimmune ILDs (Kim et al., 2010; Kelly et al., 2014). Radiological fibrosis score or extent of fibrosis on HRCT was also reported to predict outcome in chronic HP (Mooney et al., 2013), pulmonary sarcoidosis (Walsh et al., 2014a) and unclassifiable ILD (Ryerson et al., 2013). A relevant study demonstrated that CT honeycombing uniquely identified a progressive fibrotic ILD phenotype with a high mortality similar to that of IPF (Adegunsoye et al., 2019). Little data are available regarding the indicators of mortality in PF-ILD cases other than FVC and HRCT. This single-center cohort study aims to identify risk factors from demographic information, clinical features, imaging data and blood biomarkers for mortality in Chinese PF-ILD population.

METHODS

Patients diagnosed with ILD between Jan 2013 to Dec 2014 in Shanghai Pulmonary Hospital were eligible for this study, and their electronic medical records were retrospectively reviewed. Those who met at least one of the following criteria were considered as having a progressive fibrosing phenotype, within 24 months before screening, despite standard treatment in clinical practice: a relative decline in FVC≥10% of the predicted value; a relative decline in 5 ≤ FVC <10% of the predicted value and worsening of respiratory symptoms; a relative decline in 5 ≤ FVC <10% of the predicted value and increased extent of fibrosis on HRCT; worsening of respiratory symptoms and increased extent of fibrosis on HRCT (Wells et al., 2018; Flaherty et al., 2019).

Baseline characteristics of recruited patients, including age, gender, date of final diagnosis, laboratory test results, and treatment regimen were recorded. Patients with IPF or malignant tumor were excluded. Pulmonary function data were obtained, including FVC and diffusion capacity of carbon monoxide (DLCO) with % predicted values using standards (Miller et al., 2005). Echocardiographic estimate of systolic pulmonary artery pressure (SPAP) at baseline was noted. HRCT scan was independently reviewed by two expert thoracic radiologists (Dong Yu and Bing Jie) who were blinded to clinical status and demographics of subjects. Any disagreement was resolved through consensus. CT scans were classified as showing a UIP pattern or not (Kekevian et al., 2014) and the extent of fibrosis was further calculated using a 4-point scale as follows: 0 = no involvement, 1 = 1–25% involvement, 2 = 26–50% involvement, 3 = 51–75% involvement, and 4 = 76–100% involvement (Lynch et al., 2005). Main pulmonary artery diameter (MPAD) and ascending aorta diameter (AAD) were also assessed on HRCT, MPAD/AAD ratio was calculated to predict pulmonary arterial hypertension (PAH) (Jeny et al., 2020).

Primary endpoints in the present study included death or lung transplantation. Survival rate was calculated based on date of the last visit, date of death, or transplantation. The last follow-up time was November 2020. Ethical approval was waived by the Ethics Committee of Shanghai Pulmonary Hospital in view of the retrospective nature of the study (No. k21-023) and all the procedures being performed were part of the routine care.

Statistical analysis was performed using SPSS 26.0 package software (IBM). Continuous variables were expressed as mean ± standard deviation (SD) or mean (range). Chi-square test was used to analyze the composition ratio between groups. Subgroup differences were compared using One-way ANOVA, followed by Tukey's post hoc test. Receiver Operating Characteristic (ROC) curves were depicted for identifying cut-off values. Multivariate logistics regression was performed to identify risk factors and those with $p < 0.2$ were further included in a Cox proportional hazards regression model using the forward log rank (LR) method. Kaplan-Meier survival analysis was performed, followed by Log-rank test for comparing difference between curves. $p < 0.05$ considered statistically significant.

RESULTS

Of the 608 patients with ILD seen over a 2-year period at Shanghai Pulmonary Hospital, 169 were identified as the progressive fibrosing phenotype. Thirty-seven patients were excluded, including 7 cases with lung cancer, 12 with insufficient information, and 18 lost of follow-up. Finally, 132 PF-ILD patients and 392 non-progressive ILD (control group) were recruited (**Figure 1**). The number of cases corresponding to different diagnostic criteria is shown in **Table 1**. Compared with non- PF-ILD group, patients in PF-ILD group were significantly older (63 vs 58 years, $p < 0.001$), and the male-to-female proportion was higher ($p = 0.023$). Clinical characteristics of PF-ILD patients were listed in **Table 2**. There were 85 males and 47 females in PF-ILD group, with a median age at diagnosis of 63 years (24–86 years). The median time from symptoms onset to diagnosis of ILD was 21.2 months (0–120 months), and the median time from diagnosis of ILD to PF-ILD was 22.6 months (0–85 months). 88/132 (66.7%) patients with PF-ILD underwent echocardiography and the mean SPAP value was (42.6 ± 11.6) mmHg.

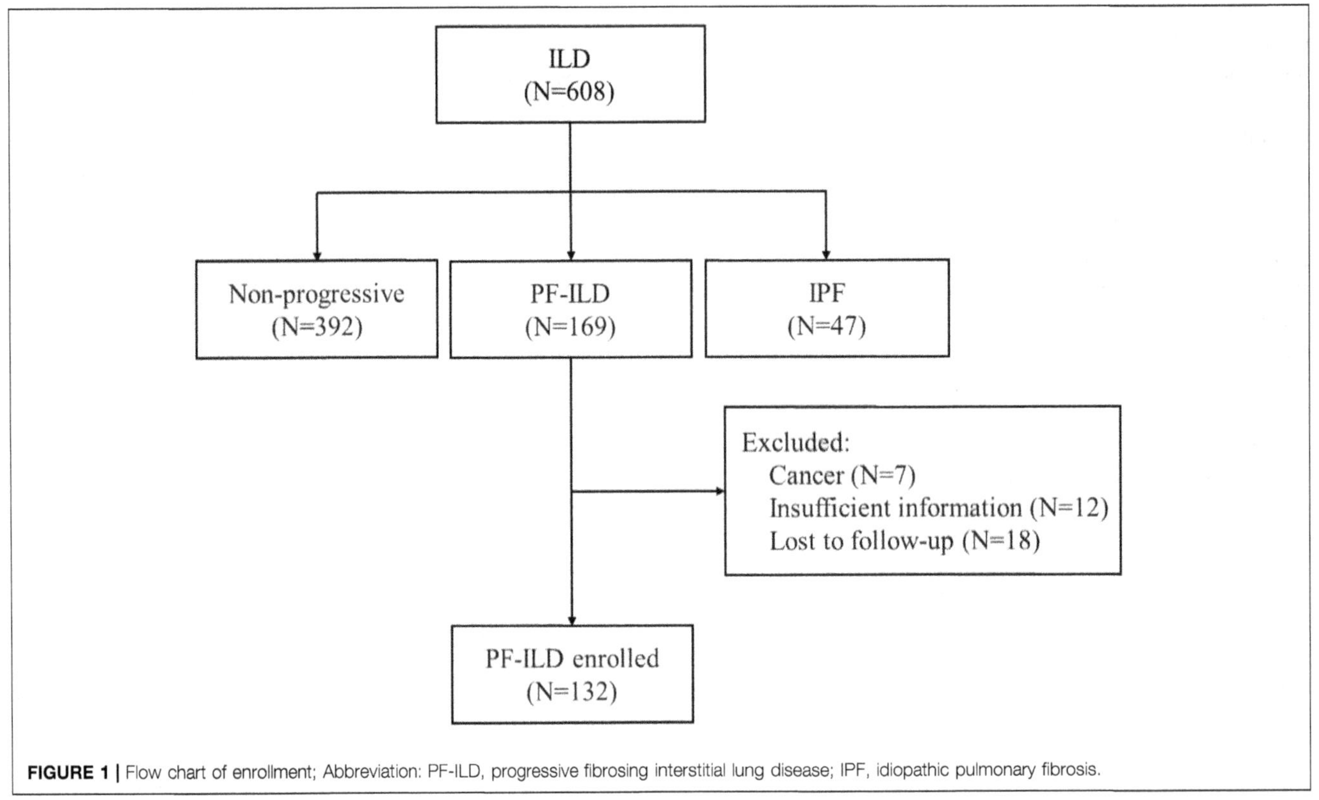

FIGURE 1 | Flow chart of enrollment; Abbreviation: PF-ILD, progressive fibrosing interstitial lung disease; IPF, idiopathic pulmonary fibrosis.

TABLE 1 | Diagnostic criteria.

Diagnostic criteria	No. (%)
a relative decline in FVC≥10% of the predicted value	6 (4.5)
a relative decline in 5 ≤ FVC <10% of the predicted value and worsening of respiratory symptoms	2 (1.5)
a relative decline in 5 ≤ FVC <10% of the predicted value and increased extent of fibrosis on HRCT	3 (2.3)
worsening of respiratory symptoms and increased extent of fibrosis on HRCT	121 (91.7)

Abbreviations: FVC, forced vital capacity; HRCT, high-resolution computed tomography.

87/132 (65.9%) patients with PF-ILD had confirmed ILD classification, including connective tissue disease-associated interstitial lung disease (CTD-ILD), interstitial pneumonia with autoimmune features (IPAF), NSIP, combined pulmonary fibrosis and emphysema (CPFE), HP, pneumoconiosis, pulmonary alveolar proteinosis (PAP) and respiratory bronchiolitis-associated interstitial lung disease (RBILD); and the remaining 45/132 (34.1%) had unclassifiable ILDs. ILD classification of all 132 patients with PF-ILD was summarized in **Figure 2**. It is showed that CTD-ILD (38.6%) was the most common subtype of PF-ILD, followed by unclassifiable ILDs (34.1%) and IPAF (8.3%). All clinical data of PF-ILD and subgroups collected and analyzed were listed in Online Resource 1.

Patients were followed up for a median time of 53.7 months (1–130 months) after ILD diagnosis. During this time, 81/132 (61.4%) patients underwent either lung transplantations (N = 4, 3.0%) or died (N = 79, 59.8%) from disease. The median survival times were 58 and 54 months in PF-ILD and IPF groups, respectively. Kaplan-Meier survival curves calculated that the 1, 3 and 5-years survival rates were 90.9, 58.8 and 48.1% respectively, which were similar to those in IPF group (89.4, 68.1 and 43.9%, respectively), and significantly worse than those of non- PF-ILD group (p < 0.001) (**Figure 3A** and **Table 3**). In PF-ILD subgroups, the median survival times of CTD-ILD + IPAF, unclassifiable ILD, NSIP and other ILDs groups were 108, 39, 25, 48 months respectively. The 3 and 5-years survival rates of CTD-ILD + IPAF patients were 67.2 and 62.3%, respectively, which were significantly higher than that of NSIP subgroup (20 and 10%, respectively) (p = 0.001), shown in **Figure 3B** and **Table 3**.

Univariate survival analysis of potential risk factors for the mortality of PF-ILD was shown in **Table 4**. The cutoff values calculated by ROC curves were used for classifying continuous variables. Logistics univariate analysis revealed that the age >67 years, time from the symptom onset to the diagnosis of ILD >23.5 months, time from the diagnosis of ILD to PF-ILD < 34.5 months, FVC% predicted ranged 40–59%, DLCO% predicted <60%, HRCT score and UIP pattern, MPAD/AAD >0.81, SPAP >36.5 mmHg, differential arterial oxygen partial

TABLE 2 | Baseline characteristics of patients with PF-ILD.

Characteristics	PF-ILD (*N* = 132)
Age at diagnosis of ILD, median (range), y	63 (24–86)
Gender	
Male/Female	85/47
BMI ($kg \cdot m^{-2}$)	24.8 ± 3.7
Smoking history (current/past/never)	26/34/72
Therapy after diagnosis of ILD (current/past/never)	
Prednisone	77/21/34
Immunosuppressant	4/3/125
Pirfenidone	8/2/122
Acetylcysteine	79/27/26
Lung transplantation	4 (3.0%)
Death during follow-up	79 (59.8%)
Time from symptoms onset to diagnosis of ILD, median (range), month	21.2 (0–120)
Time from diagnosis of ILD to PF-ILD, median (range), month	22.6 (0–85)
Median duration of follow-up, median (range), month	53.7 (1–130)
HRCT scores (1/2/3/4)	19/42/43/28
UIP pattern on HRCT	51 (38.6%)
MPAD/AAD	0.91 ± 0.16
Pulmonary function[a]	
FVC (% predicted)	68.0 ± 19.5
DLCO (% predicted)	63.6 ± 19.2
SPAP (mmHg)	42.6 ± 11.6
Arterial blood gas analysis at time of diagnosis of ILD	
PO_2 (mmHg)	78.2 ± 13.5
SaO_2 (%)	95.1 ± 4.3
P (A-a) O_2 (mm Hg)	25.7 ± 15.8

Abbreviations: ILD, interstitial lung disease; BMI, body mass index ; HRCT, high-resolution computed tomography; UIP, usual interstitial pneumonitis; MPAD, main pulmonary artery diameter; AAD, ascending aorta diameter; FVC, forced vital capacity; DLCO, diffusion capacity for carbon monoxide; SPAP, systolic pulmonary artery pressure; PaO_2, oxygen partial pressure; SaO_2, oxygen saturation; P(A-a) O_2, differential arterial oxygen partial pressure.

[a]Not all patients had pulmonary function records.

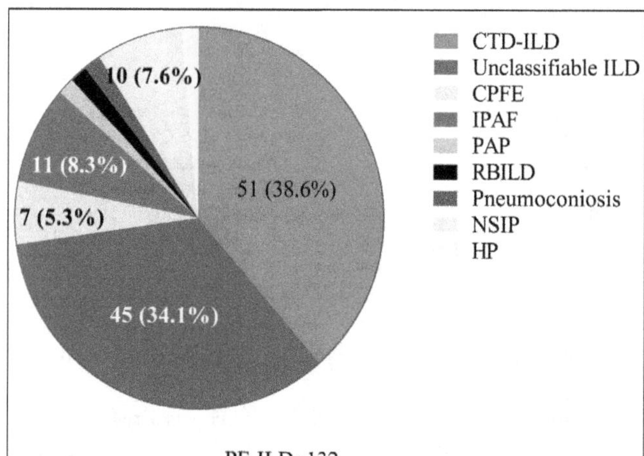

FIGURE 2 | Classifications of PF-ILD in this study; Abbreviations: PF-ILD, progressive fibrosing interstitial lung disease; CTD-ILD, connective tissue disease-associated interstitial lung disease; CPFE, combined pulmonary fibrosis and emphysema; IPAF, interstitial pneumonia with autoimmune features; PAP, pulmonary alveolar proteinosis; RBILD, respiratory bronchiolitis-associated interstitial lung disease; NSIP, nonspecific interstitial pneumonia; HP, Hypersensitivity pneumonitis. Number of cases: CTD-ILD = 51, Unclassifiable ILD = 45, IPAF = 11, NSIP = 10, CPFE = 7, PAP = 2, RBILD = 2, Pneumoconiosis = 2, HP = 2.

pressure [P (A-a) O_2] > 34.95 mmHg, soluble interleukin-2 receptor (SIL-2R) > 525 U/ml and increased level of carbohydrate antigen 199 (CA199) (>26.75 U/ml) were all risk factors for the mortality of PF-ILD (all $p < 0.05$). The impact of systemic therapy on univariate survival was also summarized, and there was no significant difference in the survival of patients treated with prednisone, immunosuppressants or antifibrotic drugs.

Cox regression analysis was performed on significant factors obtained from univariate analysis with p value <0.2, including male, prednisone treatment (current or past), and above risk factors. It is shown that SPAP >36.5 mmHg (HR 3.619, 95%CI 1.170–11.194, $p = 0.026$) and HRCT scores (HR 1.684, 95% CI 1.017–2.788, $p = 0.043$) were independent risk factors for the mortality of PF-ILD (**Figure 4**).

Kaplan-Meier survival curves consistently obtained the independent risk factors for the mortality of PF-ILD (**Figures 5A,B**). PF-ILD patients with SPAP >36.5 mmHg had a worse prognosis ($p \le 0.001$), and obviously decreases in 3-years and 5-years survival (**Table 3**). With the increase of HRCT scores, the prognosis of patients with PF-ILD became significantly worse ($p < 0.001$). The 3-years survival of PF-ILD patients with 3 and 4 HRCT scores were only about 50 and 21.4%, respectively, and their 5-years survival were 38.2 and 10.7%, respectively.

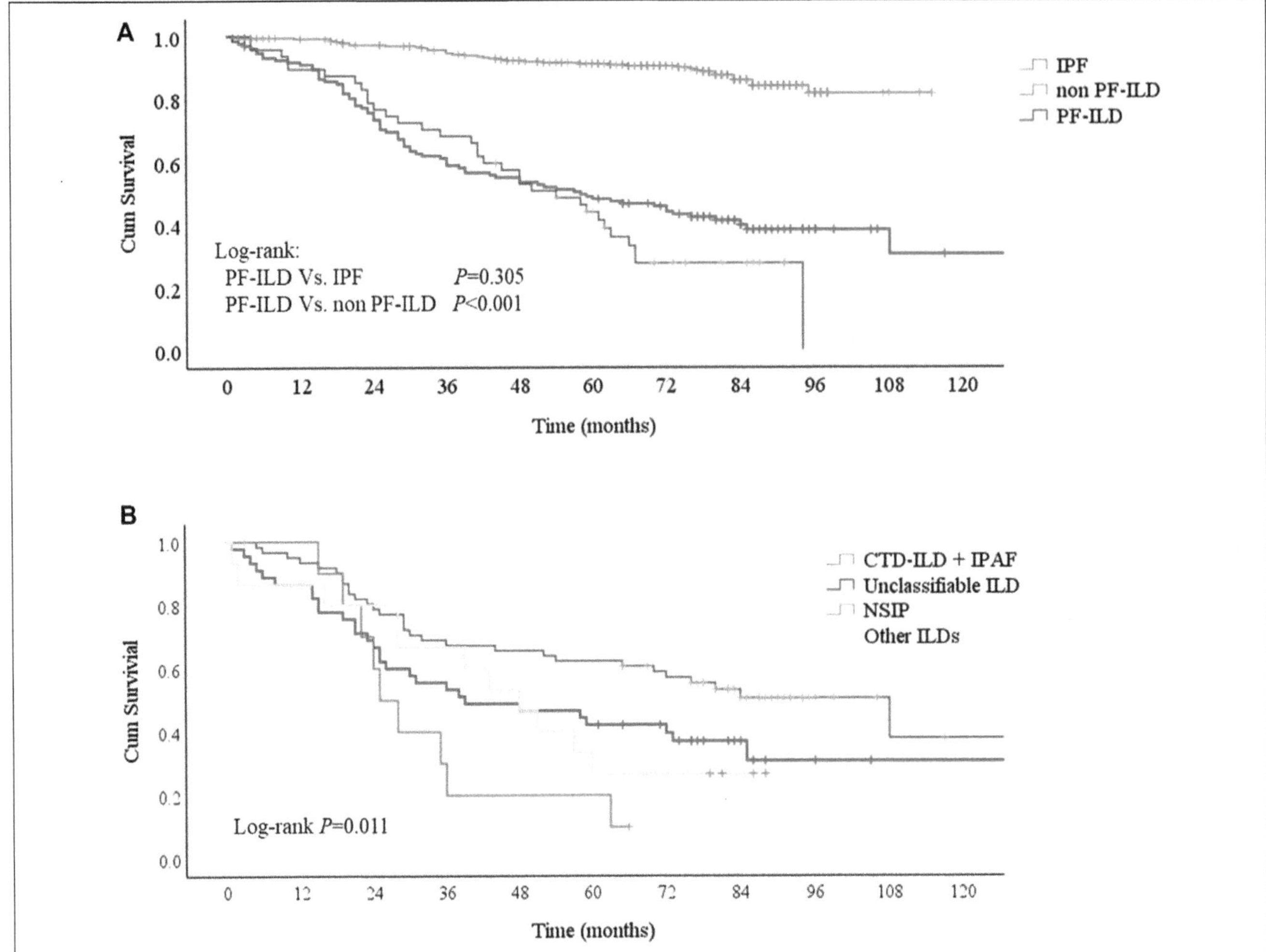

FIGURE 3 | Survival curves of PF-ILD **(A)** Survival curves of PF-ILD, non PF-ILD and IPF. Kaplan-Meier survival analysis showed no difference between PF-ILD and IPF group ($p = 0.305$). But significant difference was seen in PF-ILD group and non PF-ILD group ($p < 0.001$). The median survival times were 54 (95%CI: 39-69) and 58 (95%CI: 37-79) months in IPF and PF-ILD group respectively, NA in non PF-ILD group **(B)** Survival curves of subgroups of PF-ILD. Kaplan-Meier survival analysis showing a significant difference between groups ($p = 0\ 001$), a higher mortality in NSIP subgroup and a lower mortality in CTD-ILD + IPAF subgroup. The median survival times were 108 (95%CI: 64-152), 39 (95%CI: 4-74), 25 (95%CI: 19-31), 48 (95%CI: 33-63) months in CTD-ILD + IPAF, Unclassifiable ILD, NSIP and other ILDs groups respectively.; Abbreviations: PF-ILD, progressive fibrosing interstitial lung disease; IPF, idiopathic pulmonary fibrosis; CTD-ILD, connective tissue disease-associated interstitial lung disease; IPAF, interstitial pneumonia with autoimmune features; NSIP, nonspecific interstitial pneumonia.

DISCUSSION

In the present study, we retrospectively analyzed clinical characteristics of 132 patients with PF-ILD other than IPF. Most of the subjects were middle-aged and elderly, with a median age of 63 years, and they were older than non-PF-ILD patients. In our study cohort, the gender ratio was similar to IPF but different from PF-ILD population (mostly male patients). The gender ratio in this study differed from that in the recent PROGRESS® study (Nasser et al., 2021), in which males and females are equally distributed. However, Cox analysis revealed that both age and gender did not significantly influence the prognosis of PF-ILD. Autoimmune disease-related ILD in general has a relatively good prognosis, as previous studies reported (Oldham et al., 2016; Strek and Costabel, 2016). This study found that PF-ILD was an important clinical phenotype of ILDs, which usually had a poor prognosis and was similar to that of IPF.

Previous studies have reported that PAH was a risk factor for poor prognosis of IPF (Raghu et al., 2015). In a retrospective analysis of consecutive IPF patients undergoing right heart catheterization prior to transplantation, it was found that PAH was common in advanced IPF cases that significantly influenced their survival. The 1-year mortality in IPF patients with PAH was significantly higher than those without PAH (28 vs 5.5%), which was linearly correlated with mean pulmonary artery pressure (Lettieri et al., 2006). In patients with IPF undergoing serial right-sided heart catheterization prior to transplantation, nearly all of them develop PAH later in their course (38.6% at baseline and 86.4% at transplantation) (Nathan et al., 2008). Pulmonary involvement, including both ILD and PAH, are reported as the primary causes of morbidity and mortality of systemic

TABLE 3 | Accumulate survival rates.

Groups	12 months	36 months	60 months (%)
PF-ILD (*N* = 132)	90.9%	58.8%	48.1
IPF (*N* = 47)	89.4%	68.1%	43.9
Non PF-ILD (*N* = 392)	99.4%	96.4%	91.0
PF-ILD subgroups			
CTD-ILD + IPAF (*N* = 62)	93.4%	67.2%	62.3
Unclassifiable ILD (*N* = 45)	86.7%	53.3%	42.2
NSIP (*N* = 10)	90.0%	20.0%	10.0
Other ILDs (*N* = 15)	86.7%	66.7%	26.7
HRCT scores			
1 point (*N* = 19)	NA	NA	94.7
2 point (*N* = 42)	95.2%	73.8%	61.9
3 point (*N* = 43)	88.3%	50.1%	38.2
4 point (*N* = 28)	82.1%	21.4%	10.7
SPAP			
≤36.5 mmHg (*N* = 31)	96.8%	80.6%	77.4
>36.5 mmHg (*N* = 57)	89.5%	52.6%	38.6

Abbreviations: PF-ILD, progressive fibrosing interstitial lung disease; IPF, idiopathic pulmonary fibrosis; CTD-ILD, connective tissue disease-associated interstitial lung disease; IPAF, interstitial pneumonia with autoimmune features; NSIP, nonspecific interstitial pneumonia; UIP, usual interstitial pneumonitis; HRCT, high-resolution computed tomography; SPAP, systolic pulmonary artery pressure; Accumulate survival rates are estimated from Kaplan-Meier survival analysis.

sclerosis (Steen and Medsger, 2007). ILD cases with untreated PAH usually rapidly progress to respiratory failure and/or die within 2–3 years after being clinically detectable (Castro and Jimenez, 2010; Giacomelli et al., 2019). Echocardiography is an accessible method to estimate SPAP. In the present study, we also estimated PAH by calculating MPAD/AAD ratio through HRCT. Among the numerous factors we selected for analysis, both MPAD/AAD and SPAP at echocardiography were risk factors for the mortality of PF-ILD, but only SPAP was proven as an independent factor for it by Cox regression. The median survival time was 43 months (95%CI: 23-63) in SPAP >36.5 mmHg group. Until now, there have been few relevant conclusions reported in PF-ILD cohort. Our study suggested that monitoring SPAP calculated by echocardiography is important during the follow-up for all patients with progressive pulmonary fibrosis.

HRCT is a more sensitive modality for detecting ILD, which can be used to evaluate the prognosis of ILDs. The extent of honeycombing and reticulation has been reported as a predictor of the mortality in patients with IPF (Lynch et al., 2005). Besides, in patients with chronic HP and CTD-ILD, the severity of traction bronchiectasis and the extent of honeycombing have been verified as predictors of the mortality (Walsh et al., 2012; Walsh et al., 2014b). Identification the extent of fibrosis contributes to assess the poor prognosis of patients with fibrotic ILDs, including fibrotic IIP with little honeycombing (Shin et al., 2008; Edey et al., 2011; Lee et al., 2012). The prognostic value of HRCT findings has been doubted. Data from a large group of patients with IPF or CTD-ILD presenting UIP pattern showed that clinical but not radiological features are survival predictors (Moua et al., 2014). In our study, we defined the area of fibrosis to correspond to HRCT score, which was found to be an independent risk factor for the mortality of patients with PF-ILD. Our findings provided the latest evidence of the prognostic role of HRCT in PF-ILD. HRCT examination is of great significance in the initial evaluation of all ILDs, and monitoring of HRCT score is also a promising approach to assess treatment response (Hansell et al., 2008).

Several limitations associated with retrospective and monocentric design existed in this study. It was a single-center study with a small sample size, which may cause some biases. We will further expand the

TABLE 4 | Factors associated with mortality in patients of PF-ILD.

Factors	*p* Value	OR	95%CI	
			Lower limit	Upper limit
Gender (male)	0.059	2.015	0.974	4.168
Age >67 years (cutoff)	0.025	2.451	1.120	5.365
Time from symptom onset to diagnosis of ILD >23.5 months (cutoff)	0.030	2.494	1.092	5.698
Time from diagnosis of ILD to PF-ILD < 34.5 months (cutoff)	<0.001	8.991	3.206	25.217
Prednisone (current + past)	0.176	1.722	0.783	3.786
FVC %				
60–80%	0.473	1.400	0.559	3.507
40–59%	0.029	3.400	1.130	10.232
<40%	0.068	4.900	0.890	26.969
DLCO %				
60–80%	0.620	1.400	0.370	5.294
40–59%	0.003	6.800	1.942	23.810
<40%	0.003	10.200	2.257	46.091
HRCT score	<0.001	3.766	2.284	6.210
UIP pattern in HRCT	<0.001	4.639	2.049	10.507
MPAD/AAD >0.81	0.008	2.796	1.303	6.000
SPAP >36.5 mmHg (cutoff)	<0.001	5.752	2.200	15.036
P (A-a) O_2 > 34.95 mmHg (cutoff)	0.034	2.786	1.080	7.185
SIL-2R > 525 U/ml (cutoff)	<0.001	6.857	2.386	19.706
CA199 > 26.76 U/ml (cutoff)	0.002	3.850	1.638	9.051

Abbreviations: ILD, interstitial lung disease; FVC, forced vital capacity; DLCO, diffusion capacity for carbon monoxide; HRCT, high-resolution computed tomography; UIP, usual interstitial pneumonitis; MPAD, main pulmonary artery diameter; AAD, ascending aorta diameter; SPAP, systolic pulmonary artery pressure; P(A-a) O_2, differential arterial oxygen partial pressure. SIL-2R, soluble interleukin-2 receptor. CA199, carbohydrate antigen 199. Statistically significant p values are highlighted in bold.

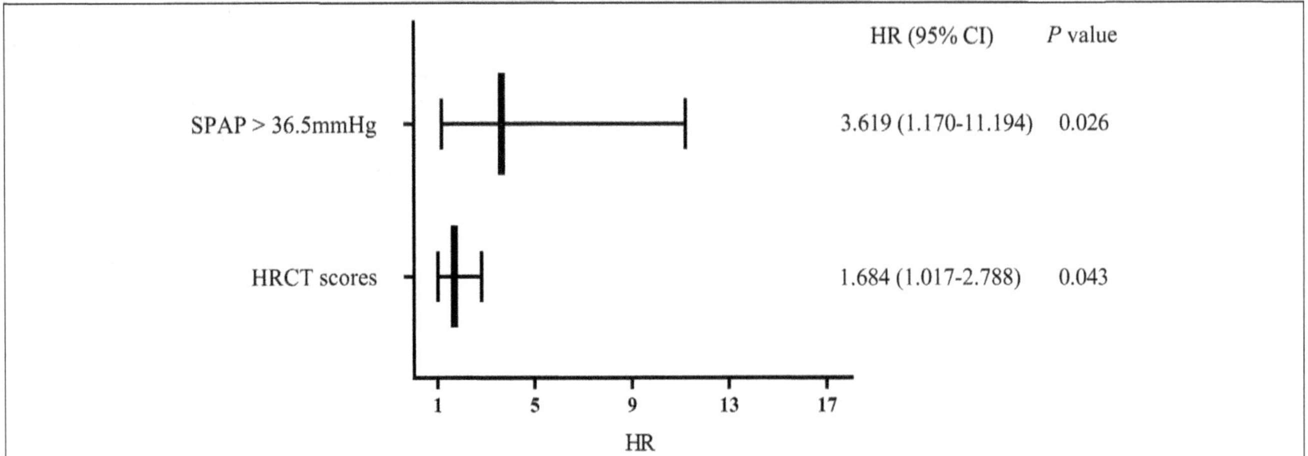

FIGURE 4 | Multivariate regression analysis of mortality; Abbreviations: SPAP, systolic pulmonary artery pressure; HRCT: high-resolution computed tomography; HR, hazard ratio. Cox regression analysis suggested that SPAP >36.5 mmHg and HRCT scores were independent risk factors for mortality in patients with PF-ILD (p = 0.026, 0.043 respectively).

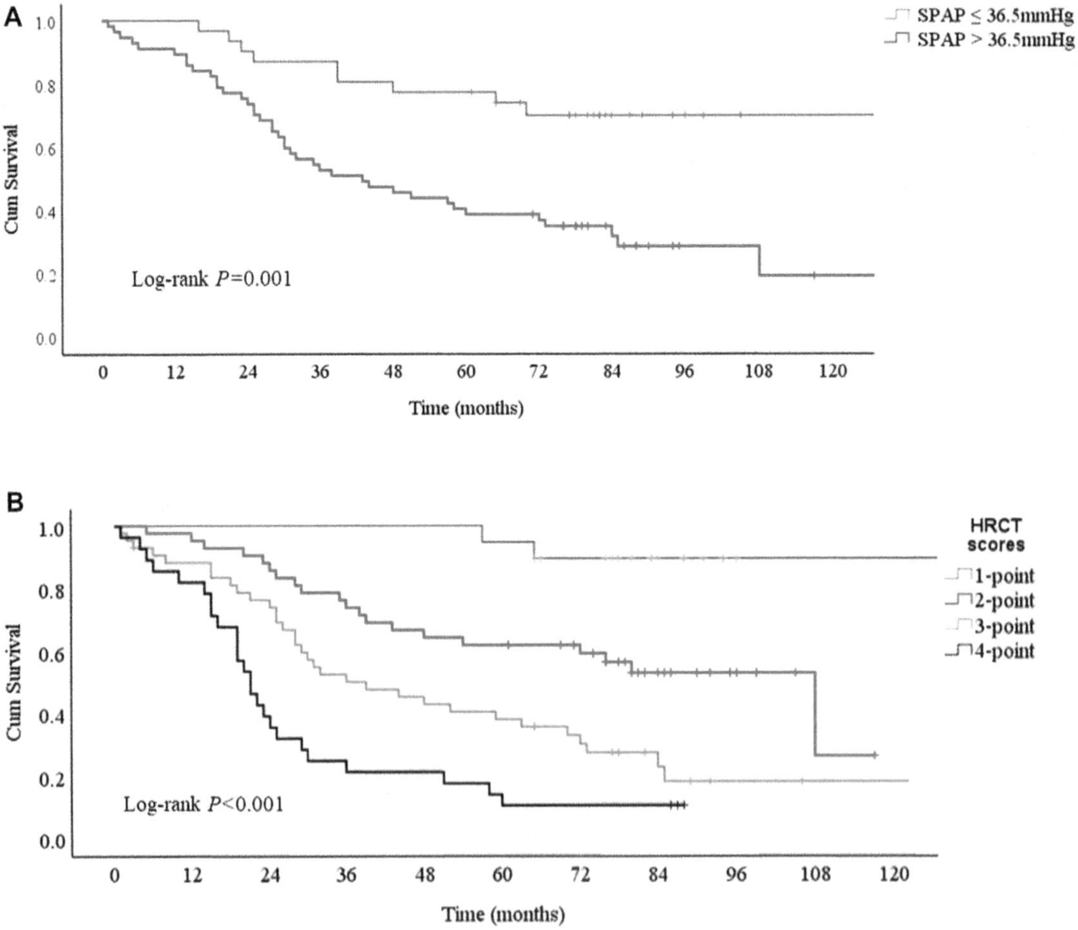

FIGURE 5 | Survival curves according to risk factors for mortality **(A)** Survival curves according to SPAP with a 36.5 mmHg threshold. Log-rank p = 0.001. The median survival times were 43 (95%CI: 23-63) months in SPAP >36.5 mmHg group and NA in SPAP ≤36.5 mmHg group **(B)** Survival curves according to HRCT scores. Log-rank p < 0.001. The median survival times were 108 (95%CI: 68-148) months in 2-point group, 39 (95%CI: 20-58) months in 3-point group, 21 (95%CI:17-25) months in 4-point group, and NA in 1-point group.; Abbreviations: SPAP, systolic pulmonary artery pressure; HRCT: high-resolution computed tomography.

cohort in the future. Secondly, due to incomplete data on lung function, the decrease in FVC was not included in the statistics, but it has been reported in the previous studies. And most of the PF-ILD cases we have diagnosed were dependent on clinical symptoms and HRCT. Thirdly, the relatively large number of patients with unclassified interstitial lung disease, due to the low percentage of surgical biopsies, may have resulted in an imprecise classification.

CONCLUSION

Patients with PF-ILD, similar to IPF cases, had worse prognosis than that of non-PF-ILD patients, but cases with an autoimmune disease-related type had a relatively good prognosis. Identifying the subtype of the disease may influence the prognosis. HRCT scores and SPAP>36.5 mmHg were independent risk factors for the mortality in patients with PF-ILD. In addition to pulmonary function, chest HRCT and echocardiography examined for monitoring SPAP are of great significance in the follow-up and the optimal time of lung transplantation of patients with PF-ILD.

AUTHOR CONTRIBUTIONS

All authors listed have made a substantial, direct, and intellectual contribution to the work and approved it for publication.

ACKNOWLEDGMENTS

The authors wish to thank the grants from Dream Mentor-Freshman Training Program of Shanghai Pulmonary Hospital (No. fkxr 1901), National Science Foundation of Shanghai, China (No.18ZR1431400), Science and Technology Innovation Research Project of Shanghai Science and Technology Commission, China (No. 20Y11902700), and Clinical Research Plan of SHDC (No. SHDC20CR40011C). And the authors wish to thank Prof. Aihong Zhang who is a statistician of Tongji University for the data analysis.

REFERENCES

Adegunsoye, A., Oldham, J. M., Bellam, S. K., Montner, S., Churpek, M. M., Noth, I., et al. (2019). Computed Tomography Honeycombing Identifies a Progressive Fibrotic Phenotype with Increased Mortality across Diverse Interstitial Lung Diseases. *Ann. Am. Thorac. Soc.* 16, 580–588. doi:10.1513/AnnalsATS.201807-443OC

Brown, K. K., Martinez, F. J., Walsh, S. L. F., Thannickal, V. J., Prasse, A., Schlenker-Herceg, R., et al. (2020). The Natural History of Progressive Fibrosing Interstitial Lung Diseases. *Eur. Respir. J.* 55, 2000085. doi:10.1183/13993003.00085-2020

Castro, S. V., and Jimenez, S. A. (2010). Biomarkers in Systemic Sclerosis. *Biomark Med.* 4, 133–147. doi:10.2217/bmm.09.79

De Sadeleer, L. J., Hermans, F., De Dycker, E., Yserbyt, J., Verschakelen, J. A., Verbeken, E. K., et al. (2019). Effects of Corticosteroid Treatment and Antigen Avoidance in a Large Hypersensitivity Pneumonitis Cohort: A Single-Centre Cohort Study. *J. Clin. Med.* 8, 14. doi:10.3390/jcm8010014

Doyle, T. J., and Dellaripa, P. F. (2017). Lung Manifestations in the Rheumatic Diseases. *Chest* 152, 1283–1295. doi:10.1016/j.chest.2017.05.015

Edey, A. J., Devaraj, A. A., Barker, R. P., Nicholson, A. G., Wells, A. U., and Hansell, D. M. (2011). Fibrotic Idiopathic Interstitial Pneumonias: HRCT Findings that Predict Mortality. *Eur. Radiol.* 21, 1586–1593. doi:10.1007/s00330-011-2098-2

Flaherty, K. R., Wells, A. U., Cottin, V., Devaraj, A., Walsh, S. L. F., Inoue, Y., et al. (2019). Nintedanib in Progressive Fibrosing Interstitial Lung Diseases. *N. Engl. J. Med.* 381, 1718–1727. doi:10.1056/NEJMoa1908681

Giacomelli, R., Afeltra, A., Alunno, A., Bartoloni-Bocci, E., Berardicurti, O., Bombardieri, M., et al. (2019). Guidelines for Biomarkers in Autoimmune Rheumatic Diseases - Evidence Based Analysis. *Autoimmun. Rev.* 18, 93–106. doi:10.1016/j.autrev.2018.08.003

Gimenez, A., Storrer, K., Kuranishi, L., Soares, M. R., Ferreira, R. G., and Pereira, C. A. C. (2018). Change in FVC and Survival in Chronic Fibrotic Hypersensitivity Pneumonitis. *Thorax* 73, 391–392. doi:10.1136/thoraxjnl-2017-210035

Guler, S. A., Ellison, K., Algamdi, M., Collard, H. R., and Ryerson, C. J. (2018). Heterogeneity in Unclassifiable Interstitial Lung Disease. A Systematic Review and Meta-Analysis. *Ann. Am. Thorac. Soc.* 15, 854–863. doi:10.1513/AnnalsATS.201801-067OC

Guler, S. A., Winstone, T. A., Murphy, D., Hague, C., Soon, J., Sulaiman, N., et al. (2018). Does Systemic Sclerosis-Associated Interstitial Lung Disease Burn Out? Specific Phenotypes of Disease Progression. *Ann. Am. Thorac. Soc.* 15, 1427–1433. doi:10.1513/AnnalsATS.201806-362OC

Hansell, D. M., Bankier, A. A., MacMahon, H., McLoud, T. C., Müller, N. L., and Remy, J. (2008). Fleischner Society: Glossary of Terms for Thoracic Imaging. *Radiology* 246, 697–722. doi:10.1148/radiol.2462070712

Jeny, F., Uzunhan, Y., Lacroix, M., Gille, T., Brillet, P. Y., Nardi, A., et al. (2020). Predictors of Mortality in Fibrosing Pulmonary Sarcoidosis. *Respir. Med.* 169, 105997. doi:10.1016/j.rmed.2020.105997

Kekevian, A., Gershwin, M. E., and Chang, C. (2014). Diagnosis and Classification of Idiopathic Pulmonary Fibrosis. *Autoimmun. Rev.* 13, 508–512. doi:10.1016/j.autrev.2014.01.037

Kelly, C. A., Saravanan, V., Nisar, M., Arthanari, S., Woodhead, F. A., Price-Forbes, A. N., et al. (2014). Rheumatoid Arthritis-Related Interstitial Lung Disease: Associations, Prognostic Factors and Physiological and Radiological Characteristics-Aa Large Multicentre UK Study. *Rheumatology* 53, 1676–1682. doi:10.1093/rheumatology/keu165

Khalil, N., Churg, A., Muller, N., and O'Connor, R. (2007). Environmental, Inhaled and Ingested Causes of Pulmonary Fibrosis. *Toxicol. Pathol.* 35, 86–96. doi:10.1080/01926230601064787

Kim, E. J., Elicker, B. M., Maldonado, F., Webb, W. R., Ryu, J. H., Van Uden, J. H., et al. (2010). Usual Interstitial Pneumonia in Rheumatoid Arthritis-Associated Interstitial Lung Disease. *Eur. Respir. J.* 35, 1322–1328. doi:10.1183/09031936.00092309

Lee, H. Y., Lee, K. S., Jeong, Y. J., Hwang, J. H., Kim, H. J., Chung, M. P., et al. (2012). High-Resolution CT Findings in Fibrotic Idiopathic Interstitial Pneumonias with Little Honeycombing: Serial Changes and Prognostic Implications. *AJR Am. J. Roentgenol* 199, 982–989. doi:10.2214/AJR.11.8192

Lettieri, C. J., Nathan, S. D., Barnett, S. D., Ahmad, S., and Shorr, A. F. (2006). Prevalence and Outcomes of Pulmonary Arterial Hypertension in Advanced Idiopathic Pulmonary Fibrosis. *Chest* 129, 746–752. doi:10.1378/chest.129.3.746

Lynch, D. A., Godwin, J. D., Safrin, S., Starko, K. M., Hormel, P., Brown, K. K., et al. (2005). High-Resolution Computed Tomography in Idiopathic Pulmonary FibrosisHigh-Resolution Computed Tomography in Idiopathic Pulmonary Fibrosis: Diagnosis and Prognosis. *Am. J. Respir. Crit. Care Med.* 172, 488–493. doi:10.1164/rccm.200412-1756oc

Miller, M. R., Hankinson, J., Brusasco, V., Burgos, F., Casaburi, R., Coates, A., et al. (2005). Standardisation of Spirometry. *Eur. Respir. J.* 26, 319–338. doi:10.1183/09031936.05.00034805

Mooney, J. J., Elicker, B. M., Urbania, T. H., Agarwal, M. R., Ryerson, C. J., Nguyen, M. L. T., et al. (2013). Radiographic Fibrosis Score Predicts Survival in Hypersensitivity Pneumonitis. *Chest* 144, 586–592. doi:10.1378/chest.12-2623

Moua, T., Zamora Martinez, A. C., Baqir, M., Vassallo, R., Limper, A. H., and Ryu, J. H. (2014). Predictors of Diagnosis and Survival in Idiopathic Pulmonary Fibrosis and Connective Tissue Disease-Related Usual Interstitial Pneumonia. *Respir. Res.* 15, 154. doi:10.1186/s12931-014-0154-6

Nasser, M., Larrieu, S., Si-Mohamed, S., Ahmad, K., Boussel, L., Brevet, M., et al. (2021). Progressive Fibrosing Interstitial Lung Disease: a Clinical Cohort (The PROGRESS(R) Study). *Eur. Respir. J.*. 57, 2002718. doi:10.1183/13993003.02718-2020

Nathan, S. D., Shlobin, O. A., Ahmad, S., Koch, J., Barnett, S. D., Ad, N., et al. (2008). Serial Development of Pulmonary Hypertension in Patients with Idiopathic Pulmonary Fibrosis. *Respiration* 76, 288–294. doi:10.1159/000114246

Oldham, J. M., Adegunsoye, A., Valenzi, E., Lee, C., Witt, L., Chen, L., et al. (2016). Characterisation of Patients with Interstitial Pneumonia with Autoimmune Features. *Eur. Respir. J.* 47, 1767–1775. doi:10.1183/13993003.01565-2015

Olson, A. L., Gifford, A. H., Inase, N., Fernández Pérez, E. R., and Suda, T. (2018). The Epidemiology of Idiopathic Pulmonary Fibrosis and Interstitial Lung Diseases at Risk of a Progressive-Fibrosing Phenotype. *Eur. Respir. Rev.* 27, 180077. doi:10.1183/16000617.0077-2018

Raghu, G., Amatto, V. C., Behr, J., and Stowasser, S. (2015). Comorbidities in Idiopathic Pulmonary Fibrosis Patients: a Systematic Literature Review. *Eur. Respir. J.* 46, 1113–1130. doi:10.1183/13993003.02316-2014

Ryerson, C. J., Urbania, T. H., Richeldi, L., Mooney, J. J., Lee, J. S., Jones, K. D., et al. (2013). Prevalence and Prognosis of Unclassifiable Interstitial Lung Disease. *Eur. Respir. J.* 42, 750–757. doi:10.1183/09031936.00131912

Shin, K. M., Lee, K. S., Chung, M. P., Han, J., Bae, Y. A., Kim, T. S., et al. (2008). Prognostic Determinants Among Clinical, Thin-Section CT, and Histopathologic Findings for Fibrotic Idiopathic Interstitial Pneumonias: Tertiary Hospital Study. *Radiology* 249, 328–337. doi:10.1148/radiol.2483071378

Solomon, J. J., Chung, J. H., Cosgrove, G. P., Demoruelle, M. K., Fernandez-Perez, E. R., Fischer, A., et al. (2016). Predictors of Mortality in Rheumatoid Arthritis-Associated Interstitial Lung Disease. *Eur. Respir. J.* 47, 588–596. doi:10.1183/13993003.00357-2015

Steen, V. D., and Medsger, T. A. (2007). Changes in Causes of Death in Systemic Sclerosis, 1972-2002. *Ann. Rheum. Dis.* 66, 940–944. doi:10.1136/ard.2006.066068

Strek, M. E., and Costabel, U. (2016). Interstitial Pneumonia with Autoimmune Features: a Critical Appraisal of the New Definition. *Curr. Opin. Pulm. Med.* 22, 442–449. doi:10.1097/MCP.0000000000000298

Walsh, S. L., Sverzellati, N., Devaraj, A., Keir, G. J., Wells, A. U., and Hansell, D. M. (2014). Connective Tissue Disease Related Fibrotic Lung Disease: High Resolution Computed Tomographic and Pulmonary Function Indices as Prognostic Determinants. *Thorax* 69, 216–222. doi:10.1136/thoraxjnl-2013-203843

Walsh, S. L., Sverzellati, N., Devaraj, A., Wells, A. U., and Hansell, D. M. (2012). Chronic Hypersensitivity Pneumonitis: High Resolution Computed Tomography Patterns and Pulmonary Function Indices as Prognostic Determinants. *Eur. Radiol.* 22, 1672–1679. doi:10.1007/s00330-012-2427-0

Walsh, S. L., Wells, A. U., Sverzellati, N., Keir, G. J., Calandriello, L., Antoniou, K. M., et al. (2014). An Integrated Clinicoradiological Staging System for Pulmonary Sarcoidosis: a Case-Cohort Study. *Lancet Respir. Med.* 2, 123–130. doi:10.1016/S2213-2600(13)70276-5

Wells, A. U., Brown, K. K., Flaherty, K. R., Kolb, M., Thannickal, V. J., and Group, I. P. F. C. W. (2018). What's in a Name? that Which We Call IPF, by Any Other Name Would Act the Same. *Eur. Respir. J.* 51, 1800692. doi:10.1183/13993003.00692-2018

Wijsenbeek, M., Kreuter, M., Olson, A., Fischer, A., Bendstrup, E., Wells, C. D., et al. (2019). Progressive Fibrosing Interstitial Lung Diseases: Current Practice in Diagnosis and Management. *Curr. Med. Res. Opin.* 35, 2015–2024. doi:10.1080/03007995.2019.1647040

Zamora-Legoff, J. A., Krause, M. L., Crowson, C. S., Ryu, J. H., and Matteson, E. L. (2017). Progressive Decline of Lung Function in Rheumatoid Arthritis-Associated Interstitial Lung Disease. *Arthritis Rheumatol.* 69, 542–549. doi:10.1002/art.39971

18

Autoimmune Progressive Fibrosing Interstitial Lung Disease: Predictors of Fast Decline

Alexandra Nagy[1†], Tamas Nagy[1†], Abigel Margit Kolonics-Farkas[1], Noemi Eszes[1], Krisztina Vincze[1], Eniko Barczi[1], Adam Domonkos Tarnoki[2], David Laszlo Tarnoki[2], György Nagy[3,4], Emese Kiss[5,6], Pal Maurovich-Horvat[2], Aniko Bohacs[1†] and Veronika Müller[1†]*

[1]Department of Pulmonology, Semmelweis University, Budapest, Hungary, [2]Medical Imaging Centre, Semmelweis University, Budapest, Hungary, [3]Department of Genetics, Cell- and Immunobiology, Semmelweis University, Budapest, Hungary, [4]Department of Rheumatology and Clinical Immunology, Semmelweis University, Budapest, Hungary, [5]Department of Clinical Immunology, Adult and Pediatric Rheumatology, National Institute of Locomotor Diseases and Disabilities, Budapest, Hungary, [6]3rd Department of Internal Medicine and Haematology, Semmelweis University, Budapest, Hungary

***Correspondence:**
Veronika Müller
muller.veronika@med.semmelweis-univ.hu

[†]These authors have contributed equally to this work and share first and last authorship

A subset of interstitial lung diseases (ILDs) with autoimmune traits—including connective tissue disease-associated ILD (CTD-ILD) and interstitial pneumonia with autoimmune features (IPAF)—develops progressive fibrosing (PF)-ILD. The aim of our study was to evaluate the clinical characteristics and predictors of longitudinal lung function (LF) changes in autoimmune PF-ILD patients in a real-world setting. All ILD cases with confirmed or suspected autoimmunity discussed by a multidisciplinary team (MDT) between January 2017 and June 2019 (n = 511) were reviewed, including 63 CTD-ILD and 44 IPAF patients. Detailed medical history, LF test, diffusing capacity of the lung for carbon monoxide (DLCO), 6-min walk test (6MWT), blood gas analysis (BGA), and high-resolution computer tomography (HRCT) were performed. Longitudinal follow-up for functional parameters was at least 2 years. Women were overrepresented (70.1%), and the age of the IPAF group was significantly higher as compared to the CTD-ILD group ($p < 0.001$). Dyspnea, crackles, and weight loss were significantly more common in the IPAF group as compared to the CTD-ILD group (84.1% vs. 58.7%, $p = 0.006$; 72.7% vs. 49.2%, $p = 0.017$; 29.6% vs. 4.8%, $p = 0.001$). Forced vital capacity (FVC) yearly decline was more pronounced in IPAF (53.1 ± 0.3 vs. 16.7 ± 0.2 ml; $p = 0.294$), while the majority of patients (IPAF: 68% and CTD-ILD 82%) did not deteriorate. Factors influencing progression included malignancy as a comorbidity, anti-SS-A antibodies, and post-exercise pulse increase at 6MWT. Antifibrotic therapy was administered significantly more often in IPAF as compared to CTD-ILD patients (n = 13, 29.5% vs. n = 5, 7.9%; $p = 0.007$), and importantly, this treatment reduced lung function decline when compared to non-treated patients. Majority of patients improved or were stable regarding lung function, and autoimmune-associated PF-ILD was more common in patients having IPAF. Functional decline predictors were anti-SS-A antibodies and marked post-exercise pulse increase at 6MWT. Antifibrotic treatments reduced progression in progressive fibrosing CTD-ILD and IPAF, emphasizing the need for guidelines including optimal treatment start and combination therapies in this special patient group.

Keywords: autoimmune disease, progressive fibrosing interstitial lung disease (PF-ILD), connective tissue disease (CTD), interstitial pneumonia with autoimmune features (IPAF), treatment, antifibrotics

INTRODUCTION

Interstitial lung diseases (ILDs) are a heterogeneous group of lung disorders, with diffuse parenchymal involvement also associated with a relevant morbidity and mortality. The spectrum of ILD is very diverse and the etiology is often idiopathic; however, a significant proportion of patients present with confirmed or possible autoimmune characteristics (Antoniou et al., 2014; Fischer et al., 2015; Martin et al., 2016). Connective tissue diseases (CTDs) are often associated with ILD. Lung involvement may occur in the initial phase of the systemic autoimmune disorder; however, ILD can manifest even before the diagnosis of CTD (Fischer and Du Bois, 2012). The term "interstitial pneumonia with autoimmune features" (IPAF) describes a type of interstitial pneumonias that are clinically and serologically associated with autoimmune characteristics but do not correspond completely to the diagnostic criteria of CTD (Sambataro et al., 2018).

Continuous monitoring of patients is essential to recognize progression (Fisher et al., 2020). The phenotype of progressive fibrosing (PF)-ILD, regardless of the underlying disease, shows common clinical features of lung function decline (Johannson et al., 2021). Worsening of symptoms—mainly dyspnea and cough—is often associated with progression of fibrosis on high-resolution computer tomography (HRCT); however, the definition for PF-ILD is not unitary (Cottin et al., 2018; Cottin et al., 2019; Brown et al., 2020; Kolb and Flaherty, 2021). PF-ILD results in the deterioration of quality of life and leads to early mortality. Forced vital capacity (FVC) and diffusing capacity of the lung for carbon monoxide (DLCO) decline are important and most frequently accepted markers of progression and are predictive factors of mortality (Brown et al., 2020), (Volkmann et al., 2019; Solomon et al., 2016; George et al., 2020).

A multidisciplinary approach is crucial for proper ILD diagnosis and treatment (Grewal et al., 2019). Considering the wide spectrum of disorders among autoimmune ILDs including different CTD-ILDs and even IPAF, it is essential to outline the best therapeutic possibilities for these patients. In addition to immunosuppressive therapy being extensively used, new antifibrotic agents—nintedanib and pirfenidone—also impact on the disease course; however, data on the interaction between these medications are lacking (Johannson et al., 2021; Wollin et al., 2019; Maher et al., 2020; Gao and Moua, 2020). It is challenging to find the best time for the introduction of certain drugs as well as choosing the optimal treatment course and combination for autoimmune-mediated ILDs (Cottin et al., 2019; Flaherty et al., 2019; George et al., 2020).

Our goal was to assess the clinical course of autoimmune ILDs—regarding the PF-ILD phenotype—and to confirm risk factors for progression and potential beneficial therapies in a real-word setting.

MATERIALS AND METHODS

Study Population

Our study is based on retrospective data analysis of ILD patients. Each case was presented and diagnosed by our multidisciplinary team (MDT) including pulmonologists, rheumatologists, radiologists, and pathologists. The ILD-MDT evaluation of the patients was performed at the Department of Pulmonology Semmelweis University between January 2017 and June 2019 (Richeldi et al., 2019).

The diagnosis of CTD was based on the internationally accepted American College of Rheumatology/European League Against Rheumatism Collaborative Initiative (EULAR-ACR) clinical and serologic criteria by rheumatology specialists working at one of the two rheumatology centers in Central Hungary. CTDs included rheumatoid arthritis (RA), systemic sclerosis (SSc), systemic lupus erythematosus (SLE), vasculitis, idiopathic inflammatory myopathies including polymyositis/dermatomyositis (IIM; PM/DM), and other categories [mixed connective tissue disease (MCTD) and undifferentiated connective tissue disease (UCTD)] (Kay and Upchurch, 2012; Van Den Hoogen et al., 2013; Petri et al., 2012; Aringer, 2019; Yates et al., 2016; Lundberg et al., 2017; Ortega-Hernandez and Shoenfeld, 2012; Mosca et al., 2014). The diagnosis of IPAF consisted of clinical, serological, and morphological domains based on the classification criteria proposed by the European Respiratory Society/American Thoracic Society (ERS/ATS) in 2015 (Fischer et al., 2015). All patients were consulted by rheumatologists to exclude manifestations of CTD at the time of diagnosis or in case of clinical suspicion thereafter. None of the IPAF patients developed CTD during follow-up.

At baseline and every follow-up, physical examination was performed, and a detailed medical history was taken with special emphasis on symptoms (dry/productive cough, sputum, and chest pain), respiratory infections, and comorbidities (Barczi et al., 2020). In our clinical routine, studied autoantibodies were anti-nuclear antibodies (ANA), rheumatoid factor (RF), anti-cyclic citrullinated peptide antibodies (ACPA), anti-RNA polymerase, anti-centromere, anti-proliferating cell nuclear antigen (APCNA), anti-Ku, anti-P-ribosomal, anti-cytoplasmatic, anti-cytoskeleton, anti-chromatin, anti-Smith, anti-myeloperoxidase, anti-proteinase-3, anti-Jo-1, anti-SS-A, anti-SS-B, anti-SCL-70, anti-ribonucleoprotein (RNP), and anti-neutrophil cytoplasmic antibodies (ANCA).

Baseline lung HRCT scans, pulmonary function test (PFT), blood gas analysis (BGA), and 6-min walk test (6MWT) were implemented at the time of the ILD diagnosis. Gender-age-physiology (GAP) score was used for clinical severity prediction in CTD-ILD and IPAF (Ryerson et al., 2014).

Confirmed ILDs were classified into four main groups: ILDs with known etiology including mainly confirmed CTD-ILD and hypersensitive pneumonitis (HP) cases; idiopathic interstitial pneumonia (IIP) including idiopathic pulmonary fibrosis (IPF), idiopathic non-specific interstitial pneumonia (iNSIP), and other IIPs; granulomatous diseases; and other rare forms of ILDs according to current guidelines (Travis et al., 2013), (Raghu et al., 2011). IPAF was considered a separate entity; nevertheless, it was included in the first group. The study population selection is summarized in **Figure 1**. Patients with autoimmune characteristics were divided into two subgroups: CTD-ILD and IPAF patients.

The long-term care included pulmonary and rheumatology controls defined by patients' disease requirements.

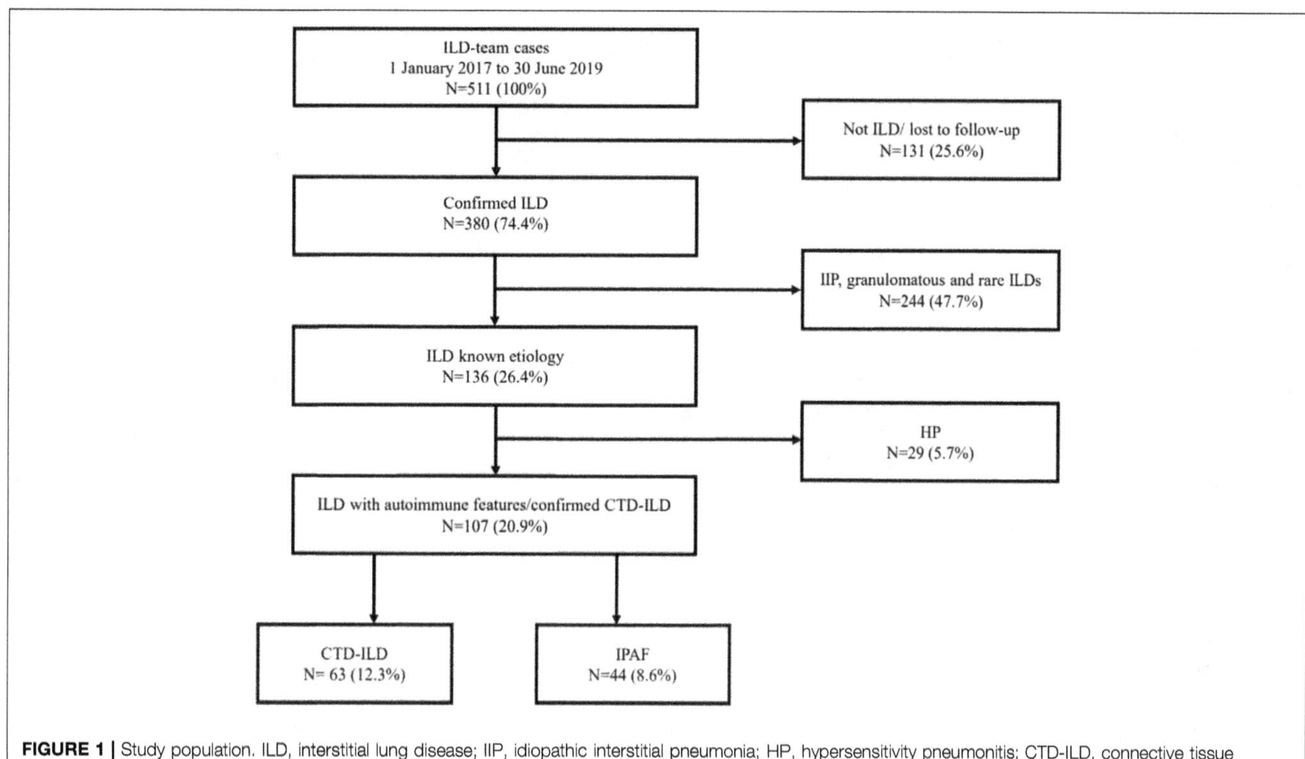

FIGURE 1 | Study population. ILD, interstitial lung disease; IIP, idiopathic interstitial pneumonia; HP, hypersensitivity pneumonitis; CTD-ILD, connective tissue disease-associated interstitial lung disease; IPAF, interstitial pneumonia with autoimmune features.

Pulmonary Evaluation and Functional Measurements and Radiological Patterns

PFT, including the analysis of FVC, forced expiratory volume in 1 s (FEV1), FEV1/FVC, total lung capacity (TLC), was performed according to the standardized protocol at the Department of Pulmonology. Lung diffusion capacity was measured for DLCO using the single-breath CO method, and transfer coefficient of the lung for CO (KLCO) was calculated (PDD-301/s, Piston, Budapest, Hungary). Exercise tolerance was established using the 6MWT. Distance in meters (m), baseline and post-exercise oxygen saturation (SpO_2), heart rate, and Borg scale referring to dyspnea were assessed. Arterialized capillary BGA were evaluated at room air temperature (Cobas b 221, Roche, Hungary).

HRCT scan was performed in both inspiration and expiration positions using Philips Ingenuity Core 64 and Philips Brilliance 16 CT scanners. NSIP pattern was divided into cellular and fibrotic subtypes by radiologist experts according to HRCT scans. Radiologic features typically include cellular variant with ground-glass opacities and fine reticular opacities; besides, the fibrotic subtype is characterized predominantly by traction bronchiectasis (Kligerman et al., 2009). In case of usual interstitial pneumonia (UIP), honeycombing with subpleural and basal predominance can be observed. Traction bronchiectasis might be associated with ground-glass opacification. The pattern of probable UIP (pUIP) is characterized by the same abnormalities without honeycombing (Raghu et al., 2011).

Pulmonary follow-up of at least 24 months after ILD diagnosis included measurements of lung function parameters, diffusion capacity, laboratory testing, and BGA controls. At this time point, we recorded the immunosuppressive and/or antifibrotic therapies between the visit intervals. All CTD patients were followed at the respective rheumatology centers.

In our study, PF-ILD was defined as FVC relative yearly decline ≥5% and either deterioration of clinical symptoms or progression of fibrosis on HRCT (Cottin et al., 2018).

Statistical Analysis

Analysis was performed using the GraphPad software (GraphPad Prism 5.0 Software, Inc., La Jolla, CA, United States) and SPSS v25 (IBM Corporation, Armonk, NY, United States). Continuous variables were expressed as mean ± standard deviation. Normality of the data was determined using Kolmogorov–Smirnov test. Differences between groups for continuous data were evaluated in normally distributed data with Student's *t*-test; otherwise, Mann–Whitney U-test was used. Chi-squared test and two-tailed Fisher's exact test were applied for comparing categorical variables. Predictors of progression were analyzed using Cox proportional hazards regression model. All percentage values are expressed for the whole study population or respective subgroups as indicated. A p-value <0.05 was defined as statistically significant.

TABLE 1 | Patient characteristics.

Parameters	All patients (n = 107)	CTD-ILD (n = 63)	IPAF (n = 44)	p-value
Age (years)	63.78 ± 13.88	59.73 ± 14.08	69.57 ± 11.45	**<0.001**
Sex (male/female), n	32:75	13:50	19:25	**0.018**
Ever smoker, n (%)	44 (41.12)	22 (34.92)	22 (50.0)	0.162
Non-smoker, n (%)	63 (58.87)	41 (65.08)	22 (50.0)	
BMI (kg/m^2)	25.60 ± 6.22	25.87 ± 4.83	25.27 ± 7.10	0.604
Symptoms, n (%)	–	–	–	–
Dyspnea	74 (69.16)	37 (58.73)	37 (84.09)	**0.006**
Cough	63 (58.57)	34 (53.97)	29 (65.91)	0.237
Dry cough	38 (35.51)	19 (30.16)	19 (43.18)	0.218
Sputum	25 (23.36)	15 (23.81)	10 (22.73)	1.000
Chest pain	20 (18.69)	10 (15.87)	10 (22.73)	0.452
Joint pain	57 (53.27)	36 (57.14)	21 (47.73)	0.431
Clubbing	12 (11.21)	4 (6.35)	8 (18.18)	0.068
Weight loss	16 (14.95)	3 (4.76)	13 (29.55)	**0.001**
Crackles	63 (58.88)	31 (49.21)	32 (72.73)	**0.017**
Raynaud's phenomenon	32 (29.91)	27 (42.86)	5 (11.36)	**<0.001**
CTD subtype, n (%)	–	–	–	–
RA	–	13 (20.63)	–	–
SSc	–	32 (50.79)	–	–
SLE	–	6 (9.52)	–	–
Vasculitis	–	2 (3.17)	–	–
DM/PM	–	4 (6.35)	–	–
Others (MCTD and UCTD)	–	6 (9.52)	–	–

CTD-ILD, connective tissue disease-associated interstitial lung disease; IPAF, interstitial pneumonia with autoimmune features; BMI, body mass index; RA, rheumatoid arthritis; SSc, systemic sclerosis; SLE, systemic lupus erythematosus; PM/DM, polymyositis/dermatomyositis; MCTD, mixed connective tissue disease; UCTD, undifferentiated connective tissue disease.

Statistically significant values were highlighted with bold in the tables.

TABLE 2 | Functional parameters.

Parameters	All patients (n = 107)	CTD-ILD (n = 63)	IPAF (n = 44)	p-value
Lung function	–	–	–	–
FEV1/FVC	0.84 ± 0.08	0.84 ± 0.06	0.82 ± 0.10	0.287
FVC (L)	2.50 ± 0.86	2.49 ± 0.89	2.52 ± 0.83	0.951
FVC (%)	84.41 ± 23.86	85.51 ± 26.93	82.82 ± 18.72	0.577
FEV1 (L)	2.08 ± 0.72	2.09 ± 0.73	2.07 ± 0.71	0.819
FEV1 (%)	85.64 ± 24.67	86.82 ± 26.26	83.93 ± 22.36	0.562
TLC (L)	4.31 ± 1.43	4.39 ± 1.54	4.19 ± 1.26	0.683
TLC (%)	80.64 ± 24.82	83.86 ± 26.54	76.13 ± 21.73	0.133
Diffusion parameters	–	–	–	–
DLCO (mmol/min/kPa)	5.52 ± 1.87	5.55 ± 1.84	5.47 ± 1.94	0.899
DLCO (%)	70.92 ± 20.88	70.53 ± 20.07	71.48 ± 22.21	0.823
KLCO (mmol/min/kPa/l)	1.26 ± 0.38	1.27 ± 0.37	1.24 ± 0.39	0.943
KLCO (%)	66.19 ± 18.54	65.25 ± 18.12	67.50 ± 19.26	0.551
BGA	–	–	–	–
pH	7.42 ± 0.04	7.43 ± 0.05	7.42 ± 0.02	0.204
pCO2	40.10 ± 11.13	41.13 ± 11.87	38.86 ± 10.19	0.859
pO2	66.69 ± 11.82	65.63 ± 13.85	67.96 ± 8.80	0.859
6MWT	–	–	–	–
Distance (m)	400.73 ± 108.15	403.45 ± 120.96	397.61 ± 93.02	0.822
SpO_2 baseline	94.51 ± 4.15	95.00 ± 3.35	93.91 ± 4.94	0.490
SpO_2 post-exercise	90.12 ± 8.97	90.69 ± 6.74	89.47 ± 11.06	0.223
Pulse baseline	84.05 ± 14.50	84.75 ± 12.88	83.24 ± 16.37	0.658
Pulse post-exercise	106.71 ± 19.83	109.84 ± 19.56	103.21 ± 19.82	0.158
Borg scale baseline	2.01 ± 11.46	3.23 ± 15.42	0.55 ± 1.25	0.253
Borg scale post-exercise	4.05 ± 11.05	5.33 ± 14.86	2.56 ± 2.15	0.223

CTD-ILD, connective tissue disease-associated interstitial lung disease; IPAF, interstitial pneumonia with autoimmune features; FVC, forced vital capacity; FEV1, forced expiratory volume in 1 s; TLC, total lung capacity; DLCO, diffusing capacity for carbon monoxide; KLCO, transfer coefficient of the lung for carbon monoxide; BGA, blood gas analysis; 6MWT, 6-min walk test.

TABLE 3 | HRCT morphological domain.

HRCT pattern	All patients (*n* = 107)	CTD-ILD (*n* = 63)	IPAF (*n* = 44)	*p*-value
pUIP, *n* (%)	27 (25.23)	8 (12.70)	19 (43.18)	**0.001**
UIP, *n* (%)	20 (18.69)	10 (15.87)	10 (22.73)	0.370
NSIP, *n* (%)	46 (42.99)	38 (60.32)	8 (18.18)	**<0.001**

HRTC, high-resolution computed tomography; CTD-ILD, connective tissue disease-associated interstitial lung disease; IPAF, interstitial pneumonia with autoimmune features; pUIP, probable usual interstitial pneumonia; UIP, usual interstitial pneumonia; NSIP, non-specific interstitial pneumonia.
Statistically significant values were highlighted with bold in the tables.

TABLE 4 | Autoimmune serology.

Autoantibodies	All patients (*n* = 107)	CTD-ILD (*n* = 63)	IPAF (*n* = 44)	*p*-value
ANA, *n* (%)	71 (66.36)	43 (68.25)	28 (63.64)	0.330
RF, *n* (%)	22 (20.56)	11 (17.46)	11 (25.00)	0.466
ACPA, *n* (%)	10 (9.35)	5 (7.94)	5 (11.36)	0.738
Anti-RNA-polymerase, *n* (%)	0	0	0	–
Anti-centromere, *n* (%)	1 (0.93)	1 (1.59)	0	–
Anti-PCNA, *n* (%)	2 (1.87)	1 (1.59)	1 (2.27)	1.000
Anti-Ku, *n* (%)	0	0	0	0
Anti-P-ribosomal, *n* (%)	0	0	0	0
Anti-cytoplasmatic, *n* (%)	27 (25.23)	17 (26.98)	10 (22.73)	0.658
Anti-cytoskeleton, *n* (%)	0	0	0	0
Anti-chromatin, *n* (%)	32 (29.90)	19 (30.16)	13 (29.55)	1.000
Anti-Smith, *n* (%)	4 (3.73)	2 (3.17)	2 (4.55)	1.000
Anti-myeloperoxidase, *n* (%)	2 (1.87)	2 (3.17)	0	–
Anti-proteinase-3, *n* (%)	1 (0.93)	1 (1.59)	0	–
Anti-Jo-1, *n* (%)	3 (2.80)	2 (3.17)	1 (2.27)	1.000
Anti-SS-A, *n* (%)	18 (16.82)	12 (19.05)	6 (13.64)	0.602
Anti-SS-B, *n* (%)	5 (4.67)	3 (4.76)	2 (4.55)	1.000
Anti-SCL-70, *n* (%)	17 (15.88)	17 (26.98)	0	–
Anti-RNP, *n* (%)	10 (9.34)	8 (12.70)	2 (4.55)	0.192
ANCA, *n* (%)	8 (7.48)	4 (6.35)	4 (9.09)	0.714

CTD-ILD, connective tissue disease-associated interstitial lung disease; IPAF, interstitial pneumonia with autoimmune features; ANA, anti-nuclear antibodies; RF, rheumatoid factor; ACPA, anti-cyclic citrullinated peptide antibodies; APCNA, anti-proliferating cell nuclear antigen; ANCA, anti-neutrophil cytoplasmic antibodies.

RESULTS

Patient characteristics are summarized in **Table 1**. The study population included mainly women. Patients in the IPAF subgroup were significantly older compared to the CTD subgroup. Dyspnea, crackles, and weight loss were significantly more common in the IPAF group as compared to the CTD-ILD group. Subtypes of CTD ($n = 63$) were, by order of prevalence, SSc (50.8%) RA (20.6%), SLE (9.5%), others (MCTD and UCTD) (9.5%), PM/DM (6.4%), and vasculitis (3.2%). Raynaud's phenomenon occurred significantly more often in patients with known CTD. LF at baseline is summarized in **Table 2**. Patients were characterized by mild restrictive functional impairment. There was a slight decrease in TLC and CO diffusion parameters. No differences in LF, 6MWT, or BGA were noted between the two groups.

The most common radiological pattern was NSIP; however, significantly more pUIP was noted in IPAF patients. HRCT data are summarized in **Table 3**. Most frequently confirmed auto-antibodies were ANA, followed by anti-chromatin antibodies and RF, with no differences among the two groups (**Table 4**).

Fifty-nine patients had functional data during the 24-month follow-up including 34 CTD-ILD (23.5% males; mean age 58.42 ± 13.01 years) and 25 IPAF (48.0% males; mean age 69.02 ± 12.51 years) patients. Baseline data of CTD-ILD [SSc (55.9%), RA (20.6%), PM/DM (11.8%), SLE (5.9%), and other MCTD and UCTD (5.9%)] and IPAF patients with available functional follow-up did not differ in any parameter from the whole respective group. To estimate mortality, we applied the GAP risk prediction model, which is also validated for non-IPF ILDs (Ryerson et al., 2014). Values were markedly better in the CTD group compared to the IPAF group (1.82 vs. 2.48, $p = 0.07$).

FVC yearly decline was more dominant in the IPAF group than in the CTD-ILD group (53.1 ± 0.3 ml vs. 16.7 ± 0.2 ml; $p = 0.294$) (**Figure 2A**). It is important to note that 68.0% (out of the followed 25 patients) did not deteriorate in the IPAF group as compared to 82.4% (out of followed 34 patients) in the CTD-ILD group ($p = 0.200$). PF-ILD criteria were met by 14 patients. We also determined the prevalence of PF-ILD in each entity of CTD-ILD: RA ($n = 3$), SSc ($n = 2$), other ($n = 1$), and IPAF ($n = 8$).

Factors influencing rapid progression qualifying as PF-ILD included malignancy as a comorbidity, ANA, anti-SS-A antibodies, and post-exercise pulse increase at the 6MWT (**Table 5**). Malignancy was diagnosed in seven patients (two males and five females) including CML (1), lung (2), ovarian (1), breast (1), esophageal (1), and laryngeal cancer (1). There was

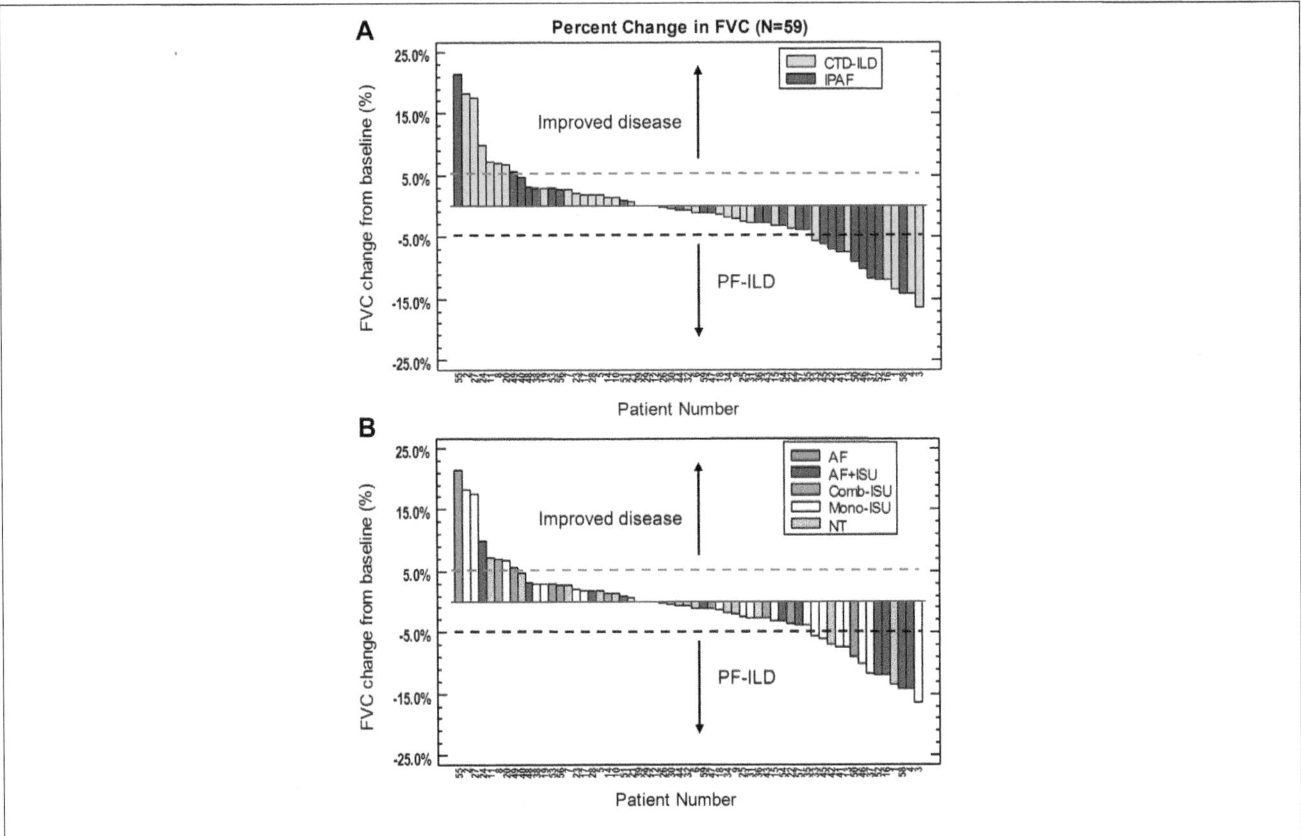

FIGURE 2 | Longitudinal follow-up of CTD-ILD and IPAF patients: percent change in FVC. **(A)** Changes according to treatment; **(B)** respective patients according to underlying disease. CTD-ILD, connective tissue disease-associated interstitial lung disease; IPAF, interstitial pneumonia with autoimmune features; FVC, forced vital capacity; PF-ILD, [progressive fibrosing ILD; AF, antifibrotic treatment; AF + ISU, antifibrotic treatment with immunosuppressive agent; Comb-ISU, combined immunosuppressive treatment; Mono-ISU, one immunosuppressive agent; NT, no treatment].

no correlation between HRCT pattern (UIP, pUIP, fibrotic, or cellular NSIP) and progression. Detailed data were not included, as no relationship was present.

During the follow-up period, 16 patients (CTD-ILD n = 11; IPAF n = 5) did not receive any treatment. Conventional immunosuppressive (ISU) therapies including corticosteroids, rituximab, mycophenolate mofetil, azathioprine, cyclophosphamide, and methotrexate were the initial medical treatment in 36 cases (CTD-ILD n = 22; IPAF n = 14). Mono or combined ISU therapies were appropriate during follow-up period for 25 patients (CTD-ILD n = 18; IPAF n = 7). In some cases, when antifibrotic therapy was given, progressive phenotype was observed. Patients showing progressive phenotype are those whose ISU therapy was supplemented with antifibrotic therapies such as nintedanib and pirfenidone. Antifibrotic drugs were administered significantly more often in IPAF as compared to CTD-ILD (n = 13 vs. n = 5; p = 0.007). The majority of these patients (72.2% on antifibrotic treatment) represented stable lung function or improvement following treatment introduction. Individual functional change according to therapy is summarized in **Figure 2B**. Antifibrotic treatment (pirfenidone 801 mg tid n = 2; nintedanib 150 mg bid n = 17, including one patient who switched to pirfenidone due to elevated liver enzymes)-related adverse events—all grade 1 and transient—included gastrointestinal symptoms, mainly nausea and vomiting, diarrhea, and heartburn. Most of them were solved by dosage reduction and supportive medications. Elevated liver enzymes were only observed in one patient and was resolved after changing to another antifibrotic drug. Unfortunately, during follow-up, nine patients with mono or combined ISU therapy developed PF-ILD according to our criteria, four (CTD-ILD n = 2; IPAF n = 2) of them had anti-SS-A antibody positivity and five patients (CTD-ILD n = 3; IPAF n = 2) had post-exercise pulse increase.

DISCUSSION

We presented the first single-center real-life data analyzing the functional progression of autoimmune ILDs. A small proportion of CTD-ILD and IPAF patients deteriorated (13.1% of the whole population) over the observed period, which is similar to other international data (Simpson et al., 2021). Most of the patients were stable, and remarkably, eight patients had even ≥5% FVC improvement due to therapy out of 59 followed.

Our data are the first to show ILD distribution of cases from an Eastern European country. Out of the 511 cases presented to the

TABLE 5 | Factors influencing progression of autoimmune ILDs.

Factor	HR	95% CI	*p*-value
Patient comorbidities	–	–	–
Hypertension	1.27	0.34 to 4.68	0.721
Thyroid disorder	11.90	0.77 to 182.80	0.076
Malignancy	8.17	1.31 to 50.81	**0.024**
PAH	1.52	0.34 to 6.84	0.584
Smoking	1.11	0.26 to 4.70	0.891
BMI	0.92	0.80 to 1.05	0.21
BGA	–	–	–
pH	21.82	0.00	0.936
pCO_2	0.10	0.83 to 1.20	0.990
pO_2	0.93	0.80 to 1.09	0.366
6MWT	–	–	–
Distance (m)	0.99	0.98 to 1.01	0.309
SpO_2 baseline	1.69	0.79 to 3.60	0.173
SpO_2 post-exercise	0.87	0.61 to 1.26	0.474
Pulse baseline	0.98	0.87 to 1.11	0.783
Pulse post-exercise	1.14	1.00 to 1.29	**0.043**
Borg scale baseline	0.72	0.12 to 4.37	0.722
Borg scale post-exercise	0.64	0.22 to 1.84	0.403
HRCT pattern	1.20	0.58 to 2.48	0.632
Autoantibodies	–	–	–
ANA	0.13	0.02 to 0.92	**0.041**
RF	3.27	0.23 to 45.95	0.380
ACPA	1.55	0.13 to 18.23	0.730
Anti-PCNA	0.00	0.00	0.992
Anti-cytoplasmatic	5.36	0.60 to 48.12	0.134
Anti-chromatin	0.47	0.08 to 2.83	0.411
Anti-Jo-1	6.13	0.08 to 482.05	0.416
Anti-SS-A	13.11	1.71 to 100.45	**0.013**
Anti-SS-B	2.23	0.02 to 279.51	0.745
Anti-SCL-70	0.97	0.07 to 12.94	0.980
Anti-RNP N	2.08	0.16 to 27.61	0.579
ANCA	0.00	0.00	0.997

HR, hazard ratio; CI, confidence interval; PAH, pulmonary arterial hypertension; BMI, body mass index; BGA, blood gas analysis; 6MWT, 6-min walk test; HRTC, high-resolution computed tomography; ANA, anti-nuclear antibodies; RF, rheumatoid factor; ACPA, anti-cyclic citrullinated peptide antibodies; APCNA, anti-proliferating cell nuclear antigen; ANCA, anti-neutrophil cytoplasmic antibodies.
Statistically significant values were highlighted with bold in the tables.

ILD team, 20.9% were CTD-ILD or IPAF, which is very similar to international data (Oldham et al., 2016; Sambataro et al., 2019). CTD-ILD did mainly include SSc (50.8%) and RA (20.6%) patients, also in line with previously published numbers (Oliveira et al., 2020; Sambataro et al., 2018).

IPAF is mainly considered as a research entity with an autoimmune profile and affected 25 patients in our study. Assessment by rheumatology specialists and serological testing were always performed to confirm or exclude CTD in these cases (Fischer et al., 2015; Sambataro et al., 2018; Raghu et al., 2018). However, there is no international agreement on which serological tests are required at the first encounter with the patient (Jee et al., 2017). The serological pattern in IPAF patients was consistent with the current classification criteria (Fischer et al., 2015; Sambataro et al., 2018).

The most common radiological pattern among IPAF patients was pUIP, which correlates with the data of Oldham et al. (2016); however, it contradicts prospective international data where NSIP was the most frequent pattern (Ahmad et al., 2017; Sambataro et al., 2018). In a retrospective study, UIP and non-UIP IPAF had a similar chance to transform into specific autoimmune diseases; thus, the role of the morphological domain of IPAF is questionable (Sambataro et al., 2020). HRCT evaluation is not homogenous among ILD expert radiologists and might have contributed partially to these differences (Walsh et al., 2016), (Widell and Lidén, 2020). Additionally, IPAF is not a homogenous entity, as it may be very similar to CTD-ILD or in contrast to IPF (Oldham et al., 2016; Ferri et al., 2016).

Treatment resulted in lung function improvement, especially in CTD-ILD. Variation of disease course is well known in SSc, where patients can have a rapid progression, stability of disease, and even improvement. Our data confirmed that most patients' lung function remained stable over the 2-year period; some of them even improved similarly to the Scleroderma Lung Study (SLS) I and II trials and SENSCIS (Volkmann et al., 2017), (Vonk et al., 2021).

An important new finding and interesting consideration of our study is the identification of new possible prognostic factors for PF-ILD in autoimmune-mediated ILDs including ANA and anti-SS-A antibodies, post-exercise pulse increase at 6MWT, and malignancy. Anti-SS-A antibodies such as Ro52 and Ro60 are often used in autoimmune disease diagnosis. Based on literature data, isolated anti-SS-A/Ro60+ is independently associated with SLE. Detection of anti-SS-A/Ro52+ has a prognostic importance in SSc-associated ILD and diagnostic value in PM/DM (Robbins et al., 2019; Hudson et al., 2012; Dugar et al., 2010; Menéndez et al., 2013). Previous small cohort studies have proven that in anti-synthetase syndrome or inflammatory myopathy, anti-SS-A antibody-positive individuals develop more severe ILD including more extensive pulmonary fibrosis and decreased LF. Additionally, these patients are less responsive to immunosuppressive therapies (La Corte et al., 2006; Váncsa et al., 2009). Literature about the diagnostic utility of separated anti-SS-A antibodies is heterogeneous (Hervier et al., 2009; Langguth et al., 2007; Robbins et al., 2019). According to the official recommendation for IPAF by ATS/ERS, in serological domain, Ro60 and Ro52 antibodies are not separated (Fischer et al., 2015). Therefore, we analyzed mixed anti-SS-A level.

Another predictor of progression was post-exercise pulse increase at the 6MWT. The connection between heart rate and 6MWT has not been studied profoundly before in CTD-ILD and IPAF patients; however an association has been found to be a prognostic marker in IPF (Holland et al., 2013). Although, chronotropic response abnormality cannot be certainly established due to various comorbidities and medication history regarding beta blockers being inaccessible (Sanges et al., 2017). The third variable for confirmed faster progression of PF-ILD in our patients was malignancy. Malignancy as a comorbidity is a serious complication associated with ILDs, especially in those showing progression as published previously in our previous study (Barczi et al., 2020).

Defining progression is a difficult task, as for CTD patients several treatment possibilities are open for their underlying disease. According to recent studies in IPF and CTD-ILD patients, a decrease in DLCO is proposed in the definition of PF-ILD (Khanna et al., 2015; Volkmann et al., 2019; Wong et al., 2020; Cottin et al., 2018). Inclusion criteria for PF-ILD subjects in the INBUILD (Efficacy and Safety of Nintedanib in Patients With

PF-ILD) trial included DLCO of at least 30% and less than 80% predicted (Brown et al., 2020; Flaherty et al., 2019). Low baseline DLCO is also a clinically meaningful risk factor for acute exacerbations (Wong et al., 2020). In our study, patients had decreased DLCO; however, we did not find any correlation between progression and DLCO change.

We provided real-world data on the treatment and functional outcome for these special patient groups. Therapy in CTD-ILD changes according to underlying disease, while no therapy guidance for IPAF is available (Sambataro et al., 2018; Gao and Moua, 2020). PF-ILD is much more of a disease phenotype than a diagnosis. Timely initiation of antifibrotic therapy slows the progression of the disease (Johannson et al., 2021). In our study, the ILD team recommended antifibrotic treatment to patients with a rapid progression and to those with IPF characteristics. More patients with IPAF and progression were offered this therapy than CTD-ILD patients showing PF-ILD phenotype, mainly due to the fact that the antifibrotic nintedanib was only approved for PF-ILD based on the data of the INBUILD trial in 2020 (Flaherty et al., 2019; Wells et al., 2020; European Medicines Agency, 2019).

Antifibrotic treatment did stabilize lung function in the majority of our patients. PF-ILD was detected in nine patients (CTD-ILD n = 4; IPAF n = 5) who did not receive antifibrotics including 44.4% with anti-SS-A positivity and 55.5% with post-exercise pulse increase, emphasizing the need for possible extension of antifibrotic treatment. Data on the effectivity of combination therapy using different immunosuppressive treatments with antifibrotics is lacking. In real life, patients under immunosuppressive or immunomodulatory therapy are not excluded from additional antifibrotic therapy. However, in the INBUILD study, restricted therapies were only applied after 6 months of deterioration (Cottin et al., 2021). Similarly, SSc-ILD treatment outcome of SENSCIS secondary analysis showed that mycophenolate mofetil and nintedanib co-treated patients did benefit the most from treatment; however, the study was not powered for combination treatment effectivity (Distler et al., 2019; Highland et al., 2021). After applying the combination of different immunosuppressive treatments with antifibrotics, two-thirds of patients experienced mild adverse events in our cohort. Safety and tolerability profile was consistent with the product label and similar to our previously published data (Barczi et al., 2019). In our patients, 67% experienced an adverse event, similar to the INBUILD trial, where diarrhea was observed in 67%, followed by nausea (29%) (Flaherty et al., 2019). The single grade 3 adverse event of liver enzyme increase needing drug discontinuation was resolved by changing to another antifibrotic agent. Acute exacerbations are serious complications of ILDs (Suzuki et al., 2020; Kolb et al., 2018). Unfortunately, our data were not available to analyze these effects on progression.

In conclusion, the majority of autoimmune-associated ILDs including CTD-ILD and IPAF might be stable or even improve due to proper combination therapy. Patients receiving antifibrotic treatment were less likely to deteriorate and fulfill criteria for PF-ILD. Progression was associated with anti-SS-A antibodies, post-exercise pulse increase at 6MWT, and concomitant malignancies—patients presenting with these parameters should be followed more closely. Antifibrotic treatment was effective in stabilizing functional decline, and the drugs confirmed a safety and tolerability profile consistent with the product label. More data is needed in a real-world setting to identify optimal combination therapies and timing for initiation of antifibrotics in CTD-ILD and IPAF patients. Stable lung function might be a result of the relatively short observation period, and more longitudinal data are awaited.

The main limitation of our study includes the retrospective single-center design and limited number of patients. Further prospective studies need to evaluate this special subgroup of ILD patients to develop guidelines for optimal treatment start and combination therapies.

On the other hand, our data are the first to represent ILD distribution of cases from an Eastern European country. Our study is based on long-term longitudinal follow-up of ILD patients with autoimmune characteristics. Disease population covered the two main rheumatology centers in the region of Central Hungary.

AUTHOR CONTRIBUTIONS

AN, TN, and VM contributed to the conception and design of the study, organized the database, performed the statistical analysis, and wrote the manuscript. All the included authors were treating physicians or radiologists, also members of the multidisciplinary ILD team at Semmelweis University and contributed with data, drafting and review of the manuscript. All authors contributed to the article and approved the submitted version.

REFERENCES

Ahmad, K., Barba, T., Gamondes, D., Ginoux, M., Khouatra, C., Spagnolo, P., et al. (2017). Interstitial Pneumonia with Autoimmune Features: Clinical, Radiologic, and Histological Characteristics and Outcome in a Series of 57 Patients. *Respir. Med.* 123, 56–62. doi:10.1016/j.rmed.2016.10.017

Antoniou, K. M., Margaritopoulos, G. A., Tomassetti, S., Bonella, F., Costabel, U., and Poletti, V. (2014). Interstitial Lung Disease. *Eur. Respir. Rev.* 23, 40–54. doi:10.1183/09059180.00009113

Aringer, M. (2019). EULAR/ACR Classification Criteria for SLE. *Semin. Arthritis Rheum.* 49, S14–S17. doi:10.1016/j.semarthrit.2019.09.009

Barczi, E., Nagy, T., Starobinski, L., Kolonics-Farkas, A., Eszes, N., Bohacs, A., et al. (2020). Impact of Interstitial Lung Disease and Simultaneous Lung Cancer on Therapeutic Possibilities and Survival. *Thorac. Cancer* 11, 1911–1917. doi:10.1111/1759-7714.13481

Barczi, E., Starobinski, L., Kolonics-Farkas, A., Eszes, N., Bohacs, A., Vasakova, M., et al. (2019). Long-Term Effects and Adverse Events of Nintedanib Therapy in Idiopathic Pulmonary Fibrosis Patients with Functionally Advanced Disease. *Adv. Ther.* 36, 1221–1232. doi:10.1007/s12325-019-00906-9

Brown, K. K., Martinez, F. J., Walsh, S. L. F., Thannickal, V. J., Prasse, A., Schlenker-Herceg, R., et al. (2020). The Natural History of Progressive Fibrosing Interstitial Lung Diseases. *Eur. Respir. J.* 55. doi:10.1183/13993003.00085-2020

Cottin, V., Hirani, N. A., Hotchkin, D. L., Nambiar, A. M., Ogura, T., Otaola, M., et al. (2018). Presentation, Diagnosis and Clinical Course of the Spectrum of Progressive-Fibrosing Interstitial Lung Diseases. *Eur. Respir. Rev.* 27. doi:10.1183/16000617.0076-2018

Cottin, V., Wollin, L., Fischer, A., Quaresma, M., Stowasser, S., and Harari, S. (2019). Fibrosing Interstitial Lung Diseases: Knowns and Unknowns. *Eur. Respir. Rev.* 28, 1–9. doi:10.1183/16000617.0100-2018

Cottin, V., Richeldi, L., Rosas, I., Otaola, M., Song, J. W., Tomassetti, S., et al. (2021). Nintedanib and Immunomodulatory Therapies in Progressive Fibrosing Interstitial Lung Diseases. *Respir. Res.* 22, 1–9. doi:10.1186/s12931-021-01668-1

Distler, O., Highland, K. B., Gahlemann, M., Azuma, A., Fischer, A., Mayes, M. D., et al. (2019). Nintedanib for Systemic Sclerosis-Associated Interstitial Lung Disease. *N. Engl. J. Med.* 380, 2518–2528. doi:10.1056/nejmoa1903076

Dugar, M., Cox, S., Limaye, V., Gordon, T. P., and Roberts-Thomson, P. J. (2010). Diagnostic Utility of Anti-ro52 Detection in Systemic Autoimmunity. *Postgrad. Med. J.* 86, 79–82. doi:10.1136/pgmj.2009.089656

European Medicines Agency (2019). Assessment Report - OFEV. Proced. No. EMEA/H/C/003821/II/0027 31, 16–33. doi:10.4324/9781351201117-4

Ferri, C., Manfredi, A., Sebastiani, M., Colaci, M., Giuggioli, D., Vacchi, C., et al. (2016). Interstitial Pneumonia with Autoimmune Features and Undifferentiated Connective Tissue Disease: Our Interdisciplinary Rheumatology-Pneumology Experience, and Review of the Literature. *Autoimmun. Rev.* 15, 61–70. doi:10.1016/j.autrev.2015.09.003

Fischer, A., Antoniou, K. M., Brown, K. K., Cadranel, J., Corte, T. J., Du Bois, R. M., et al. (2015). An Official European Respiratory Society/American Thoracic Society Research Statement: Interstitial Pneumonia with Autoimmune Features. *Eur. Respir. J.* 46, 976–987. doi:10.1183/13993003.00150-2015

Fischer, A., and Du Bois, R. (2012). Interstitial Lung Disease in Connective Tissue Disorders. *Lancet* 380, 689–698. doi:10.1016/S0140-6736(12)61079-4

Fisher, J. H., Johannson, K. A., Assayag, D., Morisset, J., Boer, K. d., Manganas, H., et al. (2020). Long-term Monitoring of Patients with Fibrotic Interstitial Lung Disease: A Canadian Thoracic Society Position Statement. *Can. J. Respir. Crit. Care Sleep Med.* 4, 147–155. doi:10.1080/24745332.2020.1796206

Flaherty, K. R., Wells, A. U., Cottin, V., Devaraj, A., Walsh, S. L. F., Inoue, Y., et al. (2019). Nintedanib in Progressive Fibrosing Interstitial Lung Diseases. *N. Engl. J. Med.* 381, 1718–1727. doi:10.1056/nejmoa1908681

Gao, Y., and Moua, T. (2020). Treatment of the Connective Tissue Disease-Related Interstitial Lung Diseases: A Narrative Review. *Mayo Clin. Proc.* 95, 554–573. doi:10.1016/j.mayocp.2019.07.007

George, P. M., Spagnolo, P., Kreuter, M., Altinisik, G., Bonifazi, M., Martinez, F. J., et al. (2020). Progressive Fibrosing Interstitial Lung Disease: Clinical Uncertainties, Consensus Recommendations, and Research Priorities. *Lancet Respir. Med.* 8, 925–934. doi:10.1016/S2213-2600(20)30355-6

Grewal, J. S., Morisset, J., Fisher, J. H., Churg, A. M., Bilawich, A. M., Ellis, J., et al. (2019). Role of a Regional Multidisciplinary Conference in the Diagnosis of Interstitial Lung Disease. *Ann. Am. Thorac. Soc.* 16, 455–462. doi:10.1513/AnnalsATS.201811-794OC

Hervier, B., Rimbert, M., Colonna, F., Hamidou, M. A., and Audrain, M. (2009). Clinical Significance of Anti-Ro/SSA-52 kDa Antibodies: a Retrospective Monocentric Study. *Rheumatology (Oxford)* 48, 964–967. doi:10.1093/rheumatology/kep145

Highland, K. B., Distler, O., Kuwana, M., Allanore, Y., Assassi, S., Azuma, A., et al. (2021). Efficacy and Safety of Nintedanib in Patients with Systemic Sclerosis-Associated Interstitial Lung Disease Treated with Mycophenolate: a Subgroup Analysis of the SENSCIS Trial. *Lancet Respir. Med.* 9, 96–106. doi:10.1016/S2213-2600(20)30330-1

Holland, A. E., Hill, C. J., Glaspole, I., Goh, N., Dowman, L., and McDonald, C. F. (2013). Impaired Chronotropic Response to 6-min Walk Test and Reduced Survival in Interstitial Lung Disease. *Respir. Med.* 107, 1066–1072. doi:10.1016/j.rmed.2013.04.002

Hudson, M., Pope, J., Mahler, M., Tatibouet, S., Steele, R., Baron, M., et al. (2012). Clinical Significance of Antibodies to Ro52/TRIM21 in Systemic Sclerosis. *Arthritis Res. Ther.* 14, R50. doi:10.1186/ar3763

Jee, A. S., Adelstein, S., Bleasel, J., Keir, G. J., Nguyen, M., Sahhar, J., et al. (2017). Role of Autoantibodies in the Diagnosis of Connective-Tissue Disease ILD (CTD-ILD) and Interstitial Pneumonia with Autoimmune Features (IPAF). *J. Clin. Med.* 6, 51. doi:10.3390/jcm6050051

Johannson, K. A., Chaudhuri, N., Adegunsoye, A., and Wolters, P. J. (2021). Series Interstitial Lung Disease 2021 3 Treatment of Fibrotic Interstitial Lung Disease : Current Approaches and Future Directions. *Lancet* 6736, 1–11. doi:10.1016/S0140-6736(21)01826-2

Kay, J., and Upchurch, K. S. (2012). ACR/EULAR 2010 Rheumatoid Arthritis Classification Criteria. *Rheumatology (Oxford)* 51 Suppl 6, vi5–9. doi:10.1093/rheumatology/kes279

Khanna, D., Mittoo, S., Aggarwal, R., Proudman, S. M., Dalbeth, N., Matteson, E. L., et al. (2015). Connective Tissue Disease-Associated Interstitial Lung Diseases (CTD-ILD) - Report from OMERACT CTD-ILD Working Group. *J. Rheumatol.* 42, 2168–2171. doi:10.3899/jrheum.141182

Kligerman, S. J., Groshong, S., Brown, K. K., and Lynch, D. A. (2009). Nonspecific Interstitial Pneumonia: Radiologic, Clinical, and Pathologic Considerations. *Radiographics* 29, 73–87. doi:10.1148/rg.291085096

Kolb, M., Bondue, B., Pesci, A., Miyazaki, Y., Song, J. W., Bhatt, N. Y., et al. (2018). Acute Exacerbations of Progressive-Fibrosing Interstitial Lung Diseases. *Eur. Respir. Rev.* 27, 1–8. doi:10.1183/16000617.0071-2018

Kolb, M. R., and Flaherty, K. R. (2021, The Justification for the Progressive Fibrotic Phenotype, 27). 363–367. doi:doi:10.1097/MCP.0000000000000803

La Corte, R., Lo Mo Naco, A., Locaputo, A., Dolzani, F., and Trotta, F. (2006). In Patients with Antisynthetase Syndrome the Occurrence of Anti-ro/SSA Antibodies Causes a More Severe Interstitial Lung Disease. *Autoimmunity* 39, 249–253. doi:10.1080/08916930600623791

Langguth, D. M., Morris, S., Clifford, L., Wilson, R. J., Neil, J., Hogan, P. G., et al. (2007). Specific Testing for "isolated" Anti-52 kDa SSA/Ro Antibodies during Standard Anti-extractable Nuclear Antigen Testing Is of Limited Clinical Value. *J. Clin. Pathol.* 60, 670–673. doi:10.1136/jcp.2006.040360

Lundberg, I. E., Tjärnlund, A., Bottai, M., Werth, V. P., Pilkington, C., Visser, M., et al. (2017). 2017 European League against Rheumatism/American College of Rheumatology Classification Criteria for Adult and Juvenile Idiopathic Inflammatory Myopathies and Their Major Subgroups. *Ann. Rheum. Dis.* 76, 1955–1964. doi:10.1136/annrheumdis-2017-211468

Maher, T. M., Corte, T. J., Fischer, A., Kreuter, M., Lederer, D. J., Molina-Molina, M., et al. (2020). Pirfenidone in Patients with Unclassifiable Progressive Fibrosing Interstitial Lung Disease: a Double-Blind, Randomised, Placebo-Controlled, Phase 2 Trial. *Lancet Respir. Med.* 8, 147–157. doi:10.1016/S2213-2600(19)30341-8

Martin, M. D., Chung, J. H., and Kanne, J. P. (2016). Idiopathic Pulmonary Fibrosis. *J. Thorac. Imaging* 31, 127–139. doi:10.1097/RTI.0000000000000204

Menéndez, A., Gómez, J., Escanlar, E., Caminal-Montero, L., and Mozo, L. (2013). Clinical Associations of Anti-SSA/Ro60 and Anti-Ro52/TRIM21 Antibodies: Diagnostic Utility of Their Separate Detection. *Autoimmunity* 46, 32–39. doi:10.3109/08916934.2012.732131

Mosca, M., Tani, C., Vagnani, S., Carli, L., and Bombardieri, S. (2014). The Diagnosis and Classification of Undifferentiated Connective Tissue Diseases. *J. Autoimmun.* 48-49, 50–52. doi:10.1016/j.jaut.2014.01.019

Oldham, J. M., Adegunsoye, A., Valenzi, E., Lee, C., Witt, L., Chen, L., et al. (2016). Characterisation of Patients with Interstitial Pneumonia with Autoimmune Features. *Eur. Respir. J.* 47, 1767–1775. doi:10.1183/13993003.01565-2015

Oliveira, R. P., Ribeiro, R., Melo, L., Grima, B., Oliveira, S., and Alves, J. D. (2020). Connective Tissue Disease-Associated Interstitial Lung Disease. *Pulmonology*, 6–11. doi:10.1016/j.pulmoe.2020.01.004

Ortega-Hernandez, O. D., and Shoenfeld, Y. (2012). Mixed Connective Tissue Disease: An Overview of Clinical Manifestations, Diagnosis and Treatment. *Best Pract. Res. Clin. Rheumatol.* 26, 61–72. doi:10.1016/j.berh.2012.01.009

Petri, M., Orbai, A. M., Alarcón, G. S., Gordon, C., Merrill, J. T., Fortin, P. R., et al. (2012). Derivation and Validation of the Systemic Lupus International Collaborating Clinics Classification Criteria for Systemic Lupus Erythematosus. *Arthritis Rheum.* 64, 2677–2686. doi:10.1002/art.34473

Raghu, G., Collard, H. R., Egan, J. J., Martinez, F. J., Behr, J., Brown, K. K., et al. (2011). An Official ATS/ERS/JRS/ALAT Statement: Idiopathic Pulmonary Fibrosis: Evidence-Based Guidelines for Diagnosis and Management. *Am. J. Respir. Crit. Care Med.* 183, 788–824. doi:10.1164/rccm.2009-040GL

Raghu, G., Remy-Jardin, M., Myers, J. L., Richeldi, L., Ryerson, C. J., Lederer, D. J., et al. (2018). Diagnosis of Idiopathic Pulmonary Fibrosis. An Official ATS/ERS/JRS/ALAT Clinical Practice Guideline. *Am. J. Respir. Crit. Care Med.* 198, e44–68. doi:10.1164/rccm.201807-1255ST

Richeldi, L., Launders, N., Martinez, F., Walsh, S. L. F., Myers, J., Wang, B., et al. (2019). The Characterisation of Interstitial Lung Disease Multidisciplinary Team Meetings: A Global Study. *ERJ Open Res.* 5. doi:10.1183/23120541.00209-2018

Robbins, A., Hentzien, M., Toquet, S., Didier, K., Servettaz, A., Pham, B. N., et al. (2019). Diagnostic Utility of Separate Anti-ro60 and Anti-Ro52/TRIM21 Antibody Detection in Autoimmune Diseases. *Front. Immunol.* 10, 444. doi:10.3389/fimmu.2019.00444

Ryerson, C. J., Vittinghoff, E., Ley, B., Lee, J. S., Mooney, J. J., Jones, K. D., et al. (2014). Predicting Survival across Chronic Interstitial Lung Disease: The ILD-GAP Model. *Chest* 145, 723–728. doi:10.1378/chest.13-1474

Sambataro, G., Sambataro, D., Torrisi, S. E., Vancheri, A., Colaci, M., Pavone, M., et al. (2019). Clinical, Serological and Radiological Features of a Prospective Cohort of Interstitial Pneumonia with Autoimmune Features (IPAF) Patients. *Respir. Med.* 150, 154–160. doi:10.1016/j.rmed.2019.03.011

Sambataro, G., Sambataro, D., Torrisi, S. E., Vancheri, A., Pavone, M., Rosso, R., et al. (2018). State of the Art in Interstitial Pneumonia with Autoimmune Features: A Systematic Review on Retrospective Studies and Suggestions for Further Advances. *Eur. Respir. Rev.* 27. doi:10.1183/16000617.0139-2017

Sambataro, G., Vancheri, A., Torrisi, S. E., Colaci, M., Pavone, M., Libra, A., et al. (2020). The Morphological Domain Does Not Affect the Rate of Progression to Defined Autoimmune Diseases in Patients with Interstitial Pneumonia with Autoimmune Features. *Chest* 157, 238–242. doi:10.1016/j.chest.2019.08.2175

Sanges, S., Giovannelli, J., Sobanski, V., Morell-Dubois, S., Maillard, H., Lambert, M., et al. (2017). Factors Associated with the 6-minute Walk Distance in Patients with Systemic Sclerosis. *Arthritis Res. Ther.* 19, 279–289. doi:10.1186/s13075-017-1489-4

Simpson, T., Barratt, S. L., Beirne, P., Chaudhuri, N., Crawshaw, A., Crowley, L. E., et al. (2021). The burden of Progressive Fibrotic Interstitial Lung Disease across the UK. *Eur. Respir. J.* 58. doi:10.1183/13993003.00221-2021

Solomon, J. J., Chung, J. H., Cosgrove, G. P., Demoruelle, M. K., Fernandez-Perez, E. R., Fischer, A., et al. (2016). Predictors of Mortality in Rheumatoid Arthritis-Associated Interstitial Lung Disease. *Eur. Respir. J.* 47, 588–596. doi:10.1183/13993003.00357-2015

Suzuki, A., Kondoh, Y., Brown, K. K., Johkoh, T., Kataoka, K., Fukuoka, J., et al. (2020). Acute Exacerbations of Fibrotic Interstitial Lung Diseases. *Respirology* 25, 525–534. doi:10.1111/resp.13682

Travis, W. D., Costabel, U., Hansell, D. M., King, T. E., Lynch, D. A., Nicholson, A. G., et al. (2013). An Official American Thoracic Society/European Respiratory Society Statement: Update of the International Multidisciplinary Classification of the Idiopathic Interstitial Pneumonias. *Am. J. Respir. Crit. Care Med.* 188, 733–748. doi:10.1164/rccm.201308-1483ST

Van Den Hoogen, F., Khanna, D., Fransen, J., Johnson, S. R., Baron, M., Tyndall, A., et al. (2013). 2013 Classification Criteria for Systemic Sclerosis: An American College of Rheumatology/European League against Rheumatism Collaborative Initiative. *Ann. Rheum. Dis.* 72, 1747–1755. doi:10.1002/art.3809810.1136/annrheumdis-2013-204424

Váncsa, A., Csípo, I., Németh, J., Dévényi, K., Gergely, L., and Dankó, K. (2009). Characteristics of Interstitial Lung Disease in SS-A positive/Jo-1 Positive Inflammatory Myopathy Patients. *Rheumatol. Int.* 29, 989–994. doi:10.1007/s00296-009-0884-9

Volkmann, E. R., Tashkin, D. P., Li, N., Roth, M. D., Khanna, D., Hoffmann-Vold, A. M., et al. (2017). Mycophenolate Mofetil versus Placebo for Systemic Sclerosis-Related Interstitial Lung Disease: An Analysis of Scleroderma Lung Studies I and II. *ARTHRITIS Rheumatol.* 69, 1451–1460. doi:10.1002/art.40114

Volkmann, E. R., Tashkin, D. P., Sim, M., Li, N., Goldmuntz, E., Keyes-Elstein, L., et al. (2019). Short-term Progression of Interstitial Lung Disease in Systemic Sclerosis Predicts Long-Term Survival in Two Independent Clinical Trial Cohorts. *Ann. Rheum. Dis.* 78, 122–130. doi:10.1136/annrheumdis-2018-213708

Vonk, M. C., Walker, U. A., Volkmann, E. R., Kreuter, M., Johnson, S. R., and Allanore, Y. (2021). Natural Variability in the Disease Course of SSC-ILD: Implications for Treatment. *Eur. Respir. Rev.* 30. doi:10.1183/16000617.0340-2020

Walsh, S. L., Calandriello, L., Sverzellati, N., Wells, A. U., and Hansell, D. M. (2016). Interobserver Agreement for the ATS/ERS/JRS/ALAT Criteria for a UIP Pattern on CT. *Thorax* 71, 45–51. doi:10.1136/thoraxjnl-2015-207252

Wells, A. U., Flaherty, K. R., Brown, K. K., Inoue, Y., Devaraj, A., Richeldi, L., et al. (2020). Nintedanib in Patients with Progressive Fibrosing Interstitial Lung Diseases-Subgroup Analyses by Interstitial Lung Disease Diagnosis in the INBUILD Trial: a Randomised, Double-Blind, Placebo-Controlled, Parallel-Group Trial. *Lancet Respir. Med.* 8, 453–460. doi:10.1016/S2213-2600(20)30036-9

Widell, J., and Lidén, M. (2020). Interobserver Variability in High-Resolution CT of the Lungs. *Eur. J. Radiol. Open* 7, 100228. doi:10.1016/j.ejro.2020.100228

Wollin, L., Distler, J. H. W., Redente, E. F., Riches, D. W. H., Stowasser, S., Schlenker-Herceg, R., et al. (2019). Potential of Nintedanib in Treatment of Progressive Fibrosing Interstitial Lung Diseases. *Eur. Respir. J.* 54. doi:10.1183/13993003.00161-2019

Wong, A. W., Ryerson, C. J., and Guler, S. A. (2020). Progression of Fibrosing Interstitial Lung Disease. *Respir. Res.* 21, 32–10. doi:10.1186/s12931-020-1296-3

Yates, M., Watts, R. A., Bajema, I. M., Cid, M. C., Crestani, B., Hauser, T., et al. (2016). EULAR/ERA-EDTA Recommendations for the Management of ANCA-Associated Vasculitis. *Ann. Rheum. Dis.* 75, 1583–1594. doi:10.1136/annrheumdis-2016-209133

Permissions

All chapters in this book were first published by Frontiers; hereby published with permission under the Creative Commons Attribution License or equivalent. Every chapter published in this book has been scrutinized by our experts. Their significance has been extensively debated. The topics covered herein carry significant findings which will fuel the growth of the discipline. They may even be implemented as practical applications or may be referred to as a beginning point for another development.

The contributors of this book come from diverse backgrounds, making this book a truly international effort. This book will bring forth new frontiers with its revolutionizing research information and detailed analysis of the nascent developments around the world.

We would like to thank all the contributing authors for lending their expertise to make the book truly unique. They have played a crucial role in the development of this book. Without their invaluable contributions this book wouldn't have been possible. They have made vital efforts to compile up to date information on the varied aspects of this subject to make this book a valuable addition to the collection of many professionals and students.

This book was conceptualized with the vision of imparting up-to-date information and advanced data in this field. To ensure the same, a matchless editorial board was set up. Every individual on the board went through rigorous rounds of assessment to prove their worth. After which they invested a large part of their time researching and compiling the most relevant data for our readers.

The editorial board has been involved in producing this book since its inception. They have spent rigorous hours researching and exploring the diverse topics which have resulted in the successful publishing of this book. They have passed on their knowledge of decades through this book. To expedite this challenging task, the publisher supported the team at every step. A small team of assistant editors was also appointed to further simplify the editing procedure and attain best results for the readers.

Apart from the editorial board, the designing team has also invested a significant amount of their time in understanding the subject and creating the most relevant covers. They scrutinized every image to scout for the most suitable representation of the subject and create an appropriate cover for the book.

The publishing team has been an ardent support to the editorial, designing and production team. Their endless efforts to recruit the best for this project, has resulted in the accomplishment of this book. They are a veteran in the field of academics and their pool of knowledge is as vast as their experience in printing. Their expertise and guidance has proved useful at every step. Their uncompromising quality standards have made this book an exceptional effort. Their encouragement from time to time has been an inspiration for everyone.

The publisher and the editorial board hope that this book will prove to be a valuable piece of knowledge for researchers, students, practitioners and scholars across the globe.

List of Contributors

Qi Fang, Shaoyu Liu, Ruiyue Zhao, Peng Hou, Youcai Li, Jie Lv, Xiaoyao Zhang and Xinlu Wang
Department of Nuclear Medicine, The First Affiliated Hospital of Guangzhou Medical University, Guangzhou, China

Jiangyu Cui, Qian Han and Qun Luo
State Key Laboratory of Respiratory Diseases, Guangzhou Institute of Respiratory Diseases, The First Affiliated Hospital of Guangzhou Medical University, Guangzhou, China

Lili Gao, Haiying Tang, Huanyu He, Jia Liu and Taihua Wu
Department of Respiratory Medicine, The First Affiliated Hospital of Dalian Medical University, Dalian, China

Jingwei Mao
Department of Gastroenterology, The First Affiliated Hospital of Dalian Medical University, Dalian, China

Hong Ji
Department of Pediatrics, The First Affiliated Hospital of Dalian Medical University, Dalian, China

Hongli Lin
Department of Nephrology, The First Affiliated Hospital of Dalian Medical University, Dalian, China

Mengmeng Shen, Lan Zhang, Liming Di, Shuangshuang He and Yu Li
School of Traditional Chinese Medicine, Beijing University of Chinese Medicine, Beijing, China

Yanan Nan and Yadong Li
School of Life Sciences, Beijing University of Chinese Medicine, Beijing, China

Hailong Li, Rui Liu, Ruotong Zhang, Yiying Wei, Honggang Zhou and Cheng Yang
The State Key Laboratory of Medicinal Chemical Biology, College of Pharmacy and Key Laboratory of Molecular Drug Research, Nankai University, Tianjin, China
High-Throughput Molecular Drug Screening Centre, Tianjin International Joint Academy of Biomedicine, Tianjin, China

Shanshan Zhang
The State Key Laboratory of Medicinal Chemical Biology, College of Pharmacy and Key Laboratory of Molecular Drug Research, Nankai University, Tianjin, China

Liang Zhang
Department of Thoracic Surgery, Tian Jin First Central Hospital, Tianjin, China

Wei Li
Department of Dermatology and The Norris Comprehensive Cancer Centre, University of Southern California Keck Medical Centre, Los Angeles, CA, United States

Suqing Liu, Ming Li, Shan He and Jinfeng Wu
Department of Dermatology, Huashan Hospital, Fudan University, Shanghai, China

Qingqing Yang
Department of Dermatology, Huashan Hospital, Fudan University, Shanghai, China
Shanghai Public Health Clinical Center, Fudan University, Shanghai, China

Binbin Dong
Department of Pediatrics, Huashan Hospital North, Fudan University, Shanghai, China

Chunhui Qi
Department of Respiratory Medicine, Qingpu District Traditional Chinese Medicine Hospital, Institute of Integrative Medicine, Fudan University, Shanghai, China

Tao Yang
Department of Cardiovascular Disease, Institute of Cardiovascular Disease of Integrated Traditional Chinese and Western Medicine, Shuguang Hospital Affiliated to Shanghai University of Traditional Chinese Medicine, Shanghai, China

Baojun Liu
Department of Integrative Medicine, Huashan Hospital, Fudan University, Shanghai, China

Suh-Young Lee
Molecular Microbiology and Immunology, Brown University, 185 Meeting St., Providence, RI, United States
Devision of Allergy and Clinical Immunology, Department of Internal Medicine, Seoul National University Hospital, Seoul, South Korea

Chang-Min Lee, Bing Ma, Suchitra Kamle, Jack A. Elias, Yang Zhou and Chun Geun Lee
Molecular Microbiology and Immunology, Brown University, 185 Meeting St., Providence, RI, United States

Yuanyuan Liu, Wenshan Zhong, Jinming Zhang, Weimou Chen, Ye lu, Yujie Qiao, Zhaojin Zeng, Haohua Huang, Hangming Dong, Xuan Wan and Shaoxi Cai
Department of Respiratory and Critical Care Medicine, Chronic Airways Diseases Laboratory, Nanfang Hospital, Southern Medical University, Guangzhou, China

Xingxing Hu, Menglin Zou, Lan Ni, Mingyang Zhang, Weishuai Zheng and Bing Liu
Department of Respiratory and Critical Care Medicine, Zhongnan Hospital of Wuhan University, Wuhan, China

Zhenshun Cheng
Department of Respiratory and Critical Care Medicine, Zhongnan Hospital of Wuhan University, Wuhan, China
Wuhan Research Center for Infectious Diseases and Cancer, Chinese Academy of Medical Sciences, Wuhan, China

Xiaojing Meng and Fei Zou
Guangdong Provincial Key Laboratory of Tropical Disease Research, Department of Occupational Health and Medicine, School of Public Health, Southern Medical University, Guangzhou, China

Qianru Mei, Zhe Liu, He Zuo, Zhenhua Yang and Jing Qu
School of Basic Medicine, Tongji Medical College, Huazhong University of Science and Technology, Wuhan, China

De-wei Zhu, Qun Yu and Yun-hui Shen
School of Pharmacy, Shanghai University of Traditional Chinese Medicine, Shanghai, China

Mei-fang Jiang and Dan-dan Wang
SPH Xing Ling Sci. & Tech. Pharmaceutical Co., Ltd., Shanghai, China

Cailing Gan, Hongyao Liu and Tinghong Ye
Sichuan University-University of Oxford Huaxi Joint Centre for Gastrointestinal Cancer, Frontiers Science Center for Disease- Related Molecular Network, State Key Laboratory of Biotherapy, West China Hospital, Sichuan University, Chengdu, China

Yali Li
Sichuan University-University of Oxford Huaxi Joint Centre for Gastrointestinal Cancer, Frontiers Science Center for Disease- Related Molecular Network, State Key Laboratory of Biotherapy, West China Hospital, Sichuan University, Chengdu, China
West China School of Public Health and West China Fourth Hospital, Sichuan University, Chengdu, China
Prenatal Diagnosis Center, The Third Affiliated Hospital of Zhengzhou University—Maternal and Child Health Hospital of Henan Province, Zhengzhou, China

Liqun Wang, Qianyu Zhang, Li Tian and Wenya Yin
West China School of Public Health and West China Fourth Hospital, Sichuan University, Chengdu, China

Yanhong Liu, Yan Ding, Yapeng Hou, Tong Yu and Hongguang Nie
Department of Stem Cells and Regenerative Medicine, College of Basic Medical Science, China Medical University, Shenyang, China

Yong Cui
Departments of Anesthesiology, The First Hospital of China Medical University, Shenyang, China

Xiang Tong, Shijie Zhang, Dongguang Wang, Li Zhang, Jizheng Huang, Tianli Zhang and Hong Fan
Department of Respiratory Medicine and Critical Care Medicine, West China Hospital/West China School of Medicine, Sichuan University, Chengdu, China

Dongxin Chen, Huirong Tang, Hongchao Jiang, Lei Sun and Wenjuan Zhao
Engineering Research Center of Cell and Therapeutic Antibody, Ministry of Education, School of Pharmacy, Shanghai Jiao Tong University, Shanghai, China

Feng Qian
Engineering Research Center of Cell and Therapeutic Antibody, Ministry of Education, School of Pharmacy, Shanghai Jiao Tong University, Shanghai, China
Anhui Province Key Laboratory of Translational Cancer Research, Bengbu Medical College, Bengbu, China

Xianqiu Chen
Department of Respiratory Medicine, Shanghai Pulmonary Hospital, Tongji University School of Medicine, Shanghai, China

Jian Guo
Department of Pulmonary Function Test, Shanghai Pulmonary Hospital, Tongji University School of Medicine, Shanghai, China

Dong Yu and Bing Jie
Department of Radiology, Shanghai Pulmonary Hospital, Tongji University School of Medicine, Shanghai, China

Ying Zhou
Department of Respiratory Medicine and Clinical Research Center, Shanghai Pulmonary Hospital, Tongji University School of Medicine, Shanghai, China

Alexandra Nagy, Tamas Nagy, Abigel Margit Kolonics-Farkas, Noemi Eszes, Krisztina Vincze, Eniko Barczi, Aniko Bohacs and Veronika Müller
Department of Pulmonology, Semmelweis University, Budapest, Hungary

Adam Domonkos Tarnoki, David Laszlo Tarnoki and Pal Maurovich-Horvat
Medical Imaging Centre, Semmelweis University, Budapest, Hungary

György Nagy
Department of Genetics, Cell- and Immunobiology, Semmelweis University, Budapest, Hungary
Department of Rheumatology and Clinical Immunology, Semmelweis University, Budapest, Hungary

Emese Kiss
Department of Clinical Immunology, Adult and Pediatric Rheumatology, National Institute of Locomotor Diseases and Disabilities, Budapest, Hungary
3rd Department of Internal Medicine and Haematology, Semmelweis University, Budapest, Hungary

Index

Printed in the USA
CPSIA information can be obtained
at www.ICGtesting.com
JSHW051624061123
51533JS00005B/90